Bruce Lansky

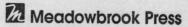

Meadowbrook Press
Distributed by Simon & Schuster
New York

Library of Congress Cataloging-in-Publication Data

Lansky, Bruce.
　45,000+ baby names / Bruce Lansky.
　　　p. cm.
　ISBN 0-88166-478-2 (Meadowbrook) ISBN 0-684-03089-6 (Simon
　& Schuster)
　1. Names, Personal—Dictionaries. I. Title: forty-five thousand plus baby
　names. II. Title.
CS2377L354　2004
929.4'4'03—dc22

　　　　　　　　　　　　　　　　　　　　　　　　　　　2004009357

Editorial Director: Christine Zuchora-Walske
Editors: Liya Lev Oertel, Megan McGinnis, Angela Wiechmann
Proofreader: Joseph Gredler
Production Manager: Paul Woods
Graphic Design Manager: Tamara Peterson
Cover Design: Tamara Peterson, Erik Broberg
Cover Photography: Comstock Images, Corbis, Getty Images

© 2004 by Bruce Lansky

Published by Meadowbrook Press, 5451 Smetana Drive,
Minnetonka, MN 55343

www.meadowbrookpress.com

BOOK TRADE DISTRIBUTION by Simon & Schuster,
a division of Simon and Schuster, Inc., 1230 Avenue
of the Americas, New York, NY 10020

09 08 07 06 05 04　　　10 9 8 7 6 5 4 3 2 1

Printed in the United States of America

Contents

Introduction

When you think about names for your baby, you'll find yourself daydreaming about what he or she may look like and be like. And you'll find yourself thinking about your hopes and dreams for the newest member of your family.

As you consider and discuss names, you'll find that they conjure up pictures in your mind. Scarlett may bring to mind Scarlett O'Hara of Margaret Mitchell's *Gone with the Wind*. Ronald may call to mind Ronald Reagan or Ronald McDonald.

You'll find yourself putting first, middle, and last names together and saying them out loud. Someone watching you may think you're talking to yourself. You probably are!

You'll also find yourself fascinated by all the names you read in the birth announcements section of the newspaper; names of students in your local day care center, school, church, or favorite team; names you see or hear in the news; and names you see in books, movies, on television, or on the Internet.

Don't be surprised to discover that you've developed a "fashion sense" about which names are currently "in" and which names are currently "out." As a result, you may find yourself considering:

- names from other countries and ethnic groups;
- names that have been recently created (perhaps a name you've made up yourself);
- names that feature new spellings of familiar names;
- names for a girl that once were more often used for boys;
- names that are traditional surnames.

The reasons you'll probably consider some names that your parents never did are simple. Pick up the sports section of your local newspaper and you'll read about Shaquille, Kobe, and LeBron on the basketball court or Andre, Gustavo, and Lleyton on the tennis court. Turn on the television and you'll see Shania, Beyoncé, and Alanis perform. Go to the movies and you can watch Uma, Charlize, and Angelina. Interesting, unusual names from all around the world surround you.

This book was designed to open up the whole world of names to you. I scoured the world for popular and unusual names that just might work for your child. Here are a few of the unusual names I find intriguing:

Native American: Cheyenne and Dakotah
Spanish: Nevada and Sierra
French: Brie and Chardonnay
African: Saki and Simba
Welsh: Bryn and Rhett
Russian: Sasha and Tamara
Gypsy: Chik and Tawny
Italian: Giulia and Matteo
Japanese: Kimiko and Ringo

I could go on for pages.

I created this book to give you the choice of a lifetime—more interesting and unusual names from all around the world than any other book.

My best advice is to:

a) Rate the names you're considering on the rating sheet that follows. It will help you make the very subjective process of selecting a name a little more objective.

b) "Go public" with the naming process. "Test" names you're considering on your friends and relatives. Find out how the names you're considering are perceived and received. What positive or negative associations come to mind?* How do your friends and relatives feel about the names?

Chances are, if a name survives this process, it may well be a name both you and your child can live with happily ever after.

Happy hunting,

Bruce Lansky

---

*If this factor intrigues you, consult *The Baby Name Survey Book* to find how 1,700 popular names are perceived by a sample of 100,000 parents.

Ten Guidelines for Naming Your Baby

A Comparative Scoring System

If you have a name you like, you already know how pleasant it is going through life with a name that "fits" or "feels right." If you don't, you know how unpleasant it is to go through life with a name that, for whatever reason, doesn't work for you.

It may help to test each name you're considering against the list of factors that could affect the way a name will work for your child. This will help make the subjective process of selecting a name more objective for you.

In the chart on the following page, give each name two points for a positive rating on any criterion, one point for a medium rating, and no points for a negative rating.

I realize that this scoring system has a built-in bias toward names that are relatively common and familiar—and therefore easy to spell and pronounce. However, you're free to give extra weight to any factor you like. If, for example, you love exotic names that are unfamiliar (and potentially hard to spell and pronounce), you might want to double the weight of the "uniqueness" and/or "sound/rhythm" factors—in other words, give four points for a positive rating and two points for a medium rating.

Factors	Positive	Medium	Negative
1. Spelling	❏ easy	❏ medium	❏ hard
2. Pronunciation	❏ easy	❏ medium	❏ hard
3. Gender ID	❏ clear		❏ confusing
4. Stereotypes	❏ positive	❏ ok	❏ negative
5. Sound/Rhythm	❏ pleasing	❏ ok	❏ unpleasant
6. Nicknames	❏ appealing	❏ ok	❏ unappealing
7. Meaning	❏ positive	❏ ok	❏ negative
8. Popularity	❏ *not* too popular		❏ too popular
9. Uniqueness	❏ *not* too strange		❏ too strange
10. Initials	❏ pleasing	❏ ok	❏ unpleasant

Top Five Girls' Names

Name 1: _____ Score_____

Name 2: _____ Score_____

Name 3: _____ Score_____

Name 4: _____ Score_____

Name 5: _____ Score_____

Top Five Boys' Names

Name 1: _____ Score_____

Name 2: _____ Score_____

Name 3: _____ Score_____

Name 4: _____ Score_____

Name 5: _____ Score_____

Where in the World?

45,000+ Baby Names includes names from over 150 different languages. Some of these languages are quite familiar, while others may be more obscure or exotic. In order to help identify where each language comes from, the following language chart has been provided.

In this chart, the languages used in *45,000+ Baby Names* have been divided up into general geographical categories. Upon encountering a name entry with an unfamiliar language citation, please refer to the chart below to discover what part of the world the name in question originated from.

Languages used in
45,000+ Baby Names:

African
Abaluhya
African
Afrikaans
Akan
Ateso
Bambara
Benin
Egyptian
Ethiopian
Ewe
Fante
Ghanaian
Hausa
Ibo
Kakwa
Kikuyu
Lomwe
Luganda
Luo
Musoga
Mwera

Nguni
Nigerian
North African
Nyakyusa
Ochi
Rhodesian
Rukiga
Runyankore
Runyoro
Rutooro
Shona
Somali
Swahili
Tanzanian
Tiv
Tswana
Twi
Ugandan
Umbundu
Uset
Xhosa
Yao

Yoruba
Zimbabwean
Zulu

Native American
Algonquin
Apache
Arapaho
Ashanti
Blackfoot
Carrier
Cherokee
Cheyenne
Choctaw
Comanche
Coos
Dakota
Dene
Eskimo
Fox
Hopi

Iroquois
Kiowa
Lakota
Mahona
Moquelumnan
Native American
Navajo
Ojibwa
Omaha
Osage
Pawnee
Pomo
Ponca
Quiché
Sauk
Shoshone
Taos
Tupi-Guarani
Watamare
Winnebago
Zuni

East Asian and Pacific
Australian
Burmese
Cambodian
Chinese
Filipino
Fijian
Hawaiian
Japanese
Korean
Malayan
Maori
Polynesian
Tai
Tibetan
Vietnamese

West Australian Aboriginal

East European and North Asian
Armenian
Basque
Bulgarian
Czech
Estonian
Hungarian
Latvian
Lithuanian
Mongolian
Polish
Romanian
Russian
Slavic
Turkish
Ukrainian

West European
Cornish
Danish
Dutch
English
Finnish
French
German
Gypsy
Icelandic
Irish
Italian
Norwegian
Portugese
Scandinavian
Scottish
Spanish
Swedish
Swiss

Welsh
Yiddish

Middle and Near Eastern
Afghan
Arabic
Hebrew
Hindi
Pakistani
Persian
Punjabi
Tamil
Todas
Urdu

South and North American
American
Peruvian

Historical
Aramaic
Assyrian
Babylonian
Greek
Latin
Phoenician
Sanskrit
Syrian
Teutonic

Girls

A

Aaleyah (Hebrew) a form of Aliya.
Aalayah, Aalayaha, Aalea, Aaleah, Aaleaha, Aaleeyah, Aaleyiah, Aaleyyah

Aaliah (Hebrew) a form of Aliya.
Aaliaya, Aaliayah

Aalisha (Greek) a form of Alisha.
Aaleasha, Aaliesha

Aaliyah (Hebrew) a form of Aliya.
Aahliyah, Aailiyah, Aailyah, Aalaiya, Aaleah, Aalia, Aalieyha, Aaliya, Aaliyaha, Aaliyha, Aalliah, Aalliyah, ·Aalyah, Aalyiah

Abagail (Hebrew) a form of Abigale.
Abagael, Abagaile, Abagale, Abagayle, Abageal, Abagil, Abaigael, Abaigeal

Abbagail (Hebrew) a form of Abigale.
Abbagale, Abbagayle, Abbegail, Abbegale, Abbegayle

Abbey, Abbie, Abby
(Hebrew) familiar forms of Abigail.
Aabbee, Abbe, Abbea, Abbeigh, Abbi, Abbye, Abeey, Abey, Abi, Abia, Abie, Aby

Abbygail (Hebrew) a form of Abigale.
Abbeygale, Abbygale, Abbygayl, Abbygayle

Abegail (Hebrew) a form of Abigail.
Abegale, Abegaile, Abegayle

Abelina (American) a combination of Abbey + Lina.
Abilana, Abilene

Abia (Arabic) great.
Abbia, Abbiah, Abiah, Abya

Abianne (American) a combination of Abbey + Ann.
Abena, Abeni, Abian, Abinaya

Abida (Arabic) worshiper.
Abedah, Abidah

Abigail (Hebrew) father's joy. Bible: one of the wives of King David. See also Gail.
Abagail, Abbagail, Abbey, Abbiegail, Abbiegayle, Abbigael, Abbigail, Abbigal, Abbigale, Abbigayl, Abbigayle, Abbygail, Abegail, Abgail, Abgale, Abgayle, Abigael, Abigaile, Abigaill, Abigal, Abigale, Abigayil, Abigayl, Abigayle, Abigel, Abigial, Abugail, Abygail, Avigail

Abinaya (American) a form of Abiann.
Abenaa, Abenaya, Abinaa, Abinaiya, Abinayan

Abira (Hebrew) my strength.
Abbira, Abeer, Abeerah, Abeir,
Abera, Aberah, Abhira, Abiir,
Abir

Abra (Hebrew) mother of
many nations.
Abree, Abri, Abria

Abria (Hebrew) a form of
Abra.
Abréa, Abrea, Abreia, Abriah,
Abriéa, Abrya

Abrial (French) open; secure,
protected.
Abrail, Abreal, Abreale, Abriale,
Abrielle

Abriana (Italian) a form of
Abra.
Abbrienna, Abbryana, Abreana,
Abreanna, Abreanne, Abreeana,
Abreona, Abreonia, Abriann,
Abrianna, Abriannah, Abrieana,
Abrien, Abrienna, Abrienne,
Abrietta, Abrion, Abrionée,
Abrionne, Abriunna, Abryann,
Abryanna, Abryona

Abrielle (French) a form of
Abrial.
Aabriella, Abriel, Abriell, Abryell

Abril (French) a form of
Abrial.
Abrilla, Abrille

Abygail (Hebrew) a form of
Abigail.
Abygael, Abygale, Abygayle

Acacia (Greek) thorny.
Mythology: the acacia tree
symbolizes immortality and
resurrection. See also Casey.
Acasha, Acatia, Accassia, Acey,
Acie, Akacia, Cacia, Casia,
Kasia

Ada (German) a short form of
Adelaide. (English) prosper-
ous; happy.
Adabelle, Adah, Adan, Adaya,
Adda, Auda

Adah (Hebrew) ornament.
Ada, Addah

Adair (Greek) a form of
Adara.
Adaire

Adalene (Spanish) a form of
Adalia.
Adalane, Adalena, Adalin,
Adalina, Adaline, Adalinn,
Adalyn, Adalynn, Adalynne,
Addalyn, Addalynn

Adalia (German, Spanish)
noble.
Adal, Adala, Adalea, Adaleah,
Adalee, Adalene, Adali, Adalie,
Adaly, Addal, Addala, Addaly

Adama (Phoenician, Hebrew)
a form of Adam (see Boys'
Names).

Adamma (Ibo) child of
beauty.

Adana (Spanish) a form of
Adama.

Adanna (Nigerian) her father's
daughter.
Adanya

Adara (Greek) beauty. (Arabic)
virgin.
*Adair, Adaira, Adaora, Adar,
Adarah, Adare, Adaria, Adarra,
Adasha, Adauré, Adra*

Adaya (American) a form of
Ada.
*Adaija, Adaijah, Adaja, Adajah,
Adayja, Adayjah, Adejah*

Addie (Greek, German) a
familiar form of Adelaide,
Adrienne.
*Aday, Adde, Addee, Addey,
Addi, Addia, Addy, Ade, Adee,
Adei, Adey, Adeye, Adi, Adie,
Ady, Atti, Attie, Atty*

Addison, Addyson (English)
child of Adam.
*Addis, Addisen, Addisson,
Adison*

Adela (English) a short form
of Adelaide.
Adelae, Adelia, Adelista, Adella

Adelaide (German) noble and
serene. See also Ada, Adela,
Adeline, Adelle, Ailis, Delia,
Della, Ela, Elke, Heidi.
*Adelade, Adelaid, Adelaida,
Adelei, Adelheid, Adeliade,
Adelka, Aley, Laidey, Laidy*

Adele (English) a form of
Adelle.
Adel, Adelie, Adile

Adelina (English) a form of
Adeline.
*Adalina, Adeleana, Adelena,
Adellyna, Adeliana, Adellena,
Adileena, Adlena*

Adeline (English) a form of
Adelaide.
*Adaline, Adelaine, Adelin,
Adelina, Adelind, Adelita,
Adeliya, Adelle, Adelyn,
Adelynn, Adelynne, Adilene,
Adlin, Adline, Adlyn, Adlynn,
Aline*

Adelle (German, English) a
short form of Adelaide,
Adeline.
Adele, Adell

Adena (Hebrew) noble;
adorned.
*Adeana, Adeen, Adeena, Aden,
Adene, Adenia, Adenna, Adina*

Adia (Swahili) gift.
Addia, Adéa, Adea, Adiah

Adila (Arabic) equal.
*Adeala, Adeela, Adela, Adelah,
Adeola, Adilah, Adileh, Adilia,
Adyla*

Adilene (English) a form of
Adeline.
*Adilen, Adileni, Adilenne,
Adlen, Adlene*

Adina (Hebrew) a form of
Adena. See also Dina.
*Adeana, Adiana, Adiena,
Adinah, Adine, Adinna, Adyna*

Adira (Hebrew) strong.
Ader, Adera, Aderah, Aderra, Adhira, Adirah, Adirana

Adison, Adyson (English) forms of Addison, Addyson.
Adis, Adisa, Adisen, Adisynne, Adysen

Aditi (Hindi) unbound. Religion: the mother of the Hindu sun gods.
Adithi, Aditti

Adleigh (Hebrew) my ornament.
Adla, Adleni

Adonia (Spanish) beautiful.
Adonica, Adonis, Adonna, Adonnica, Adonya

Adora (Latin) beloved. See also Dora.
Adore, Adoree, Adoria

Adra (Arabic) virgin.
Adara

Adreana, Adreanna (Latin) forms of Adrienne.
Adrean, Adreanne, Adreauna, Adreeanna, Adreen, Adreena, Adreeyana, Adrena, Adrene, Adrenea, Adréona, Adreonia, Adreonna

Adria (English) a short form of Adriana, Adriene.
Adrea, Adriani, Adrya

Adriana, Adrianna (Italian) forms of Adrienne.
Addrianna, Addriyanna, Adreiana, Adreinna, Adria, Adriannea, Adriannia, Adrionna

Adriane, Adrianne (English) forms of Adrienne.
Addrian, Adranne, Adria, Adrian, Adreinne, Adriann, Adriayon, Adrion

Adrielle (Hebrew) member of God's flock.
Adriel, Adrielli, Adryelle

Adrien, Adriene (English) forms of Adrienne.

Adrienna (Italian) a form of Adrienne. See also Edrianna.
Adreana, Adrieanna, Adrieaunna, Adriena, Adrienia, Adriennah, Adrieunna

Adrienne (Greek) rich. (Latin) dark. See also Hadriane.
Addie, Adrien, Adriana, Adriane, Adrianna, Adrianne, Adrie, Adrieanne, Adrien, Adrienna, Adriyanna

Adrina (English) a short form of Adriana.
Adrinah, Adrinne

Adriyanna (American) a form of Adrienne.
Adrieyana, Adriyana, Adryan, Adryana, Adryane, Adryanna, Adryanne

Adya (Hindi) Sunday.
Adia

Aerial, Aeriel (Hebrew) forms of Ariel.
Aeriale, Aeriela, Aerielle, Aeril, Aerile, Aeryal

Afi (African) born on Friday.
Affi, Afia, Efi, Efia

Afra (Hebrew) young doe. (Arabic) earth color. See also Aphra.
Affery, Affrey, Affrie, Afraa

Africa (Irish) pleasant. Geography: one of the seven continents.
Affrica, Afric, Africah, Africaya, Africia, Africiana, Afrika, Aifric

Afrika (Irish) a form of Africa.
Afrikah

Afrodite, Aphrodite (Greek) Mythology: the goddess of love and beauty.
Afrodita

Afton (English) from Afton, England.
Aftan, Aftine, Aftinn, Aftyn

Agate (English) a semiprecious stone.
Aggie

Agatha (Greek) good, kind. Literature: Agatha Christie was a British writer of more than seventy detective novels. See also Gasha.
Agace, Agaisha, Agasha, Agata, Agatah, Agathe, Agathi, Agatka, Agetha, Aggie, Ágota, Ágotha, Agueda, Atka

Agathe (Greek) a form of Agatha.

Aggie (Greek) a short form of Agatha, Agnes.
Ag, Aggy, Agi

Agnes (Greek) pure. See also Aneesa, Anessa, Anice, Anisha, Ina, Inez, Necha, Nessa, Nessie, Neza, Nyusha, Una, Ynez.
Aganetha, Aggie, Agna, Agne, Agneis, Agnelia, Agnella, Agnés, Agnesa, Agnesca, Agnese, Agnesina, Agness, Agnessa, Agnesse, Agneta, Agneti, Agnetta, Agnies, Agnieszka, Agniya, Agnola, Agnus, Aignéis, Aneska, Anka

Ahava (Hebrew) beloved.
Ahivia

Ahliya (Hebrew) a form of Aliya.
Ahlai, Ahlaia, Ahlaya, Ahleah, Ahleeyah, Ahley, Ahleya, Ahlia, Ahliah, Ahliyah

Aida (Latin) helpful. (English) a form of Ada.
Aidah, Aidan, Aide, Aidee

Aidan, Aiden (Latin) forms of Aida.

Aiesha (Swahili, Arabic) a form of Aisha.
Aeisha, Aeshia, Aieshia, Aieysha, Aiiesha

Aiko (Japanese) beloved.

Ailani (Hawaiian) chief.
Aelani, Ailana

Aileen (Scottish) light bearer. (Irish) a form of Helen. See also Eileen.
Ailean, Aileena, Ailen, Ailene, Aili, Ailina, Ailinn, Aillen

Aili (Scottish) a form of Alice. (Finnish) a form of Helen.
Aila, Ailee, Ailey, Ailie, Aily

Ailis (Irish) a form of Adelaide.
Ailesh, Ailish, Ailyse, Eilis

Ailsa (Scottish) island dweller. Geography: Ailsa Craig is an island in Scotland.
Ailsha

Ailya (Hebrew) a form of Aliya.
Ailiyah

Aimee (Latin) a form of Amy. (French) loved.
Aime, Aimée, Aimey, Aimi, Aimia, Aimie, Aimy

Ainsley (Scottish) my own meadow.
Ainslee, Ainsleigh, Ainslie, Ainsly, Ansley, Aynslee, Aynsley, Aynslie

Airiana (English) a form of Ariana, Arianna.
Airana, Airanna, Aireana, Aireanah, Aireanna, Aireona, Aireonna, Aireyonna, Airianna, Airianne, Airiona, Airriana, Airrion, Airryon, Airyana, Airyanna

Airiél (Hebrew) a form of Ariel.
Aieral, Aierel, Aiiryel, Aire, Aireal, Aireale, Aireel, Airel, Airele, Airelle, Airi, Airial, Airiale, Airrel

Aisha (Swahili) life. (Arabic) woman. See also Asha, Asia, Iesha, Isha, Keisha, Yiesha.
Aaisha, Aaishah, Aesha, Aeshah, Aheesha, Aiasha, Aiesha, Aieshah, Aisa, Aischa, Aish, Aishah, Aisheh, Aishia, Aishiah, Aiysha, Aiyesha, Ayesha, Aysa, Ayse, Aytza

Aislinn, Aislynn (Irish) forms of Ashlyn.
Aishellyn, Aishlinn, Aislee, Aisley, Aislin, Aisling, Aislyn, Aislynne

Aiyana (Native American) forever flowering.
Aiyhana, Aiyona, Aiyonia, Ayana

Aiyanna (Hindi) a form of Ayanna.
Aianna, Aiyannah, Aiyonna, Aiyunna

Aja (Hindi) goat.
Ahjah, Aija, Aijah, Ajá, Ajada, Ajah, Ajara, Ajaran, Ajare, Ajaree, Ajha, Ajia

Ajanae (American) a combination of the letter A + Janae.
Ajahnae, Ajahne, Ajana, Ajanaé, Ajane, Ajané, Ajanee, Ajanique, Ajena, Ajenae, Ajené

Ajia (Hindi) a form of Aja.
Aijia, Ajhia, Aji, Ajjia

Akayla (American) a combination of the letter A + Kayla.
Akaela, Akaelia, Akaila, Akailah, Akala, Akaylah, Akaylia

Akeisha (American) a combination of the letter A + Keisha.
Akaesha, Akaisha, Akasha, Akasia, Akeecia, Akeesha, Akeishia, Akeshia, Akisha

Akela (Hawaiian) noble.
Ahkayla, Ahkeelah, Akelah, Akelia, Akeliah, Akeya, Akeyla, Akeylah

Akeria (American) a form of Akira.
Akera, Akerah, Akeri, Akerra, Akerra

Aki (Japanese) born in autumn.
Akeeye

Akia (American) a combination of the letter A + Kia.
Akaja, Akeia, Akeya, Akiá, Akiah, Akiane, Akiaya, Akiea,
Akiya, Akiyah, Akya, Akyan, Akyia, Akyiah

Akiko (Japanese) bright light.

Akilah (Arabic) intelligent.
Aikiela, Aikilah, Akeela, Akeelah, Akeila, Akeilah, Akeiyla, Akiela, Akielah, Akila, Akilaih, Akilia, Akilka, Akillah, Akkila, Akyla, Akylah

Akili (Tanzanian) wisdom.

Akina (Japanese) spring flower.

Akira (American) a combination of the letter A + Kira.
Akeria, Akiera, Akierra, Akirah, Akire, Akiria, Akirrah, Akyra

Alaina, Alayna (Irish) forms of Alana.
Aalaina, Alainah, Alaine, Alainna, Alainnah, Alane, Alaynah, Alayne, Alaynna, Aleine, Alleyna, Alleynah, Alleyne

Alair (French) a form of Hilary.
Alaira, Ali, Allaire

Alamea (Hawaiian) ripe; precious.

Alameda (Spanish) poplar tree.

Alana (Irish) attractive; peaceful. (Hawaiian) offering. See also Lana.
Alaana, Alaina, Alanae, Alanah, Alane, Alanea, Alani, Alania, Alanis, Alanna, Alawna, Alayna, Allana, Allanah, Allyn, Alonna

Alandra, Alandria (Spanish) forms of Alexandra, Alexandria.
Alandrea, Alantra, Aleandra, Aleandrea

Alani (Hawaiian) orange tree. (Irish) a form of Alana.
Alaini, Alainie, Alania, Alanie, Alaney, Alannie

Alanna (Irish) a form of Alana.
Alannah

Alanza (Spanish) noble and eager.

Alaysha, Alaysia (American) forms of Alicia.
Alaysh, Alayshia

Alba (Latin) from Alba Longa, an ancient city near Rome, Italy.
Albana, Albani, Albanie, Albany, Albeni, Albina, Albine, Albinia, Albinka, Elba

Alberta (German, French) noble and bright. See also Auberte, Bertha, Elberta.
Albertina, Albertine, Albertyna, Albertyne, Alverta

Albreanna (American) a combination of Alberta + Breanna (see Breana).
Albré, Albrea, Albreona, Albreonna, Albreyon

Alcina (Greek) strong-minded.
Alceena, Alcine, Alcinia, Alseena, Alsinia, Alsyna, Alzina

Alda (German) old; elder.
Aldina, Aldine

Alden (English) old; wise protector.
Aldan, Aldon, Aldyn

Aldina, Aldine (Hebrew) forms of Alda.
Aldeana, Aldene, Aldona, Aldyna, Aldyne

Alea, Aleah (Arabic) high, exalted. (Persian) God's being.
Aileah, Aleea, Aleeah, Aleia, Aleiah, Allea, Alleah, Alleea, Alleeah

Aleasha, Aleesha (Greek) forms of Alisha.
Aleashae, Aleashea, Aleashia, Aleassa, Aleeshia

Alecia (Greek) a form of Alicia.
Aalecia, Ahlasia, Aleacia, Aleacya, Aleasia, Alecea, Aleceea, Aleceia, Aleciya, Aleciyah, Alecy, Alecya, Aleeceia, Aleecia, Aleesia, Aleesiya, Aleicia, Alesha, Alesia, Allecia, Alleecia

Aleela (Swahili) she cries.
Aleelah, Alila, Alile

Aleena (Dutch) a form of Aleene.
Ahleena, Aleana, Aleeanna

Aleene (Dutch) alone.
Aleen, Aleena, Alene, Alleen

Aleeya (Hebrew) a form of
Aliya.
*Alee, Aleea, Aleeyah, Aleiya,
Aleiyah*

Aleeza (Hebrew) a form of
Aliza. See also Leeza.
Aleiza

Alegria (Spanish) cheerful.
Aleggra, Alegra, Allegra, Allegria

Aleisha, Alesha (Greek) forms
of Alecia, Alisha.
*Aleasha, Aleashea, Aleasia,
Aleesha, Aleeshah, Aleeshia,
Aleeshya, Aleisa, Alesa, Alesah,
Aleisha, Aleshia, Aleshya,
Alesia, Alessia*

Alejandra (Spanish) a form of
Alexandra.
*Aleiandra, Alejanda, Alejandr,
Alejandrea, Alejandria,
Alejandrina, Alejandro*

Aleka (Hawaiian) a form of
Alice.
Aleeka, Alekah

Aleksandra (Greek) a form of
Alexandra.
*Alecsandra, Aleksasha,
Aleksandrija, Aleksandriya*

Alena (Russian) a form of
Helen.
*Alenah, Alene, Alenea, Aleni,
Alenia, Alenka, Alenna,
Alennah, Alenya, Alyna*

Alesia, Alessia (Greek) forms
of Alice, Alicia, Alisha.
Alessea, Alesya, Allesia

Alessa (Greek) a form of
Alice.
Alessi, Allessa

Alessandra (Italian) a form of
Alexandra.
*Alesandra, Alesandrea,
Alissandra, Alissondra, Allesand,
Allessandra*

Aleta (Greek) a form of Alida.
See also Leta.
Aletta, Alletta

Alethea (Greek) truth.
*Alathea, Alathia, Aletea, Aletha,
Aletheia, Alethia, Aletia,
Alithea, Alithia*

Alette (Latin) wing.

Alex (Greek) a short form of
Alexander, Alexandra.
*Aleix, Aleks, Alexe, Alexx,
Allex, Allexx*

Alexa (Greek) a short form of
Alexandra.
*Aleixa, Alekia, Aleksa, Aleksha,
Aleksi, Alexah, Alexsa, Alexssa,
Alexxa, Allexa, Alyxa*

Alexandra (Greek) defender
of humankind. History: the
last czarina of Russia. See
also Lexia, Lexie, Olesia,
Ritsa, Sandra, Sandrine,
Sasha, Shura, Sondra, Xandra,
Zandra.
*Alandra, Alaxandra,
Aleczandra, Alejandra,
Aleksandra, Alessandra, Alex,
Alexa, Alexande, Alexandera,*

Alexandre, Alexas, Alexi,
Alexina, Alexine, Alexis,
Alexsandra, Alexius, Alexsis,
Alexus, Alexxandra, Alexys,
Alexzandra, Alix, Alixandra,
Aljexi, Alla, Alyx, Alyxandra,
Lexandra

Alexandrea (Greek) a form of
Alexandria.
Alexandreana, Alexandreia,
Alexandriea, Alexandrieah,
Alexanndrea

Alexandria (Greek) a form of
Alexandra. See also Drinka,
Xandra, Zandra.
Alaxandria, Alecsandria,
Aleczandria, Alexanderia,
Alexanderine, Alexandrea,
Alexandrena, Alexandrie,
Alexandrina, Alexandrine,
Alexanndria, Alexandrya,
Alexendria, Alexendrine, Alexia,
Alixandrea, Alyxandria

Alexandrine (Greek) a form
of Alexandra.
Alexandrina

Alexanne (American) a com-
bination of Alex + Anne.
Alexan, Alexanna, Alexane,
Alexann, Alexanna, Alexian,
Alexiana

Alexas, Alexes (Greek) short
forms of Alexandra.
Alexess

Alexi, Alexie (Greek) short
forms of Alexandra.
Aleksey, Aleksi, Alexey, Alexy

Alexia (Greek) a short form of
Alexandria. See also Lexia.
Aleksia, Aleska, Alexcia, Alexea,
Alexsia, Alexsiya, Allexia,
Alyxia

Alexis (Greek) a short form of
Alexandra.
Aalexis, Ahlexis, Alaxis, Alecsis,
Alecxis, Aleexis, Aleksis, Alexcis,
Alexias, Alexiou, Alexiss,
Alexiz, Alexxis, Alixis, Allexis,
Elexis, Lexis

Alexius, Alexus (Greek) short
forms of Alexandra.
Aalexus, Aalexxus, Aelexus,
Ahlexus, Alecsus, Alexsus,
Alexuss, Alexxus, Alixus,
Allexius, Allexus, Elexus, Lexus

Alexsandra (Greek) a form of
Alexandra.
Alexsandria, Alexsandro,
Alixsandra

Alexsis, Alexxis (Greek) short
forms of Alexandra.
Alexxiz

Alexys (Greek) a short form of
Alexandra.
Alexsys, Alexyes, Alexyis,
Alexyss, Allexys

Alexzandra, Alexzandra
(Greek) forms of Alexandra.
Alexzand, Alexzandrea,
Alexzandriah, Alexzandrya,
Alixzandria

Aleya, Aleyah (Hebrew) forms of Aliya.
Alayah, Aleayah, Aleeya, Aléyah, Aleyia, Aleyiah

Alfie (English) a familiar form of Alfreda.
Alfi, Alfy

Alfreda (English) elf counselor; wise counselor. See also Effie, Elfrida, Freda, Frederica.
Alfie, Alfredda, Alfredia, Alfreeda, Alfreida, Alfrieda

Ali, Aly (Greek) familiar forms of Alice, Alicia, Alisha, Alison.
Allea, Alli, Allie, Ally

Alia, Aliah (Hebrew) forms of Aliya. See also Aaliyah, Alea.
Aelia, Allia, Alya

Alice (Greek) truthful. (German) noble. See also Aili, Aleka, Alie, Alisa, Alison, Alli, Alysa, Alyssa, Alysse, Elke.
Adelice, Alecia, Aleece, Alesia, Alicie, Aliece, Alise, Alix, Alize, Alla, Alleece, Allice, Allis, Allise, Allix

Alicia (English) a form of Alice. See also Elicia, Licia.
Aelicia, Alaysha, Alecea, Alecia, Aleecia, Ali, Alicea, Alicha, Alichia, Aliciah, Alician, Alicja, Alicya, Aliecia, Alisha, Allicea, Allicia, Alycia, Ilysa

Alida (Latin) small and winged. (Spanish) noble. See also Aleta, Lida, Oleda.
Aleda, Aleida, Alidia, Alita, Alleda, Allida, Allidah, Alyda, Alydia, Elida, Elidia

Alie, Allie (Greek) familiar forms of Alice.

Aliesha (Greek) a form of Alisha.
Alieshai, Alieshia, Alliesha

Alika (Hawaiian) truthful. (Swahili) most beautiful.
Aleka, Alica, Alikah, Alike, Alikee, Aliki

Alima (Arabic) sea maiden; musical.

Alina, Alyna (Slavic) bright. (Scottish) fair. (English) short forms of Adeline. See also Alena.
Aliana, Alianna, Alinah, Aline, Alinna, Allyna, Alynna, Alyona

Aline (Scottish) a form of Alina.
Alianne, Allene, Alline, Allyn, Allyne, Alyne, Alynne

Alisa, Alissa (Greek) a form of Alice. See also Elisa, Ilisa.
Aalissah, Aaliysah, Aleessa, Alisah, Alisea, Alisia, Alisza, Alisza, Aliysa, Allissa, Alyssa

Alise, Allise (Greek) forms of Alice.
Alics, Aliese, Alis, Aliss, Alisse, Alisse, Alles, Allesse, Allis, Allisse

Alisha (Greek) truthful.
(German) noble. (English) a
form of Alicia. See also
Elisha, Ilisha, Lisha.
*Aalisha, Aleasha, Aleesha,
Aleisha, Alesha, Ali, Aliesha,
Aliscia, Alishah, Alishay,
Alishaye, Alishia, Alishya,
Alitsha, Allisha, Allysha, Alysha*

Alishia, Alisia, Alissia
(English) forms of Alisha.
*Alishea, Alisheia, Alishiana,
Alyssaya, Alisea, Alissya,
Alisyia, Allissia*

Alison, Allison (English)
forms of Alice. See also
Lissie.
*Ali, Alicen, Alicyn, Alisan,
Alisann, Alisanne, Alisen,
Alisenne, Alisin, Alision,
Alisonn, Alisson, Alisun, Alles,
Allesse, Alleyson, Allie, Allisson,
Allisyn, Allix, Allsun*

Alita (Spanish) a form of
Alida.
Allita

Alivia (Latin) a form of Olivia.
Alivah

Alix (Greek) a short form of
Alexandra, Alice.
Alixe, Alixia, Allix, Alyx

Alixandra, Alixandria (Greek)
forms of Alexandria.
*Alixandriya, Allixandra,
Allixandria, Allixandrya*

Aliya (Hebrew) ascender.
*Aaleyah, Aaliyah, Aeliyah,
Ahliya, Ailya, Alea, Aleya, Alia,
Alieya, Alieyah, Aliyah, Aliyiah,
Aliyyah, Allia, Alliyah, Aly,
Alyah*

Aliye (Arabic) noble.
Aliyeh

Aliza (Hebrew) joyful. See also
Aleeza, Eliza.
*Alieza, Aliezah, Alitza, Aliz,
Alizah, Alize, Alizee*

Alizabeth (Hebrew) a form of
Elizabeth.
Alyzabeth

Allana, Allanah (Irish) forms
of Alana.
Allanie, Allanna, Allauna

Allegra (Latin) cheerful.
Legra

Allena (Irish) a form of Alana.
Alleen, Alleyna, Alleynah

Alli, Ally (Greek) familiar
forms of Alice.
Ali, Alley

Allia, Alliah (Hebrew) forms
of Aliya.

Allissa (Greek) a form of
Alyssa.
Allisa

Alliyah (Hebrew) a form of
Aliya.
*Alliya, Alliyha, Alliyia,
Alliyyah, Allya, Allyah*

Allysa, Allyssa (Greek) a form of Alyssa.
Allissa, Allyisa, Allysa, Allysah, Allyssah

Allysha (English) a form of Alisha.
Alishia, Allysia

Allyson, Alyson (English) forms of Alison.
Allysen, Allyson, Allysonn, Allysson, Allysun, Alyson

Alma (Arabic) learned. (Latin) soul.
Almah

Almeda (Arabic) ambitious.
Allmeda, Allmedah, Allmeta, Allmita, Almea, Almedah, Almeta, Almida, Almita

Almira (Arabic) aristocratic, princess; exalted. (Spanish) from Almeíra, Spain. See also Elmira, Mira.
Allmeera, Allmeria, Allmira, Almeera, Almeeria, Almeira, Almeria, Almire

Aloha (Hawaiian) loving, kindhearted, charitable.
Alohi

Aloisa (German) famous warrior.
Aloisia, Aloysia

Aloma (Latin) a short form of Paloma.

Alondra (Spanish) a form of Alexandra.
Allandra, Alonda

Alonna (Irish) a form of Alana.
Alona, Alonnah, Alonya, Alonyah

Alonza (English) noble and eager.

Alora (American) a combination of the letter A + Lora.
Alorah, Alorha, Alorie, Aloura, Alouria

Alpha (Greek) first-born. Linguistics: the first letter of the Greek alphabet.
Alphia

Alta (Latin) high; tall.
Allta, Altah, Altana, Altanna, Altea, Alto

Althea (Greek) wholesome; healer. History: Althea Gibson was the first African American to win a major tennis title. See also Thea.
Altha, Altheda, Altheya, Althia, Elthea, Eltheya, Elthia

Alva (Latin, Spanish) white; light skinned. See also Elva.
Alvana, Alvanna, Alvannah

Alvina (English) friend to all; noble friend; friend to elves. See also Elva, Vina.
Alveanea, Alveen, Alveena, Alveenia, Alvenea, Alvie, Alvinae, Alvincia, Alvine,

Alvinea, Alvinesha, Alvinia,
Alvinna, Alvita, Alvona,
Alvyna, Alwin, Alwina, Alwyn

Alyah, Alyiah (Hebrew) forms
of Aliya.
Aly, Alya, Aleah, Alyia

Alycia, Alyssia (English) forms
of Alicia.
Allyce, Alycea, Alyciah, Alyse,
Lycia

Alysa, Alyse, Alysse (Greek)
forms of Alice.
Allys, Allyse, Allyss, Alys, Alyss

Alysha, Alysia (Greek) forms
of Alisha.
Allysea, Allyscia, Alysea,
Alyshia, Alyssha, Alyssia

Alyssa (Greek) rational.
Botany: alyssum is a flower-
ing herb. See also Alice,
Elissa.
Ahlyssa, Alissa, Allissa, Allyssa,
Alyesa, Alyessa, Alyissa, Alysah,
Ilyssa, Lyssa, Lyssah

Alysse (Greek) a form of
Alice.
Allyce, Allys, Allyse, Allyss, Alys,
Alyss

Alyx, Alyxis (Greek) short
forms of Alexandra.

Alyxandra, Alyxandria
(Greek) forms of Alexandria.
Alyxandrea, Alyxzandrya

Am (Vietnamese) lunar; female.

Ama (African) born on Saturday.

Amabel (Latin) lovable. See
also Bel, Mabel.

Amada (Spanish) beloved.
Amadea, Amadi, Amadia,
Amadita

Amairani (Greek) a form of
Amara.
Amairaine, Amairane,
Amairanie, Amairany

Amal (Hebrew) worker.
(Arabic) hopeful.
Amala

Amalia (German) a form of
Amelia.
Ahmalia, Amalea, Amaleah,
Amaleta, Amalija, Amalina,
Amalisa, Amalita, Amaliya,
Amalya, Amalyn

Amalie (German) a form of
Amelia.
Amalee, Amali, Amaly

Aman, Amani (Arabic) forms
of Imani.
Aamani, Ahmani, Amane,
Amanee, Amaney, Amanie,
Ammanu

Amanada (Latin) a form of
Amanda.

Amanda (Latin) lovable. See
also Manda.
Amada, Amanada, Amandah,
Amandalee, Amandalyn,
Amandi, Amandie, Amandine,
Amandy

Amandeep (Punjabi) peaceful light.

Amara (Greek) eternally beautiful. See also Mara.
Amar, Amaira, Amairani, Amarah, Amari, Amaria, Amariah

Amaranta (Spanish) a flower that never fades.

Amari (Greek) a form of Amara.
Amaree, Amarie, Amarii, Amarri

Amaris (Hebrew) promised by God.
Amarissa, Amarys, Maris

Amaryllis (Greek) fresh; flower.
Amarillis, Amarylis

Amaui (Hawaiian) thrush.

Amaya (Japanese) night rain.

Ambar (French) a form of Amber.

Amber (French) amber.
Aamber, Ahmber, Ambar, Amberia, Amberise, Amberly, Ambria, Ambur, Ambyr, Ambyre, Ammber, Ember

Amberly (American) a familiar form of Amber.
Amberle, Amberlea, Amberlee, Amberleigh, Amberley, Amberli, Amberlie, Amberlly, Amberlye

Amberlyn, Amberlynn (American) combinations of Amber + Lynn.
Amberlin, Amberlina, Amberlyne, Amberlynne

Ambria (American) a form of Amber.
Ambrea, Ambra, Ambriah

Amelia (German) hard working. (Latin) a form of Emily. History: Amelia Earhart, an American aviator, was the first woman to fly solo across the Atlantic Ocean. See also Ima, Melia, Millie, Nuela, Yamelia.
Aemilia, Aimilia, Amalia, Amalie, Amaliya, Ameila, Ameilia, Amelie, Amelina, Ameline, Amelisa, Amelita, Amella, Amilia, Amilina, Amilisa, Amilita, Amilyn, Amylia

Amelie (German) a familiar form of Amelia.
Amaley, Amalie, Amelee, Ameleigh, Ameley, Amélie, Amely, Amilie

America (Teutonic) industrious.
Americana, Amerika

Ami, Amie (French) forms of Amy.
Aami, Amiee, Amii, Amiiee, Ammee, Ammie, Ammiee

Amilia, Amilie (Latin, German) forms of Amelia.
Amilee, Amili, Amillia, Amily, Amilya

Amina (Arabic) trustworthy, faithful. History: the mother of the prophet Muhammad.
Aamena, Aamina, Aaminah, Ameena, Ameenah, Aminah, Aminda, Amindah, Aminta, Amintah

Amira (Hebrew) speech; utterance. (Arabic) princess. See also Mira.
Ameera, Ameerah, Amirah

Amissa (Hebrew) truth.
Amissah

Amita (Hebrew) truth.
Amitha

Amity (Latin) friendship.
Amitie

Amlika (Hindi) mother.
Amlikah

Amma (Hindi) god, godlike. Religion: another name for the Hindu goddess Shakti.

Amorie (German) industrious leader.

Amparo (Spanish) protected.

Amrit (Sanskrit) nectar.
Amrita

Amy (Latin) beloved. See also Aimee, Emma, Esmé.
Amata, Ame, Amey, Ami, Amia, Amie, Amio, Ammy, Amye, Amylyn

An (Chinese) peaceful.

Ana (Hawaiian, Spanish) a form of Hannah.
Anai, Anaia

Anaba (Native American) she returns from battle.

Anabel, Anabelle (English) forms of Annabel.
Anabela, Anabele, Anabell, Anabella

Anahita (Persian) a river and water goddess.
Anahai, Anahi, Anahit, Anahy

Anais (Hebrew) gracious.
Anaise, Anaïse

Anala (Hindi) fine.

Analisa, Analise (English) combinations of Ana + Lisa.
Analice, Analicia, Analis, Analisha, Analisia, Analissa

Anamaria (English) a combination of Ana + Maria.
Anamarie, Anamary

Ananda (Hindi) blissful.

Anastacia (Greek) a form of Anastasia.
Anastace, Anastacie

Anastasia (Greek) resurrection. See also Nastasia, Stacey, Stacia, Stasya.
Anastacia, Anastase, Anastascia, Anastasha, Anastashia, Anastasie, Anastasija, Anastassia, Anastassya, Anastasya, Anastatia, Anastaysia, Anastazia, Anastice, Annastasia,

Anastasia *(cont.)*
Annastasija, Annastaysia,
Annastazia, Annstás

Anatola (Greek) from the
east.

Anci (Hungarian) a form of
Hannah.
Annus, Annushka

Andee, Andi, Andie
(American) short forms of
Andrea, Fernanda.
Ande, Andea, Andy

Andrea (Greek) strong; coura-
geous. See also Ondrea.
Aindrea, Andee, Andera,
Anderea, Andra, Andrah,
Andraia, Andraya, Andreah,
Andreaka, Andreana, Andreane,
Andree, Andrée, Andreea,
Andreia, Andreja, Andreka,
Andrel, Andrell, Andrelle,
Andreo, Andressa, Andrette,
Andreya, Andria, Andriana,
Andrieka, Andrietta, Andris,
Aundrea

Andreana, Andreanna
'Greek) forms of Andrea.
Ahndrianna, Andreina,
Andrena, Andreyana,
Andreyonna, Andrina,
Andriona, Andrionna

Andreane, Andreanne
(Greek) forms of Andrea.
Andrean, Andreeanne, Andree
Anne, Andrene, Andrian,
Andrienne

Andria (Greek) a form of
Andrea.
Andri, Andriea

Andriana, Andrianna (Greek)
forms of Andrea.

Aneesa, Aneesha (Greek)
forms of Agnes.
Ahnesha, Ahnesia, Ahnesshia,
Anee, Aneesah, Aneese,
Aneeshah, Aneesia, Aneisa,
Aneisha, Anessa, Anessia

Aneko (Japanese) older sister.

Anela (Hawaiian) angel.
Anel, Anelle

Anessa (Greek) a form of Agnes.
Anesha, Aneshia, Anesia,
Anessia, Annessa

Anetra (American) a form of
Annette.
Anitra

Anezka (Czech) a form of
Hannah.

Angel (Greek) a short form of
Angela.
Angele, Angéle, Angell, Angelle,
Angil, Anjel

Angela (Greek) angel; messen-
ger.
Angala, Anganita, Angel,
Angelanell, Angelanette,
Angelee, Angeleigh, Angeles,
Angeli, Angelia, Angelica,
Angelina, Angelique, Angelita,
Angella, Angellita, Angie,
Anglea, Anjela, Anjelica

Angelia (Greek) a form of
Angela.
Angelea, Angeleah, Angelie

Angelica, Angelika (Greek)
forms of Angela.
*Angalic, Angelic, Angelici,
Angelicia, Angelike, Angeliki,
Angellica, Angilica*

Angelina, Angeline (Russian)
forms of Angela.
*Angalena, Angalina, Angeleen,
Angelena, Angelene, Angeliana,
Angeleana, Angellina, Angelyn,
Angelyna, Angelyne, Angelynn,
Angelynne, Anhelina, Anjelina*

Angelique (French) a form of
Angela.
*Angeliqua, Angélique, Angilique,
Anjelique*

Angeni (Native American)
spirit.

Angie (Greek) a familiar form
of Angela.
Ange, Angee, Angey, Angi, Angy

Ani (Hawaiian) beautiful.
Aany, Aanye

Ania (Polish) a form of
Hannah.
Ahnia, Anaya, Aniah

Anica, Anika (Czech) familiar
forms of Anna.
*Aanika, Anaka, Aneeky, Aneka,
Anekah, Anicka, Anik, Anikah,
Anike, Anikka, Anikke, Aniko,
Anneka, Annik, Annika,
Anouska, Anuska*

Anice (English) a form of
Agnes.
*Anesse, Anis, Anise, Annes,
Annice, Annis, Annus*

Anila (Hindi) Religion: an
attendant of the Hindu god
Vishnu.
Anilla

Anisa, Anisah (Arabic) friendly.
Annissah

Anissa, Anisha (English)
forms of Agnes, Ann.
*Aanisha, Aeniesha, Anis, Anisa,
Anissah, Anise, Annisa,
Annisha, Annissa, Anyssa*

Anita (Spanish) a form of
Ann, Anna. See also Nita.
*Aneeta, Aneetah, Aneethah,
Anetha, Anitha, Anithah,
Anitia, Anitra, Anitte*

Anjelica (Greek) a form of
Angela.
Anjelika

Anka (Polish) a familiar form
of Hannah.
Anke

Ann, Anne (English) gracious.
*Anissa, Anita, Annchen,
Annette, Annie, Annik, Annika,
Annze, Anouche*

Anna (German, Italian, Czech,
Swedish) gracious. Culture:
Anna Pavlova was a famous
Russian ballerina. See also
Anica, Anissa, Nina.
Ahnna, Ana, Anah, Anica,

Anna *(cont.)*
Anita, Annah, Annina, Annora, Anona, Anya, Anyu, Aska

Annabel (English) a combination of Anna + Bel.
Amabel, Anabel, Annabal, Annabelle

Annabelle (English) a form of Annabel.
Anabelle, Annabell, Annabella

Annalie (Finnish) a form of Hannah.
Analee, Annalea, Annaleah, Annalee, Annaleigh, Annaleigha, Annali, Anneli, Annelie

Annalisa, Annalise (English) combinations of Anna + Lisa.
Analisa, Analise, Annaliesa, Annaliese, Annalissa, Annalisse

Annamarie, Annemarie, Annmarie, Anne-Marie (English) combinations of Anne + Marie.
Annamaria, Anna-Maria, Anna-Marie, Annmaria

Anneka (Swedish) a form of Hannah.
Annaka, Anneke, Annika, Anniki, Annikki

Annelisa (English) a combination of Ann + Lisa.
Analiese, Anelisa, Anelise, Anneliese, Annelise

Annette (French) a form of Ann. See also Anetra, Nettie.
Anet, Aneta, Anetra, Anett, Anetta, Anette, Anneth, Annett, Annetta

Annie (English) a familiar form of Ann.
Anni, Anny

Annik, Annika (Russian) forms of Ann.
Aneka, Anekah, Annick, Annicka, Annike, Annikka, Anninka, Anouk

Annjanette (American) a combination of Ann + Janette (see Janett).
Angen, Angenett, Angenette, Anjane, Anjanetta, Anjani

Anona (English) pineapple.

Anouhea (Hawaiian) cool, soft fragrance.

Ansley (Scottish) forms of Ainsley.
Anslea, Anslee, Ansleigh, Anslie

Anthea (Greek) flower.
Antha, Anthe, Anthia, Thia

Antionette (French) a form of Antonia.
Antionet, Antionett, Anntionett

Antoinette (French) a form of Antonia. See also Netti, Toinette, Toni.
Anta, Antanette, Antoinella, Antoinet, Antonella, Antonetta,

Antonette, Antonice, Antonieta,
Antonietta, Antonique

Antonia (Greek) flourishing.
(Latin) praiseworthy. See also
Toni, Tonya, Tosha.
Ansonia, Ansonya, Antania,
Antinia, Antionette, Antoinette,
Antona, Antoñía, Antonice,
Antonie, Antonina, Antonine,
Antoniya, Antonnea, Antonnia,
Antonya

Antonice (Latin) a form of
Antonia.
Antanise, Antanisha, Antonesha,
Antoneshia, Antonise, Antonisha

Anya (Russian) a form of
Anna.
Aaniyah, Aniya, Aniyah, Anja

Anyssa (English) a form of
Anissa.
Anysa, Anysha

'Aolani (Hawaiian) heavenly
cloud.

Aphra (Hebrew) young doe.
See also Afra.

April (Latin) opening. See also
Avril.
Aprele, Aprelle, Apriell, Aprielle,
Aprila, Aprile, Aprilette, Aprili,
Aprill, Apryl

Apryl (Latin) a form of April.
Apryle

Aquene (Native American)
peaceful.

Ara (Arabic) opinionated.
Ahraya, Aira, Arae, Arah, Araya,
Arayah

Arabella (Latin) beautiful altar.
See also Belle, Orabella.
Arabela, Arabele, Arabelle

Araceli, Aracely (Latin) heav-
enly altar.
Aracele, Aracelia, Aracelli,
Araseli, Arasely, Arcelia, Arceli

Ardelle (Latin) warm; enthusiastic.
Ardelia, Ardelis, Ardella

Arden (English) valley of the
eagle. Literature: in
Shakespeare, a romantic place
of refuge.
Ardeen, Ardeena, Ardena,
Ardene, Ardenia, Ardi, Ardin,
Ardina, Ardine

Ardi (Hebrew) a short form of
Arden, Ardice, Ardith.
Ardie, Arti, Artie

Ardice (Hebrew) a form of
Ardith.
Ardis, Artis, Ardiss, Ardyce, Ardys

Ardith (Hebrew) flowering
field.
Ardath, Ardi, Ardice, Ardyth

Areli, Arely (American) forms
of Oralee.
Areil, Areile, Arelee, Areli, Arelis,
Arelli, Arellia, Arelly

Arella (Hebrew) angel; messenger.
Arela, Arelle, Orella, Orelle

Aretha (Greek) virtuous. See also Oretha.
Areatha, Areetha, Areta, Aretina, Aretta, Arette, Arita, Aritha, Retha, Ritha

Ari, Aria, Arie (Hebrew) short forms of Ariel.
Ariah, Ariea, Aryia

Ariadne (Greek) holy. Mythology: the daughter of King Minos of Crete.

Ariana, Arianna (Greek) holy.
Aeriana, Aerianna, Aerionna, Ahreanna, Ahriana, Ahrianna, Airiana, Arieana, Ariona, Arionna, Aryonna

Ariane (French), Arianne (English) forms of Ariana, Arianna.
Aerian, Aeriann, Aerion, Aerionne, Airiann, Ari, Arianie, Ariann, Ariannie, Arieann, Arien, Ariene, Arienne, Arieon, Arionne, Aryane, Aryann, Aryanne

Arica (Scandinavian) forms of Erica.
Aerica, Aericka, Aeryka, Aricca, Aricka, Arika, Arike, Arikka

Ariel (Hebrew) lion of God.
Aerial, Aeriale, Aeriel, Aeriela, Aeryal, Ahriel, Aire, Aireal, Airial, Ari, Aria, Arial, Ariale,

Arieal, Ariela, Arielle, Arrieal, Arriel, Aryel, Auriel

Arielle (French) a form of Ariel.
Aeriell, Ariella, Arriele, Arriell, Arrielle, Aryelle, Aurielle

Arin (Hebrew) enlightened. (Arabic) messenger. See also Erin.
Aaren, Aerin, Aieron, Aieren, Arinn, Aryn

Arista (Greek) best.
Aris, Arissa, Aristana, Aristen

Arla (German) a form of Carla.

Arleigh (English) a form of Harley.
Arlea, Arlee, Arley, Arlie, Arly

Arlene (Irish) pledge. See also Lena, Lina.
Airlen, Arlana, Arleen, Arleene, Arlen, Arlena, Arlenis, Arlette, Arleyne, Arliene, Arlina, Arlinda, Arline, Arlis

Arlette (English) a form of Arlene.
Arleta, Arletta, Arletty

Arlynn (American) a combination of Arlene + Lynn.
Arlyn, Arlyne, Arlynne

Armani (Persian) desire, goal.
Armahni, Arman, Armanee, Armanii

Armine (Latin) noble. (German) soldier. (French) a

form of Herman (see Boys'
Names).
Armina

Arnelle (German) eagle.
Arnell, Arnella

Artha (Hindi) wealthy, prosperous.
Arthi, Arti, Artie

Artis (Irish) noble; lofty hill.
(Scottish) bear. (English)
rock. (Icelandic) follower of
Thor.
*Arthea, Arthelia, Arthene,
Arthette, Arthurette, Arthurina,
Arthurine, Artina, Artice*

Aryana, Aryanna (Italian)
forms of Ariana.
Aryan, Aryanah, Aryannah

Aryn (Hebrew) a form of
Arin.
*Aerryn, Aeryn, Airyn, Aryne,
Arynn, Arynne*

Asa (Japanese) born in the
morning.

Asha (Arabic, Swahili) a form
of Aisha, Ashia.

Ashanti (Swahili) from a tribe
in West Africa.
*Achante, Achanti, Asante,
Ashanta, Ashantae, Ashante,
Ashanté, Ashantee, Ashantie,
Ashaunta, Ashauntae,
Ashauntee, Ashaunti, Ashonti,
Ashuntae, Ashunti*

Ashely (English) form of
Ashley.
*Ashelee, Ashelei, Asheley,
Ashelie, Ashelley, Ashelly*

Ashia (Arabic) life.
*Asha, Ashya, Ashyah, Ashyia,
Ayshia*

Ashlee, Ashli, Ashlie, Ashly
(English) forms of Ashley.
*Ashle, Ashlea, Ashleah, Ashleeh,
Ashliee*

Ashleigh (English) a form of
Ashley.
*Ahsleigh, Asheleigh, Ashlei,
Ashliegh*

Ashley (English) ash tree
meadow. See also Lee.
*Ahslee, Aishlee, Ashala, Ashalee,
Ashalei, Ashaley, Ashely, Ashla,
Ashlay, Ashleay, Ashlee,
Ashleigh, Ashleye, Ashli, Ashlie,
Ashly, Ashlye*

Ashlin (English) a form of
Ashlyn.
*Ashlean, Ashliann, Ashlianne,
Ashline*

Ashlyn, Ashlynn (English) ash
tree pool. (Irish) vision,
dream.
*Ashlan, Ashleann, Ashleen,
Ashleene, Ashlen, Ashlene,
Ashlin, Ashling, Ashlyne,
Ashlynne*

Ashten, Ashtin (English)
forms of Ashton.
Ashtine

Ashton (English) ash-tree *settlement.*
Ashten, Ashtyn

Ashtyn (English) a form of Ashton.
Ashtynne

Asia (Greek) resurrection. (English) eastern sunrise. (Swahili) a form of Aisha.
Ahsia, Aisia, Aisian, Asiah, Asian, Asianae, Asya, Aysia, Aysiah, Aysian, Ayzia

Aspen (English) aspen tree.
Aspin, Aspyn

Aster (English) a form of Astra.
Astera, Asteria, Astyr

Astra (Greek) star.
Asta, Astara, Aster, Astraea, Astrea

Astrid (Scandinavian) divine strength.
Astri, Astrida, Astrik, Astrud, Atti, Estrid

Atalanta (Greek) mighty huntress. Mythology: an athletic young woman who refused to marry any man who could not outrun her in a footrace. See also Lani.
Atalaya, Atlanta, Atlante, Atlee

Atara (Hebrew) crown.
Atarah, Ataree

Athena (Greek) wise. Mythology: the goddess of wisdom.
Athenea, Athene, Athina, Atina

Atira (Hebrew) prayer.

Auberte (French) a form of Alberta.
Auberta, Aubertha, Auberthe, Aubine

Aubree, Aubrie (French) forms of Aubrey.
Auberi, Aubre, Aubrei, Aubreigh, Aubri, Aubrielle

Aubrey (German) noble; bear-like. (French) blond ruler; elf ruler.
Aubary, Aubery, Aubray, Aubrea, Aubreah, Aubree, Aubrette, Aubria, Aubrie, Aubry, Aubury, Avery

Aubriana, Aubrianna (English) combinations of Aubrey + Anna.
Aubreyana, Aubreyanna, Aubreyanne, Aubreyena, Aubrianne

Audey (English) a familiar form of Audrey.
Aude, Audi, Audie

Audra (French) a form of Audrey.
Audria, Audriea

Audreanne (English) a combination of Audrey + Anne.
Audrea, Audreen, Audrianne, Audrienne

Audree, Audrie (English) forms of Audrey.
Audre, Audri

Audrey (English) noble strength.
Adrey, Audey, Audra, Audray, Audree, Audrie, Audrin, Audriya, Audry, Audrye

Audriana, Audrianna (English) combinations of Audrey + Anna.
Audreanna, Audrienna, Audrina

Audris (German) fortunate, wealthy.
Audrys

Augusta (Latin) a short form of Augustine. See also Gusta.
Agusta, August, Auguste, Augustia, Augustus, Austina

Augustine (Latin) majestic. Religion: Saint Augustine was the first archbishop of Canterbury. See also Tina.
Agustina, Augusta, Augustina, Augustyna, Augustyne, Austin

'Aulani (Hawaiian) royal messenger.
Lani, Lanie

Aundrea (Greek) a form of Andrea.
Aundreah

Aura (Greek) soft breeze. (Latin) golden. See also Ora.

Aurelia (Latin) golden. See also Oralia.
Auralea, Auralia, Aurea, Aureal, Aurel, Aurele, Aurelea, Aureliana, Aurelie, Auria, Aurie, Aurilia, Aurita

Aurelie (Latin) a form of Aurelia.
Auralee, Auralei, Aurelee, Aurelei, Aurelle

Aurora (Latin) dawn. Mythology: Aurora was the goddess of dawn.
Aurore, Ora, Ori, Orie, Rora

Austin (Latin) a short form of Augustine.
Austen, Austin, Austyn, Austynn

Autumn (Latin) autumn.
Autum

Ava (Greek) a form of Eva.
Avada, Avae, Ave, Aveen

Avalon (Latin) island.
Avallon

Avery (English) a form of Aubrey.
Aivree, Averi, Averie, Avry

Avis (Latin) bird.
Avais, Avi, Avia, Aviana, Avianca, Aviance, Avianna

Aviva (Hebrew) springtime. See also Viva.
Aviv, Avivah, Avivi, Avivice, Avni, Avnit, Avri, Avrit, Avy

Avril (French) a form of April.
*Averil, Averyl, Avra, Avri,
Avrilia, Avrill, Avrille, Avrillia,
Avy*

Axelle (Latin) axe. (German)
small oak tree; source of life.
Aixa

Aya (Hebrew) bird; fly swiftly.
Aia, Aiah, Aiya, Aiyah

Ayanna (Hindi) innocent.
*Ahyana, Aiyanna, Ayan, Ayana,
Ayania, Ayannica, Ayna*

Ayesha (Persian) a form of
Aisha.
*Ayasha, Ayeshah, Ayessa,
Ayisha, Ayishah, Aysha,
Ayshah, Ayshe, Ayshea, Aysia*

Ayita (Cherokee) first in the
dance.

Ayla (Hebrew) oak tree.
*Aylana, Aylee, Ayleen, Aylene,
Aylie, Aylin*

Aza (Arabic) comfort.
Aiza, Aizha, Aizia, Azia

Aziza (Swahili) precious.
Azize

B

Baba (African) born on
Thursday.
Aba

Babe (Latin) a familiar form
of Barbara. (American) a
form of Baby.
Babby

Babette (French, German) a
familiar form of Barbara.
Babita, Barbette

Babs (American) a familiar
form of Barbara.
Bab

Baby (American) baby.
Babby, Babe, Bebe

Bailee, Bailie (English) forms
of Bailey.
*Baelee, Baeli, Bailea, Bailei,
Baillee, Baillie, Bailli*

Baileigh, Baleigh (English)
forms of Bailey.
Baeleigh

Bailey (English) bailiff.
*Baeley, Bailee, Baileigh, Bailley,
Bailly, Baily, Bali, Balley,
Baylee, Bayley*

Baka (Hindi) crane.

Bakula (Hindi) flower.

Bambi (Italian) child.
Bambee, Bambie, Bamby

Bandi (Punjabi) prisoner.
Banda, Bandy

Baptista (Latin) baptizer.
*Baptiste, Batista, Battista,
Bautista*

Bara, Barra (Hebrew) chosen.
Bára, Bari

Barb (Latin) a short form of
Barbara.
Barba, Barbe

Barbara (Latin) stranger, for-
eigner. See also Bebe, Varvara,
Wava.
*Babara, Babb, Babbie, Babe,
Babette, Babina, Babs, Barb,
Barbara-Ann, Barbarit,
Barbarita, Barbary, Barbeeleen,
Barbera, Barbie, Barbora,
Barborah, Barborka, Barbra,
Barbraann, Barbro, Barùska,
Basha, Bebe, Bobbi, Bobbie*

Barbie (American) a familiar
form of Barbara.
*Barbee, Barbey, Barbi, Barby,
Baubie*

Barbra (American) a form of
Barbara.
Barbro

Barrett (German) strong as a
bear.

Barrie (Irish) spear;
markswoman.
Bari, Barri, Berri, Berrie, Berry

Basia (Hebrew) daughter of
God.
*Basya, Bathia, Batia, Batya,
Bitya, Bithia*

Bathsheba (Hebrew) daugh-
ter of the oath; seventh
daughter. Bible: a wife of
King David. See also Sheba.
*Bathshua, Batsheva, Bersaba,
Bethsabee, Bethsheba*

Batini (Swahili) inner
thoughts.

Baylee, Bayleigh, Baylie
(English) forms of Bailey.
*Bayla, Bayle, Baylea, Bayleah,
Baylei, Bayli, Bayliee, Bayliegh*

Bayley (English) a form of
Bailey.
Bayly

Bayo (Yoruba) joy is found.

Bea, Bee (American) short
forms of Beatrice.

Beata (Latin) a short form of
Beatrice.
Beatta

Beatrice (Latin) blessed;
happy; bringer of joy. See
also Trish, Trixie.
*Bea, Beata, Beatrica, Béatrice,
Beatricia, Beatriks, Beatrisa,
Beatrise, Beatrissa, Beatriz,
Beattie, Beatty, Bebe, Bee, Trice*

Beatriz (Latin) a form of
Beatrice.
Beatris, Beatriss, Beatrix, Beitris

Bebe (Spanish) a form of
Barbara, Beatrice.
BB, Beebee, Bibi

Becca (Hebrew) a short form
of Rebecca.
Beca, Becka, Bekah, Bekka

Becky (American) a familiar
form of Rebecca.
Beckey, Becki, Beckie

Bedelia (Irish) a form of
Bridget.
Bedeelia, Biddy, Bidelia

Bel (Hindi) sacred wood of
apple trees. A short form of
Amabel, Belinda, Isabel.

Bela (Czech) white.
(Hungarian) bright.
Belah, Biela

Belen (Greek) arrow. (Spanish)
Bethlehem.
Belina

Belicia (Spanish) dedicated to
God.
Beli, Belia, Belica

Belinda (Spanish) beautiful.
Literature: a name coined by
English poet Alexander Pope
in *The Rape of the Lock*. See
also Blinda, Linda.
Bel, Belindra, Belle, Belynda

Bella (Latin) beautiful.
Bellah

Belle (French) beautiful. A
short form of Arabella,
Belinda, Isabel. See also
Billie.
Belita, Bell, Belli, Bellina

Belva (Latin) beautiful view.
Belvia

Bena (Native American)
pheasant. See also Bina.
Benea

Benecia (Latin) a short form
of Benedicta.
*Beneisha, Benicia, Benish,
Benisha, Benishia, Bennicia*

Benedicta (Latin) blessed.
*Bendite, Benecia, Benedetta,
Benedicte, Benedikta, Bengta,
Benita, Benna, Benni, Bennicia,
Benoîte, Binney*

Benedicte (Latin) a form of
Benedicta.

Benita (Spanish) a form of
Benedicta.
*Beneta, Benetta, Benitta,
Bennita, Neeta*

Bennett (Latin) little blessed
one.
Bennet, Bennetta

Benni (Latin) a familiar form
of Benedicta.
Bennie, Binni, Binnie, Binny

Bente (Latin) blessed.

Berenice (Greek) a form of
Bernice.
*Berenise, Berenisse, Bereniz,
Berenize*

Berget (Irish) a form of
Bridget.
Bergette, Bergit

Berit (German) glorious.
Beret, Berette, Berta

Berkley (Scottish, English)
birch-tree meadow.
Berkeley, Berkly

Berlynn (English) a combination of Bertha + Lynn.
Berla, Berlin, Berlinda, Berline, Berling, Berlyn, Berlyne, Berlynne

Bernadette (French) a form of Bernadine. See also Nadette.
Bera, Beradette, Berna, Bernadet, Bernadete, Bernadett, Bernadetta, Bernarda, Bernardette, Bernedet, Bernedette, Bernessa, Berneta

Bernadine (English, German) brave as a bear.
Bernadene, Bernadette, Bernadin, Bernadina, Bernardina, Bernardine, Berni

Berneta (French) a short form of Bernadette.
Bernatta, Bernetta, Bernette, Bernita

Berni (English) a familiar form of Bernadine, Bernice.
Bernie, Berny

Bernice (Greek) bringer of victory. See also Bunny, Vernice.
Berenice, Berenike, Bernessa, Berni, Bernicia, Bernise, Nixie

Bertha (German) bright; illustrious; brilliant ruler. A short form of Alberta. See also Birdie, Peke.
Barta, Bartha, Berta, Berthe, Bertille, Bertita, Bertrona, Bertus, Birtha

Berti (German, English) a familiar form of Gilberte, Bertina.
Berte, Bertie, Berty

Bertille (French) a form of Bertha.

Bertina (English) bright, shining.
Bertine

Beryl (Greek) sea green jewel.
Beryle

Bess, Bessie (Hebrew) familiar forms of Elizabeth.
Bessi, Bessy

Beth (Hebrew, Aramaic) house of God. A short form of Bethany, Elizabeth.
Betha, Bethe, Bethia

Bethani, Bethanie (Aramaic) forms of Bethany.
Bethanee, Bethania, Bethannie, Bethni, Bethnie

Bethann (English) a combination of Beth + Ann.
Beth-Ann, Bethan, Bethane, Bethanne, Beth-Anne

Bethany (Aramaic) house of figs. Bible: the site of Lazarus's resurrection.
Beth, Bethaney, Bethani, Bethanney, Bethanny, Bethena, Betheny, Bethia, Bethina, Bethney, Bethny, Betthany

Betsy (American) a familiar
form of Elizabeth.
Betsey, Betsi, Betsie

Bette (French) a form of Betty.
Beta, Beti, Betka, Bett, Betta

Bettina (American) a combination of Beth + Tina.
Betina, Betine, Betti, Bettine

Betty (Hebrew) consecrated to
God. (English) a familiar
form of Elizabeth.
*Bette, Bettey, Betti, Bettie,
Bettye, Bettyjean, Betty-Jean,
Bettyjo, Betty-Jo, Bettylou,
Betty-Lou, Bety, Boski, Bözsi*

Betula (Hebrew) girl, maiden.

Beulah (Hebrew) married.
Bible: Beulah is a name for
Israel.
Beula, Beulla, Beullah

Bev (English) a short form of
Beverly.

Bevanne (Welsh) child of Evan.
Bevan, Bevann, Bevany

Beverly (English) beaver field.
See also Buffy.
*Bev, Bevalee, Beverle, Beverlee,
Beverley, Beverlie, Beverlly,
Bevlyn, Bevlynn, Bevlynne,
Bevvy, Verly*

Beverlyann (American) a
combination of Beverly +
Ann.
*Beverliann, Beverlianne,
Beverlyanne*

Bian (Vietnamese) hidden;
secretive.

Bianca (Italian) white. See also
Blanca, Vianca.
*Biancca, Biancha, Biancia,
Bianco, Bianey, Bianica, Bianka,
Biannca, Binney, Bionca,
Blanca, Blanche, Byanca*

Bianka (Italian) a form of
Bianca.
Beyanka, Biannka

Bibi (Latin) a short form of
Bibiana. (Arabic) lady.
(Spanish) a form of Bebe.

Bibiana (Latin) lively.
Bibi

Biddy (Irish) a familiar form
of Bedelia.
Biddie

Billi, Billy (English) forms of
Billie.
Billye

Billie (English) strong willed.
(German, French) a familiar
form of Belle, Wilhelmina.
*Bilee, Bileigh, Bili, Bilie, Billee,
Billi, Billy, Billye*

Billie-Jean (American) a combination of Billie + Jean.
Billiejean, Billyjean, Billy-Jean

Billie-Jo (American) a combination of Billie + Jo.
Billiejo, Billyjo, Billy-Jo

Bina (Hebrew) wise; understanding. (Swahili) dancer.

(Latin) a short form of
Sabina. See also Bena.
Binah, Binney, Binta, Bintah

Binney (English) a familiar
form of Benedicta, Bianca,
Bina.
Binnee, Binni, Binnie, Binny

Bionca (Italian) a form of
Bianca.
*Beonca, Beyonca, Beyonka,
Bioncha, Bionica, Bionka,
Bionnca*

Birdie (English) bird.
(German) a familiar form of
Bertha.
*Bird, Birdee, Birdella, Birdena,
Birdey, Birdi, Birdy, Byrd,
Byrdey, Byrdie, Byrdy*

Birgitte (Swedish) a form of
Bridget.
Birgit, Birgita, Birgitta

Blaine (Irish) thin.
Blane, Blayne

Blair (Scottish) plains dweller.
Blaire

Blaire (Scottish) a form of
Blair.
Blare, Blayre

Blaise (French) one who
stammers.
*Blaize, Blasha, Blasia, Blaza,
Blaze, Blazena*

Blake (English) dark.
Blaque, Blayke

Blakely (English) dark
meadow.
*Blakelea, Blakelee, Blakeleigh,
Blakeley, Blakeli, Blakelyn,
Blakelynn, Blakesley, Blakley,
Blakli*

Blanca (Italian) a form of
Bianca.
Bellanca, Blancka, Blanka

Blanche (French) a form of
Bianca.
Blanch, Blancha, Blinney

Blinda (American) a short
form of Belinda.
Blynda

Bliss (English) blissful, joyful.
Blisse, Blyss, Blysse

Blodwyn (Welsh) flower. See
also Wynne.
Blodwen, Blodwynne, Blodyn

Blondelle (French) blond, fair
haired.
Blondell, Blondie

Blondie (American) a familiar
form of Blondell.
Blondee, Blondey, Blondy

Blossom (English) flower.

Blum (Yiddish) flower.
Bluma

Blythe (English) happy, cheerful.
Blithe, Blyss, Blyth

Bo (Chinese) precious.

Boacha (Hebrew) blessed.

Bobbette (American) a familiar form of Roberta.
Bobbet, Bobbetta

Bobbi, Bobbie (American) familiar forms of Barbara, Roberta.
Baubie, Bobbe, Bobbey, Bobbisue, Bobby, Bobbye, Bobi, Bobie, Bobina, Bobbie-Jean, Bobbie-Lynn, Bobbie-Sue

Bobbi-Ann, Bobbie-Ann (American) combinations of Bobbi + Ann.
Bobbiann, Bobbi-Anne, Bobbianne, Bobbie-Anne, Bobby-Ann, Bobbyann, Bobby-Anne, Bobbyanne

Bobbi-Jo (American) a combination of Bobbi + Jo.
Bobbiejo, Bobbie-Jo, Bobbijo, Bobby-Jo, Bobijo

Bobbi-Lee (American) a combination of Bobbi + Lee.
Bobbie-Lee, Bobbilee, Bobbylee, Bobby-Leigh, Bobile

Bonita (Spanish) pretty.
Bonesha, Bonetta, Bonnetta, Bonnie, Bonny

Bonnie, Bonny (English, Scottish) beautiful, pretty. (Spanish) familiar forms of Bonita.
Boni, Bonie, Bonne, Bonnee, Bonnell, Bonney, Bonni, Bonnin

Bonnie-Bell (American) a combination of Bonnie + Belle.
Bonnebell, Bonnebelle, Bonnibell, Bonnibelle, Bonniebell, Bonniebelle, Bonnybell, Bonnybelle

Bradley (English) broad meadow.
Bradlee, Bradleigh, Bradlie

Brady (Irish) spirited.
Bradee, Bradey, Bradi, Bradie, Braedi, Braidee, Braidi, Braidie, Braidey, Braidy, Braydee

Braeden (English) broad hill.
Bradyn, Bradynn, Braedan, Braedean, Braedyn, Braidan, Braiden, Braidyn, Brayden, Braydn, Braydon

Braelyn (American) a combination of Braeden + Lynn.
Braelee, Braeleigh, Braelin, Braelle, Braelon, Braelynn, Braelynne, Brailee, Brailenn, Brailey, Braili, Brailyn, Braylee, Brayley, Braylin, Braylon, Braylyn, Braylynn

Branda (Hebrew) blessing.

Brandee (Dutch) a form of Brandy.
Brande, Brandea, Brendee

Branden (English) beacon valley.
Brandan, Brandon, Brendan, Brandyn, Brennan

Brandi, Brandie (Dutch) forms of Brandy.
Brandei, Brandice, Brandiee,

*Brandii, Brandily, Brandin,
Brandis, Brandise, Brani,
Branndie, Brendi*

Brandy (Dutch) an after-din-
ner drink made from distilled
wine.
*Brand, Brandace, Brandaise,
Brandala, Brandee, Brandeli,
Brandell, Brandi, Brandye,
Brandylee, Brandy-Lee, Brandy-
Leigh, Brann, Brantley,
Branyell, Brendy*

Brandy-Lynn (American) a
combination of Brandy +
Lynn.
*Brandalyn, Brandalynn,
Brandelyn, Brandelynn,
Brandelynne, Brandilyn,
Brandilynn, Brandilynne,
Brandlin, Brandlyn, Brandlynn,
Brandlynne, Brandolyn,
Brandolynn, Brandolynne,
Brandylyn, Brandy-Lyn,
Brandylynne, Brandy-Lynne*

Braxton (English) Brock's
town.
Braxten, Braxtyn

Brea, Bria (Irish) short forms
of Breana, Briana.
Breah, Breea, Briah, Brya

Breana, Breanna (Irish) forms
of Briana.
*Brea, Breanah, Breanda, Bre-
Anna, Breannah, Breannea,
Breannia, Breasha, Breawna,
Breeanna, Breila*

Breann, Breanne (Irish) short
forms of Briana.
*Breane, Bre-Ann, Bre-Anne,
Breaunne, Bree, Breean,
Breeann, Breeanne, Breelyn,
Breeon, Breiann, Breighann,
Breyenne, Brieann, Brieon*

Breasha (Russian) a familiar
form of Breana.

Breauna, Breunna, Briauna
(Irish) forms of Briana.
*Breaunna, Breeauna, Breuna,
Breuna, Briaunna*

Breck (Irish) freckled.
Brecken

Bree (English) broth. (Irish) a
short form of Breann. See
also Brie.
Breay, Brei, Breigh

Breeana, Breeanna (Irish)
forms of Briana.
Breeanah, Breeannah

Breena (Irish) fairy palace. A
form of Brina.
Breenea, Breene, Breina, Brina

Breiana, Breianna (Irish)
forms of Briana.
Breiane, Breiann, Breianne

Brenda (Irish) little raven.
(English) sword.
*Brendell, Brendelle, Brendette,
Brendie, Brendyl, Brenna*

Brenda-Lee (American) a
combination of Brenda +
Lee.
*Brendalee, Brendaleigh,
Brendali, Brendaly, Brendalys,
Brenlee, Brenley*

Brenna (Irish) a form of
Brenda.
*Bren, Brenie, Brenin, Brenn,
Brennah, Brennaugh, Brenne*

Brennan (English) a form of
Brendan (see Boys' Names).
*Brennea, Brennen, Brennon,
Brennyn*

Breona, Breonna (Irish)
forms of Briana.
*Breeona, Breiona, Breionna,
Breonah, Breonia, Breonie,
Breonne*

Brett (Irish) a short form of
Brittany. See also Brita.
Bret, Brette, Brettin, Bretton

Breyana, Breyann, Breyanna
(Irish) forms of Briana.
*Breyan, Breyane, Breyannah,
Breyanne*

Breyona, Breyonna (Irish)
forms of Briana.
Breyonia

Briana, Brianna (Irish) strong;
virtuous, honorable.
*Bhrianna, Brana, Brea, Breana,
Breann, Breauna, Breeana,
Breiana, Breona, Breyana,
Breyona, Bria, Briahna,
Brianah, Briand, Brianda,*
*Briannah, Brianne, Brianni,
Briannon, Brienna, Brina,
Briona, Briyana, Bryanna,
Bryona*

Brianne (Irish) a form of
Briana.
*Briane, Briann, Brienne,
Bryanne*

Briar (French) heather.
Brear, Brier, Bryar

Bridey (Irish) a familiar form
of Bridget.
Bridi, Bridie, Brydie

Bridget (Irish) strong. See also
Bedelia, Bryga, Gitta.
*Berget, Birgitte, Bride, Bridey,
Bridger, Bridgete, Bridgett,
Bridgette, Bridgid, Bridgot,
Brietta, Brigada, Briget, Brigid,
Brigida, Brigitte, Brita*

Bridgett, Bridgette (Irish)
forms of Bridget.
*Bridgitte, Brigette, Bridggett,
Briggitte, Bridgitt, Brigitta*

Brie (French) a type of cheese.
Geography: a region in
France known for its cheese.
See also Bree.
*Briea, Brielle, Briena, Brieon,
Brietta, Briette*

Brieana, Brieanna
(American) combinations of
Brie + Anna.
Brieannah

Brieann, Brieanne
(American) combinations of

Brie + Ann. See also Briana.
Brie-Ann, Brie-Anne

Brielle (French) a form of
Brie.
Briel, Briele, Briell, Briella

Brienna, Brienne (Irish)
forms of Briana.
*Briene, Brieon, Brieona,
Brieonna*

Brienne (French) a form of
Briana.
Brienn

Brigette (French) a form of
Bridget.
*Briget, Brigett, Brigetta,
Brigettee, Brigget*

Brigitte (French) a form of
Bridget.
Briggitte, Brigit, Brigita

Brina (Latin) a short form of
Sabrina. (Irish) a familiar
form of Briana.
*Brin, Brinan, Brinda, Brindi,
Brindy, Briney, Brinia, Brinlee,
Brinly, Brinn, Brinna, Brinnan,
Briona, Bryn, Bryna*

Briona (Irish) a form of
Briana.
*Brione, Brionna, Brionne,
Briony, Briunna, Bryony*

Brisa (Spanish) beloved.
Mythology: Briseis was the
Greek name of Achilles's
beloved.
*Breezy, Breza, Brisha, Brishia,
Brissa, Bryssa*

Brita (Irish) a form of Bridget.
(English) a short form of
Britany.
*Bretta, Brieta, Brietta, Brit,
Britta*

Britaney, Brittaney (English)
forms of Britany, Brittany.
*Britanee, Britanny, Britenee,
Briteny, Britianey, British,
Britkney, Britley, Britlyn,
Britney, Briton*

Britani, Brittani, Brittanie
(English) forms of Britany.
*Brit, Britania, Britanica,
Britanie, Britanii, Britanni,
Britannia, Britatani, Britia,
Britini, Brittane, Brittanee,
Brittanni, Brittannia, Brittannie,
Brittenie, Brittiani, Brittianni*

Britany, Brittany (English)
from Britain. See also Brett.
*Brita, Britana, Britaney, Britani,
Britanna, Britlyn, Britney, Britt,
Brittainny, Brittainy, Brittamy,
Brittana, Brittaney, Brittani,
Brittania, Brittanica, Brittanny,
Brittany-Ann, Brittanyne,
Brittell, Britteny, Brittiany,
Brittini, Brittlin, Brittlynn,
Brittnee, Brittony, Bryttany*

Britin, Brittin (English) from
Britain.
*Britann, Brittan, Brittin,
Brittina, Brittine, Brittini,
Brittiny*

Britney, Brittney, Brittny
(English) forms of Britany.
Bittney, Bridnee, Bridney,
Britnay, Britne, Britnee, Britnei,
Britni, Britny, Britnye, Brittnay,
Brittnaye, Brytnea, Brytni

Britni, Brittni, Brittnie
(English) forms of Britney,
Britney.
Britnie

Briton, Brittin (English) forms
of Britin, Brittin.
Britton

Britt, Britta (Latin) short
forms of Britany, Brittany.
(Swedish) strong.
Brett, Briet, Brit, Brita, Britte

Britteny (English) a form of
Britany, Brittany.
Britten, Brittenay, Brittenee,
Britteney, Brittenie

Brittini, Brittiny (English)
forms of Britany, Brittany.
Brittinee, Brittiney, Brittinie,
Brittiny

Brittnee (English) a form of
Britany, Brittany.
Brittne, Brittnea, Brittnei,
Brittneigh

Briyana, Briyanna (Irish)
forms of Briana.

Brodie (Irish) ditch; canal
builder.
Brodee, Brodi, Brody

Bronnie (Welsh) a familiar
form of Bronwyn.
Bron, Bronia, Bronney, Bronny,
Bronya

Bronwyn (Welsh) white
breasted.
Bronnie, Bronwen, Bronwin,
Bronwynn, Bronwynne

Brook, Brooke (English)
brook, stream.
Bhrooke, Brookelle, Brookie,
Brooks, Brooky

Brooklyn, Brooklynn
(American) combinations of
Brook + Lynn.
Brookellen, Brookelyn,
Brookelyne, Brookelynn,
Brooklen, Brooklin, Brooklyne,
Brooklynne

Bruna (German) a short form
of Brunhilda.
Brona

Brunhilda (German) armored
warrior.
Brinhilda, Brinhilde, Bruna,
Brunhilde, Brünnhilde,
Brynhild, Brynhilda, Brynhilde,
Hilda

Bryana, Bryanna, Bryanne
(Irish) short forms of Bryana.
Bryann, Bryanni

Bryce (Welsh) alert; ambitious.

Bryga (Polish) a form of
Bridget.
Brygid, Brygida, Brygitka

Brylie (American) a combination of the letter B + Riley.
Brylee, Brylei, Bryley, Bryli

Bryn, Brynn (Latin) from the boundary line. (Welsh) mound.
Brinn, Brynee, Brynne

Bryna (Latin, Irish) a form of Brina.
Brynan, Brynna, Brynnan

Bryona, Bryonna (Irish) forms of Briana.
Bryonia, Bryony

Bryttani, Bryttany (English) forms of Britany.
Brytani, Brytanie, Brytanny, Brytany, Brytnee, Brytnie, Bryton, Bryttanee, Bryttanie, Bryttine, Bryttney, Bryttnie, Brytton

Buffy (American) buffalo; from the plains.
Buffee, Buffey, Buffie, Buffye

Bunny (Greek) a familiar form of Bernice. (English) little rabbit. See also Bonnie.
Bunni, Bunnie

Burgundy (French) Geography: a region of France known for its Burgundy wine.
Burgandi, Burgandie, Burgandy, Burgunde

C

Cachet (French) prestigious; desirous.
Cachae, Cache, Cachea, Cachee, Cachée

Cadence (Latin) rhythm.
Cadena, Cadenza, Kadena

Cady (English) a form of Kady.
Cade, Cadee, Cadey, Cadi, Cadie, Cadine, Cadye

Caeley, Cailey, Cayley (American) forms of Kaylee, Kelly.
Caela, Caelee, Caeleigh, Caeley, Caeli, Caelie, Caelly, Caely, Cailee, Caileigh, Caili, Cailie, Cailley, Caillie, Caily, Caylee

Caelin, Caelyn (American) forms of Kaelyn.
Caelan, Caelinn, Caelynn, Cailan, Caylan

Cai (Vietnamese) feminine.
Cae, Cay, Caye

Cailida (Spanish) adoring.
Kailida

Cailin, Cailyn (American) forms of Caitlin.
Caileen, Cailene, Cailine, Cailynn, Cailynne, Calen, Cayleen, Caylen, Caylene, Caylin, Cayline, Caylyn, Caylyne, Caylynne

Caitlan (Irish) a form of Caitlin.
Caitland, Caitlandt

Caitlin (Irish) pure. See also Kaitlin, Katalina, Katelin, Katelyn, Kaytlyn.
Caetlin, Cailin, Caitlan, Caitleen, Caitlen, Caitlene, Caitlenn, Caitline, Caitlinn, Caitlon, Caitlyn, Catlee, Catleen, Catleene, Catlin

Caitlyn, Caitlynn (Irish) forms of Caitlin. See also Kaitlyn.
Caitlyne, Caitlynne, Catelyn, Catlyn, Catlynn, Catlynne

Cala (Arabic) castle, fortress. See also Callie, Kala.
Calah, Calan, Calla, Callah

Calandra (Greek) lark.
Calan, Calandrea, Calandria, Caleida, Calendra, Calendre, Kalandra, Kalandria

Caleigh, Caley (American) forms of Caeley.
Caileigh, Caleah

Cali, Calli (Greek) forms of Calie. See also Kali.
Calee

Calida (Spanish) warm; ardent.
Calina, Calinda, Callida, Callinda, Kalida

Callie (Greek, Arabic) a familiar form of Cala, Callista. See also Kalli.
Cal, Cali, Calie, Callee, Calley, Calli, Cally, Caly

Callista (Greek) most beautiful. See also Kallista.
Calesta, Calista, Callie, Calysta

Calvina (Latin) bald.
Calvine, Calvinetta, Calvinette

Calypso (Greek) concealer. Botany: a pink orchid native to northern regions. Mythology: the sea nymph who held Odysseus captive for seven years.
Caly, Lypsie, Lypsy

Cam (Vietnamese) sweet citrus.
Kam

Camara (American) a form of Cameron.
Camera, Cameri, Cameria, Camira, Camry

Camberly (American) a form of Kimberly.
Camber, Camberlee, Camberleigh

Cambria (Latin) from Wales. See also Kambria.
Camberry, Cambreia, Cambie, Cambrea, Cambree, Cambrie, Cambrina, Cambry, Cambrya, Cami

Camden (Scottish) winding valley.
Camdyn

Camellia (Italian) Botany: a camellia is an evergreen tree or shrub with fragrant rose-like flowers.
Camala, Camalia, Camallia,

*Camela, Camelia, Camelita,
Camella, Camellita, Cami,
Kamelia, Kamellia*

Cameo (Latin) gem or shell
on which a portrait is
carved.
Cami, Kameo

Cameron (Scottish) crooked
nose. See also Kameron,
Kamryn.
*Camara, Cameran, Cameren,
Camira, Camiran, Camiron,
Camryn*

Cami (French) a short form of
Camille. See also Kami.
*Camey, Camie, Cammi,
Cammie, Cammy, Cammye,
Camy*

Camila, Camilla (Italian)
forms of Camille. See also
Kamila, Mila.
*Camia, Camilia, Camillia,
Camilya, Cammilla, Chamelea,
Chamelia, Chamika, Chamila,
Chamilia*

Camille (French) young cere-
monial attendant. See also
Millie.
*Cam, Cami, Camiel, Camielle,
Camil, Camila, Camile,
Camill, Cammille, Cammillie,
Cammilyn, Cammyl, Cammyll,
Camylle, Chamelle, Chamille,
Kamille*

Camisha (American) a combination of Cami + Aisha.
Cameasha, Cameesha,

*Cameisha, Camesa, Camesha,
Cameshaa, Cameshia,
Camiesha, Camyeshia*

Camri, Camrie (American)
short forms of Camryn. See
also Kamri.
*Camrea, Camree, Camrey,
Camry*

Camryn (American) a form of
Cameron. See also Kamryn.
*Camri, Camrin, Camron,
Camrynn*

Camylle (French) a form of
Camille.
Camyle, Camyll

Candace (Greek) glittering
white; glowing. History: the
title of the queens of ancient
Ethiopia. See also Dacey,
Kandace.
*Cace, Canace, Canda, Candas,
Candece, Candelle, Candi,
Candiace, Candice, Candyce*

Candi, Candy (American)
familiar forms of Candace,
Candice, Candida. See also
Kandi.
Candee, Candie

Candice, Candis (Greek)
forms of Candace.
*Candes, Candi, Candias,
Candies, Candise, Candiss,
Candus*

Candida (Latin) bright white.
*Candeea, Candi, Candia,
Candide, Candita*

Candra (Latin) glowing. See also Kandra.
Candrea, Candria

Candyce (Greek) a form of Candace.
Candys, Candyse, Cyndyss

Cantara (Arabic) small crossing.
Cantarah

Cantrelle (French) song.
Cantrella

Capri (Italian) a short form of Caprice. Geography: an island off the west coast of Italy. See also Kapri.
Capria, Caprie, Capry

Caprice (Italian) fanciful.
Cappi, Caprece, Caprecia, Capresha, Capricia, Capriese, Caprina, Capris, Caprise, Caprisha, Capritta

Cara (Latin) dear. (Irish) friend. See also Karah.
Caira, Caragh, Carah, Caralee, Caranda, Carey, Carra

Caralee (Irish) a form of Cara.
Caralea, Caraleigh, Caralia, Caralie, Carely

Caralyn (English) a form of Caroline.
Caralin, Caraline, Caralynn, Caralynna, Caralynne

Caressa (French) a form of Carissa.
Caresa, Carese, Caresse,
Carissa, Charessa, Charesse, Karessa

Carey (Welsh) a familiar form of Cara, Caroline, Karen, Katherine. See also Carrie, Kari.
Caree, Cari, Carrey, Cary

Cari, Carie (Welsh) forms of Carey, Kari.

Carina (Italian) dear little one. (Swedish) a form of Karen. (Greek) a familiar form of Cora.
Carena, Carinah, Carine, Carinna

Carine (Italian) a form of Carina.
Carin, Carinn, Carinne

Carisa, Carrisa (Greek) forms of Carissa.
Carise, Carisha, Carisia, Charisa

Carissa (Greek) beloved. See also Karissa.
Caressa, Carisa, Carrissa, Charissa

Carita (Latin) charitable.
Caritta, Karita, Karitta

Carla (German) farmer. (English) strong. (Latin) a form of Carol, Caroline.
Carila, Carilla, Carleta, Carlia, Carliqua, Carliyle, Carlonda, Carlyjo, Carlyle, Carlysle

Carlee, Carleigh, Carley
(English) forms of Carly. See
also Karlee.
Carle, Carlea, Carleah, Carleh

Carleen, Carlene (English)
forms of Caroline. See also
Karlene.
*Carlaen, Carlaena, Carleena,
Carlen, Carlena, Carlenna,
Carline, Carlyn, Carlyne*

Carli, Carlie (English) forms
of Carly. See also Karli.

Carlin (Irish) little champion.
(Latin) a short form of
Caroline.
*Carlan, Carlana, Carlandra,
Carlina, Carlinda, Carline,
Carling, Carllan, Carlyn,
Carllen, Carrlin*

Carlisa (American) a form of
Carlissa.
*Carilis, Carilise, Carilyse,
Carleesia, Carlesia, Carletha,
Carlethe, Carlicia, Carlis,
Carlise, Carlisha, Carlisia,
Carlyse*

Carlissa (American) a combi-
nation of Carla + Lissa.
*Carleeza, Carlisa, Carliss,
Carlissah, Carlisse, Carlissia,
Carlista*

Carlotta (Italian) a form of
Charlotte.
Carletta, Carlita, Carlota

Carly (English) a familiar form
of Caroline, Charlotte. See

also Karli.
Carlee, Carli, Carlie, Carlye

Carlyn, Carlynn (Irish) forms
of Carlin.
Carlyna, Carlynne

Carmela, Carmella (Hebrew)
garden; vineyard. Bible:
Mount Carmel in Israel is
often thought of as paradise.
See also Karmel.
*Carma, Carmalla, Carmarit,
Carmel, Carmeli, Carmelia,
Carmelina, Carmelit, Carmelle,
Carmellia, Carmellina,
Carmesa, Carmesha, Carmi,
Carmie, Carmiel, Carmil,
Carmila, Carmile, Carmilla,
Carmille, Carmisha, Leeta, Lita*

Carmelit (Hebrew) a form of
Carmela.
*Carmaletta, Carmalit,
Carmalita, Carmelita,
Carmelitha, Carmelitia,
Carmellit, Carmellita,
Carmellitha, Carmellitia*

Carmen (Latin) song.
Religion: Nuestra Señora del
Carmen—Our Lady of
Mount Carmel—is one of
the titles of the Virgin Mary.
See also Karmen.
*Carma, Carmaine, Carman,
Carmelina, Carmencita,
Carmene, Carmi, Carmia,
Carmin, Carmina, Carmine,
Carmita, Carmon, Carmynn,
Charmaine*

Carol (German) farmer.
(French) song of joy.
(English) strong. See also
Charlene, Kalle, Karoll.
*Carel, Cariel, Caro, Carola,
Carole, Carolenia, Carolinda,
Caroline, Caroll, Carrie, Carrol,
Carroll, Caryl*

**Carolane, Carolann,
Carolanne** (American) com-
binations of Carol + Ann.
Forms of Caroline.
*Carolan, Carol Ann, Carole-
Anne*

Carole (English) a form of
Carol.
Carolee, Karole, Karrole

Carolina (Italian) a form of
Caroline. See also Karolina.
*Carilena, Carlena, Carlina,
Caroleena, Caroleina, Carolena,
Carrolena*

Caroline (French) little and
strong. See also Carla,
Carleen, Carlin, Karolina.
*Caralin, Caraline, Carileen,
Carilene, Carilin, Cariline,
Carling, Carly, Caro, Carolann,
Caroleen, Carolin, Carolina,
Carolyn, Carrie, Carroleen,
Carrolene, Carrolin, Carroline,
Cary, Charlene*

Carolyn (English) a form of
Caroline. See also Karolyn.
*Carilyn, Carilynn, Carilynne,
Carlyn, Carlynn, Carlynne,
Carolyne, Carolynn, Carolynne,*

*Carrolyn, Carrolynn,
Carrolynne*

Caron (Welsh) loving, kindhearted, charitable.
Caronne, Carron, Carrone

Carra (Irish) a form of Cara.
Carrah

Carrie (English) a familiar
form of Carol, Caroline. See
also Carey, Kari, Karri.
*Carree, Carrey, Carri, Carria,
Carry, Cary*

Carson (English) child of
Carr.
Carsen, Carsyn

Carter (English) cart driver.

Caryl (Latin) a form of Carol.
Caryle, Caryll, Carylle

Caryn (Danish) a form of
Karen.
*Caren, Carren, Carrin, Carryn,
Caryna, Caryne, Carynn*

Carys (Welsh) love.
Caris, Caryse, Ceris, Cerys

Casandra (Greek) a form of
Cassandra.
*Casandera, Casandre,
Casandrea, Casandrey,
Casandri, Casandria,
Casanndra, Casaundra,
Casaundre, Casaundri,
Casaundria, Casondra,
Casondre, Casondri, Casondria*

Casey (Irish) brave. (Greek) a
familiar form of Acacia. See

also Kasey.
*Cacy, Cascy, Casie, Casse,
Cassee, Cassey, Cassye, Casy,
Cayce, Cayse, Caysee, Caysy*

Casidy (Irish) a form of
Cassidy.
Casidee, Casidi

Casie (Irish) a form of Casey.
*Caci, Caesi, Caisie, Casci,
Cascie, Casi, Cayci, Caysi,
Caysie, Cazzi*

Cass (Greek) a short form of
Cassandra.

Cassady (Irish) a form of
Cassidy.
*Casadee, Casadi, Casadie,
Cassaday, Cassadee, Cassadey,
Cassadi, Cassadie, Cassadina*

Cassandra (Greek) helper of
men. Mythology: a prophet-
ess of ancient Greece whose
prophesies were not believed.
See also Kassandra, Sandra,
Sandy, Zandra.
*Casandra, Cass, Cassandre,
Cassandri, Cassandry,
Cassaundra, Cassie, Cassondra*

Cassaundra (Greek) a form of
Cassandra.
*Cassaundre, Cassaundri,
Cassundra, Cassundre,
Cassundri, Cassundria*

Cassia (Greek) a cinnamon-
like spice. See also Kasia.
Casia, Cass, Casya

Cassidy (Irish) clever. See also
Kassidy.
*Casidy, Cassady, Casseday,
Cassiddy, Cassidee, Cassidi,
Cassidie, Cassity*

Cassie, Cassey, Cassi (Greek)
familiar forms of Cassandra,
Catherine. See also Kassie.
Cassee, Cassii, Cassy, Casy

Cassiopeia (Greek) clever.
Mythology: the wife of the
Ethiopian king Cepheus; the
mother of Andromeda.
Cassio

Cassondra (Greek) a form of
Cassandra.
*Cassondre, Cassondri,
Cassondria*

Catalina (Spanish) a form of
Catherine. See also Katalina.
*Cataleen, Catalena, Catalene,
Catalin, Catalyn, Catalyna,
Cateline*

Catarina (German) a form of
Catherine.
*Catarena, Catarin, Catarine,
Caterin, Caterina, Caterine*

Catelyn (Irish) a form of
Caitlin.
*Catelin, Cateline, Catelyne,
Catelynn*

Catharine (Greek) a form of
Catherine.
*Catharen, Catharin, Catharina,
Catharyn*

Catherine (Greek) pure.
(English) a form of
Katherine.
*Cat, Catalina, Catarina, Cate,
Cathann, Cathanne, Catharine,
Cathenne, Catheren, Catherene,
Catheria, Catherin, Catherina,
Catheryn, Catheryne, Cathi,
Cathleen, Cathrine, Cathryn,
Cathy, Catlaina, Catreeka,
Catrelle, Catrice, Catricia,
Catrika, Catrina*

Cathi, Cathy (Greek) familiar
forms of Catherine,
Cathleen. See also Kathy.
*Catha, Cathe, Cathee, Cathey,
Cathie*

Cathleen (Irish) a form of
Catherine. See also Caitlin,
Kathleen.
*Caithlyn, Cathaleen, Cathelin,
Cathelina, Cathelyn, Cathi,
Cathleana, Cathleene, Cathlene,
Cathleyn, Cathlin, Cathline,
Cathlyn, Cathlyne, Cathlynn,
Cathy*

Cathrine (Greek) a form of
Catherine.

Cathryn (Greek) forms of
Catherine.
Cathryne, Cathrynn, Catryn

Catrina (Slavic) a form of
Catherine, Katrina.
*Caitriana, Caitriona, Catina,
Catreen, Catreena, Catrene,
Catrenia, Catrin, Catrine,
Catrinia, Catriona, Catroina*

Cayla (Hebrew) a form of
Kayla.
Caylea, Caylia

Caylee, Caylie (American)
forms of Caeley, Cailey,
Cayley.
Cayle, Cayleigh, Cayli, Cayly

Ceara (Irish) a form of Ciara.
*Ceaira, Ceairah, Ceairra,
Cearaa, Cearie, Cearah, Cearra,
Cera*

Cecelia (Latin) a form of
Cecilia. See also Sheila.
*Caceli, Cacelia, Cece, Ceceilia,
Ceceli, Cecelia, Cecelie, Cecely,
Cecelyn, Cecette, Cescelia,
Cescelie*

Cecilia (Latin) blind. See also
Cicely, Cissy, Secilia, Selia,
Sissy.
*Cacilia, Caecilia, Cecelia, Cecil,
Cecila, Cecile, Cecilea, Cecilija,
Cecilla, Cecille, Cecillia, Cecily,
Cecilya, Ceclia, Cecylia, Cee,
Ceil, Ceila, Ceilagh, Ceileh,
Ceileigh, Ceilena, Celia,
Cesilia, Cicelia*

Cecily (Latin) a form of
Cecilia.
*Cacilie, Cecilee, Ceciley, Cecilie,
Cescily, Cicely, Cilley*

Ceil (Latin) a short form of
Cecilia.
Ceel, Ciel

Ceira, Ceirra (Irish) forms of
Ciara.
Ceire

Celena (Greek) a form of
Selena.
*Celeena, Celene, Celenia,
Celine, Cena*

Celene (Greek) a form of
Celena.
Celeen

Celeste (Latin) celestial, heav-
enly.
*Cele, Celeeste, Celense, Celes,
Celesia, Celesley, Celest,
Celesta, Celestia, Celestial,
Celestin, Celestina, Celestine,
Celestinia, Celestyn, Celestyna,
Cellest, Celleste, Selestina*

Celia (Latin) a short form of
Cecilia.
Ceilia, Celie

Celina (Greek) a form of
Celena. See also Selina.
*Caleena, Calena, Calina,
Celena, Celinda, Celinka,
Celinna, Celka, Cellina*

Celine (Greek) a form of
Celena.
*Caline, Celeen, Celene, Céline,
Cellinn*

Cera (French) a short form of
Cerise.
Cerea, Ceri, Ceria, Cerra

Cerella (Latin) springtime.
Cerelisa, Ceres

Cerise (French) cherry; cherry
red.
*Cera, Cerese, Cerice, Cericia,
Cerissa, Cerria, Cerrice,
Cerrina, Cerrita, Cerryce,
Ceryce, Cherise*

Cesilia (Latin) a form of Cecilia.
Cesia, Cesya

Chablis (French) a dry, white
wine. Geography: a region in
France where wine grapes
are grown.
*Chabeli, Chabelly, Chabely,
Chablee, Chabley, Chabli*

Chadee (French) from Chad,
a country in north-central
Africa. See also Sade.
*Chaday, Chadday, Chade,
Chadea, Chadi*

Chai (Hebrew) life.
*Chae, Chaela, Chaeli, Chaella,
Chaena, Chaia*

Chaka (Sanskrit) a form of
Chakra. See also Shaka.
*Chakai, Chakia, Chakka,
Chakkah*

Chakra (Sanskrit) circle of
energy.
*Chaka, Chakara, Chakaria,
Chakena, Chakina, Chakira,
Chakrah, Chakria, Chakriya,
Chakyra*

Chalice (French) goblet.
*Chalace, Chalcie, Chalece,
Chalicea, Chalie, Chaliese,
Chalis, Chalisa, Chalise,*

Chalice (cont.)
  Chalisk, Chalissa, Chalisse,
  Challa, Challaine, Challis,
  Challisse, Challysse, Chalsey,
  Chalyce, Chalyn, Chalyse,
  Chalyssa, Chalysse

Chalina (Spanish) a form of
  Rose.
  Chaline, Chalini

Chalonna (American) a com-
  bination of the prefix Cha +
  Lona.
  Chalon, Chalona, Chalonda,
  Chalonn, Chalonne, Chalonte,
  Shalon

Chambray (French) a light-
  weight fabric.
  Chambrae, Chambre, Chambree,
  Chambrée, Chambrey, Chambria,
  Chambrie

Chan (Cambodian) sweet-
  smelling tree.

Chana (Hebrew) a form of
  Hannah.
  Chanae, Chanai, Chanay,
  Chanea, Chanie

Chancey (English) chancellor;
  church official.
  Chance, Chancee, Chancie,
  Chancy

Chanda (Sanskrit) short tem-
  pered. Religion: the demon
  defeated by the Hindu goddess
  Chamunda. See also Shanda.
  Chandee, Chandey, Chandi,
  Chandie, Chandin

Chandelle (French) candle.
  Chandal, Chandel, Shandal,
  Shandel

Chandler (Hindi) moon. (Old
  English) candlemaker.
  Chandlar, Chandlier, Chandlor,
  Chandlyr

Chandra (Sanskrit) moon.
  Religion: the Hindu god of
  the moon. See also Shandra.
  Chandrae, Chandray, Chandre,
  Chandrea, Chandrelle,
  Chandria

Chanel (English) channel. See
  also Shanel.
  Chanal, Chaneel, Chaneil,
  Chanele, Chanell, Channal,
  Channel, Chenelle

Chanell, Chanelle (English)
  forms of Chanel.
  Channell, Shanell

Chanise (American) a form of
  Shanice.
  Chanisse, Chenice, Chenise

Channa (Hindi) chickpea.
  Channah

Chantal (French) song.
  Chandal, Chantaal, Chantael,
  Chantala, Chantale, Chantall,
  Chantalle, Chantara, Chantarai,
  Chantasia, Chante, Chanteau,
  Chantel, Chantle, Chantoya,
  Chantrill, Chauntel

Chante (French) a short form
of Chantal.
*Chanta, Chantae, Chantai,
Chantay, Chantaye, Chanté,
Chantéa, Chantee, Chanti,
Chantia, Chaunte, Chauntea,
Chauntéa, Chauntee*

Chantel, Chantell, Chantelle
(French) forms of Chantal.
See also Shantel.
*Chanteese, Chantela, Chantele,
Chantella, Chanter, Chantey,
Chantez, Chantrel, Chantrell,
Chantrelle, Chatell*

Chantilly (French) fine lace.
See also Shantille.
*Chantiel, Chantielle, Chantil,
Chantila, Chantilée, Chantill,
Chantille*

Chantrea (Cambodian)
moon; moonbeam.
*Chantra, Chantrey, Chantri,
Chantria*

Chantrice (French) singer. See
also Shantrice.
Chantreese, Chantress

Chardae, Charde (Punjabi)
charitable. (French) short
forms of Chardonnay. See
also Shardae.
*Charda, Chardai, Charday,
Chardea, Chardee, Chardée,
Chardese, Chardey, Chardie*

Chardonnay (French) a dry
white wine.
*Char, Chardae, Chardnay,
Chardney, Chardon, Chardonae,*
*Chardonai, Chardonay,
Chardonaye, Chardonee,
Chardonna, Chardonnae,
Chardonnai, Chardonnee,
Chardonnée, Chardonney,
Shardonay, Shardonnay*

Charis (Greek) grace;
kindness.
*Charece, Chareece, Chareeze,
Charese, Chari, Charice,
Charie, Charish, Charisse*

Charissa, Charisse (Greek)
forms of Charity.
*Charesa, Charese, Charessa,
Charesse, Charis, Charisa,
Charise, Charisha, Charissee,
Charista, Charyssa*

Charity (Latin) charity,
kindness.
*Chariety, Charis, Charissa,
Charisse, Charista, Charita,
Chariti, Charitie, Sharity*

Charla (French, English) a
short form of Charlene,
Charlotte.
Char, Charlea

Charlaine (English) a form of
Charlene.
*Charlaina, Charlane,
Charlanna, Charlayna,
Charlayne*

Charlee, Charley (German,
English) forms of Charlie.
Charle, Charleigh

Charlene (English) a form of
Caroline. See also Carol,
Karla, Sharlene.
*Charla, Charlaine, Charlean,
Charleen, Charleene, Charleesa,
Charlena, Charlenae,
Charlesena, Charline, Charlyn,
Charlyne, Charlynn, Charlynne,
Charlzina, Charoline*

Charlie (German, English)
strong.
*Charlee, Charley, Charli,
Charyl, Chatty, Sharli, Sharlie*

Charlotte (French) a form of
Caroline. Literature:
Charlotte Brontë was a
British novelist and poet best
known for her novel *Jane
Eyre*. See also Karlotte, Lotte,
Sharlotte, Tottie.
*Carlotta, Carly, Chara, Charil,
Charl, Charla, Charlet,
Charlett, Charletta, Charlette,
Charlisa, Charlita, Charlott,
Charlotta, Charlottie, Charlotty,
Charolet, Charolette, Charolot,
Charolotte*

Charmaine (French) a form
of Carmen. See also
Sharmaine.
*Charamy, Charma, Charmae,
Charmagne, Charmaigne,
Charmain, Chamaine,
Charmalique, Charman,
Charmane, Charmar,
Charmara, Charmayane,
Charmayne, Charmeen,
Charmeine, Charmene,*

*Charmese, Charmian,
Charmin, Charmine,
Charmion, Charmisa,
Charmon, Charmyn,
Charmyne, Charmynne*

Charnette (American) a com-
bination of Charo +
Annette.
Charnetta, Charnita

Charnika (American) a com-
bination of Charo + Nika.
*Charneka, Charniqua,
Charnique*

Charo (Spanish) a familiar
form of Rosa.
Charyanna (American) a
combination of Charo +
Anna.
Charian, Charyian, Cheryn

Chasidy, Chassidy (Latin)
forms of Chastity.
*Chasa Dee, Chasadie, Chasady,
Chasidee, Chasidey, Chasidie,
Chassedi, Chassidi, Chasydi*

Chasity (Latin) a form of
Chastity.
*Chasiti, Chasitie, Chasitty,
Chassey, Chassie, Chassiti,
Chassity, Chassy*

Chastity (Latin) pure.
*Chasidy, Chasity, Chasta,
Chastady, Chastidy, Chastin,
Chastitie, Chastney, Chasty*

Chauntel (French) a form of
Chantal.
Chaunta, Chauntae, Chauntay,

Chaunte, Chauntell,
Chauntelle, Chawntel,
Chawntell, Chawntelle,
Chontelle

Chava (Hebrew) life. (Yiddish)
bird. Religion: the original
name of Eve.
Chabah, Chavae, Chavah,
Chavalah, Chavarra, Chavarria,
Chave, Chavé, Chavette,
Chaviva, Chavvis, Hava, Kaÿa

Chavella (Spanish) a form of
Isabel.
Chavel, Chaveli, Chavell,
Chavelle, Chevelle, Chavely,
Chevie

Chavi (Gypsy) girl.
Chavali

Chavon (Hebrew) a form of
Jane.
Chavona, Chavonda, Chavonn,
Chavonne, Shavon

Chavonne (Hebrew) a form
of Chavon. (American) a
combination of the prefix
Cha + Yvonne.
Chavondria, Chavonna,
Chevon, Chevonn, Chevonna

Chaya (Hebrew) life; living.
Chaike, Chaye, Chayka,
Chayla, Chaylah, Chaylea,
Chaylee, Chaylene, Chayra

Chelci, Chelcie (English)
forms of Chelsea.
Chelce, Chelcee, Chelcey, Chelcy

Chelsea (English) seaport. See
also Kelsi, Shelsea.
Chelci, Chelese, Chelesia,
Chelsa, Chelsae, Chelsah,
Chelse, Chelseah, Chelsee,
Chelsey, Chelsia, Chelsie,
Chesea, Cheslee, Chessea

Chelsee (English) a form of
Chelsea.
Chelsei, Chelseigh

Chelsey, Chelsy (English)
forms of Chelsea. See also
Kelsey.
Chelcy, Chelsay, Chelssy,
Chelssey, Chelsye, Chesley

Chelsie (English) a form of
Chelsea.
Chelli, Chellie, Chellise,
Chellsie, Chelsi, Chelssie,
Cheslie, Chessie

Chenelle (English) a form of
Chanel.
Chenel, Chenell

Chenoa (Native American)
white dove.
Chenee, Chenika, Chenita,
Chenna, Chenoah

Cher (French) beloved, dear-
est. (English) a short form of
Cherilyn.
Chere, Cheri, Cherie, Sher

Cherelle, Cherrelle (French)
forms of Cheryl. See also
Sherelle.
Charell, Charelle, Cherell,
Cherrel, Cherrell

Cherese (Greek) a form of
Cherish.
*Chereese, Cheresa, Cheresse,
Cherice*

Cheri, Cherie (French) famil-
iar forms of Cher.
*Cheree, Chérie, Cheriee, Cherri,
Cherrie*

Cherilyn (English) a combina-
tion of Cheryl + Lynn.
*Cher, Cheralyn, Chereen,
Chereena, Cherilynn, Cherlyn,
Cherlynn, Cherralyn, Cherrilyn,
Cherrylyn, Cherylene, Cherylin,
Cheryline, Cheryl-Lyn, Cheryl-
Lynn, Cheryl-Lynne, Cherylyn,
Cherylynn, Cherylynne, Sherilyn*

Cherise (French) a form of
Cherish. See also Sharice,
Sherice.
*Charisa, Charise, Cherece,
Chereese, Cheresa, Cherice,
Cheriss, Cherissa, Cherisse,
Cherrise*

Cherish (English) dearly held,
precious.
*Charish, Charisha, Cheerish,
Cherise, Cherishe, Cherrish,
Sherish*

Cherokee (Native American)
a tribal name.
*Cherika, Cherkita, Cherrokee,
Sherokee*

Cherry (Latin) a familiar form
of Charity. (French) cherry;
cherry red.
Chere, Cheree, Cherey, Cherida,

*Cherita, Cherrey, Cherrita,
Cherry-Ann, Cherry-Anne,
Cherrye, Chery, Cherye*

Cheryl (French) beloved. See
also Sheryl.
*Charel, Charil, Charyl,
Cherelle, Cherrelle, Cheryl-
Ann, Cheryl-Anne, Cheryle,
Cherylee, Cheryll, Cherylle,
Cheryl-Lee*

Chesarey (American) a form
of Desiree.
Chesarae, Chessa

Chesna (Slavic) peaceful.
*Chesnee, Chesney, Chesnie,
Chesny*

Chessa (American) a short
form of Chesarey.
Chessi, Chessie, Chessy

Cheyanne (Cheyenne) a form
of Cheyenne.
*Cheyan, Cheyana, Cheyane,
Cheyann, Cheyanna,
Cheyeana, Cheyeannna,
Cheyeannne*

Cheyenne (Cheyenne) a tribal
name. See also Shaianne,
Sheyenne, Shianne, Shyann.
*Cheyanne, Cheyeene, Cheyena,
Cheyene, Cheyenna, Cheyna,
Chi, Chi-Anna, Chie, Chyanne*

Cheyla (American) a form of
Sheila.
Cheylan, Cheyleigh, Cheylo

Cheyna (American) a short form of Cheyenne.
Chey, Cheye, Cheyne, Cheynee, Cheyney, Cheynna

Chiara (Italian) a form of Clara.
Cheara, Chiarra

Chika (Japanese) near and dear.
Chikaka, Chikako, Chikara, Chikona

Chiku (Swahili) chatterer.

China (Chinese) fine porcelain. Geography: a country in eastern Asia. See also Ciana, Shina.
Chinaetta, Chinah, Chinasa, Chinda, Chinea, Chinesia, Chinita, Chinna, Chinwa, Chyna, Chynna

Chinira (Swahili) God receives.
Chinara, Chinarah, Chinirah

Chinue (Ibo) God's own blessing.

Chiquita (Spanish) little one. See also Shiquita.
Chaqueta, Chaquita, Chica, Chickie, Chicky, Chikata, Chikita, Chiqueta, Chiquila, Chiquite, Chiquitha, Chiquithe, Chiquitia, Chiquitta

Chiyo (Japanese) eternal.
Chiya

Chloe (Greek) blooming, verdant. Mythology: another name for Demeter, the goddess of agriculture.
Chloé, Chlöe, Chloee, Chloie, Cloe, Kloe

Chloris (Greek) pale. Mythology: the only daughter of Niobe to escape the vengeful arrows of Apollo and Artemis. See also Loris.
Cloris, Clorissa

Cho (Korean) beautiful.
Choe

Cholena (Native American) bird.

Chriki (Swahili) blessing.

Chris (Greek) a short form of Christina. See also Kris.
Chrys, Cris

Chrissa (Greek) a short form of Christina. See also Khrissa.
Chrysa, Chryssa, Crissa, Cryssa

Chrissy (English) a familiar form of Christina.
Chrisie, Chrissee, Chrissie, Crissie, Khrissy

Christa (German) a short form of Christina. History: Christa McAuliffe, an American school teacher, was the first civilian on a U. S. space flight. See also Krista.
Chrysta, Crista, Crysta

Christabel (Latin, French)
beautiful Christian.
Christabell, Christabella,
Christabelle, Christable,
Cristabel, Kristabel

Christain (Greek) a form of
Christina.
Christana, Christann,
Christanna

Christal (Latin) a form of
Crystal. (Scottish) a form of
Christina.
Christalene, Christalin,
Christaline, Christall, Christalle,
Christalyn, Christelle, Christle,
Chrystal

Christelle (French) a form of
Christal.
Christel, Christele, Christell,
Chrystel, Chrystelle

Christen, Christin (Greek)
forms of Christina. See also
Kristen.
Christan, Christyn, Chrystan,
Chrysten, Chrystyn, Crestienne

Christena, Christen (Greek)
forms of Christina.

Christi, Christie (Greek)
short forms of Christina,
Christine. See also Kristi.
Christy, Chrysti, Chrystie,
Chrysty, Kristi

Christian, Christiana,
Christianna (Greek) forms
of Christina. See also

Kristian, Krystian.
Christiane, Christiann, Christi-
Ann, Christianne, Christi-
Anne, Christianni, Christiaun,
Christiean, Christien,
Christiena, Christienne,
Christinan, Christy-Ann,
Christy-Anne, Crystian,
Chrystyann, Chrystyanne,
Crystiann, Crystianne

Christin (Greek) a short form
of Christina.
Christen, Chrystin

Christina (Greek) Christian;
anointed. See also Khristina,
Kristina, Stina, Tina.
Chris, Chrissa, Chrissy, Christa,
Christain, Christal, Christeena,
Christella, Christen, Christena,
Christi, Christian, Christie,
Christin, Christinaa, Christine,
Christinea, Christinia,
Christinna, Christinnah,
Christna, Christy, Christyn,
Christyna, Christynna,
Chrystina, Chrystyna,
Cristeena, Cristena, Cristina,
Crystina, Chrystena, Cristena

Christine (French, English) a
form of Christina. See also
Kirsten, Kristen, Kristine.
Chrisa, Christeen, Christen,
Christene, Christi, Christie,
Christy, Chrystine, Cristeen,
Cristene, Cristine, Crystine

Christophe (Greek) Christ-
bearer.

Christy (English) a short form of Christina, Christine.
Cristy

Christyn (Greek) a form of Christina.
Christyne

Chrys (English) a form of Chris.
Krys

Chrystal (Latin) a form of Christal.
Chrystale, Chrystalla, Chrystallina, Chrystallynn,

Chu Hua (Chinese) chrysanthemum.

Chumani (Lakota) dewdrops.
Chumany

Chun (Burmese) nature's renewal.

Chyanne, Chyenne (Cheyenne) forms of Cheyenne.
Chyan, Chyana, Chyane, Chyann, Chyanna, Chyeana, Chyenn, Chyenna, Chyennee

Chyna, Chynna (Chinese) forms of China.

Ciana (Chinese) a form of China. (Italian) a form of Jane.
Cian, Ciandra, Ciann, Cianna

Ciara, Ciarra (Irish) black. See also Sierra.
Ceara, Chiairah, Ciaara, Ciaera, Ciaira, Ciarah, Ciaria, Ciarrah, Cieara, Ciearra, Ciearria, Ciera, Cierra, Cioria, Cyarra

Cicely (English) a form of Cecilia. See also Sissy.
Cicelia, Cicelie, Ciciley, Cicilia, Cicilie, Cicily, Cile, Cilka, Cilla, Cilli, Cillie, Cilly

Cidney (French) a form of Sydney.
Cidnee, Cidni, Cidnie

Ciera, Cierra (Irish) forms of Ciara.
Ceira, Cierah, Ciere, Cieria, Cierrah, Cierre, Cierria, Cierro

Cinderella (French, English) little cinder girl. Literature: a fairy tale heroine.
Cindella

Cindy (Greek) moon. (Latin) a familiar form of Cynthia. See also Sindy.
Cindee, Cindi, Cindie, Cyndi

Cinthia, Cinthya (Greek) forms of Cynthia.
Cinthiya, Cintia

Cira (Spanish) a form of Cyrilla.

Cissy (American) a familiar form of Cecelia, Cicely.
Cissey, Cissi, Cissie

Claire (French) a form of Clara.
Clair, Klaire, Klarye

Clairissa (Greek) a form of
Clarissa.
Clairisa, Clairisse, Claraissa

Clara (Latin) clear; bright.
Music: Clara Shumann was a
famous nineteenth-century
German composer. See also
Chiara, Klara.
*Claira, Claire, Clarabelle, Clare,
Claresta, Clarice, Clarie,
Clarina, Clarinda, Clarine,
Clarissa, Clarita*

Clarabelle (Latin) bright and
beautiful.
Clarabella, Claribel, Claribell

Clare (English) a form of
Clara.

Clarie (Latin) a familiar form
of Clara.
Clarey, Clari, Clary

Clarice (Italian) a form of
Clara.
*Claris, Clarise, Clarisse,
Claryce, Cleriese, Klarice,
Klarise*

Clarisa (Greek) a form of
Clarissa.
Claresa, Clarise, Clarisia

Clarissa (Greek) brilliant.
(Italian) a form of Clara. See
also Klarissa.
*Clairissa, Clarecia, Claressa,
Claresta, Clarisa, Clarissia,
Claritza, Clarizza, Clarrisa,
Clarrissa, Clerissa*

Clarita (Spanish) a form of
Clara.
*Clairette, Clareta, Claretta,
Clarette, Claritza*

Claudette (French) a form of
Claudia.
Clauddetta

Claudia (Latin) lame. See also
Gladys, Klaudia.
*Claudeen, Claudel, Claudelle,
Claudette, Claudex, Claudiana,
Claudiane, Claudie, Claudie-
Anne, Claudina, Claudine*

Claudie (Latin) a form of
Claudia.
Claudee

Clea (Greek) a form of Cleo,
Clio.

Clementine (Latin) merciful.
*Clemence, Clemencia,
Clemencie, Clemency,
Clementia, Clementina,
Clemenza, Clemette*

Cleo (Greek) a short form of
Cleopatra.
Chleo, Clea

Cleone (Greek) famous.
Cleonie, Cleonna, Cliona

Cleopatra (Greek) her father's
fame. History: a great
Egyptian queen.
Cleo

Cleta (Greek) illustrious.

Clio (Greek) proclaimer; glorifier. Mythology: the Muse of history.
Clea

Cloe (Greek) a form of Chloe.
Clo, Cloei, Cloey, Cloie

Clotilda (German) heroine.

Coco (Spanish) coconut. See also Koko.

Codi, Cody (English) cushion. See also Kodi.
Coady, Codee, Codey, Codia, Codie

Colby (English) coal town. Geography: a region in England known for cheese-making. See also Kolby.
Cobi, Cobie, Colbi, Colbie

Colette (Greek, French) a familiar form of Nicole.
Coe, Coetta, Coletta, Collet, Collete, Collett, Colletta, Collette, Kolette, Kollette

Colleen (Irish) girl. See also Kolina.
Coe, Coel, Cole, Coleen, Colene, Coley, Coline, Colleene, Collen, Collene, Collie, Collina, Colline, Colly

Collina (Irish) a form of Colleen.
Colena, Colina, Colinda

Concetta (Italian) pure.
Concettina, Conchetta

Conchita (Spanish) conception.
Chita, Conceptia, Concha, Conciana

Concordia (Latin) harmonious. Mythology: the goddess governing the peace after war.
Con, Cordae, Cordaye

Connie (Latin) a familiar form of Constance.
Con, Connee, Conni, Conny, Konnie, Konny

Connor (Scottish) wise. (Irish) praised; exhalted.
Connar, Conner, Connery, Conor

Constance (Latin) constant; firm. History: Constance Motley was the first African-American woman to be appointed as a U. S. federal judge. See also Konstance, Kosta.
Connie, Constancia, Constancy, Constanta, Constantia, Constantina, Constantine, Constanza, Constynse

Constanza (Spanish) a form of Constance.
Constanz, Constanze

Consuelo (Spanish) consolation. Religion: Nuestra Señora del Consuelo—Our Lady of Consolation—is a name for the Virgin Mary.
Consolata, Consuela, Consuella, Consula, Conzuelo, Konsuela, Konsuelo

Cora (Greek) maiden.
Mythology: Kore is another
name for Persephone, the
goddess of the underworld.
See also Kora.
*Corah, Coralee, Coretta,
Corissa, Corey, Corra*

Corabelle (American) a combination of Cora + Belle.
Corabel, Corabella

Coral (Latin) coral. See also
Koral.
Coraal, Corral

Coralee (American) a combi-
nation of Cora + Lee.
*Coralea, Cora-Lee, Coralena,
Coralene, Coraley, Coralie,
Coraline, Coraly, Coralyn,
Corella, Corilee, Koralie*

Coralie (American) a form of
Coralee.
*Corali, Coralia, Coralina,
Coralynn, Coralynne*

Corazon (Spanish) heart.

Corbin (Latin) raven.
*Corbe, Corbi, Corby, Corbyn,
Corbynn*

Cordasha (American) a combination of Cora + Dasha.

Cordelia (Latin) warm-
hearted. (Welsh) sea jewel.
See also Delia, Della.
*Cordae, Cordelie, Cordett,
Cordette, Cordi, Cordilia,
Cordilla, Cordula, Kordelia,
Kordula*

Cordi (Welsh) a short form of
Cordelia.
Cordey, Cordia, Cordie, Cordy

Coretta (Greek) a familiar
form of Cora.
*Coreta, Corette, Correta,
Corretta, Corrette, Koretta,
Korretta*

Corey, Cory (Irish) from the
hollow. (Greek) familiar
forms of Cora. See also Kori.
*Coree, Cori, Correy, Correye,
Corry*

Cori, Corie, Corrie (Irish)
forms of Corey.

Coriann, Corianne
(American) combinations of
Cori + Ann, Cori + Anne.
*Corian, Coriane, Cori-Ann,
Corri, Corrie-Ann, Corrianne,
Corrie-Anne*

Corina, Corinna (Greek)
familiar forms of Corinne.
See also Korina.
*Coreena, Coriana, Corianna,
Corinda, Correna, Corrinna,
Coryna*

Corinne (Greek) maiden.
*Coreen, Coren, Corin, Corina,
Corine, Corinee, Corinn,
Corinna, Corrina, Coryn,
Corynn, Corynne*

Corissa (Greek) a familiar
form of Cora.
*Coresa, Coressa, Corisa,
Coryssa, Korissa*

Corliss (English) cheerful; goodhearted.
Corlisa, Corlise, Corlissa, Corly, Korliss

Cornelia (Latin) horn colored. See also Kornelia, Nelia, Nellie.
Carna, Carniella, Corneilla, Cornela, Cornelie, Cornella, Cornelle, Cornie, Cornilear, Cornisha, Corny

Corrina, Corrine (Greek) forms of Corinne.
Correen, Corren, Corrin, Corrinn, Corrinna, Corrinne, Corrinne, Corryn

Cortney (English) a form of Courtney.
Cortne, Cortnea, Cortnee, Cortneia, Cortni, Cortnie, Cortny, Cortnye, Corttney

Cosette (French) a familiar form of Nicole.
Cosetta, Cossetta, Cossette, Cozette

Courtenay (English) a form of Courtney.
Courtaney, Courtany, Courteney, Courteny

Courtnee, Courtnie (English) forms of Courtney.
Courtne, Courtnée, Courtnei, Courtneigh, Courtni, Courtnii

Courtney (English) from the court. See also Kortney, Kourtney.
Cortney, Courtena, Courtenay,
Courtene, Courtnae, Courtnay, Courtnee, Courtny, Courtonie

Crisbell (American) a combination of Crista + Belle.
Crisbel, Cristabel

Crista, Crysta (Italian) forms of Christa.
Cristah

Cristal (Latin) a form of Crystal.
Cristalie, Cristalina, Cristalle, Cristel, Cristela, Cristelia, Cristella, Cristelle, Cristhie, Cristle

Cristen, Cristin (Irish) forms of Christen, Christin. See also Kristin.
Cristan, Cristyn, Crystan, Crysten, Crystin, Crystyn

Cristina, Cristine (Greek) forms of Christina. See also Kristina.
Cristiona, Cristy

Cristy (English) a familiar form of Cristina. A form of Christy. See also Kristy.
Cristey, Cristi, Cristie, Crysti, Crystie, Crysty

Crystal (Latin) clear, brilliant glass. See also Kristal, Krystal.
Christal, Chrystal, Chrystal-Lynn, Chrystel, Cristal, Crystala, Crystale, Crystalee, Crystalin, Crystall, Crystalle, Crystaly, Crystel, Crystela, Crystelia, Crystelle, Crysthelle, Crystl, Crystle, Crystol, Crystole, Crystyl

Crystalin (Latin) crystal pool.
*Crystal-Ann, Cristalanna,
Crystal-Anne, Cristalina,
Cristallina, Cristalyn,
Crystallynn, Crystallynne,
Cristilyn, Crystalina, Crystal-
Lee, Crystal-Lynn, Crystalyn,
Crystalynn*

Crystina (Greek) a form of
Christina.
*Crystin, Crystine, Crystyn,
Crystyna, Crystyne*

Curran (Irish) heroine.
Cura, Curin, Curina, Curinna

Cybele (Greek) a form of
Sybil.
Cybel, Cybil, Cybill, Cybille

Cydney (French) a form of
Sydney.
*Cydne, Cydnee, Cydnei,
Cydni, Cydnie*

Cyerra (Irish) a form of Ciara.
Cyera, Cyerria

Cyndi (Greek) a form of Cindy.
*Cynda, Cyndal, Cyndale,
Cyndall, Cyndee, Cyndel,
Cyndia, Cyndie, Cyndle, Cyndy*

Cynthia (Greek) moon.
Mythology: another name
for Artemis, the moon god-
dess. See also Hyacinth,
Kynthia.
*Cindy, Cinthia, Cyneria,
Cynethia, Cynithia, Cynthea,
Cynthiana, Cynthiann,
Cynthie, Cynthria, Cynthy,*
*Cynthya, Cyntia, Cyntreia,
Cythia, Synthia*

Cyrilla (Greek) noble.
*Cerelia, Cerella, Cira, Cirilla,
Cyrella, Cyrille*

D

Dacey (Irish) southerner.
(Greek) a familiar form of
Candace.
*Dacee, Dacei, Daci, Dacia,
Dacie, Dacy, Daicee, Daici,
Daicie, Daicy, Daycee, Daycie,
Daycy*

Dacia (Irish) a form of Dacey.
Daciah

Dae (English) day. See also
Dai.

Daeja (French) a form of
Déja.
Daejah, Daejia

Daelynn (American) a combi-
nation of Dae + Lynn.
*Daeleen, Daelena, Daelin,
Daelyn, Daelynne*

Daeshandra (American) a
combination of Dae +
Shandra.
*Daeshandria, Daeshaundra,
Daeshaundria, Daeshawndra,
Daeshawndria, Daeshondra,
Daeshondria*

Daeshawna (American) a
combination of Dae +
Shawna.
Daeshan, Daeshaun,
Daeshauna, Daeshavon,
Daeshawn, Daeshawntia,
Daeshon, Daeshona

Daeshonda (American) a
combination of Dae +
Shonda.
Daeshanda, Daeshawnda

Dafny (American) a form of
Daphne.
Dafany, Daffany, Daffie, Daffy,
Dafna, Dafne, Dafney, Dafnie

Dagmar (German) glorious.
Dagmara

Dagny (Scandinavian) day.
Dagna, Dagnanna, Dagne,
Dagney, Dagnie

Dahlia (Scandinavian) valley.
Botany: a perennial flower.
See also Daliah.
Dahliah, Dahlya, Dahlye

Dai (Japanese) great. See also
Dae.
Day, Daye

Daija, Daijah (French) forms
of Déja.
Daijaah, Daijea, Daijha,
Daijhah, Dayja

Daisha (American) a form of
Dasha.
Daesha, Daishae, Daishia,
Daishya, Daisia

Daisy (English) day's eye.
Botany: a white and yellow
flower.
Daisee, Daisey, Daisi, Daisia,
Daisie, Dasey, Dasi, Dasie,
Dasy, Daysi, Deisy

Daja, Dajah (French) forms of
Déja.
Dajae, Dajai, Daje, Dajha,
Dajia

Dakayla (American) a combi-
nation of the prefix Da +
Kayla.
Dakala, Dakila

Dakira (American) a combina-
tion of the prefix Da + Kira.
Dakara, Dakaria, Dakarra,
Dakirah, Dakyra

Dakota (Native American) a
tribal name.
Dakkota, Dakoda, Dakotah,
Dakotha, Dakotta, Dekoda,
Dekota, Dekotah, Dekotha

Dale (English) valley.
Dael, Dahl, Daile, Daleleana,
Dalena, Dalina, Dayle

Dalia, Daliah (Hebrew)
branch. See also Dahlia.
Daelia, Dailia, Daleah, Daleia,
Dalialah, Daliyah

Dalila (Swahili) gentle.
Dalela, Dalida, Dalilah, Dalilia

Dalisha (American) a form of
Dallas.
Dalisa, Dalishea, Dalishia,
Dalishya, Dalisia, Dalissia

Dallas (Irish) wise.
Dalis, Dalise, Dalisha, Dalisse, Dallace, Dallis, Dallise, Dallus, Dallys, Dalyce, Dalys

Damaris (Greek) gentle girl. See also Maris.
Dama, Damar, Damara, Damarius, Damary, Damarylis, Damarys, Dameress, Dameris, Damiris, Dammaris, Dammeris, Damris, Demaras, Demaris

Damiana (Greek) tamer, soother.
Daimenia, Daimiona, Damia, Damiann, Damianna, Damianne, Damien, Damienne, Damiona, Damon, Demion

Damica (French) friendly.
Damee, Dameeka, Dameka, Damekah, Damicah, Damicia, Damicka, Damie, Damieka, Damika, Damikah, Damyka, Demeeka, Demeka, Demekah, Demica, Demicah

Damita (Spanish) small noblewoman.
Damee, Damesha, Dameshia, Damesia, Dametia, Dametra, Dametrah

Damonica (American) a combination of the prefix Da + Monica.
Damonec, Damoneke, Damonik, Damonika, Damonique, Diamoniqua, Diamonique

Dana (English) from Denmark; bright as day.
Daina, Dainna, Danah, Danaia, Danan, Danarra, Dane, Danean, Danna, Dayna

Danae (Greek) Mythology: the mother of Perseus.
Danaë, Danay, Danayla, Danays, Danai, Danea, Danee, Dannae, Denae, Denee

Danalyn (American) a combination of Dana + Lynn.
Danalee, Donaleen

Daneil (Hebrew) a form of Danielle.
Daneal, Daneala, Daneale, Daneel, Daneela, Daneila

Danella (American) a form of Danielle.
Danayla, Danela, Danelia, Danelle, Danna, Donella, Donnella

Danelle (Hebrew) a form of Danielle.
Danael, Danalle, Danel, Danele, Danell, Danella, Donelle, Donnelle

Danesha, Danisha (American) forms of Danessa.
Daneisha, Daneshia, Daniesha, Danishia

Danessa (American) a combination of Danielle + Vanessa. See also Doneshia.
Danasia, Danesa, Danesha, Danessia, Daniesa, Danisa, Danissa

Danessia (American) a form
of Danessa.
*Danesia, Danieshia, Danisia,
Danissia*

Danette (American) a form of
Danielle.
*Danetra, Danett, Danetta,
Donnita*

Dani (Hebrew) a familiar form
of Danielle.
*Danee, Danie, Danne, Dannee,
Danni, Dannie, Danny,
Dannye, Dany*

Dania, Danya (Hebrew) short
forms of Danielle.
*Daniah, Danja, Dannia,
Danyae*

Danica, Danika (Slavic)
morning star. (Hebrew)
forms of Danielle.
*Daneca, Daneeka, Daneekah,
Danicah, Danicka, Danieka,
Danikah, Danikla, Danneeka,
Dannica, Dannika, Dannikah,
Danyka, Denica, Donica,
Donika, Donnaica, Donnica,
Donnika*

Danice (American) a combination of Danielle + Janice.
Donice

Daniela (Italian) a form of
Danielle.
Daniellah, Dannilla, Danijela

Danielan (Spanish) a form of
Danielle.

Daniella (English) a form of
Dana.
Danka, Danniella, Danyella

Danielle (Hebrew, French)
God is my judge.
*Daneen, Daneil, Daneille,
Danelle, Dani, Danial,
Danialle, Danica, Daniel,
Daniela, Danielan, Daniele,
Danielka, Daniell, Daniella,
Danilka, Danille, Danit,
Dannielle, Danyel, Donniella*

Danille (American) a form of
Danielle.
*Danila, Danile, Danilla,
Dannille*

Danit (Hebrew) a form of
Danielle.
*Danett, Danis, Danisha,
Daniss, Danita, Danitra,
Danitrea, Danitria, Danitza,
Daniz*

Danna (Hebrew) a short form
of Danella.
Dannah

Dannielle (Hebrew, French) a
form of Danielle.
Danniel, Danniele, Danniell

Danyel, Danyell, Danyelle
(American) forms of
Danielle.
*Daniyel, Danyae, Danyail,
Danyaile, Danyal, Danyale,
Danyea, Danyele, Danyiel,
Danyielle, Danyle, Donnyale,
Donnyell, Donyale, Donyell*

Daphne (Greek) laurel tree.
Dafny, Daphane, Daphany,
Dapheney, Daphna, Daphnee,
Daphnique, Daphnit, Daphny

Daphnee (Greek) a form of
Daphne.
Daphaney, Daphanie, Daphney,
Daphni, Daphnie

Dara (Hebrew) compassionate.
Dahra, Daira, Dairah, Darah,
Daraka, Daralea, Daralee,
Daraleigh, Daralie, Daravie,
Darda, Darice, Darisa, Darissa,
Darja, Darra, Darrah

Darby (Irish) free.
(Scandinavian) deer estate.
Darb, Darbe, Darbee, Darbi,
Darbie, Darbra, Darbye

Darcelle (French) a form of
Darci.
Darcel, Darcell, Darcella,
Darselle

Darci, Darcy (Irish) dark.
(French) fortress.
Darcee, Darcelle, Darcey, Darcie,
Darsey, Darsi, Darsie

Daria (Greek) wealthy.
Dari, Dariya, Darria, Darya,
Daryia

Darian, Darrian (Greek)
forms of Daron.
Dariana, Dariane, Dariann,
Darianna, Darianne, Dariyan,
Dariyanne, Darriana, Darriane,
Darriann, Darrianna,
Darrianne, Derrian, Driana

Darielle (French) a form of
Daryl.
Dariel, Dariela, Dariell, Darriel,
Darrielle

Darien, Darrien (Greek)
forms of Daron.
Dariene, Darienne, Darriene

Darilynn (American) a form
of Darlene.
Daralin, Daralyn, Daralynn,
Daralynne, Darilin, Darilyn,
Darilynne, Darlin, Darlyn,
Darlynn, Darlynne, Darylin,
Darylyn, Darylynn, Darylynne

Darion, Darrion (Irish) forms
of Daron.
Dariona, Darione, Darionna,
Darionne, Darriona, Darrionna

Darla (English) a short form
of Darlene.
Darlecia, Darli, Darlice, Darlie,
Darlis, Darly, Darlys

Darlene (French) little darling.
See also Daryl.
Darilynn, Darla, Darlean, Darlee,
Darleen, Darleene, Darlena,
Darlenia, Darlenne, Darletha,
Darlin, Darline, Darling, Darlyn,
Darlynn, Darlynne

Darnee (Irish) a familiar form
of Darnelle.

Darnelle (English) hidden place.
Darnee, Darnel, Darnell,
Darnella, Darnesha, Darnetta,
Darnette, Darnice, Darniece,
Darnita, Darnyell

Darnesha, Darnisha
(American) forms of Darnelle.
*Darneisha, Darneishia,
Darneshea, Darneshia,
Darnesia, Darniesha, Darnishia,
Darnisia, Darrenisha*

Daron (Irish) great.
*Darian, Darien, Darion,
Daronica, Daronice, Darron,
Daryn*

Darselle (French) a form of
Darcelle.
Darsel, Darsell, Darsella

Daru (Hindi) pine tree.

Daryl (English) beloved.
(French) a short form of
Darlene.
*Darelle, Darielle, Daril,
Darilynn, Darrel, Darrell,
Darrelle, Darreshia, Darryl,
Darryll, Daryll, Darylle*

Daryn (Greek) gifts. (Irish) great.
*Daron, Daryan, Daryne,
Darynn, Darynne*

Dasha, Dasia (Russian) forms
of Dorothy.
*Daisha, Dashae, Dashenka,
Dashia, Dashiah, Dasiah,
Daysha*

Dashawna (American) a com-
bination of the prefix Da +
Shawna.
*Dashawn, Dashawnna, Dashay,
Dashell, Dayshana,
Dayshawnna, Dayshona,
Deshawna*

Dashiki (Swahili) loose-fitting
shirt worn in Africa.
*Dashi, Dashika, Dashka,
Desheka, Deshiki*

Dashonda (American) a com-
bination of the prefix Da +
Shonda.
Dashawnda, Dishante

Davalinda (American) a com-
bination of Davida + Linda.
*Davalynda, Davelinda,
Davilinda, Davylinda*

Davalynda (American) a form
of Davalinda.
*Davelynda, Davilynda,
Davylynda*

Davalynn (American) a com-
bination of Davida + Lynn.
*Davalin, Davalyn, Davalynne,
Davelin, Davelyn, Davelynn,
Davelynne, Davilin, Davilyn,
Davilynn, Davilynne, Dayleen,
Devlyn*

Davida (Hebrew) beloved.
Bible: David was the second
king of Israel. See also Vida.
*Daveta, Davetta, Davette,
Davika, Davita*

Davina (Scottish) a form of
Davida. See also Vina.
*Dava, Davannah, Davean, Davee,
Daveen, Daveena, Davene,
Daveon, Davey, Davi, Daviana,
Davie, Davin, Davinder, Davine,
Davineen, Davinia, Davinna,
Davonna, Davria, Devean,
Deveen, Devene, Devina*

Davisha (American) a combination of the prefix Da + Aisha.
Daveisha, Davesia, Davis, Davisa

Davonna (Scottish, English) a form of Davina, Devonna.
Davion, Daviona, Davionna, Davon, Davona, Davonda, Davone, Davonia, Davonne, Davonnia

Dawn (English) sunrise, dawn.
Dawana, Dawandrea, Dawanna, Dawin, Dawna, Dawne, Dawnee, Dawnetta, Dawnisha, Dawnlynn, Dawnn, Dawnrae

Dawna (English) a form of Dawn.
Dawnna, Dawnya

Dawnyelle (American) a combination of Dawn + Danielle.
Dawnele, Dawnell, Dawnelle, Dawnyel, Dawnyella

Dawnisha (American) a form of Dawn.
Dawnesha, Dawni, Dawniell, Dawnielle, Dawnisia, Dawniss, Dawnita, Dawnnisha, Dawnysha, Dawnysia

Dayana (Latin) a form of Diana.
Dayanara, Dayani, Dayanna, Dayanne, Dayanni, Deyanaira, Dyani, Dyanna, Dyia

Dayle (English) a form of Dale.
Dayla, Daylan, Daylea, Daylee

Dayna (Scandinavian) a form of Dana.
Daynah, Dayne, Daynna, Deyna

Daysha (American) a form of Dasha.
Daysa, Dayshalie, Daysia, Deisha

Daysi, Deysi (English) forms of Daisy.
Daysee, Daysia, Daysie, Daysy, Deysia, Deysy

Dayton, Daytona (English) day town; bright, sunny town.
Daytonia

Deana (Latin) divine. (English) valley.
Deanah, Deane, Deanielle, Deanisha, Deanna, Deeana, Deeann, Deeanna, Deena

Deandra (American) a combination of Dee + Andrea.
Dandrea, Deandre, Deandré, Deandrea, Deandree, Deandreia, Deandria, Deanndra, Deaundra, Deaundria, Deeandra, Deyaneira, Deondra, Diandra, Diandre, Diandrea, Diondria, Dyandra

Deangela (Italian) a combination of the prefix De + Angela.
Deangala, Deangalique, Deangle

Deanna (Latin) a form of
Deana, Diana.
Deaaana, Deahana, Deandra,
Deandre, Déanna, Deannia,
Deeanna, Deena

Deanne (Latin) a form of
Diane.
Deahanne, Deane, Deann,
Déanne, Deeann, Dee-Ann,
Deeanne

Debbie (Hebrew) a short
form of Deborah.
Debbee, Debbey, Debbi, Debby,
Debee, Debi, Debie

Deborah (Hebrew) bee. Bible:
a great Hebrew prophetess.
Deb, Debbie, Debbora,
Debborah, Deberah, Debor,
Debora, Deboran, Deborha,
Deborrah, Debra, Debrena,
Debrina, Debroah, Devora,
Dobra

Debra (American) a form of
Deborah.
Debbra, Debbrah, Debrah,
Debrea, Debria

Dedra (American) a form of
Deirdre.
Deeddra, Deedra, Deedrea,
Deedrie

Dedriana (American) a combination of Dedra + Adriana.
Dedranae

Dee (Welsh) black, dark.
De, Dea, Deah, Dede, Dedie,
Deea, Deedee, Dee Dee, Didi

Deena (American) a form of
Deana, Dena, Dinah.

Deidra, Deidre (Irish) forms
of Deirdre.
Deidrah, Deidrea, Deidrie,
Diedra, Diedre, Dierdra

Deirdre (Irish) sorrowful;
wanderer.
Dedra, Deerdra, Deerdre,
Deidra, Deidre, Deidree, Didi,
Diedra, Dierdre, Diérdre,
Dierdrie

Deisy (English) a form of
Daisy.
Deisi, Deissy

Deitra (Greek) a short form
of Demetria.
Deetra, Detria

Déja (French) before.
Daeja, Daija, Deejay, Dejae,
Déjah, Dejai, Dejanae,
Dejanelle, Dejon

Dejanae (French) a form of
Déja.
Dajahnae, Dajona, Dejana,
Dejanah, Dejanae, Dejanai,
Dejanay, Dejane, Dejanea,
Dejanee, Dejanna, Dejannaye,
Dejena, Dejonae

Dejon (French) a form of
Déja.
Daijon, Dajan, Dejone,
Dejonee, Dejonelle, Dejonna

Deka (Somali) pleasing.
Dekah

Delacy (American) a combination of the prefix De +
Lacy.
Delaceya

Delainey (Irish) a form of
Delaney.
Delaine, Delainee, Delaini,
Delainie, Delainy

Delana (German) noble protector.
Dalanna, Dalayna, Daleena,
Dalena, Dalenna, Dalina,
Dalinda, Dalinna, Delaina,
Delania, Delanya, Delayna,
Deleena, Delena, Delenya,
Delina, Dellaina

Delaney (Irish) descendant of
the challenger. (English) a
form of Adeline.
Dalaney, Dalania, Dalene,
Daleney, Daline, Del, Delainey,
Delane, Delanee, Delanie,
Delany, Delayne, Delayney,
Delaynie, Deleani, Déline,
Della, Dellaney

Delanie (Irish) a form of
Delaney.
Delani

Delfina (Greek) a form of
Delphine. (Spanish) dolphin.
Delfeena, Delfine

Delia (Greek) visible; from
Delos, Greece. (German,
Welsh) a short form of
Adelaide, Cordelia.
Mythology: a festival of
Apollo held in ancient
Greece.
Dehlia, Delea, Deli, Deliah,
Deliana, Delianne, Delinda,
Dellia, Dellya, Delya

Delicia (English) delightful.
Delecia, Delesha, Delice, Delisa,
Delise, Delisha, Delishia,
Delisiah, Delya, Delys, Delyse,
Delysia, Doleesha

Delilah (Hebrew) brooder.
Bible: the companion of
Samson. See also Lila.
Dalialah, Dalila, Daliliah,
Delila, Delilia

Della (English) a short form
of Adelaide, Cordelia,
Delaney.
Del, Dela, Dell, Delle, Delli,
Dellie, Dells

Delores (Spanish) a form of
Dolores.
Delora, Delore, Deloria,
Delories, Deloris, Delorise,
Delorita, Delsie

Delphine (Greek) from
Delphi, Greece. See also
Delfina.
Delpha, Delphe, Delphi,
Delphia, Delphina, Delphinia,
Delvina

Delsie (English) a familiar
form of Delores.
Delsa, Delsey, Delza

Delta (Greek) door.
Linguistics: the fourth letter
in the Greek alphabet.

Geography: a triangular land mass at the mouth of a river.
Delte, Deltora, Deltoria, Deltra

Demetria (Greek) cover of the earth. Mythology: Demeter was the Greek goddess of the harvest.
Deitra, Demeta, Demeteria, Demetra, Demetriana, Demetrianna, Demetrias, Demetrice, Demetriona, Demetris, Demetrish, Demetrius, Demi, Demita, Demitra, Demitria, Dymitra

Demi (French) half. (Greek) a short form of Demetria.
Demia, Demiah, Demii, Demmi, Demmie, Demy

Dena (English, Native American) valley. (Hebrew) a form of Dinah. See also Deana.
Deane, Deena, Deeyn, Denae, Denah, Dene, Denea, Deney, Denna, Deonna

Denae (Hebrew) a form of Dena.
Denaé, Denay, Denee, Deneé

Deni (French) a short form of Denise.
Deney, Denie, Denni, Dennie, Denny, Dinnie, Dinny

Denica, Denika (Slavic) forms of Danica.
Denikah, Denikia

Denise (French) Mythology: follower of Dionysus, the god of wine.
Danice, Danise, Denese, Deni, Denice, Denicy, Deniece, Denisha, Denisse, Denize, Dennise, Dennys, Denyce, Denys, Denyse

Denisha (American) a form of Denise.
Deneesha, Deneichia, Deneisha, Deneishea, Denesha, Deneshia, Deniesha, Denishia

Denisse (French) a form of Denise.
Denesse, Denissa

Deonna (English) a form of Dena.
Deon, Deona, Deonah, Deondra, Deonne

Derika (German) ruler of the people.
Dereka, Derekia, Derica, Dericka, Derrica, Derricka, Derrika

Derry (Irish) redhead.
Deri, Derie

Deryn (Welsh) bird.
Derien, Derienne, Derion, Derin, Deron, Derren, Derrin, Derrine, Derrion, Derriona, Deryne

Desarae (French) a form of
Desiree.
*Desara, Desarai, Desaraie,
Desaray, Desare, Desaré,
Desarea, Desaree, Desarie,
Dezarae*

Deserae, Desirae (French)
forms of Desiree.
*Desera, Deserai, Deseray,
Desere, Deseree, Deseret, Deseri,
Deserie, Deserrae, Deserray,
Deserré, Dessirae, Dezeray,
Dezere, Dezerea, Dezrae,
Dezyrae*

Deshawna (American) a com-
bination of the prefix De +
Shawna.
*Dashawna, Deshan, Deshane,
Deshaun, Deshawn, Desheania,
Deshona, Deshonna*

Deshawnda (American) a
combination of the prefix
De + Shawnda.
*Deshanda, Deshandra,
Deshaundra, Deshawndra,
Deshonda*

Desi (French) a short form of
Desiree.
*Désir, Desira, Dezi, Dezia,
Dezzia, Dezzie*

Desiree (French) desired,
longed for. See also Dessa.
*Chesarey, Desarae, Deserae,
Desi, Desirae, Desirah, Desirai,
Desiray, Desire, Desirea,
Desireah, Desirée, Désirée,
Desirey, Desiri, Desray, Desree,*

*Dessie, Dessire, Dezarae,
Dezirae, Deziree*

Dessa (Greek) wanderer.
(French) a form of Desiree.
Desta (Ethiopian) happy.
(French) a short form of
Destiny.
Desti, Destie, Desty

Destany (French) a form of
Destiny.
*Destanee, Destaney, Destani,
Destanie, Destannee, Destannie*

Destinee, Destini, Destinie
(French) forms of Destiny.
*Desteni, Destiana, Destine,
Destinée, Destnie*

Destiney (French) a form of
Destiny.

Destiny (French) fate.
*Desnine, Desta, Destany,
Destenee, Destenie, Desteny,
Destin, Destinee, Destiney,
Destini, Destinie, Destonie,
Destynee, Dezstany*

Destynee, Destyni (French)
forms of Destiny.
*Desty, Destyn, Destyne,
Destyne, Destynie*

Deva (Hindi) divine.
Deeva

Devan (Irish) a form of
Devin.
*Devana, Devane, Devanee,
Devaney, Devani, Devanie,
Devann, Devanna, Devannae,
Devanne, Devany*

Devi (Hindi) goddess.
Religion: the Hindu goddess
of power and destruction.

Devin (Irish) poet.
*Devan, Deven, Devena,
Devenje, Deveny, Devine,
Devinn, Devinne, Devyn*

Devon (English) a short form
of Devonna. (Irish) a form of
Devin.
*Deaven, Devion, Devione,
Devionne, Devone, Devoni,
Devonne*

Devonna (English) from
Devonshire.
*Davonna, Devon, Devona,
Devonda, Devondra, Devonia*

Devora (Hebrew) a form of
Deborah.
Deva, Devorah, Devra, Devrah

Devyn (Irish) a form of
Devin.
*Deveyn, Devyne, Devynn,
Devynne*

Dextra (Latin) adroit, skillful.
Dekstra, Dextria

Dezarae, Dezirae, Deziree
(French) forms of Desiree.
*Dezaraee, Dezarai, Dezaray,
Dezare, Dezaree, Dezarey,
Dezerie, Deziray, Dezirea,
Dezirée, Dezorae, Dezra*

Di (Latin) a short form of
Diana, Diane.
Dy

Dia (Latin) a short form of
Diana, Diane.

Diamond (Latin) precious
gem.
*Diamantina, Diamon,
Diamonda, Diamonde,
Diamonia, Diamonique,
Diamonte, Diamontina,
Dyamond*

Diana (Latin) divine.
Mythology: the goddess of
the hunt, the moon, and fer-
tility. See also Deanna,
Deanne, Dyan.
*Daiana, Daianna, Dayana,
Dayanna, Di, Dia, Dianah,
Dianalyn, Dianarose, Dianatris,
Dianca, Diandra, Diane,
Dianelis, Diania, Dianielle,
Dianita, Dianna, Dianys, Didi*

Diane, Dianne (Latin) short
forms of Diana.
*Deane, Deanne, Deeane,
Deeanne, Di, Dia, Diahann,
Dian, Diani, Dianie, Diann*

Dianna (Latin) a form of
Diana.
Diahanna, Diannah

Diantha (Greek) divine
flower.
Diandre, Dianthe

Diedra (Irish) a form of
Deirdre.
Didra, Diedre

Dillan (Irish) loyal, faithful.
Dillon, Dillyn

Dilys (Welsh) perfect; true.

Dina (Hebrew) a form of Dinah.
Dinna, Dyna

Dinah (Hebrew) vindicated. Bible: a daughter of Jacob and Leah.
Dina, Dinnah, Dynah

Dinka (Swahili) people.

Dionna (Greek) an alternative form of Dionne.
Deona, Deondra, Deonia, Deonna, Deonyia, Diona, Diondra, Diondrea

Dionne (Greek) divine queen. Mythology: Dione was the mother of Aphrodite, the goddess of love.
Deonne, Dion, Dione, Dionee, Dionis, Dionna, Dionte

Dior (French) golden.
Diora, Diore, Diorra, Diorre

Dita (Spanish) a form of Edith.
Ditka, Ditta

Divinia (Latin) divine.
Devina, Devinae, Devinia, Devinie, Devinna, Diveena, Divina, Divine, Diviniea, Divya

Dixie (French) tenth. (English) wall; dike. Geography: a nickname for the American South.
Dix, Dixee, Dixi, Dixy

Diza (Hebrew) joyful.
Ditza, Ditzah, Dizah

Dodie (Hebrew) beloved. (Greek) a familiar form of Dorothy.
Doda, Dode, Dodee, Dodi, Dody

Dolly (American) a short form of Dolores, Dorothy.
Dol, Doll, Dollee, Dolley, Dolli, Dollie, Dollina

Dolores (Spanish) sorrowful. Religion: Nuestra Señora de los Dolores—Our Lady of Sorrows—is a name for the Virgin Mary. See also Lola.
Delores, Deloria, Dolly, Dolorcitas, Dolorita, Doloritas

Dominica, Dominika (Latin) belonging to the Lord. See also Mika.
Domenica, Domenika, Domineca, Domineka, Dominga, Domini, Dominick, Dominicka, Dominique, Dominixe, Domino, Dominyika, Domka, Domnicka, Domonica, Domonice, Domonika

Dominique, Domonique (French) forms of Dominica, Dominika.
Domanique, Domeneque, Domenique, Domineque, Dominiqua, Domino, Dominoque, Dominque, Dominuque, Domique, Domminique, Domoniqua

Domino (English) a short
form of Dominica,
Dominique.

Dona (English) world leader;
proud ruler. (Italian) a form
of Donna.
*Donae, Donah, Donalda,
Donaldina, Donelda, Donellia,
Doni*

Doña (Italian) a form of
Donna.
*Donail, Donalea, Donalisa,
Donay, Doni, Donia, Donie,
Donise, Donitrae*

Donata (Latin) gift.
*Donatha, Donato, Donatta,
Donetta, Donette, Donita,
Donnette, Donnita, Donte*

Dondi (American) a familiar
form of Donna.
Dondra, Dondrea, Dondria

Doneshia, Donisha
(American) forms of
Danessa.
*Donasha, Donashay, Doneisha,
Doneishia, Donesha, Donisa,
Donisha, Donishia, Donneshia,
Donnisha*

Donna (Italian) lady.
*Doña, Dondi, Donnae,
Donnalee, Donnalen, Donnay,
Donne, Donnell, Donni,
Donnie, Donnise, Donny,
Dontia, Donya*

Donniella (American) a form
of Danielle.
*Donella, Doniele, Doniell,
Doniella, Donielle, Donnella,
Donnielle, Donnyella, Donyelle*

Dora (Greek) gift. A short
form of Adora, Eudora,
Pandora, Theodora.
*Dorah, Doralia, Doralie,
Doralisa, Doraly, Doralynn,
Doran, Dorchen, Dore, Dorece,
Doree, Doreece, Doreen, Dorelia,
Dorella, Dorelle, Doresha,
Doressa, Doretta, Dori, Dorielle,
Dorika, Doriley, Dorilis,
Dorinda, Dorion, Dorita, Doro,
Dory*

Doralynn (English) a combi-
nation of Dora + Lynn.
*Doralin, Doralyn, Doralynne,
Dorlin*

Doreen (Irish) moody, sullen.
(French) golden. (Greek) a
form of Dora.
*Doreena, Dorena, Dorene,
Dorina, Dorine*

Doretta (American) a form of
Dora, Dorothy.
Doretha, Dorette, Dorettie

Dori, Dory (American) famil-
iar forms of Dora, Doria,
Doris, Dorothy.
*Dore, Dorey, Dorie, Dorree,
Dorri, Dorrie, Dorry*

Doria (Greek) a form of
Dorian.
Dori

Dorian (Greek) from Doris,
Greece.
*Dorean, Doriana, Doriane,
Doriann, Dorianna, Dorianne,
Dorin, Dorina, Dorriane*

Dorinda (Spanish) a form of
Dora.

Doris (Greek) sea. Mythology:
wife of Nereus and mother
of the Nereids or sea
nymphs.
*Dori, Dorice, Dorisa, Dorise,
Dorris, Dorrise, Dorrys, Dory,
Dorys*

Dorothea (Greek) a form of
Dorothy. See also Thea.
*Dorethea, Dorotea, Doroteya,
Dorotha, Dorothia, Dorotthea,
Dorthea, Dorthia*

Dorothy (Greek) gift of God.
See also Dasha, Dodie,
Lolotea, Theodora.
*Dasya, Do, Doa, Doe, Dolly,
Doortje, Dorathy, Dordei, Dordi,
Doretta, Dori, Dorika, Doritha,
Dorka, Dorle, Dorlisa, Doro,
Dorolice, Dorosia, Dorota,
Dorothea, Dorothee, Dorothi,
Dorothie, Dorottya, Dorte,
Dortha, Dorthy, Dory, Dosi,
Dossie, Dosya, Dottie*

Dorrit (Greek) dwelling.
(Hebrew) generation.
Dorit, Dorita, Doritt

Dottie, Dotty (Greek) familiar
forms of Dorothy.
Dot, Dottee

Drew (Greek) courageous;
strong. (Latin) a short form
of Drusilla.
Dru, Drue

Drinka (Spanish) a form of
Alexandria.
Dreena, Drena, Drina

Drusi (Latin) a short form of
Drusilla.
*Drucey, Druci, Drucie, Drucy,
Drusey, Drusie, Drusy*

Drusilla (Latin) descendant of
Drusus, the strong one. See also
Drew.
*Drewsila, Drucella, Drucill,
Drucilla, Druscilla, Druscille, Drusi*

Dulce (Latin) sweet.
*Delcina, Delcine, Douce, Doucie,
Dulcea, Dulcey, Dulci, Dulcia,
Dulciana, Dulcibel, Dulcibella,
Dulcie, Dulcine, Dulcinea,
Dulcy, Dulse, Dulsea*

Dulcinea (Spanish) sweet.
Literature: Don Quixote's
love interest.

Duscha (Russian) soul; sweetheart; term of endearment.
Duschah, Dusha, Dushenka

Dusti, Dusty (English) familiar
forms of Dustine.
Dustee, Dustie

Dustine (German) valiant
fighter. (English) brown rock
quarry.
*Dusteena, Dusti, Dustin,
Dustina, Dustyn*

Dyamond, Dymond (Latin)
forms of Diamond.
*Dyamin, Dyamon, Dyamone,
Dymin, Dymon, Dymonde,
Dymone, Dymonn*

Dyana (Latin) a form of
Diana. (Native American)
deer.
*Dyan, Dyane, Dyani, Dyann,
Dyanna, Dyanne*

Dylan (Welsh) sea.
*Dylaan, Dylaina, Dylana,
Dylane, Dylanee, Dylanie,
Dylann, Dylanna, Dylen,
Dylin, Dyllan, Dylynn*

Dyllis (Welsh) sincere.
Dilys, Dylis, Dylys

Dynasty (Latin) powerful
ruler.
Dynastee, Dynasti, Dynastie

Dyshawna (American) a com-
bination of the prefix Dy +
Shawna.
*Dyshanta, Dyshawn,
Dyshonda, Dyshonna*

E

Earlene (Irish) pledge.
(English) noblewoman.
*Earla, Earlean, Earlecia,
Earleen, Earlena, Earlina,
Earlinda, Earline, Erla, Erlana,
Erlene, Erlenne, Erlina, Erlinda,
Erline, Erlisha*

Eartha (English) earthy.
Ertha

Easter (English) Easter
time. History: a name for a child
born on Easter.
Eastan, Eastlyn, Easton

Ebone, Ebonee (Greek) forms
of Ebony.
*Abonee, Ebanee, Eboné,
Ebonea, Ebonne, Ebonnee*

Eboni, Ebonie (Greek) forms
of Ebony.
Ebanie, Ebeni, Ebonni, Ebonnie

Ebony (Greek) a hard, dark
wood.
*Abony, Eban, Ebanie, Ebany,
Ebbony, Ebone, Eboney, Eboni,
Ebonie, Ebonique, Ebonisha,
Ebonye, Ebonyi*

Echo (Greek) repeated sound.
Mythology: the nymph who
pined for the love of
Narcissus until only her
voice remained.
Echoe, Ecko, Ekko, Ekkoe

Eda (Irish, English) a short
form of Edana, Edith.

Edana (Irish) ardent; flame.
Eda, Edan, Edanna

Edda (German) a form of
Hedda.
Etta

Eddy (American) a familiar
form of Edwina.
Eady, Eddi, Eddie, Edy

Edeline (English) noble; kind.
Adeline, Edelyne, Ediline,
Edilyne

Eden (Babylonian) a plain.
(Hebrew) delightful. Bible:
the earthly paradise.
Eaden, Ede, Edena, Edene,
Edenia, Edin, Edyn

Edie (English) a familiar form
of Edith.
Eadie, Edi, Edy, Edye, Eyde,
Eydie

Edith (English) rich gift. See
also Dita.
Eadith, Eda, Ede, Edetta,
Edette, Edie, Edit, Edita, Edite,
Editha, Edithe, Editta, Ediva,
Edyta, Edyth, Edytha, Edythe

Edna (Hebrew) rejuvenation.
Religion: the wife of Enoch,
according to the Book of
Enoch.
Adna, Adnisha, Ednah,
Edneisha, Edneshia, Ednisha,
Ednita, Edona

Edrianna (Greek) a form of
Adrienne.
Edria, Edriana, Edrina

Edwina (English) prosperous
friend. See also Winnie.
Eddy, Edina, Edweena,
Edwena, Edwine, Edwyna,
Edwynn

Effia (Ghanaian) born on
Friday.

Effie (Greek) spoken well of.
(English) a short form of
Alfreda, Euphemia.
Effi, Effia, Effy, Ephie

Eileen (Irish) a form of Helen.
See also Aileen, Ilene.
Eilean, Eileena, Eileene, Eilena,
Eilene, Eiley, Eilie, Eilieh,
Eilina, Eiline, Eilleen, Eillen,
Eilyn, Eleen, Elene

Ekaterina (Russian) a form of
Katherine.
Ekaterine, Ekaterini

Ela (Polish) a form of
Adelaide.

Elaina (French) a form of
Helen.
Elainea, Elainia, Elainna

Elaine (French) a form of
Helen. See also Lainey, Laine.
Eilane, Elain, Elaina, Elaini,
Elan, Elana, Elane, Elania,
Elanie, Elanit, Elauna, Elayna,
Ellaine

Elana (Greek) a short form of
Eleanor. See also Ilana, Lana.
Elan, Elanee, Elaney, Elani,
Elania, Elanie, Elanna, Elanni

Elayna (French) a form of
Elaina.
Elayn, Elaynah, Elayne, Elayni

Elberta (English) a form of
Alberta.
Elbertha, Elberthina, Elberthine,
Elbertina, Elbertine

Eldora (Spanish) golden, gilded.
Eldoree, Eldorey, Eldori,
Eldoria, Eldorie, Eldory

Eleanor (Greek) light. History:
Anna Eleanor Roosevelt was a
U.S. delegate to the United
Nations, a writer, and the
thirty-second First Lady of the
United States. See also Elana,
Ella, Ellen, Leanore, Lena,
Lenore, Leonore, Leora, Nellie,
Nora, Noreen.
Elana, Elanor, Elanore, Eleanora,
Eleanore, Elena, Eleni, Elenor,
Elenorah, Elenore, Eleonor,
Eleonore, Elianore, Elinor, Elinore,
Elladine, Ellenor, Ellie, Elliner,
Ellinor, Ellinore, Elna, Elnore,
Elynor, Elynore

Eleanora (Greek) a form of
Eleanor. See also Lena.
Elenora, Eleonora, Elianora,
Ellenora, Ellenorah, Elnora,
Elynora

Electra (Greek) shining; brilliant. Mythology: the daughter of Agamemnon, leader of
the Greeks in the Trojan War.
Elektra

Elena (Greek) a form of Eleanor.
(Italian) a form of Helen.
Eleana, Eleen, Eleena, Elen, Elene,
Elenitsa, Elenka, Elenna, Elenoa,
Elenola, Elina, Ellena, Lena

Eleni (Greek) a familiar form
of Eleanor.
Elenie, Eleny

Eleora (Hebrew) the Lord is
my light.
Eliora, Elira, Elora

Elexis (Greek) a form of Alexis.
Elexas, Elexes, Elexess, Elexeya,
Elexia, Elexiah

Elexus (Greek) a form of
Alexius, Alexus.
Elexius, Elexsus, Elexxus, Elexys

Elfrida (German) peaceful. See
also Freda.
Elfrea, Elfreda, Elfredda,
Elfreeda, Elfreyda, Elfrieda,
Elfryda

Elga (Norwegian) pious.
(German) a form of Helga.
Elgiva

Elia (Hebrew) a short form of
Eliana.
Eliah

Eliana (Hebrew) my God has
answered me. See also Iliana.
Elia, Eliane, Elianna, Ellianna,
Liana, Liane

Eliane (Hebrew) a form of Eliana.
Elianne, Elliane, Ellianne

Elicia (Hebrew) a form of
Elisha. See also Alicia.
Elecia, Elica, Elicea, Elicet,
Elichia, Eliscia, Elisia, Elissia,
Ellecia, Ellicia

Elida, Elide (Latin) forms of
Alida.
Elidee, Elidia, Elidy

Elisa (Spanish, Italian, English) a short form of Elizabeth. See also Alisa, Ilisa.
Elecea, Eleesa, Elesa, Elesia, Elisia, Elisya, Ellisa, Ellisia, Ellissa, Ellissia, Ellissya, Ellisya, Elysa, Elysia, Elyssia, Elyssya, Elysya, Lisa

Elisabeth (Hebrew) a form of Elizabeth.
Elisabet, Elisabeta, Elisabethe, Elisabetta, Elisabette, Elisabith, Elisebet, Elisheba, Elisheva

Elise (French, English) a short form of Elizabeth, Elysia. See also Ilise, Liese, Lisette, Lissie.
Eilis, Eilise, Elese, Élise, Elisee, Elisie, Elisse, Elizé, Ellice, Ellise, Ellyce, Ellyse, Ellyze, Elsey, Elsie, Elsy, Elyce, Elyci, Elyse, Elyze, Lisel, Lisl, Lison

Elisha (Hebrew) consecrated to God. (Greek) a form of Alisha. See also Ilisha, Lisha.
Eleacia, Eleasha, Eleesha, Eleisha, Elesha, Eleshia, Eleticia, Elicia, Elishah, Elisheva, Elishia, Elishua, Eliska, Ellesha, Ellexia, Ellisha, Elsha, Elysha, Elyshia

Elissa, Elyssa (Greek, English) forms of Elizabeth. Short forms of Melissa. See also Alissa, Alyssa, Lissa.
Elissah, Ellissa, Ellyssa, Ilissa, Ilyssa

Elita (Latin, French) chosen. See also Lida, Lita.
Elitia, Elitia, Elitie, Ellita, Ellitia, Ellitie, Ilida, Ilita, Litia

Eliza (Hebrew) a short form of Elizabeth. See also Aliza.
Eliz, Elizaida, Elizalina, Elize, Elizea

Elizabet (Hebrew) a form of Elizabeth.
Elizabete, Elizabette

Elizabeth (Hebrew) consecrated to God. Bible: the mother of John the Baptist. See also Bess, Beth, Betsy, Betty, Elsa, Ilse, Libby, Liese, Liesel, Lisa, Lisbeth, Lisette, Lissa, Lissie, Liz, Liza, Lizabeta, Lizabeth, Lizbeth, Lizina, Lizzy, Veta, Yelisabeta, Zizi.
Alizabeth, Eliabeth, Elisa, Elisabeth, Elise, Elissa, Eliza, Elizabee, Elizabet, Elizaveta, Elizebeth, Elka, Elsabeth, Elsbeth, Elschen, Elspeth, Elysabeth, Elzbieta, Elzsébet, Helsa, Ilizzabet, Lusa

Elizaveta (Polish, English) a form of Elizabeth.
Elisavet, Elisaveta, Elisavetta, Elisveta, Elizavet, Elizavetta, Elizveta, Elsveta, Elzveta

Elka (Polish) a form of Elizabeth.
Ilka

Elke (German) a form of
Adelaide, Alice.
Elki, Ilki

Ella (English) elfin; beautiful
fairy-woman. (Greek) a short
form of Eleanor.
Ellah, Ellamae, Ellia, Ellie

Elle (Greek) a short form of
Eleanor. (French) she.
El, Ele, Ell

Ellen (English) a form of
Eleanor, Helen.
*Elen, Elenee, Eleny, Elin, Elina,
Elinda, Ellan, Ellena, Ellene,
Ellie, Ellin, Ellon, Ellyn,
Ellynn, Ellynne, Elyn*

Ellice (English) a form of Elise.
Ellecia, Ellyce, Elyce

Ellie, Elly (English) short
forms of Eleanor, Ella, Ellen.
Ele, Elie, Ellee, Elleigh, Elli

Elma (Turkish) sweet fruit.

Elmira (Arabic, Spanish) a
form of Almira.
*Elmeera, Elmera, Elmeria,
Elmyra*

Elnora (American) a combination of Ella + Nora.

Elodie (American) a form of
Melody. (English) a form of
Alodie.
Elodee, Elodia, Elody

Eloise (French) a form of
Louise.
Elois, Eloisa, Eloisia

Elora (American) a short form
of Elnora.
Ellora, Elloree, Elorie

Elsa (German) noble.
(Hebrew) a short form of
Elizabeth. See also Ilse.
*Ellsa, Ellse, Else, Elsia, Elsie,
Elsje*

Elsbeth (German) a form of
Elizabeth.
Elsbet, Elzbet, Elzbieta

Elsie (German) a familiar form
of Elsa, Helsa.
Ellsie, Ellsie, Ellsy, Elsi, Elsy

Elspeth (Scottish) a form of
Elizabeth.
Elspet, Elspie

Elva (English) elfin. See also
Alva, Alvina.
Elvia, Elvie

Elvina (English) a form of
Alvina.
*Elvenea, Elvinea, Elvinia,
Elvinna*

Elvira (Latin) white; blond.
(German) closed up. (Spanish)
elfin. Geography: the town in
Spain that hosted a Catholic
synod in 300 A.D.
Elva, Elvera, Elvire, Elwira, Vira

Elyse (Latin) a form of Elysia.
Ellysa, Ellyse, Elyce, Elys,
Elysee, Elysse

Elysia (Greek) sweet; blissful.
Mythology: Elysium was the
dwelling place of happy
souls.
Elise, Elishia, Ellicia, Elycia,
Elyssa, Ilysha, Ilysia

Elyssa (Latin) a form of Elysia.
Ellyssa

Emalee (Latin) a form of
Emily.
Emaili, Emalea, Emaleigh,
Emali, Emalia, Emalie

Emani (Arabic) a form of
Iman.
Eman, Emane, Emaneé,
Emanie, Emann

Emanuelle (Hebrew) a form
of Emmanuelle.
Emanual, Emanuel, Emanuela,
Emanuella

Ember (French) a form of
Amber.
Emberlee, Emberly

Emelia, Emelie (Latin) forms
of Emily.
Emellie

Emely (Latin) a form of Emily.
Emelly

Emerald (French) bright
green gemstone.
Emelda, Esmeralda

Emery (German) industrious
leader.
Emeri, Emerie

Emilee, Emilie (English) forms
of Emily.
Emile, Emilea, Emileigh, Émi-
lie, Emiliee, Emillee, Emillie,
Emmélie, Emmilee, Emylee

Emilia (Italian) a form of
Amelia, Emily.
Emalia, Emelia, Emila

Emily (Latin) flatterer.
(German) industrious. See
also Amelia, Emma, Millie.
Eimile, Em, Emaily, Emalee,
Emeli, Emelia, Emelie, Emelita,
Emely, Emilee, Emiley, Emili,
Emilia, Emilie, Émilie, Emilis,
Emilka, Emillie, Emilly,
Emmaline, Emmaly, Emmélie,
Emmey, Emmi, Emmie,
Emmilly, Emmily, Emmy,
Emmye, Emyle

Emilyann (American) a com-
bination of Emily + Ann.
Emileane, Emileann,
Emileanna, Emileanne,
Emiliana, Emiliann, Emilianna,
Emilianne, Emillyane,
Emillyann, Emillyanna,
Emillyanne, Emliana, Emliann,
Emlianna, Emlianne

Emma (German) a short form
of Emily. See also Amy.
Em, Ema, Emmah, Emmy

Emmalee (American) a combination of Emma + Lee. A

form of Emily.
Emalea, Emalee, Emilee,
Emmalea, Emmalei,
Emmaleigh, Emmaley, Emmali,
Emmalia, Emmalie, Emmaliese,
Emmalyse, Emylee

Emmaline (French) a form of
Emily.
Emalina, Emaline, Emelina,
Emeline, Emilienne, Emilina,
Emiline, Emmalina, Emmalene,
Emmeline, Emmiline

Emmalynn (American) a
combination of Emma +
Lynn.
Emelyn, Emelyne, Emelynne,
Emilyn, Emilynn, Emilynne,
Emlyn, Emlynn, Emlynne,
Emmalyn, Emmalynne

Emmanuelle (Hebrew) God is
with us.
Emanuelle, Emmanuela,
Emmanuella

Emmy (German) a familiar
form of Emma.
Emi, Emie, Emiy, Emmi,
Emmie, Emmye, Emy

Emmylou (American) a com-
bination of Emmy + Lou.
Emlou, Emmalou, Emmelou,
Emmilou, Emylou

Ena (Irish) a form of Helen.
Enna

Enid (Welsh) life; spirit.

Enrica (Spanish) a form of
Henrietta. See also Rica.
Enrieta, Enrietta, Enrika,
Enriqua, Enriqueta, Enriquetta,
Enriquette

Eppie (English) a familiar
form of Euphemia.
Effie, Effy, Eppy

Erica (Scandinavian) ruler of
all. (English) brave ruler. See
also Arica, Rica, Ricki.
Ericca, Ericha, Ericka, Errica

Ericka, Erika (Scandanavian)
forms of Erica.
Erickah, Erikaa, Erikah,
Erikka, Erricka, Errika, Eyka,
Erykka, Eyrika

Erin (Irish) peace. History:
another name for Ireland.
See also Arin.
Earin, Earrin, Eran, Eren,
Erena, Erene, Ereni, Eri, Erian,
Erina, Erine, Erinetta, Erinn,
Errin, Eryn

Erinn (Irish) a form of Erin.
Erinna, Erinne

Erma (Latin) a short form of
Ermine, Hermina. See also
Irma.
Ermelinda

Ermine (Latin) a form of
Hermina.
Erma, Ermin, Ermina,
Erminda, Erminia, Erminie

Erna (English) a short form of
Ernestine.

Ernestine (English) earnest, sincere.
Erna, Ernaline, Ernesia, Ernesta, Ernestina, Ernesztina

Eryn (Irish) a form of Erin.
Eiryn, Eryne, Erynn, Erynne

Eshe (Swahili) life.
Eisha, Esha

Esmé (French) a familiar form of Esmeralda. A form of Amy.
Esma, Esme, Esmëe

Esmeralda (Greek, Spanish) a form of Emerald.
Emelda, Esmé, Esmerelda, Esmerilda, Esmiralda, Ezmerelda, Ezmirilda

Esperanza (Spanish) hope. See also Speranza.
Esparanza, Espe, Esperance, Esperans, Esperansa, Esperanta, Esperanz, Esperenza

Essence (Latin) life; existence.
Essa, Essenc, Essencee, Essences, Essenes, Essense, Essynce

Essie (English) a short form of Estelle, Esther.
Essa, Essey, Essie, Essy

Estee (English) a short form of Estelle, Esther.
Esta, Estée, Esti

Estefani, Estefania, Estefany (Spanish) forms of Stephanie.
Estafania, Estafana, Estefane, Estefanie

Estelle (French) a form of Esther. See also Stella, Trella.
Essie, Estee, Estel, Estela, Estele, Esteley, Estelina, Estelita, Estell, Estella, Estellina, Estellita, Esthella

Estephanie (Spanish) a form of Stephanie.
Estephania, Estephani, Estephany

Esther (Persian) star. Bible: the Jewish captive whom Ahasuerus made his queen. See also Hester.
Essie, Estee, Ester, Esthur, Eszter, Eszti

Estrella (French) star.
Estrela, Estrelinha, Estrell, Estrelle, Estrellita

Ethana (Hebrew) strong; firm.

Ethel (English) noble.
Ethelda, Ethelin, Etheline, Ethelle, Ethelyn, Ethelynn, Ethelynne, Ethyl

Étoile (French) star.

Etta (German) little. (English) a short form of Henrietta.
Etka, Etke, Etti, Ettie, Etty, Itke, Itta

Eudora (Greek) honored gift. See also Dora.

Eugenia (Greek) born to nobility. See also Gina.
Eugenie, Eugenina, Eugina, Evgenia

Eugenie (Greek) a form of
Eugenia.
Eugenee, Eugénie

Eulalia (Greek) well spoken.
See also Ula.
*Eula, Eulalee, Eulalie, Eulalya,
Eulia*

Eun (Korean) silver.

Eunice (Greek) happy; victori-
ous. Bible: the mother of
Saint Timothy. See also
Unice.
Euna, Eunique, Eunise, Euniss

Euphemia (Greek) spoken
well of, in good repute.
History: a fourth-century
Christian martyr.
*Effam, Effie, Eppie, Eufemia,
Euphan, Euphemie, Euphie*

Eurydice (Greek) wide, broad.
Mythology: the wife of
Orpheus.
Euridice, Euridyce, Eurydyce

Eustacia (Greek) productive.
(Latin) stable; calm. See also
Stacey.
Eustasia

Eva (Greek) a short form of
Evangelina. (Hebrew) a form
of Eve. See also Ava, Chava.
*Éva, Evah, Evalea, Evalee,
Evike*

Evaline (French) a form of
Evelyn.
Evalin, Evalina, Evalyn,

*Evalynn, Eveleen, Evelene,
Evelina, Eveline*

Evangelina (Greek) bearer of
good news.
*Eva, Evangelene, Evangelia,
Evangelica, Evangeline,
Evangelique, Evangelyn,
Evangelynn*

Evania (Irish) young warrior.
*Evan, Evana, Evanka, Evann,
Evanna, Evanne, Evany,
Eveania, Evvanne, Evvunea,
Evyan*

Eve (Hebrew) life. Bible: the
first woman created by God.
(French) a short form of
Evonne. See also Chava,
Hava, Naeva, Vica, Yeva.
*Eva, Evie, Evita, Evuska,
Evyn, Ewa, Yeva*

Evelin (English) a form of
Evelyn.
Evelina, Eveline

Evelyn (English) hazelnut.
*Avalyn, Aveline, Evaleen,
Evalene, Evaline, Evalyn,
Evalynn, Evalynne, Eveleen,
Evelin, Evelyna, Evelyne,
Evelynn, Evelynne, Evline,
Ewalina*

Everett (German) courageous
as a boar.

Evette (French) a form of
Yvette. A familiar form of
Evonne. See also Ivette.
Evett

Evie (Hungarian) a form of
Eve.
Evey, Evi, Evicka, Evike, Evka,
Evuska, Evvie, Evvy, Evy, Ewa

Evita (Spanish) a form of Eve.

Evline (English) a form of
Evelyn.
Evleen, Evlene, Evlin, Evlina,
Evlyn, Evlynn, Evlynne

Evonne (French) a form of
Yvonne. See also Ivonne.
Evanne, Eve, Evenie, Evenne,
Eveny, Evette, Evin, Evon,
Evona, Evone, Evoni, Evonna,
Evonnie, Evony, Evyn, Evynn,
Eyona, Eyvone

Ezri (Hebrew) helper; strong.
Ezra, Ezria

F

Fabia (Latin) bean grower.
Fabiana, Fabienne, Fabiola,
Fabra, Fabria

Fabiana (Latin) a form of Fabia.
Fabyana

Fabienne (Latin) a form of
Fabia.
Fabian, Fabiann, Fabianne,
Fabiene, Fabreanne

Fabiola, Faviola (Latin) forms
of Fabia.
Fabiole, Fabyola, Faviana,
Faviolha

Faith (English) faithful; fidelity.
See also Faye, Fidelity.
Fayth, Faythe

Faizah (Arabic) victorious.

Falda (Icelandic) folded wings.
Faida, Fayda

Faline (Latin) catlike.
Faleen, Falena, Falene, Falin,
Falina, Fallyn, Fallyne, Faylina,
Fayline, Faylyn, Faylynn,
Faylynne, Felenia, Felina

Fallon (Irish) grandchild of the
ruler.
Falan, Falen, Fallan, Fallen,
Fallonne, Falon, Falyn, Falynn,
Falynne, Phalon

Fancy (French) betrothed.
(English) whimsical; decora-
tive.
Fanchette, Fanchon, Fanci,
Fancia, Fancie

Fannie, Fanny (American)
familiar forms of Frances.
Fan, Fanette, Fani, Fania,
Fannee, Fanney, Fanni, Fannia,
Fany, Fanya

Fantasia (Greek) imagination.
Fantasy, Fantasya, Fantaysia,
Fantazia, Fiantasi

Farah, Farrah (English) beautiful; pleasant.
Fara, Farra, Fayre

Faren, Farren (English) wanderer.
Faran, Fare, Farin, Faron,

*Farrahn, Farran, Farrand, Farrin,
Farron, Farryn, Farye, Faryn,
Feran, Ferin, Feron, Ferran,
Ferren, Ferrin, Ferron, Ferryn*

Fatima (Arabic) daughter of
the Prophet. History: the
daughter of Muhammad.
*Fatema, Fathma, Fatimah,
Fatime, Fatma, Fatmah, Fatme,
Fattim*

Fawn (French) young deer.
Faun, Fawna, Fawne

Fawna (French) a form of Fawn.
Fauna, Fawnia, Fawnna

Faye (French) fairy; elf.
(English) a form of Faith.
*Fae, Fay, Fayann, Fayanna,
Fayette, Fayina, Fey*

Fayola (Nigerian) lucky.
Fayla, Feyla

Felecia (Latin) a form of Felicia.
Flecia

Felica (Spanish) a short form
of Felicia.
*Falisa, Felisa, Felisca, Felissa,
Feliza*

Felice (Latin) a short form of
Felicia.
*Felece, Felicie, Felise, Felize,
Felyce, Felysse*

Felicia (Latin) fortunate;
happy. See also Lecia,
Phylicia.
*Falecia, Faleshia, Falicia, Fela,
Felecia, Felica, Felice, Felicidad,*

*Feliciona, Felicity, Felicya,
Felisea, Felisha, Felisia,
Felisiana, Felissya, Felita,
Felixia, Felizia, Felka, Fellcia,
Felycia, Felysia, Felyssia,
Fleasia, Fleichia, Fleishia,
Flichia*

Felicity (English) a form of
Felicia.
*Falicity, Felicita, Felicitas,
Félicité, Feliciti, Felisita, Felisity*

Felisha (Latin) a form of
Felicia.
*Faleisha, Falesha, Falisha,
Falleshia, Feleasha, Feleisha,
Felesha, Felishia, Fellishia,
Felysha, Flisha*

Femi (French) woman.
(Nigerian) love me.
Femie, Femmi, Femmie, Femy

Feodora (Greek) gift of God.
Fedora, Fedoria

Fern (English) fern. (German)
a short form of Fernanda.
*Ferne, Ferni, Fernlee, Fernleigh,
Fernley, Fernly*

Fernanda (German) daring,
adventurous. See also Andee,
Nan.
*Ferdie, Ferdinanda, Ferdinande,
Fern, Fernande, Fernandette,
Fernandina, Nanda*

Fiala (Czech) violet

Fidelia (Latin) a form of
Fidelity.
Fidela, Fidele, Fidelina

Fidelity (Latin) faithful, true.
See also Faith.
Fidelia, Fidelita

Fifi (French) a familiar form of
Josephine.
Feef, Feefee, Fifine

Filippa (Italian) a form of
Philippa.
Felipa, Filipa, Filippina, Filpina

Filomena (Italian) a form of
Philomena.
Fila, Filah, Filemon

Fiona (Irish) fair, white.
Fionna

Fionnula (Irish) white shoul-
dered. See also Nola, Nuala.
*Fenella, Fenula, Finella, Finola,
Finula*

Flair (English) style; verve.
Flaire, Flare

Flannery (Irish) redhead.
Literature: Flannery
O'Connor was a renowned
American writer.
Flan, Flann, Flanna

Flavia (Latin) blond, golden
haired.
*Flavere, Flaviar, Flavie, Flavien,
Flavienne, Flaviere, Flavio,
Flavyere, Fulvia*

Flavie (Latin) a form of Flavia.
Flavi

Fleur (French) flower.
Fleure, Fleuree, Fleurette

Flo (American) a short form
of Florence.

Flora (Latin) flower. A short
form of Florence. See also
Lore.
*Fiora, Fiore, Fiorenza, Flor,
Florann, Florella, Florelle,
Floren, Floria, Floriana,
Florianna, Florica, Florimel*

Florence (Latin) blooming;
flowery; prosperous. History:
Florence Nightingale, a
British nurse, is considered
the founder of modern nurs-
ing. See also Florida.
*Fiorenza, Flo, Flora, Florance,
Florencia, Florency, Florendra,
Florentia, Florentina,
Florentyna, Florenza, Floretta,
Florette, Florie, Florina, Florine,
Floris, Flossie*

Floria (Basque) a form of
Flora.
Flori, Florria

Florida (Spanish) a form of
Florence.
Floridia, Florinda, Florita

Florie (English) a familiar
form of Florence.
*Flore, Flori, Florri, Florrie,
Florry, Flory*

Floris (English) a form of
Florence.
Florisa, Florise

Flossie (English) a familiar
form of Florence.
Floss, Flossi, Flossy

Fola (Yoruba) honorable.

Fonda (Latin) foundation.
(Spanish) inn.
Fondea, Fonta

Fontanna (French) fountain.
*Fontaine, Fontana, Fontane,
Fontanne, Fontayne*

Fortuna (Latin) fortune; fortunate.
Fortoona, Fortune

Fran (Latin) a short form of
Frances.
Frain, Frann

Frances (Latin) free; from
France. See also Paquita.
*Fanny, Fran, Franca, France,
Francee, Francena, Francesca,
Francess, Francesta, Franceta,
Francetta, Francette, Francine,
Francis, Francisca, Françoise,
Frankie, Frannie, Franny*

Francesca (Italian) a form of
Frances.
*Franceska, Francessca, Francesta,
Franchesca, Franzetta*

Franchesca (Italian) a form of
Francesca.
*Cheka, Chekka, Chesca,
Cheska, Francheca, Francheka,
Franchelle, Franchesa,
Francheska, Franchessca,
Franchesska*

Franci (Hungarian) a familiar
form of Francine.
Francey, Francie, Francy

Francine (French) a form of
Frances.
*Franceen, Franceine, Franceline,
Francene, Francenia, Franci,
Francin, Francina, Francyne*

Francis (Latin) a form of
Frances.
Francise, Franncia, Francys

Francisca (Italian) a form of
Frances.
*Franciska, Franciszka,
Frantiska, Franziska*

Françoise (French) a form of
Frances.
Frankie (American) a familiar
form of Frances.
*Francka, Francki, Franka,
Frankey, Franki, Frankia,
Franky, Frankye*

Frannie, Franny (English)
familiar forms of Frances.
*Frani, Frania, Franney, Franni,
Frany*

Freda, Freida, Frida
(German) short forms of
Alfreda, Elfrida, Frederica,
Sigfreda.
*Frayda, Fredda, Fredella, Fredia,
Fredra, Freeda, Freeha, Freia,
Frida, Frideborg, Frieda*

Freddi, Freddie (English)
familiar forms of Frederica,
Winifred.
*Fredda, Freddy, Fredi, Fredia,
Fredy, Frici*

Frederica (German) peaceful
ruler. See also Alfreda, Rica,
Ricki.
*Farica, Federica, Freda,
Fredalena, Fredaline, Freddi,
Freddie, Frederickina, Frederika,
Frederike, Frederina, Frederine,
Frederique, Fredith, Fredora,
Fredreca, Fredrica, Fredricah,
Fredricia, Freida, Fritzi,
Fryderica*

Frederika (German) a form of
Frederica.
*Fredericka, Fredreka, Fredricka,
Fredrika, Fryderyka*

Frederike (German) a form of
Frederica.
Fredericke, Friederike

Frederique (French) a form of
Frederica.
Frédérique, Rike

Freja (Scandinavian) a form of
Freya.

Freya (Scandinavian) noble-
woman. Mythology: the
Norse goddess of love.
Fraya, Freya

Fritzi (German) a familiar
form of Frederica.
*Friezi, Fritze, Fritzie, Fritzinn,
Fritzline, Fritzy*

G

Gabriel, Gabriele (French)
forms of Gabrielle.
*Gabbriel, Gabbryel, Gabreal,
Gabreale, Gabreil, Gabrial,
Gabryel*

Gabriela, Gabriella (Italian)
forms of Gabrielle.
*Gabriala, Gabrialla, Gabrielia,
Gabriellia, Gabrila, Gabrilla,
Gabryella*

Gabrielle (French) devoted to
God.
*Gabbrielle, Gabielle, Gabrealle,
Gabriana, Gabriel, Gabriela,
Gabriele, Gabriell, Gabriella,
Gabrille, Gabrina, Gabriylle,
Gabryell, Gabryelle, Gaby,
Gavriella*

Gaby (French) a familiar form
of Gabrielle.
*Gabbey, Gabbi, Gabbie, Gabby,
Gabey, Gabi, Gabie, Gavi, Gavy*

Gada (Hebrew) lucky.
Gadah

Gaea (Greek) planet Earth.
Mythology: the Greek god-
dess of Earth.
Gaia, Gaiea, Gaya

Gaetana (Italian) from Gaeta.
Geography: a city in south-
ern Italy.
Gaetan, Gaétane, Gaetanne

Gagandeep (Sikh) sky's light.
Gagandip, Gagnadeep,
Gagndeep

Gail (Hebrew) a short form of
Abigail.(English) merry, lively.
Gael, Gaela, Gaelle, Gaila,
Gaile, Gale, Gayla, Gayle

Gala (Norwegian) singer.
Galla

Galen (Greek) healer; calm.
(Irish) little and lively.
Gaelen, Gaellen, Galyn,
Gaylaine, Gayleen, Gaylen,
Gaylene, Gaylyn

Galena (Greek) healer; calm.

Gali (Hebrew) hill; fountain;
spring.
Galice, Galie

Galina (Russian) a form of
Helen.
Gailya, Galayna, Galenka,
Galia, Galiana, Galiena,
Galinka, Galochka, Galya,
Galyna

Ganesa (Hindi) fortunate.
Religion: Ganesha was the
Hindu god of wisdom.

Ganya (Hebrew) garden of the
Lord. (Zulu) clever.
Gana, Gani, Gania, Ganice,
Ganit

Gardenia (English) Botany: a
sweet-smelling flower.
Deeni, Denia, Gardena,
Gardinia

Garland (French) wreath of
flowers.

Garnet (English) dark red gem.
Garnetta, Garnette

Garyn (English) spear carrier.
Garan, Garen, Garra, Garryn

Gasha (Russian) a familiar
form of Agatha.
Gashka

Gavriella (Hebrew) a form of
Gabrielle.
Gavila, Gavilla, Gavrid,
Gavrieela, Gavriela, Gavrielle,
Gavrila, Gavrilla

Gay (French) merry.
Gae, Gai, Gaye

Gayle (English) a form of Gail.
Gayla

Gayna (English) a familiar
form of Guinevere.
Gaynah, Gayner, Gaynor

Geela (Hebrew) joyful.
Gela, Gila

Geena (American) a form of
Gena.
Geania, Geeana, Geeanna

Gelya (Russian) angelic.

Gema, Gemma (Latin, Italian)
jewel, precious stone. See also
Jemma.
Gem, Gemmey, Gemmie,
Gemmy

Gemini (Greek) twin.
*Gemelle, Gemima, Gemina,
Geminine, Gemmina*

Gen (Japanese) spring. A short
form of names beginning
with "Gen."

Gena (French) a form of Gina.
A short form of Geneva,
Genevieve, Iphigenia.
*Geanna, Geena, Geenah, Gen,
Genae, Genah, Genai, Genea,
Geneja, Geni, Genia, Genie*

Geneen (Scottish) a form of
Jeanine.
*Geanine, Geannine, Gen,
Genene, Genine, Gineen,
Ginene*

Genell (American) a form of
Jenelle.

Genesis (Latin) origin; birth.
*Genes, Genese, Genesha,
Genesia, Genesiss, Genessa,
Genesse, Genessie, Genessis,
Genicis, Genises, Genysis,
Yenesis*

Geneva (French) juniper tree.
A short form of Genevieve.
Geography: a city in
Switzerland.
*Geena, Gen, Gena, Geneieve,
Geneiva, Geneive, Geneve,
Ginneva, Janeva, Jeaneva, Jeneva*

Genevieve (German, French)
a form of Guinevere. See also
Gwendolyn.
Gen, Gena, Genaveeve,

*Genaveve, Genavie, Genavieve,
Genavive, Geneva, Geneveve,
Genevie, Geneviéve, Genevievre,
Genevive, Genovieve, Genvieve,
Ginette, Gineveve, Ginevieve,
Ginevive, Guinevieve,
Guinivive, Gwenevieve,
Gwenivive, Jennavieve*

Genevra (French, Welsh) a
form of Guinevere.
*Gen, Genever, Genevera,
Ginevra*

Genice (American) a form of
Janice.
*Gen, Genece, Geneice, Genesa,
Genesee, Genessia, Genis,
Genise*

Genita (American) a form of
Janita.
Gen, Genet, Geneta

Genna (English) a form of
Jenna.
*Gen, Gennae, Gennay, Genni,
Gennie, Genny*

Gennifer (American) a form
of Jennifer.
Gen, Genifer, Ginnifer

Genovieve (French) a form of
Genevieve.
Genoveva, Genoveve, Genovive

Georgeanna (English) a com-
bination of Georgia + Anna.
*Georgana, Georganna,
Georgeana, Georgiana,
Georgianna, Georgyanna,
Giorgianna*

Georgeanne (English) a com-
bination of Georgia + Anne.
*Georgann, Georganne,
Georgean, Georgeann, Georgie,
Georgyann, Georgyanne*

Georgene (English) a familiar
form of Georgia.
*Georgeena, Georgeina,
Georgena, Georgenia,
Georgiena, Georgienne,
Georgina, Georgine*

Georgette (French) a form of
Georgia.
*Georgeta, Georgett, Georgetta,
Georjetta*

Georgia (Greek) farmer. Art:
Georgia O'Keeffe was an
American painter known
especially for her paintings of
flowers. Geography: a south-
ern American state; a country
in Eastern Europe. See also
Jirina, Jorja.
*Georgene, Georgette, Georgie,
Giorgia*

Georgianna (English) a form
of Georgeanna.
*Georgiana, Georgiann,
Georgianne, Georgie,
Georgieann, Georgionna*

Georgie (English) a familiar
form of Georgeanne,
Georgia, Georgianna.
Georgi, Georgy, Giorgi

Georgina (English) a form of
Georgia.
*Georgena, Georgene, Georgine,
Giorgina, Jorgina*

Geraldine (German) mighty
with a spear. See also Dena,
Jeraldine.
*Geralda, Geraldina, Geraldyna,
Geraldyne, Gerhardine, Geri,
Gerianna, Gerianne, Gerrilee,
Giralda*

Geralyn (American) a combi-
nation of Geraldine + Lynn.
*Geralisha, Geralynn, Gerilyn,
Gerrilyn*

Gerardo (English) brave
spearwoman.
Gerardine

Gerda (Norwegian) protector.
(German) a familiar form of
Gertrude.
Gerta

Geri (American) a familiar
form of Geraldine. See also
Jeri.
Gerri, Gerrie, Gerry

Germaine (French) from
Germany. See also Jermaine.
*Germain, Germana, Germanee,
Germani, Germanie, Germaya,
Germine*

Gertie (German) a familiar
form of Gertrude.
Gert, Gertey, Gerti, Gerty

Gertrude (German) beloved warrior. See also Trudy.
Gerda, Gerta, Gertie, Gertina, Gertraud, Gertrud, Gertruda

Gervaise (French) skilled with a spear.

Gessica (Italian) a form of Jessica.
Gesica, Gesika, Gess, Gesse, Gessy

Geva (Hebrew) hill.
Gevah

Ghada (Arabic) young; tender.
Gada

Ghita (Italian) pearly.
Gita

Gianna (Italian) a short form of Giovanna. See also Jianna, Johana.
Geona, Geonna, Giana, Gianella, Gianetta, Gianina, Gianinna, Gianne, Giannee, Giannella, Giannetta, Gianni, Giannie, Giannina, Gianny, Gianoula

Gigi (French) a familiar form of Gilberte.
Geegee, G. G., Giggi

Gilana (Hebrew) joyful.
Gila, Gilah

Gilberte (German) brilliant; pledge; trustworthy. See also Berti.
Gigi, Gilberta, Gilbertina, Gilbertine, Gill

Gilda (English) covered with gold.
Gilde, Gildi, Gildie, Gildy

Gill (Latin, German) a short form of Gilberte, Gillian.
Gili, Gilli, Gillie, Gilly

Gillian (Latin) a form of Jillian.
Gila, Gilana, Gilenia, Gili, Gilian, Gill, Gilliana, Gilliane, Gilliann, Gillianna, Gillianne, Gillie, Gilly, Gillyan, Gillyane, Gillyann, Gillyanne, Gyllian, Lian

Gin (Japanese) silver. A short form of names beginning with "Gin."

Gina (Italian) a short form of Angelina, Eugenia, Regina, Virginia. See also Jina.
Gena, Gin, Ginah, Ginai, Ginna

Ginette (English) a form of Genevieve.
Gin, Ginata, Ginett, Ginetta, Ginnetta, Ginnette

Ginger (Latin) flower; spice. A familiar form of Virginia.
Gin, Ginja, Ginjer, Ginny

Ginia (Latin) a familiar form of Virginia.
Gin

Ginnifer (English) white; smooth; soft. (Welsh) a form of Jennifer.
Gin, Ginifer

Ginny (English) a familiar
form of Ginger, Virginia. See
also Jin, Jinny.
*Gin, Gini, Ginney, Ginni,
Ginnie, Giny, Gionni, Gionny*

Giordana (Italian) a form of
Jordana.

Giorgianna (English) a form
of Georgeanna.
Giorgina

Giovanna (Italian) a form of
Jane.
*Geovana, Geovanna, Geovonna,
Giavanna, Giavonna, Giovana,
Giovanne, Giovanni,
Giovannica, Giovonna,
Givonnie, Jeveny*

Gisa (Hebrew) carved stone.
Gazit, Gissa

Gisela (German) a form of
Giselle.
Gisella, Gissela, Gissella

Giselle (German) pledge;
hostage. See also Jizelle.
*Ghisele, Gisel, Gisela, Gisele,
Geséle, Giseli, Gisell, Gissell,
Gisselle, Gizela, Gysell*

Gissel, Gisselle (German)
forms of Giselle.
Gissell

Gita (Yiddish) good. (Polish) a
short form of Margaret.
Gitka, Gitta, Gituska

Gitana (Spanish) gypsy; wanderer.

Gitta (Irish) a short form of
Bridget.
Getta

Giulia (Italian) a form of Julia.
*Giulana, Giuliana, Giulianna,
Giulliana, Guila, Guiliana,
Guilietta*

Gizela (Czech) a form of
Giselle.
*Gizel, Gizele, Gizella, Gizelle,
Gizi, Giziki, Gizus*

Gladis (Irish) a form of Gladys.
Gladi, Gladiz

Gladys (Latin) small sword.
(Irish) princess. (Welsh) a
form of Claudia.
*Glad, Gladis, Gladness,
Gladwys, Glady, Gwladys*

Glenda (Welsh) a form of
Glenna.
Glanda, Glennda, Glynda

Glenna (Irish) valley, glen. See
also Glynnis.
*Glenda, Glenetta, Glenina,
Glenine, Glenn, Glenne,
Glennesha, Glennia, Glennie,
Glenora, Gleny, Glyn*

Glennesha (American) a form
of Glenna.
*Glenesha, Glenisha, Glennisha,
Glennishia*

Gloria (Latin) glory. History:
Gloria Steinem, a leading
American feminist, founded
Ms. magazine.
Gloresha, Gloriah, Gloribel,

Gloria *(cont.)*
Gloriela, Gloriella, Glorielle,
Gloris, Glorisha, Glorvina, Glory

Glorianne (American) a com-
bination of Gloria + Anne.
Gloriana, Gloriane, Gloriann,
Glorianna

Glory (Latin) a form of Gloria.

Glynnis (Welsh) a form of
Glenna.
Glenice, Glenis, Glenise,
Glenyse, Glennis, Glennys,
Glenwys, Glenys, Glenyss,
Glinnis, Glinys, Glynesha,
Glynice, Glynis, Glynisha,
Glyniss, Glynitra, Glynys,
Glynyss

Golda (English) gold. History:
Golda Meir was a Russian-
born politician who served
as prime minister of Israel.
Goldarina, Golden, Goldie,
Goldina

Goldie (English) a familiar
form of Golda.
Goldi, Goldy

Goma (Swahili) joyful dance.

Grace (Latin) graceful.
Engracia, Graca, Gracia, Gracie,
Graciela, Graciella, Gracinha,
Graice, Grata, Gratia, Gray,
Grayce, Grecia

Graceanne (English) a combination of Grace + Anne.
Graceann, Graceanna, Gracen,

Graciana, Gracianna, Gracin,
Gratiana

Gracia (Spanish) a form of
Grace.
Gracea, Grecia

Gracie (English) a familiar
form of Grace.
Gracee, Gracey, Graci, Gracy,
Graecie, Graysie

Grant (English) great; giving.

Grayson (English) bailiff's
child.
Graison, Graisyn, Grasien,
Grasyn, Graysen

Grazia (Latin) a form of
Grace.
Graziella, Grazielle, Graziosa,
Grazyna

Grecia (Latin) a form of
Grace.

Greer (Scottish) vigilant.
Grear, Grier

Greta (German) a short form
of Gretchen, Margaret.
Greatal, Greatel, Greeta,
Gretal, Grete, Gretel, Gretha,
Grethal, Grethe, Grethel,
Gretta, Grette, Grieta, Gryta,
Grytta

Gretchen (German) a form of
Margaret.
Greta, Gretchin, Gretchyn

Gricelda (German) a form of
Griselda.
Gricelle

Grisel (German) a short form
of Griselda.
Grisell, Griselle, Grissel,
Grissele, Grissell, Grizel

Griselda (German) gray
woman warrior. See also
Selda, Zelda.
Gricelda, Grisel, Griseldis,
Griseldys, Griselys, Grishilda,
Grishilde, Grisselda, Grissely,
Grizelda

Guadalupe (Arabic) river of
black stones. See also Lupe.
Guadalup, Guadelupe,
Guadlupe, Guadulupe,
Gudalupe

Gudrun (Scandinavian) battler.
See also Runa.
Gudren, Gudrin, Gudrinn,
Gudruna

Guillerma (Spanish) a short
form of Guillermina.
Guilla, Guillermina

Guinevere (French, Welsh)
white wave; white phantom.
Literature: the wife of King
Arthur. See also Gayna,
Genevieve, Genevra, Jennifer,
Winifred, Wynne.
Generva, Genn, Ginette,
Guenevere, Guenna, Guinivere,
Guinna, Gwen, Gwenevere,
Gwenivere, Gwynnevere

Gunda (Norwegian) female
warrior.
Gundala, Gunta

Gurit (Hebrew) innocent baby.

Gurleen (Sikh) follower of the
guru.

Gurpreet (Punjabi) religion.
Gurprit

Gusta (Latin) a short form of
Augusta.
Gus, Gussi, Gussie, Gussy,
Gusti, Gustie, Gusty

Gwen (Welsh) a short form of
Guinevere, Gwendolyn.
Gwenesha, Gweness, Gweneta,
Gwenetta, Gwenette, Gweni,
Gwenisha, Gwenita, Gwenn,
Gwenna, Gwennie, Gwenny

Gwenda (Welsh) a familiar
form of Gwendolyn.
Gwinda, Gwynda, Gwynedd

Gwendolyn (Welsh) white
wave; white browed; new
moon. Literature:
Gwendoloena was the wife
of Merlin, the magician. See
also Genevieve, Gwyneth,
Wendy.
Guendolen, Gwen, Gwendalin,
Gwenda, Gwendalee,
Gwendaline, Gwendalyn,
Gwendalynn, Gwendela,
Gwendelyn, Gwendelynn,
Gwendilyn, Gwendolen,
Gwendolene, Gwendolin,
Gwendoline, Gwendolyne,
Gwendolynn, Gwendolynne,
Gwendylan, Gwyndolyn,
Gwynndolen

Gwyn (Welsh) a short form of
Gwyneth.
*Gwinn, Gwinne, Gwynn,
Gwynne*

Gwyneth (Welsh) a form of
Gwendolyn. See also Winnie,
Wynne.
*Gweneth, Gwenith, Gwenneth,
Gwennyth, Gwenyth, Gwyn,
Gwynneth*

Gypsy (English) wanderer.
Gipsy, Gypsie, Jipsi

H

Habiba (Arabic) beloved.
Habibah, Habibeh

Hachi (Japanese) eight; good
luck.
Hachiko, Hachiyo

Hadara (Hebrew) adorned
with beauty.
Hadarah

Hadassah (Hebrew) myrtle
tree.
*Hadas, Hadasah, Hadassa,
Haddasa, Haddasah*

Hadiya (Swahili) gift.
*Hadaya, Hadia, Hadiyah,
Hadiyyah*

Hadley (English) field of
heather.
*Hadlea, Hadlee, Hadleigh,
Hadli, Hadlie, Hadly*

Hadriane (Greek, Latin) a
form of Adrienne.
*Hadriana, Hadrianna,
Hadrianne, Hadriene,
Hadrienne*

Haeley (English) a form of
Hailey.
*Haelee, Haeleigh, Haeli, Haelie,
Haelleigh, Haelli, Haellie, Haely*

Hagar (Hebrew) forsaken;
stranger. Bible: Sarah's hand-
maiden, the mother of
Ishmael.
Haggar

Haidee (Greek) modest.
*Hady, Haide, Haidi, Haidy,
Haydee, Haydy*

Haiden (English) heather-cov-
ered hill.
*Haden, Hadyn, Haeden,
Haidn, Haidyn*

Hailee (English) a form of
Hayley.
Haile, Hailei, Haileigh, Haillee

Hailey (English) a form of
Hayley.
*Haeley, Haiely, Hailea, Hailley,
Hailly, Haily*

Haili, Hailie (English) forms
of Hayley.
Haille, Hailli, Haillie

Haldana (Norwegian) half-
Danish.

Halee (English) a form of
Haley.
*Hale, Halea, Haleah, Haleh,
Halei*

Haleigh (English) a form of
Haley.

Haley (Scandinavian) heroine.
See also Hailey, Hayley.
*Halee, Haleigh, Hali, Halley,
Hallie, Haly, Halye*

Hali, Halie (English) forms of
Haley.
Haliegh

Halia (Hawaiian) in loving
memory.

Halimah (Arabic) gentle;
patient.
Halima, Halime

Halina (Hawaiian) likeness.
(Russian) a form of Helen.
*Haleen, Haleena, Halena,
Halinka*

Halla (African) unexpected
gift.
Hala, Hallah, Halle

Halley (English) a form of
Haley.
Hally, Hallye

Hallie (Scandinavian) a form
of Haley.
Hallee, Hallei, Halleigh, Halli

Halona (Native American)
fortunate.
Halonah, Haloona, Haona

Halsey (English) Hall's island.
Halsea, Halsie

Hama (Japanese) shore.

Hana, Hanah (Japanese)
flower. (Arabic) happiness.
(Slavic) forms of Hannah.
*Hanae, Hanan, Haneen,
Hanicka, Hanin, Hanita,
Hanka*

Hanako (Japanese) flower
child.

Hania (Hebrew) resting place.
*Haniya, Hanja, Hannia,
Hanniah, Hanya*

Hanna (Hebrew) a form of
Hannah.

Hannah (Hebrew) gracious.
Bible: the mother of Samuel.
See also Anci, Anezka, Ania,
Anka, Ann, Anna, Annalie,
Anneka, Chana, Nina, Nusi.
*Hana, Hanna, Hanneke,
Hannele, Hanni, Hannon,
Honna*

Hanni (Hebrew) a familiar
form of Hannah.
Hani, Hanne, Hannie, Hanny

Happy (English) happy.
Happi

Hara (Hindi) tawny. Religion:
another name for the Hindu
god Shiva, the destroyer.

Harlee, Harleigh, Harlie
(English) forms of Harley.
Harlei, Harli

Harley (English) meadow of the hare. See also Arleigh.
Harlee, Harleey, Harly

Harleyann (English) a combination of Harley + Ann.
Harlann, Harlanna, Harlanne, Harleen, Harlene, Harleyanna, Harleyanne, Harliann, Harlianna, Harlianne, Harlina, Harline

Harmony (Latin) harmonious.
Harmene, Harmeni, Harmon, Harmonee, Harmonei, Harmoni, Harmonia, Harmonie

Harpreet (Punjabi) devoted to God.
Harprit

Harriet (French) ruler of the household. (English) a form of Henrietta. Literature: Harriet Beecher Stowe was an American writer noted for her novel *Uncle Tom's Cabin*.
Harri, Harrie, Harriett, Harrietta, Harriette, Harriot, Harriott, Hattie

Haru (Japanese) spring.

Hasana (Swahili) she arrived first. Culture: a name used for the first-born female twin. See also Huseina.
Hasanna, Hasna, Hassana, Hassna, Hassona

Hasina (Swahili) good.
Haseena, Hasena, Hassina

Hateya (Moquelumnan) footprints.

Hattie (English) familiar forms of Harriet, Henrietta.
Hatti, Hatty, Hetti, Hettie, Hetty

Hausu (Moquelumnan) like a bear yawning upon awakening.

Hava (Hebrew) a form of Chava. See also Eve.
Havah, Havvah

Haven (English) a form of Heaven.
Havan, Havana, Havanna, Havannah, Havyn

Haviva (Hebrew) beloved.
Havalee, Havelah, Havi, Hayah

Hayden (English) a form of Haiden.
Hayde, Haydin, Haydn, Haydon

Hayfa (Arabic) shapely.

Haylee, Hayleigh, Haylie (English) forms of Hayley.
Hayle, Haylea, Haylei, Hayli, Haylle, Hayllie

Hayley (English) hay meadow. See also Hailey, Haley.
Hailee, Haili, Haylee, Hayly

Hazel (English) hazelnut tree; commanding authority.
Hazal, Hazaline, Haze, Hazeline, Hazell, Hazelle, Hazen, Hazyl

Heather (English) flowering heather.
Heath, Heatherlee, Heatherly

Heaven (English) place of beauty and happiness. Bible: where God and angels are said to dwell.
Haven, Heavan, Heavenly, Heavin, Heavon, Heavyn, Hevean, Heven, Hevin

Hedda (German) battler. See also Edda, Hedy.
Heda, Hedaya, Hedia, Hedvick, Hedvig, Hedvika, Hedwig, Hedwiga, Heida, Hetta

Hedy (Greek) delightful; sweet. (German) a familiar form of Hedda.
Heddey, Heddi, Heddie, Heddy, Hede, Hedi

Heidi, Heidy (German) short forms of Adelaide.
Heida, Heide, Heidee, Heidie, Heydy, Hidee, Hidi, Hidie, Hidy, Hiede, Hiedi, Hydi

Helen (Greek) light. See also Aileen, Aili, Alena, Eileen, Elaina, Elaine, Eleanor, Ellen, Galina, Ila, Ilene, Ilona, Jelena, Leanore, Leena, Lelya, Lenci, Lene, Liolya, Nellie, Nitsa, Olena, Onella, Yalena, Yelena.
Elana, Ena, Halina, Hela, Hele, Helena, Helene, Helle, Hellen, Helli, Hellin, Hellon, Hellyn, Helon

Helena (Greek) a form of Helen. See also Ilena.
Halena, Halina, Helaina, Helana, Helania, Helayna, Heleana, Heleena, Helenia, Helenka, Helenna, Helina, Hellanna, Hellena, Hellenna, Helona, Helonna

Helene (French) a form of Helen.
Helaine, Helanie, Helayne, Heleen, Heleine, Hèléne, Helenor, Heline, Hellenor

Helga (German) pious. (Scandinavian) a form of Olga. See also Elga.

Helki (Native American) touched.
Helkey, Helkie, Helky

Helma (German) a short form of Wilhelmina.
Halma, Helme, Helmi, Helmine, Hilma

Heloise (French) a form of Louise.
Héloïse, Hlois

Helsa (Danish) a form of Elizabeth.
Helse, Helsey, Helsi, Helsie, Helsy

Heltu (Moquelumnan) like a bear reaching out.

Henna (English) a familiar form of Henrietta.
Hena, Henaa, Henah, Heni, Henia, Henny, Henya

Henrietta (English) ruler of
the household. See also
Enrica, Etta, Yetta.
*Harriet, Hattie, Hatty,
Hendrika, Heneretta, Henka,
Henna, Hennrietta, Hennriette,
Henretta, Henrica, Henrie,
Henrieta, Henriete, Henriette,
Henrika, Henrique,
Henriquetta, Henryetta, Hetta,
Hettie*

Hera (Greek) queen; jealous.
Mythology: the queen of
heaven and the wife of Zeus.

Hermia (Greek) messenger.

Hermina (Latin) noble.
(German) soldier. See also
Erma, Ermine, Irma.
*Herma, Hermenia, Hermia,
Herminna*

Hermione (Greek) earthy.
*Hermalina, Hermia, Hermina,
Hermine, Herminia*

Hermosa (Spanish) beautiful.

Hertha (English) child of the
earth.
Heartha, Hirtha

Hester (Dutch) a form of
Esther.
*Hessi, Hessie, Hessye, Hesther,
Hettie*

Hestia (Persian) star.
Mythology: the Greek god-
dess of the hearth and home.
Hestea, Hesti, Hestie, Hesty

Heta (Native American) racer.

Hetta (German) a form of
Hedda. (English) a familiar
form of Henrietta.

Hettie (German) a familiar
form of Henrietta, Hester.
Hetti, Hetty

Hilary, Hillary (Greek) cheer-
ful, merry. See also Alair.
*Hilaree, Hilari, Hilaria, Hilarie,
Hilery, Hiliary, Hillaree, Hillari,
Hillarie, Hilleary, Hilleree,
Hilleri, Hillerie, Hillery,
Hillianne, Hilliary, Hillory*

Hilda (German) a short form
of Brunhilda, Hildegarde.
*Helle, Hilde, Hildey, Hildie,
Hildur, Hildy, Hulda, Hylda*

Hildegarde (German) fortress.
*Hilda, Hildagard, Hildagarde,
Hildegard, Hildred*

Hinda (Hebrew) hind; doe.
Hindey, Hindie, Hindy, Hynda

Hisa (Japanese) long lasting.
Hisae, Hisako, Hisay

Hiti (Eskimo) hyena.
Hitty

Hoa (Vietnamese) flower;
peace.
Ho, Hoai

Hola (Hopi) seed-filled club.

Holley (English) a form of
Holly.
Holleah, Hollee

Holli, Hollie (English) forms of Holly.
Holeigh, Holleigh

Hollis (English) near the holly bushes.
Hollise, Hollyce, Holyce

Holly (English) holly tree.
Holley, Holli, Hollie, Hollye

Hollyann (English) a combination of Holly + Ann.
Holliann, Hollianna, Hollianne, Hollyanne, Hollyn

Hollyn (English) a short form of Hollyann.
Holin, Holeena, Hollina, Hollynn

Honey (English) sweet. (Latin) a familiar form of Honora.
Honalee, Hunney, Hunny

Hong (Vietnamese) pink.

Honora (Latin) honorable. See also Nora, Onora.
Honey, Honner, Honnor, Honnour, Honor, Honorah, Honorata, Honore, Honoree, Honoria, Honorina, Honorine, Honour, Honoure

Hope (English) hope.
Hopey, Hopi, Hopie

Hortense (Latin) gardener. See also Ortensia.
Hortencia, Hortensia

Hoshi (Japanese) star.
Hoshie, Hoshiko, Hoshiyo

Hua (Chinese) flower.

Huata (Moquelumnan) basket carrier.

Hunter (English) hunter.
Hunta, Huntar, Huntter

Huong (Vietnamese) flower.

Huseina (Swahili) a form of Hasana.

Hyacinth (Greek) Botany: a plant with colorful, fragrant flowers. See also Cynthia, Jacinda.
Giacinta, Hyacintha, Hyacinthe, Hyacinthia, Hyacinthie, Hycinth, Hycynth

Hydi, Hydeia (German) forms of Heidi.
Hyde, Hydea, Hydee, Hydia, Hydie, Hydiea

Hye (Korean) graceful.

I

Ian (Hebrew) God is gracious.
Iaian, Iain, Iana, Iann, Ianna, Iannel, Iyana

Ianthe (Greek) violet flower.
Iantha, Ianthia, Ianthina

Icess (Egyptian) a form of Isis.
Ices, Icesis, Icesse, Icey, Icia, Icis, Icy

Ida (German) hard working.
(English) prosperous.
Idah, Idaia, Idalia, Idalis, Idaly,
Idamae, Idania, Idarina, Idarine,
Idaya, Ide, Idelle, Idette, Idys

Idalina (English) a combina-
tion of Ida + Lina.
Idaleena, Idaleene, Idalena,
Idalene, Idaline

Idalis (English) a form of Ida.
Idalesse, Idalise, Idaliz, Idallas,
Idallis, Idelis, Idelys, Idialis

Ideashia (American) a combination of Ida + Iesha.
Idasha, Idaysha, Ideesha, Idesha

Idelle (Welsh) a form of Ida.
Idell, Idella, Idil

Iesha (American) a form of
Aisha.
Ieachia, Ieaisha, Ieasha, Ieashe,
Ieesha, Ieeshia, Ieisha, Ieishia,
Iescha, Ieshah, Ieshea, Iesheia,
Ieshia, Iiesha, Iisha

Ignacia (Latin) fiery, ardent.
Ignacie, Ignasha, Ignashia,
Ignatia, Ignatzia

Ikia (Hebrew) God is my sal-
vation. (Hawaiian) a form of
Isaiah (see Boys' Names).
Ikaisha, Ikea, Ikeea, Ikeia,
Ikeisha, Ikeishi, Ikeishia, Ikesha,
Ikeshia, Ikeya, Ikeyia, Ikiea,
Ikiia

Ila (Hungarian) a form of
Helen.

Ilana (Hebrew) tree.
Ilaina, Ilane, Ilani, Ilania,
Ilainie, Illana, Illane, Illani,
Ilania, Illanie, Ilanit

Ileana (Hebrew) a form of
Iliana.
Ilea, Ileah, Ileane, Ileanna,
Ileanne, Illeana

Ilena (Greek) a form of Helena.
Ileana, Ileena, Ileina, Ilina, Ilyna

Ilene (Irish) a form of Helen.
See also Aileen, Eileen.
Ileen, Ileene, Iline, Ilyne

Iliana (Greek) from Troy.
Ileana, Ili, Ilia, Iliani, Illiana,
Illiani, Illianna, Illyana, Illyanna

Ilima (Hawaiian) flower of
Oahu.

Ilisa (Scottish, English) a form
of Alisa, Elisa.
Ilicia, Ilissa, Iliza, Illisa, Illissa,
Illysa, Illyssa, Ilycia, Ilysa, Ilysia,
Ilyssa, Ilyza

Ilise (German) a form of Elise.
Ilese, Illytse, Ilyce, Ilyse

Ilisha (Hebrew) a form of
Alisha, Elisha. See also Lisha.
Ileshia, Ilishia, Ilysha, Ilyshia

Ilka (Hungarian) a familiar
form of Ilona.
Ilke, Milka, Milke

Ilona (Hungarian) a form of
Helen.
Ilka, Illona, Illonia, Illonya,
Ilonka, Ilyona

Ilse (German) a form of
Elizabeth. See also Elsa.
Ilsa, Ilsey, Ilsie, Ilsy

Ima (Japanese) presently.
(German) a familiar form of
Amelia.

Imala (Native American)
strong-minded.

Iman (Arabic) believer.
Aman, Imana, Imane, Imani

Imani (Arabic) a form of
Iman.
*Amani, Emani, Imahni, Imanie,
Imanii, Imonee, Imoni*

Imelda (German) warrior.
Imalda, Irmhilde, Melda

Imena (African) dream.
Imee, Imene

Imogene (Latin) image, like-
ness.
*Emogen, Emogene, Imogen,
Imogenia, Imojean, Imojeen,
Innogen, Innogene*

Ina (Irish) a form of Agnes.
Ena, Inanna, Inanne

India (Hindi) from India.
*Indea, Indeah, Indee, Indeia,
Indeya, Indi, Indiah, Indian,
Indiana, Indianna, Indie,
Indieya, Indiya, Indy, Indya*

Indigo (Latin) dark blue color.
Indiga, Indygo

Indira (Hindi) splendid.
History: Indira Nehru Gandhi
was an Indian politician and
prime minister.
Indiara, Indra, Indre, Indria

Ines, Inez (Spanish) forms of
Agnes. See also Ynez.
*Inés, Inesa, Inesita, Inésita,
Inessa*

Inga (Scandinavian) a short
form of Ingrid.
*Ingaberg, Ingaborg, Inge,
Ingeberg, Ingeborg, Ingela*

Ingrid (Scandinavian) hero's
daughter; beautiful daughter.
Inga, Inger

Inoa (Hawaiian) name.

Ioana (Romanian) a form of
Joan.
Ioani, Ioanna

Iola (Greek) dawn; violet col-
ored. (Welsh) worthy of the
Lord.
Iole, Iolee, Iolia

Iolana (Hawaiian) soaring like
a hawk.

Iolanthe (English) a form of
Yolanda. See also Jolanda.
Iolanda, Iolande

Iona (Greek) violet flower.
*Ione, Ioney, Ioni, Ionia, Iyona,
Iyonna*

Iphigenia (Greek) sacrifice.
Mythology: the daughter of
the Greek leader
Agamemnon. See also Gena.

Irene (Greek) peaceful.
Mythology: the goddess of
peace. See also Orina, Rena,
Rene, Yarina.
Irén, Irien, Irina, Jereni

Irina (Russian) a form of
Irene.
*Eirena, Erena, Ira, Irana,
Iranda, Iranna, Irena, Irenea,
Irenka, Iriana, Irin, Irinia,
Irinka, Irona, Ironka, Irusya,
Iryna, Irynka, Rina*

Iris (Greek) rainbow.
Mythology: the goddess of
the rainbow and messenger
of the gods.
*Irisa, Irisha, Irissa, Irita, Irys,
Iryssa*

Irma (Latin) a form of Erma.
Irmina, Irminia

Isabeau (French) a form of
Isabel.

Isabel (Spanish) consecrated
to God. See also Bel, Belle,
Chavella, Ysabel.
*Isabal, Isabeau, Isabeli, Isabelita,
Isabella, Isabelle, Ishbel, Isobel,
Issie, Izabel, Izabele, Izabella*

Isabella (Italian) a form of
Isabel.
Isabela, Isabelia, Isabello

Isabelle (French) a form of
Isabel.
Isabele, Isabell

Isadora (Latin) gift of Isis.
Isidora

Isela (Scottish) a form of Isla.
Isel

Isha (American) a form of
Aisha.
*Ishae, Ishana, Ishanaa, Ishanda,
Ishanee, Ishaney, Ishani,
Ishanna, Ishaun, Ishawna,
Ishaya, Ishenda, Ishia, Iysha*

Ishi (Japanese) rock.
Ishiko, Ishiyo, Shiko, Shiyo

Isis (Egyptian) supreme goddess. Mythology: the goddess
of nature and fertility.
Icess, Issis, Isys

Isla (Scottish) Geography: the
River Isla is in Scotland.
Isela

Isobel (Spanish) a form of
Isabel.
Isobell, Isobella, Isobelle

Isoka (Benin) gift from god.
Soka

Isolde (Welsh) fair lady.
Literature: a princess in the
Arthurian legends; a heroine
in the medieval romance
Tristan and Isolde. See also
Yseult.
Isolda, Isolt, Izolde

Issie (Spanish) a familiar form
of Isabel.
Isa, Issi, Issy, Iza

Ita (Irish) thirsty.

Italia (Italian) from Italy.
Itali, Italie, Italy, Italya

Girls 103

Itamar (Hebrew) palm island.
*Isamar, Isamari, Isamaria,
Ithamar, Ittamar*

Itzel (Spanish) protected.
*Itcel, Itchel, Itesel, Itsel, Itssel,
Itza, Itzallana, Itzayana, Itzell,
Ixchel*

Iva (Slavic) a short form of Ivana.
Ivah

Ivana (Slavic) God is gracious.
See also Yvanna.
*Iva, Ivanah, Ivania, Ivanka,
Ivanna, Ivannia, Ivany*

Iverem (Tiv) good fortune;
blessing.

Iverna (Latin) from Ireland.
Ivernah

Ivette (French) a form of
Yvette. See also Evette.
*Ivet, Ivete, Iveth, Ivetha, Ivett,
Ivetta*

Ivonne (French) a form of
Yvonne. See also Evonne.
*Ivon, Ivona, Ivone, Ivonna,
Iwona, Iwonka, Iwonna, Iwonne*

Ivory (Latin) made of ivory.
Ivoory, Ivori, Ivorie, Ivorine, Ivree

Ivria (Hebrew) from the land
of Abraham.
Ivriah, Ivrit

Ivy (English) ivy tree.
Ivey, Ivie

Iyabo (Yoruba) mother has
returned.

Iyana, Iyanna (Hebrew) forms
of Ian.
Iyanah, Iyannah, Iyannia

Izabella (Spanish) a form of
Isabel.
*Izabela, Izabell, Izabellah,
Izabelle, Izobella*

Izusa (Native American) white
stone.

J

Jabrea, Jabria (American)
combinations of the prefix Ja
+ Brea.
*Jabreal, Jabree, Jabreea, Jabreena,
Jabrelle, Jabreona, Jabri, Jabriah,
Jabriana, Jabrie, Jabriel, Jabrielle,
Jabrienna, Jabrina*

Jacalyn (American) a form of
Jacqueline.
*Jacalynn, Jacolyn, Jacolyne,
Jacolynn*

Jacelyn (American) a form of
Jocelyn.
*Jaceline, Jacelyne, Jacelynn,
Jacilyn, Jacilyne, Jacilynn,
Jacylyn, Jacylyne, Jacylynn*

Jacey, Jacy (Greek) familiar forms of Jacinda. (American) combinations of the initials J. + C.
Jace, Jac-E, Jacee, Jaci, Jacie, Jacylin, Jaice, Jaicee

Jaci, Jacie (Greek) forms of Jacey.
Jacci, Jacia, Jacie, Jaciel, Jaici, Jaicie

Jacinda, Jacinta (Greek) beautiful, attractive. (Spanish) forms of Hyacinth.
Jacenda, Jacenta, Jacey, Jacinthe, Jacintia, Jacynthe, Jakinda, Jaxine

Jacinthe (Spanish) a form of Jacinda.
Jacinte, Jacinth, Jacintha

Jackalyn (American) a form of Jacqueline.
Jackalene, Jackalin, Jackaline, Jackalynn, Jackalynne, Jackelin, Jackeline, Jackelyn, Jackelynn, Jackelynne, Jackilin, Jackilyn, Jackilynn, Jackilynne, Jackolin, Jackoline, Jackolyn, Jackolynn, Jackolynne

Jackeline, Jackelyn (American) forms of Jacqueline.
Jackelin, Jackelline, Jackellyn, Jockeline

Jacki, Jackie (American) familiar forms of Jacqueline.
Jackee, Jackey, Jackia, Jackielee, Jacky, Jackye

Jacklyn (American) a form of Jacqueline.
Jacklin, Jackline, Jacklyne, Jacklynn, Jacklynne

Jackquel (French) a short form of Jacqueline.
Jackqueline, Jackquetta, Jackquiline, Jackquilyn, Jackquilynn, Jackquilynne

Jaclyn (American) a short form of Jacqueline.
Jacleen, Jaclin, Jacline, Jaclyne, Jaclynn

Jacobi (Hebrew) supplanter, substitute. Bible: Jacob was the son of Isaac, brother of Esau.
Coby, Jacoba, Jacobee, Jacobette, Jacobia, Jacobina, Jacoby, Jacolbi, Jacolbia, Jacolby

Jacqualine (French) a form of Jacqueline.
Jacqualin, Jacqualine, Jacqualyn, Jacqualyne, Jacqualynn

Jacquelin (French) a form of Jacqueline.
Jacquelina

Jacqueline (French) supplanter, substitute; little Jacqui.
Jacalyn, Jackalyn, Jackeline, Jacki, Jacklyn, Jackquel, Jaclyn, Jacqueena, Jacqueine, Jacquel, Jacqueleen, Jacquelene, Jacquelin, Jacquelyn, Jacquelynn, Jacquena, Jacquene, Jacquenetta, Jacquenette, Jacqui, Jacquiline, Jacquine, Jakelin, Jaquelin, Jaqueline, Jaquelyn, Jocqueline

Jacquelyn, Jacquelynn
(French) forms of Jacqueline.
Jackquelyn, Jackquelynn,
Jacquelyne, Jacquelynne

Jacqui (French) a short form
of Jacqueline.
Jacquay, Jacqué, Jacquee,
Jacqueta, Jacquete, Jacquetta,
Jacquette, Jacquie, Jacquise,
Jacquita, Jaquay, Jaqui, Jaquie,
Jaquiese, Jaquina, Jaquita

Jacqulin, Jacqulyn (American)
forms of Jacqueline.
Jackquilin, Jacqul, Jacqulin,
Jacqulyne, Jacqulynn, Jacqulynne,
Jacquoline

Jacquiline (French) a form of
Jacqueline.
Jacquil, Jacquilin, Jacquilyn,
Jacquilyne, Jacquilynn

Jacynthe (Spanish) a form of
Jacinda.
Jacynda, Jacynta, Jacynth,
Jacyntha

Jada (Spanish) a form of Jade.
Jadah, Jadda, Jadae, Jadzia,
Jadziah, Jaeda, Jaedra, Jayda

Jade (Spanish) jade.
Jada, Jadea, Jadeann, Jadee,
Jaden, Jadera, Jadi, Jadie,
Jadienne, Jady, Jadyn, Jaedra,
Jaida, Jaide, Jaiden, Jayde, Jayden

Jadelyn (American) a combi-
nation of Jade + Lynn.
Jadalyn, Jadelaine, Jadeline,
Jadelyne, Jadelynn, Jadielyn

Jaden (Spanish) a form of
Jade.
Jadeen, Jadena, Jadene, Jadeyn,
Jadin, Jadine, Jaeden, Jaedine

Jadyn (Spanish) a form of Jade.
Jadynn, Jaedyn, Jaedynn

Jae (Latin) jaybird. (French) a
familiar form of Jacqueline.
Jaea, Jaey, Jaya

Jael (Hebrew) mountain goat;
climber. See also Yael.
Jaela, Jaelee, Jaeli, Jaelie, Jaelle,
Jahla, Jahlea

Jaelyn, Jaelynn (American)
combinations of Jae + Lynn.
Jaeleen, Jaelin, Jaelinn, Jaelyn,
Jailyn, Jalyn, Jalynn, Jayleen,
Jaylyn, Jaylynn, Jaylynne

Jaffa (Hebrew) a form of Yaffa.
Jaffice, Jaffit, Jafit, Jafra

Jaha (Swahili) dignified.
Jahaida, Jahaira, Jaharra,
Jahayra, Jahida, Jahira, Jahitza

Jai (Tai) heart. (Latin) a form
of Jaye.

Jaida, Jaide (Spanish) forms of
Jade.
Jaidah, Jaidan

Jaiden, Jaidyn (Spanish) forms
of Jade.
Jaidey, Jaidi, Jaidin, Jaidon

Jailyn (American) a form of
Jaelyn.
Jaileen, Jailen, Jailene, Jailin,
Jailine

Jaime (French) I love.
*Jaima, Jaimee, Jaimey, Jaimie,
Jaimini, Jaimme, Jaimy, Jamee*

Jaimee (French) a form of
Jaime.

Jaimie (French) a form of Jaime.
Jaimi, Jaimmie

Jaira (Spanish) Jehovah
teaches.
Jairah, Jairy

Jakeisha (American) a combination of Jakki + Aisha.
Jakeisia, Jakesha, Jakisha

Jakelin (American) a form of
Jacqueline.
*Jakeline, Jakelyn, Jakelynn,
Jakelynne*

Jakki (American) a form of
Jacki.
*Jakala, Jakea, Jakeela, Jakeida,
Jakeita, Jakela, Jakelia, Jakell,
Jakena, Jaketta, Jakevia, Jaki,
Jakia, Jakiah, Jakira, Jakita,
Jakiya, Jakiyah, Jakke, Jakkia*

Jaleesa (American) a form of
Jalisa.
*Jaleasa, Jalece, Jalecea, Jaleesah,
Jaleese, Jaleesia, Jaleisa, Jaleisha,
Jaleisya*

Jalena (American) a combina-
tion of Jane + Lena.
*Jalaina, Jalana, Jalani, Jalanie,
Jalayna, Jalean, Jaleen, Jaleena,
Jaleene, Jalen, Jalene, Jalina,
Jaline, Jallena, Jalyna, Jelayna,
Jelena, Jelina, Jelyna*

Jalesa, Jalessa (American)
forms of Jalisa.
Jalese, Jalesha, Jaleshia, Jalesia

Jalia, Jalea (American) combi-
nations of Jae + Leah.
*Jaleah, Jalee, Jaleea, Jaleeya,
Jaleia, Jalitza*

Jalila (Arabic) great.
Jalile

Jalisa, Jalissa (American)
combinations of Jae + Lisa.
*Jaleesa, Jalesa, Jalise, Jalisha,
Jalisia, Jalysa*

Jalyn, Jalynn (American) com-
binations of Jae + Lynn. See
also Jaylyn.
*Jaelin, Jaeline, Jaelyn, Jaelyne,
Jaelynn, Jaelynne, Jalin, Jaline,
Jalyne, Jalynne*

Jalysa (American) a form of
Jalisa.
Jalyse, Jalyssa, Jalyssia

Jamaica (Spanish) Geography:
an island in the Caribbean.
*Jameca, Jamecia, Jameica,
Jameika, Jameka, Jamica,
Jamika, Jamoka, Jemaica,
Jemika, Jemyka*

Jamani (American) a form of
Jami.
Jamana

Jamaria (American) combina-
tions of Jae + Maria.
*Jamar, Jamara, Jamarea, Jamaree,
Jamari, Jamarie, Jameira,
Jamerial, Jamira*

Jamecia (Spanish) a form of Jamaica.

Jamee (French) a form of Jaime.

Jameika, Jameka (Spanish) forms of Jamaica.
Jamaika, Jamaka, Jamecka, Jamekia, Jamekka

Jamesha (American) a form of Jami.
Jameisha, Jamese, Jameshia, Jameshyia, Jamesia, Jamesica, Jamesika, Jamesina, Jamessa, Jameta, Jametta, Jamiesha, Jamisha, Jammesha, Jammisha

Jamey (English) a form of Jami, Jamie.

Jami, Jamie (Hebrew, English) supplanter, substitute.
Jama, Jamani, Jamay, Jamesha, Jamey, Jamia, Jamii, Jamis, Jamise, Jammie, Jamy, Jamye, Jayme, Jaymee, Jaymie

Jamia (English) a form of Jami, Jamie.
Jamea, Jamiah, Jamiea, Jamiya, Jamiyah, Jamya, Jamyah

Jamica (Spanish) a form of Jamaica.
Jamika

Jamila (Arabic) beautiful. See also Yamila.
Jahmela, Jahmelia, Jahmil, Jahmilla, Jameela, Jameelah, Jameeliah, Jameila, Jamela, Jamelia, Jameliah, Jamell, Jamella, Jamelle, Jamely, Jamelya, Jamiela,
Jamielee, Jamilah, Jamilee, Jamilia, Jamiliah, Jamilla, Jamillah, Jamille, Jamillia, Jamilya, Jamyla, Jemeela, Jemelia, Jemila, Jemilla

Jamilynn (English) a combination of Jami + Lynn.
Jamielin, Jamieline, Jamielyn, Jamielyne, Jamielynn, Jamielynne, Jamilin, Jamiline, Jamilyn, Jamilyne, Jamilynne

Jammie (American) a form of Jami.
Jammi, Jammice, Jammise

Jamonica (American) a combination of Jami + Monica.
Jamoni

Jamylin (American) a form of Jamilynn.
Jamylin, Jamyline, Jamylyn, Jamylyne, Jamylynn, Jamylynne, Jaymylin, Jaymyline, Jaymylyn, Jaymylyne, Jaymylynn, Jaymylynne

Jan (English) a short form of Jane, Janet, Janice.
Jania, Jandy

Jana (Hebrew) gracious, merciful. (Slavic) a form of Jane. See also Yana.
Janalee, Janalisa, Janna, Janne

Janae, Janay (American) forms of Jane.
Janaé, Janaea, Janaeh, Janah, Janai, Janaya, Janaye, Janea, Janee, Janée, Jannae, Jannay, Jenae, Jenay, Jenaya, Jennae, Jennay, Jennaya, Jennaye

Janai (American) a form of
Janae.
Janaiah, Janaira, Janaiya

Janalynn (American) a combi-
nation of Jana + Lynn.
*Janalin, Janaline, Janalyn,
Janalyne, Janalynne*

Janan (Arabic) heart; soul.
*Jananee, Janani, Jananie,
Janann, Jananni*

Jane (Hebrew) God is
gracious. See also Chavon,
Jean, Joan, Juanita, Seana,
Shana, Shawna, Sheena,
Shona, Shunta, Sinead,
Zaneta, Zanna, Zhana.
*Jaine, Jan, Jana, Janae, Janay,
Janelle, Janessa, Janet, Jania,
Janice, Janie, Janika, Janine,
Janis, Janka, Jannie, Jasia, Jayna,
Jayne, Jenica*

Janel, Janell (French) forms of
Janelle.
*Janiel, Jannel, Jannell, Janyll,
Jaynel, Jaynell*

Janelle (French) a form of
Jane.
*Janel, Janela, Janele, Janelis,
Janell, Janella, Janelli, Janellie,
Janelly, Janely, Janelys, Janielle,
Janille, Jannelle, Jannellies,
Jaynelle*

Janesha (American) a form of
Janessa.
*Janeisha, Janeshia, Janiesha,
Janisha, Janishia, Jannesha,*

*Jannisha, Janysha, Jenesha,
Jenisha, Jennisha*

Janessa (American) a form of
Jane.
*Janeesa, Janesa, Janesea, Janesha,
Janesia, Janeska, Janessi,
Janessia, Janiesa, Janissa,
Jannesa, Jannessa, Jannisa,
Jannissa, Janyssa, Jenesa,
Jenessa, Jenissa, Jennisa, Jennissa*

Janet (English) a form of Jane.
See also Jessie, Yanet.
*Jan, Janeta, Janete, Janeth,
Janett, Janette, Jannet, Janot,
Jante, Janyte*

Janeth (English) a form of
Janet.
Janetha, Janith, Janneth

Janette, Jannette (French)
forms of Janet.
Janett, Janetta, Jannett, Jannetta

Janice (Hebrew) God is gra-
cious. (English) a familiar
form of Jane. See also
Genice.
*Jan, Janece, Janecia, Janeice,
Janiece, Janizzette, Jannice,
Janniece, Janyce, Jenice, Jhanice,
Jynice*

Janie (English) a familiar form
of Jane.
*Janey, Jani, Janiyh, Jannie,
Janny, Jany*

Janika (Slavic) a form of Jane.
*Janaca, Janeca, Janecka, Janeika,
Janeka, Janica, Janick, Janicka,*

Janieka, Janikka, Janikke, Janique, Janka, Jankia, Jannica, Jannick, Jannika, Janyca, Jenica, Jenicka, Jenika, Jeniqua, Jenique, Jennica, Jennika, Jonika

Janine (French) a form of Jane.
Janean, Janeann, Janeanne, Janeen, Janenan, Janene, Janina, Jannen, Jannina, Jannine, Jannyne, Janyne, Jeannine, Jeneen, Jenine

Janis (English) a form of Jane.
Janees, Janese, Janesey, Janess, Janesse, Janise, Jannis, Jannise, Janys, Jenesse, Jenis, Jennise, Jennisse

Janita (American) a form of Juanita. See also Genita.
Janitra, Janitza, Janneta, Jaynita, Jenita, Jennita

Janna (Arabic) harvest of fruit. (Hebrew) a short form of Johana.
Janaya, Janaye, Jannae, Jannah, Jannai

Jannie (English) a familiar form of Jan, Jane.
Janney, Janny

Jaquana (American) a combination of Jacqueline + Anna.
Jaqua, Jaquai, Jaquanda, Jaquania, Jaquanna

Jaquelen (American) a form of Jacqueline.
Jaquala, Jaquera, Jaqulene, Jaquonna

Jaquelin, Jaqueline (French) forms of Jacqueline.
Jaqualin, Jaqualine, Jaquelina, Jaquline, Jaquella

Jaquelyn (French) a form of Jacqueline.
Jaquelyne, Jaquelynn, Jaquelynne

Jardena (Hebrew) a form of Jordan. (French, Spanish) garden.
Jardan, Jardana, Jardane, Jarden, Jardenia, Jardin, Jardine, Jardyn, Jardyne

Jarian (American) a combination of Jane + Marian.

Jarita (Arabic) earthen water jug.
Jara, Jaretta, Jari, Jaria, Jarica, Jarida, Jarietta, Jarika, Jarina, Jaritta, Jaritza, Jarixa, Jarnita, Jarrika, Jarrine

Jas (American) a short form of Jasmine.
Jase, Jass, Jaz, Jazz, Jazze, Jazzi

Jasia (Polish) a form of Jane.
Jaisha, Jasa, Jasea, Jasha, Jashae, Jashala, Jashona, Jashonte, Jasie, Jassie, Jaysa

Jasleen, Jaslyn (Latin) forms of Jocelyn.
Jaslene, Jaslien, Jaslin, Jasline, Jaslynn, Jaslynne

Jasmain (Persian) a short form of Jasmine.
Jasmaine, Jasmane, Jassmain, Jassmaine

Jasmarie (American) a combination of Jasmine + Marie.
Jasmari

Jasmin (Persian) a form of Jasmine.
Jasimin, Jasman, Jasmeen, Jasmen, Jasmon, Jassmin, Jassminn

Jasmine (Persian) jasmine flower. See also Jessamine, Yasmin.
Jas, Jasma, Jasmain, Jasme, Jasmeet, Jasmene, Jasmin, Jasmina, Jasminne, Jasmira, Jasmit, Jasmyn, Jassma, Jassmin, Jassmine, Jassmit, Jassmon, Jassmyn, Jazmin, Jazmyn, Jazzmin

Jasmyn, Jasmyne (Persian) forms of Jasmine.
Jasmynn, Jasmynne, Jassmyn

Jaspreet (Punjabi) virtuous.
Jaspar, Jasparit, Jasparita, Jasper, Jasprit, Jasprita, Jasprite

Jatara (American) a combination of Jane + Tara.
Jataria, Jatarra, Jatori, Jatoria

Javana (Malayan) from Java.
Javanna, Javanne, Javona, Javonna, Jawana, Jawanna, Jawn

Javiera (Spanish) owner of a new house. See also Xaviera.
Javeera, Viera

Javona, Javonna (Malayan) forms of Javana.
Javon, Javonda, Javone, Javoni, Javonne, Javonni, Javonya

Jaya (Hindi) victory.
Jaea, Jaia

Jaycee (American) a combination of the initials J. + C.
Jacee, Jacey, Jaci, Jacie, Jacy, Jayce, Jaycey, Jayci, Jaycie, Jaycy

Jayda (Spanish) a form of Jada.
Jaydah, Jeyda

Jayde (Spanish) a form of Jade.
Jayd

Jaydee (American) a combination of the initials J. + D.
Jadee, Jadey, Jadi, Jadie, Jady, Jaydey, Jaydi, Jaydie, Jaydy

Jayden (Spanish) a form of Jade.
Jaydeen, Jaydene, Jaydin, Jaydn, Jaydon

Jaye (Latin) jaybird.
Jae, Jay

Jayla (American) a short form of Jaylene.
Jaylaa, Jaylah, Jayli, Jaylia, Jayliah, Jaylie

Jaylene (American) forms of Jaylyn.
Jayelene, Jayla, Jaylan, Jayleana, Jaylee, Jayleen, Jayleene, Jaylen, Jaylenne

Jaylin (American) a form of Jaylyn.
Jayline, Jaylinn

Jaylyn, Jaylynn (American) combinations of Jaye +

Lynn. See also Jalyn.
Jaylene, Jaylin, Jaylyne, Jaylynne

Jayme, Jaymie (English) forms
of Jami.
Jaymi, Jaymia, Jaymine, Jaymini

Jaymee, Jaymi (English) forms
of Jami.

Jayna (Hebrew) a form of Jane.
Jaynae, Jaynah, Jaynna

Jayne (Hindi) victorious.
(English) a form of Jane.
Jayn, Jaynie, Jaynne

Jaynie (English) a familiar
form of Jayne.
Jaynee, Jayni

Jazlyn (American) a combina-
tion of Jazmin + Lynn.
*Jasleen, Jazaline, Jazalyn,
Jazleen, Jazlene, Jazlin, Jazline,
Jazlon, Jazlynn, Jazlynne,
Jazzalyn, Jazzleen, Jazzlene,
Jazzlin, Jazzline, Jazzlyn,
Jazzlynn, Jazzlynne*

Jazmin, Jazmine (Persian)
forms of Jasmine.
*Jazmaine, Jazman, Jazmen,
Jazminn, Jazmon, Jazzmit*

Jazmyn, Jazmyne (Persian)
forms of Jasmine.
*Jazmynn, Jazmynne, Jazzmyn,
Jazzmyne*

Jazzmin, Jazzmine (Persian)
forms of Jasmine.
*Jazzman, Jazzmeen, Jazzmen,
Jazzmene, Jazzmenn, Jazzmon*

Jean, Jeanne (Scottish) God is
gracious. See also Kini.
*Jeana, Jeanann, Jeancie, Jeane,
Jeaneia, Jeanette, Jeaneva,
Jeanice, Jeanie, Jeanine,
Jeanmaria, Jeanmarie, Jeanna,
Jeanné, Jeannie, Jeannita,
Jeannot, Jeantelle*

Jeana, Jeanna (Scottish) forms
of Jean.
Jeanae, Jeannae, Jeannia

Jeanette, Jeannett (French)
forms of Jean.
*Jeanet, Jeanete, Jeanett, Jeanetta,
Jeanita, Jeannete, Jeannetta,
Jeannette, Jeannita, Jenet, Jenett,
Jenette, Jennet, Jennett, Jennetta,
Jennette, Jennita, Jinetta, Jinette*

Jeanie, Jeannie (Scottish)
familiar forms of Jean.
*Jeannee, Jeanney, Jeani, Jeanny,
Jeany*

Jeanine, Jenine (Scottish)
forms of Jean. See also
Geneen.
*Jeaneane, Jeaneen, Jeanene,
Jeanina, Jeannina, Jeannine,
Jennine*

Jelena (Russian) a form of
Helen. See also Yelena.
*Jalaine, Jalane, Jalani, Jalanna,
Jalayna, Jalayne, Jaleen, Jaleena,
Jaleene, Jalena, Jalene, Jelaina,
Jelaine, Jelana, Jelane, Jelani,
Jelanni, Jelayna, Jelayne, Jelean,
Jeleana, Jeleen, Jeleena, Jelene*

Jelisa (American) a combination of Jean + Lisa.
Jalissa, Jelesha, Jelessa, Jelise, Jelissa, Jellese, Jellice, Jelysa, Jelyssa, Jillisa, Jillissa, Julissa

Jem (Hebrew) a short form of Jemima.
Gem, Jemi, Jemia, Jemiah, Jemie, Jemm, Jemmi, Jemmy

Jemima (Hebrew) dove.
Jamim, Jamima, Jem, Jemimah, Jemma

Jemma (Hebrew) a short form of Jemima. (English) a form of Gemma.
Jemmia, Jemmiah, Jemmie, Jemmy

Jena, Jenae (Arabic) forms of Jenna.
Jenah, Jenai, Jenal, Jenay, Jenaya, Jenea

Jendaya (Zimbabwean) thankful.
Daya, Jenda, Jendayah

Jenelle (American) a combination of Jenny + Nell.
Genell, Jeanell, Jeanelle, Jenall, Jenalle, Jenel, Jenela, Jenele, Jenell, Jenella, Jenille, Jennel, Jennell, Jennella, Jennelle, Jennielle, Jennille, Jinelle, Jinnell

Jenessa (American) a form of Jenisa.
Jenesa, Jenese, Jenesia, Jenessia, Jennesa, Jennese, Jennessa, Jinessa

Jenica (Romanian) a form of Jane.
Jeneca, Jenika, Jenikka, Jennica, Jennika

Jenifer, Jeniffer (Welsh) forms of Jennifer.
Jenefer

Jenilee (American) a combination of Jennifer + Lee.
Jenalea, Jenalee, Jenaleigh, Jenaly, Jenelea, Jenelee, Jeneleigh, Jenely, Jenelly, Jenileigh, Jenily, Jennalee, Jennely, Jennielee, Jennilea, Jennilee, Jennilie

Jenisa (American) a combination of Jennifer + Nisa.
Jenessa, Jenisha, Jenissa, Jenisse, Jennisa, Jennise, Jennisha, Jennissa, Jennisse, Jennysa, Jennyssa, Jenysa, Jenyse, Jenyssa, Jenysse

Jenka (Czech) a form of Jane.

Jenna (Arabic) small bird. (Welsh) a short form of Jennifer. See also Gen.
Jena, Jennae, Jennah, Jennai, Jennat, Jennay, Jennaya, Jennaye, Jhenna

Jenni, Jennie (Welsh) familiar forms of Jennifer.
Jeni, Jenne, Jenné, Jennee, Jenney, Jennia, Jennier, Jennita, Jennora, Jensine

Jennifer (Welsh) white wave; white phantom. A form of Guinevere. See also Gennifer,

Ginnifer, Yenifer.
*Jen, Jenifer, Jeniffer, Jenipher,
Jenna, Jennafer, Jenni,
Jenniferanne, Jenniferlee, Jenniffe,
Jenniffer, Jenniffier, Jennifier,
Jennilee, Jenniphe, Jennipher,
Jenny, Jennyfer*

Jennilee (American) a combi-
nation of Jenny + Lee.
*Jennalea, Jennalee, Jennielee,
Jennilea, Jennilie, Jinnalee*

Jennilyn, Jennilynn
(American) combinations of
Jenni + Lynn.
*Jennalin, Jennaline, Jennalyn,
Jenalynann, Jenelyn, Jenilyn,
Jennalyne, Jennalynn,
Jennalynne, Jennilin, Jenniline,
Jennilyne, Jennilynne*

Jenny (Welsh) a familiar form
of Jennifer.
Jenney, Jenni, Jennie, Jeny, Jinny

Jennyfer (Welsh) a form of
Jennifer.
Jenyfer

Jeraldine (English) a form of
Geraldine.
*Jeraldeen, Jeraldene, Jeraldina,
Jeraldyne, Jeralee, Jeri*

Jereni (Russian) a form of
Irene.
Jerena, Jerenae, Jerina

Jeri, Jerri, Jerrie (American)
short forms of Jeraldine. See
also Geri.
Jera, Jerae, JeRae, Jeree, Jeriel,

*Jerilee, Jerinda, Jerra, Jerrah,
Jerrece, Jerree, Jerriann, Jerrilee,
Jerrine, Jerry, Jerrylee, Jerryne,
Jerzy*

Jerica (American) a combina-
tion of Jeri + Erica.
*Jereca, Jerecka, Jerice, Jericka,
Jerika, Jerrica, Jerrice, Jeryka*

Jerilyn (American) a combina-
tion of Jeri + Lynn.
*Jeralin, Jeraline, Jeralyn, Jeralyne,
Jeralynn, Jeralynne, Jerelin,
Jereline, Jerelyn, Jerelyne,
Jerelynn, Jerelynne, Jerilin,
Jeriline, Jerilyne, Jerilynn,
Jerilynne, Jerrilin, Jerriline,
Jerrilyn, Jerrilyne, Jerrilynn,
Jerrilynne, Jerrylea*

Jermaine (French) a form of
Germaine.
*Jermain, Jerman, Jermanay,
Jermanaye, Jermane, Jermanee,
Jermani, Jermanique, Jermany,
Jermayne, Jermecia, Jermia,
Jermice, Jermicia, Jermika,
Jermila*

Jerrica (American) a form of
Jerica.
*Jerreka, Jerricah, Jerricca,
Jerricha, Jerricka, Jerrieka, Jerrika*

Jerusha (Hebrew) inheritance.
Jerushah, Yerusha

Jesenia, Jessenia (Arabic)
flower.
Jescenia, Jessennia, Jessenya

Jesica, Jesika (Hebrew) forms of Jessica.
Jesicca, Jesikah, Jesikkah

Jessa (American) a short form of Jessalyn, Jessamine, Jessica.
Jesa, Jesha, Jessah

Jessalyn (American) a combination of Jessica + Lynn.
Jesalin, Jesaline, Jesalyn, Jesalyne, Jesalynn, Jesalynne, Jesilin, Jesiline, Jesilyn, Jesilyne, Jesilynn, Jesilynne, Jessa, Jessalin, Jessaline, Jessalyne, Jessalynn, Jessalynne, Jesselin, Jesseline, Jesselyn, Jesselyne, Jesselynn, Jesselynne, Jesslyn

Jessamine (French) a form of Jasmine.
Jessa, Jessamin, Jessamon, Jessamy, Jessamyn, Jessemin, Jessemine, Jessimin, Jessimine, Jessmin, Jessmine, Jessmon, Jessmy, Jessmyn

Jesse, Jessi (Hebrew) forms of Jessie.
Jese, Jesi, Jesie

Jesseca (Hebrew) a form of Jessica.

Jessica (Hebrew) wealthy. Literature: a name perhaps invented by Shakespeare for a character in his play *The Merchant of Venice*. See also Gessica, Yessica.
Jesica, Jesika, Jessa, Jessaca, Jessca, Jesscia, Jesseca, Jessia, Jessicah, Jessicca, Jessicia, Jessicka, Jessie,

Jessika, Jessiqua, Jessy, Jessyca, Jessyka, Jezeca, Jezica, Jezika, Jezyca

Jessie, Jessy (Hebrew) short forms of Jessica. (Scottish) forms of Janet.
Jescie, Jesey, Jess, Jesse, Jessé, Jessee, Jessey, Jessi, Jessia, Jessiya, Jessye

Jessika (Hebrew) a form of Jessica.
Jessieka

Jesslyn (American) a short form of Jessalyn.
Jessilyn, Jessilynn, Jesslin, Jesslynn, Jesslynne

Jessyca, Jessyka (Hebrew) forms of Jessica.

Jésusa (Hebrew, Spanish) God is my salvation.

Jetta (English) jet black mineral. (American) a familiar form of Jevette.
Jeta, Jetia, Jetje, Jette, Jettie

Jevette (American) a combination of Jean + Yvette.
Jetta, Jeva, Jeveta, Jevetta

Jewel (French) precious gem.
Jewelann, Jewelia, Jeweliana, Jeweliann, Jewelie, Jewell, Jewelle, Jewellee, Jewellene, Jewellie, Juel, Jule

Jezebel (Hebrew) unexalted; impure. Bible: the wife of King Ahab.
Jesibel, Jessabel, Jessebel, Jez,

*Jezabel, Jezabella, Jezabelle,
Jezebell, Jezebella, Jezebelle*

Jianna (Italian) a form of
Giana.
*Jiana, Jianina, Jianine, Jianni,
Jiannini*

Jibon (Hindi) life.

Jill (English) a short form of
Jillian.
Jil, Jilli, Jillie, Jilly

Jillaine (Latin) a form of
Jillian.
*Jilaine, Jilane, Jilayne, Jillana,
Jillane, Jillann, Jillanne, Jillayne*

Jilleen (Irish) a form of Jillian.
*Jileen, Jilene, Jiline, Jillene,
Jillenne, Jilline, Jillyn*

Jillian (Latin) youthful. See
also Gillian.
*Jilian, Jiliana, Jiliann, Jilianna,
Jilianne, Jilienna, Jilienne, Jill,
Jillaine, Jilliana, Jilliane, Jilliann,
Jillianne, Jileen, Jillien, Jillienne,
Jillion, Jilliyn*

Jimi (Hebrew) supplanter, sub-
stitute.
*Jimae, Jimaria, Jimee, Jimella,
Jimena, Jimia, Jimiah, Jimie,
Jimiyah, Jimmeka, Jimmet,
Jimmi, Jimmia, Jimmie*

Jimisha (American) a combi-
nation of Jimi + Aisha.
*Jimica, Jimicia, Jimmicia,
Jimysha*

Jin (Japanese) tender.
(American) a short form of
Ginny, Jinny.

Jina (Swahili) baby with a
name. (Italian) a form of
Gina.
*Jena, Jinae, Jinan, Jinda, Jinna,
Jinnae*

Jinny (Scottish) a familiar form
of Jenny. (American) a familiar form of Virginia. See also
Ginny.
Jin, Jinnee, Jinney, Jinni, Jinnie

Jirina (Czech) a form of
Georgia.
Jirah, Jireh

Jizelle (American) a form of
Giselle.
*Jessel, Jezel, Jezell, Jezella,
Jezelle, Jisel, Jisela, Jisell, Jisella,
Jiselle, Jissel, Jissell, Jissella,
Jisselle, Jizel, Jizella, Joselle*

Jo (American) a short form of
Joanna, Jolene, Josephine.
Joangie, Joetta, Joette, Joey

Joan (Hebrew) God is
gracious. History: Joan of Arc
was a fifteenth-century hero-
ine and resistance fighter. See
also Ioana, Jean, Juanita,
Siobahn.
*Joane, Joaneil, Joanel, Joanelle,
Joanie, Joanmarie, Joann,
Joannanette, Joanne, Joannel,
Joanny, Jonni*

Joana, Joanna (English) a
form of Joan. See also
Yoanna.
*Janka, Jhoana, Jo, Jo-Ana,
Joandra, Joanka, Joananna, Jo-
Anie, Joanka, Jo-Anna,
Joannah, Jo-Annie, Joeana,
Joeanna, Johana, Johanna,
Johannah*

Joanie, Joannie (Hebrew)
familiar forms of Joan.
*Joanee, Joani, Joanni, Joenie,
Johanie, Johnnie, Joni*

Joanne (English) a form of
Joan.
*Joanann, Joananne, Joann, Jo-
Ann, Jo-Anne, Joayn, Joeann,
Joeanne*

Joanny (Hebrew) a familiar
form of Joan.
Joany

Joaquina (Hebrew) God will
establish.
Joaquine

Jobeth (English) a combination of Jo + Beth.
Joby

Joby (Hebrew) afflicted.
(English) a familiar form of
Jobeth.
*Jobey, Jobi, Jobie, Jobina, Jobita,
Jobrina, Jobye, Jobyna*

Jocacia (American) a combination of Joy + Acacia.

Jocelin, Joceline (Latin) forms
of Jocelyn.
Jocelina, Jocelinn

Jocelyn (Latin) joyous. See also
Yocelin, Yoselin.
*Jacelyn, Jasleen, Jocelin, Jocelle,
Jocelyne, Jocelynn, Joci, Jocia,
Jocilyn, Jocilynn, Jocinta, Joclyn,
Joclynn, Josalyn, Joscelin, Joselin,
Joselyn, Joshlyn, Josilin, Jossalin,
Josselyn, Joycelyn*

Jocelyne (Latin) a form of
Jocelyn.
Joceline, Jocelynne, Joclynne

Jodi, Jodie, Jody (American)
familiar forms of Judith.
*Jodee, Jodele, Jodell, Jodelle,
Jodevea, Jodey, Jodia, Jodiee,
Jodilee, Jodi-Lee, Jodilynn, Jodi-
Lynn, Joedi, Joedy*

Jodiann (American) a combi-
nation of Jodi + Ann.
*Jodene, Jodi-Ann, Jodianna,
Jodi-Anna, Jodianne, Jodi-Anne,
Jodine, Jodyann, Jody-Ann,
Jodyanna, Jody-Anna, Jodyanne,
Jody-Anne, Jodyne*

Joelle (Hebrew) God is will-
ing.
*Joela, Joele, Joelee, Joeli, Joelia,
Joelie, Joell, Joella, Joëlle, Joelli,
Joelly, Joely, Joyelle*

Joelynn (American) a combi-
nation of Joelle + Lynn.
*Joeleen, Joelene, Joeline, Joellen,
Joellyn, Joelyn, Joelyne*

Johana, Johanna, Johannah
(German) forms of Joana.
Janna, Joahna, Johanah,
Johanka, Johanne, Johnna,
Johonna, Jonna, Joyhanna,
Joyhannah

Johanie, Johannie (Hebrew)
forms of Joanie.
Johani, Johanni, Johanny, Johany

Johnna, Jonna (American)
forms of Johana, Joanna.
Jahna, Jahnaya, Jhona, Jhonna,
Johna, Johnda, Johnnielynn,
Johnnie-Lynn, Johnnquia,
Joncie, Jonda, Jondrea, Jontel,
Jutta

Johnnie (Hebrew) a form of
Joanie.
Johni, Johnie, Johnni, Johnny

Johnnessa (American) a com-
bination of Johnna + Nessa.
Jahnessa, Johneatha, Johnecia,
Johnesha, Johnetra, Johnisha,
Johnishi, Johnnise, Jonyssa

Joi (Latin) a form of Joy.
Joia, Joie

Jokla (Swahili) beautiful robe.

Jolanda (Greek) a form of
Yolanda. See also Iolanthe.
Jola, Jolan, Jolán, Jolande,
Jolander, Jolanka, Jolánta,
Jolantha, Jolanthe

Joleen, Joline (English) forms
of Jolene.
Joleena, Joleene, Jolleen, Jollene

Jolene (Hebrew) God will
add, God will increase.
(English) a form of
Josephine.
Jo, Jolaine, Jolana, Jolane,
Jolanna, Jolanne, Jolanta,
Jolayne, Jole, Jolean, Joleane,
Joleen, Jolena, Joléne, Jolenna,
Jolin, Jolina, Jolinda, Joline,
Jolinn, Jolinna, Jolleane, Jolleen,
Jolline

Jolie (French) pretty.
Jole, Jolea, Jolee, Joleigh, Joley,
Joli, Jolibeth, Jollee, Jollie, Jolly,
Joly, Jolye

Jolisa (American) a combina-
tion of Jo + Lisa.
Joleesa, Joleisha, Joleishia,
Jolieasa, Jolise, Jolisha, Jolisia,
Jolissa, Jolysa, Jolyssa, Julissa

Jolynn (American) a combination of Jo + Lynn.
Jolyn, Jolyne, Jolynne

Jonatha (Hebrew) gift of God.
Johnasha, Johnasia, Jonesha,
Jonisha

Jonelle (American) a combi-
nation of Joan + Elle.
Jahnel, Jahnell, Jahnelle, Johnel,
Johnell, Johnella, Johnelle, Jonel,
Jonell, Jonella, Jonyelle, Jynell,
Jynelle

Jonesha, Jonisha (American)
forms of Jonatha.
Joneisha, Jonesa, Joneshia,
Jonessa, Jonisa, Jonishia,
Jonneisha, Jonnesha, Jonnessia

Joni (American) a familiar
form of Joan.
*Jona, Jonae, Jonai, Jonann,
Jonati, Joncey, Jonci, Joncie,
Jonice, Jonie, Jonilee, Joni-lee,
Jonis, Jony*

Jonika (American) a form of
Janika.
*Johnica, Johnique, Johnquia,
Johnnica, Johnnika, Joneeka,
Joneika, Jonica, Joniqua, Jonique*

Jonina (Hebrew) dove. See
also Yonina.
Jona, Jonita, Jonnina

Jonita (Hebrew) a form of
Jonina. See also Yonita.
*Johnetta, Johnette, Johnita,
Johnittia, Jonati, Jonetia, Jonetta,
Jonette, Jonit, Jonnita, Jonta,
Jontae, Jontaé, Jontaya*

Jonni, Jonnie (American)
familiar forms of Joan.
Jonny

Jonquil (Latin, English) Botany:
an ornamental plant with fragrant yellow flowers.
*Jonquelle, Jonquie, Jonquill,
Jonquille*

Jontel (American) a form of
Johna.
*Jontaya, Jontell, Jontelle, Jontia,
Jontila, Jontrice*

Jora (Hebrew) autumn rain.
Jorah

Jordan (Hebrew) descending.
See also Jardena.
*Jordain, Jordaine, Jordana,
Jordane, Jordann, Jordanna,
Jordanne, Jordany, Jordea, Jordee,
Jorden, Jordi, Jordian, Jordie,
Jordin, Jordon, Jordyn, Jori, Jorie,
Jourdan*

Jordana, Jordanna (Hebrew)
forms of Jordan. See also
Giordana, Yordana.
*Jordannah, Jordina, Jordonna,
Jourdana, Jourdanna*

Jorden, Jordin, Jordon
(Hebrew) forms of Jordan.
Jordenne, Jordine

Jordyn (Hebrew) a form of
Jordan.
Jordyne, Jordynn, Jordynne

Jori, Jorie (Hebrew) familiar
forms of Jordan.
*Jorai, Jorea, Joree, Jorée, Jorey,
Jorian, Jorin, Jorina, Jorine,
Jorita, Jorre, Jorrey, Jorri, Jorrian,
Jorrie, Jorry, Jory*

Joriann (American) a combi-
nation of Jori + Ann.
*Jori-Ann, Jorianna, Jori-Anna,
Jorianne, Jori-Anne, Jorriann,
Jorrianna, Jorrianne, Jorryann,
Jorryanna, Jorryanne, Joryann,
Joryanna, Joryanne*

Jorja (American) a form of
Georgia.
*Jeorgi, Jeorgia, Jorgana, Jorgi,
Jorgia, Jorgina, Jorjana, Jorji*

Josalyn (Latin) a form of
Jocelyn.
Josalene, Josalin, Josalind,
Josaline, Josalynn, Joshalyne

Joscelin, Joscelyn (Latin)
forms of Jocelyn.
Josceline, Joscelyne, Joscelynn,
Joscelynne, Joselin, Joseline,
Joselyn, Joselyne, Joselynn,
Joselynne, Joshlyn

Josee, Josée (American)
familiar forms of Josephine.
Joesee, Josey, Josi, Josina, Josy,
Jozee

Josefina (Spanish) a form of
Josephine.
Josefa, Josefena, Joseffa, Josefine

Joselin, Joseline (Latin) forms
of Jocelyn.
Joselina, Joselinne, Josielina

Joselle (American) a form of
Jizelle.
Joesell, Jozelle

Joselyn, Joslyn (Latin) forms
of Jocelyn.
Joselene, Joselyne, Joselynn,
Joshely, Josiline, Josilyn

Josephine (French) God will
add, God will increase. See also
Fifi, Pepita, Yosepha.
Fina, Jo, Joey, Josee, Josée, Josefina,
Josepha, Josephe, Josephene,
Josephin, Josephina, Josephyna,
Josephyne, Josette, Josey, Josie,
Jozephine, Jozie, Sefa

Josette (French) a familiar
form of Josephine.
Joesette, Josetta, Joshetta, Jozette

Josey, Josie (Hebrew) familiar
forms of Josephine.
Josi, Josse, Jossee, Jossie, Josy, Josye

Joshann (American) a combination of Joshlyn + Ann.
Joshana, Joshanna, Joshanne

Joshlyn (Latin) a form of
Jocelyn. (Hebrew) God is my
salvation.
Joshalin, Joshalyn, Joshalynn,
Joshalynne, Joshelle, Joshleen,
Joshlene, Joshlin, Joshline,
Joshlyne, Joshlynn, Joshlynne

Josiane, Josianne (American)
combinations of Josie + Anne.
Josian, Josie-Ann, Josieann

Josilin, Joslin (Latin) forms of
Jocelyn.
Josielina, Josiline, Josilyn,
Josilyne, Josilynn, Josilynne,
Joslin, Josline, Joslyn, Joslyne,
Joslynn, Joslynne

Jossalin (Latin) a form of
Jocelyn.
Jossaline, Jossalyn, Jossalynn,
Jossalynne, Josselyn, Josslin, Jossline

Josselyn (Latin) a form of
Jocelyn.
Josselen, Josselin, Josseline,
Jossellen, Jossellin, Jossellyn,
Josselyne, Josselynn, Josselynne,
Josslyn, Josslyne, Josslynn,
Josslynne

Jourdan (Hebrew) a form of Jordan.
Jourdain, Jourdann, Jourdanne, Jourden, Jourdian, Jourdon, Jourdyn

Jovana (Latin) a form of Jovanna.
Jeovana, Jouvan, Jovan, Jovanah, Jovena, Jovian, Jowan, Jowana

Jovanna (Latin) majestic. (Italian) a form of Giovanna. Mythology: Jove, also known as Jupiter, was the supreme Roman god.
Jeovanna, Jovado, Joval, Jovana, Jovann, Jovannie, Jovena, Jovina, Jovon, Jovonda, Jovonia, Jovonna, Jovonnah, Jovonne, Jowanna

Jovannie (Italian) a familiar form of Jovanna.
Jovanee, Jovani, Jovanie, Jovanne, Jovanni, Jovanny, Jovonnie

Jovita (Latin) jovial.
Joveda, Joveta, Jovetta, Jovida, Jovitta

Joy (Latin) joyous.
Joe, Joi, Joya, Joye, Joyeeta, Joyella, Joyia, Joyous, Joyvina

Joyanne (American) a combination of Joy + Anne.
Joyan, Joyann, Joyanna,

Joyce (Latin) joyous. A short form of Joycelyn.
Joice, Joycey, Joycie, Joyous, Joysel

Joycelyn (American) a form of Jocelyn.
Joycelin, Joyceline, Joycelyne, Joycelynn, Joycelynne

Joylyn (American) a combination of Joy + Lynn.
Joyleen, Joylene, Joylin, Joyline, Joylyne, Joylynn, Joy-Lynn, Joylynne

Jozie (Hebrew) a familiar form of Josephine.
Jozee, Jozée, Jozi, Jozy

Juana (Spanish) a short form of Juanita.
Juanell, Juaney, Juanika, Juanit, Juanna, Juannia

Juandalyn (Spanish) a form of Juanita.
Jualinn, Juandalin, Juandaline, Juandalyne, Juandalynn, Juandalynne

Juanita (Spanish) a form of Jane, Joan. See also Kwanita, Nita, Waneta, Wanika.
Juana, Juandalyn, Juaneice, Juanequa, Juanesha, Juanice, Juanicia, Juaniqua, Juanisha, Juanishia

Juci (Hungarian) a form of Judy.
Jucika

Judith (Hebrew) praised. Mythology: the slayer of Holofernes, according to ancient Jewish legend. See also Yehudit, Yudita.
Giuditta, Ioudith, Jodi, Jodie, Jody,

Jude, Judine, Judit, Judita, Judite,
Juditha, Judithe, Judy, Judyta,
Jutka

Judy (Hebrew) a familiar form
of Judith.
Juci, Judi, Judie, Judye

Judyann (American) a combi-
nation of Judy + Ann.
*Judana, Judiann, Judianna,
Judianne, Judyanna, Judyanne*

Jula (Polish) a form of Julia.
Julca, Julcia, Juliska, Julka

Julene (Basque) a form of
Julia. See also Yulene.
*Julena, Julina, Juline, Julinka,
Juliska, Julleen, Jullena, Jullene,
Julyne*

Julia (Latin) youthful. See also
Giulia, Jill, Jillian, Sulia, Yulia.
*Iulia, Jula, Julea, Juleah, Julene,
Juliah, Juliana, Juliann, Julica,
Julie, Juliea, Juliet, Julija, Julina,
Juline, Julisa, Julissa, Julita,
Juliya, Julka, Julyssa*

Juliana, Julianna (Czech,
Spanish, Hungarian) forms of
Julia.
*Julieana, Julieanna, Juliena,
Julliana, Jullianna, Julyana,
Julyanna, Yuliana*

Juliann, Julianne (English)
forms of Julia.
*Julean, Juleann, Julian, Juliane,
Julieann, Julie-Ann, Julieanne,
Julie-Anne, Julien, Juliene,
Julienn, Julienne, Jullian*

Julie (English) a form of Julia.
*Juel, Jule, Julee, Juli, Julie-Lynn,
Julie-Mae, Julle, Jullee, Jullie,
Jully, July*

Juliet, Juliette (French) forms
of Julia.
*Julet, Julieta, Juliett, Julietta,
Jullet, Julliet, Jullietta*

Julisa, Julissa (Latin) forms of
Julia.
Julis, Julisha, Julysa, Julyssa

Julita (Spanish) a form of Julia.
Julitta, Julyta

Jumaris (American) a combination of Julie + Maris.

Jun (Chinese) truthful.

June (Latin) born in the sixth
month.
*Juna, Junea, Junel, Junell,
Junella, Junelle, Junette, Juney,
Junia, Junie, Juniet, Junieta,
Junietta, Juniette, Junina, Junita*

Juno (Latin) queen. Mythology:
the supreme Roman goddess.

Justice (Latin) just, righteous.
*Justis, Justise, Justiss, Justisse,
Justus, Justyce, Justys*

Justina (Italian) a form of
Justine.
Jestena, Jestina, Justinna, Justyna

Justine (Latin) just, righteous.
*Giustina, Jestine, Juste, Justi,
Justice, Justie, Justina, Justinn,
Justy, Justyn, Justyne, Justynn,
Justynne*

K

Kacey, Kacy (Irish) brave.
(American) forms of Casey.
Combinations of the initials
K. + C.
*K. C., Kace, Kacee, Kaci, Kacie,
Kaicee, Kaicey, Kasey, Kasie,
Kaycee, Kayci, Kaycie*

Kachina (Native American)
sacred dancer.
Kachine

Kaci, Kacie (American) forms
of Kacey, Kacy.
Kasci, Kaycie, Kaysie

Kacia (Greek) a short form of
Acacia.
Kaycia, Kaysia

Kadedra (American) a combi-
nation of Kady + Dedra.
*Kadeadra, Kadedrah, Kadedria,
Kadeedra, Kadeidra, Kadeidre,
Kadeidria*

Kadejah (Arabic) a form of
Kadijah.
*Kadeija, Kadeijah, Kadejá,
Kadejia*

Kadelyn (American) a combination of Kady + Lynn.

Kadesha (American) a combi-
nation of Kady + Aisha.
*Kadeesha, Kadeeshia, Kadeesia,
Kadeesiah, Kadeezia, Kadesa,
Kadesheia, Kadeshia, Kadesia,
Kadessa, Kadezia*

Kadie (English) a form of
Kady.
Kadi, Kadia, Kadiah

Kadijah (Arabic) trustworthy.
*Kadajah, Kadeeja, Kadeejah,
Kadija*

Kadisha (American) a form of
Kadesha.
*Kadiesha, Kadieshia, Kadishia,
Kadisia, Kadysha, Kadyshia*

Kady (English) a form of Katy.
A combination of the initials
K. + D. See also Cady.
*K. D., Kade, Kadee, Kadey,
Kadie, Kadya, Kadyn, Kaidi,
Kaidy, Kayde, Kaydee, Kaydey,
Kaydi, Kaydie, Kaydy*

Kaedé (Japanese) maple leaf.

Kaela (Hebrew, Arabic)
beloved, sweetheart. A short
form of Kalila, Kelila.
*Kaelah, Kaelea, Kaeleah,
Kaelee, Kaeli, Kayla*

Kaelee, Kaeli (American)
forms of Kaela.
*Kaelei, Kaeleigh, Kaeley,
Kaelia, Kaelie, Kaelii, Kaelly,
Kaely, Kaelye*

Kaelin (American) a form of
Kaelyn.
*Kaeleen, Kaelene, Kaelina,
Kaelinn, Kalan*

Kaelyn (American) a combination of Kae + Lynn. See also Caelin, Kaylyn.
Kaelan, Kaelen, Kaelin, Kaelynn, Kaelynne

Kaetlyn (Irish) a form of Kaitlin.
Kaetlin, Kaetlynn

Kagami (Japanese) mirror.

Kahsha (Native American) fur robe.
Kasha, Kashae, Kashia

Kai (Hawaiian) sea. (Hopi, Navaho) willow tree.
Kae, Kaie

Kaia (Greek) earth. Mythology: Gaea was the earth goddess.
Kaiah, Kaija

Kaila (Hebrew) laurel; crown.
Kailah, Kailea, Kaileah, Kailee, Kailey, Kayla

Kailee, Kailey (American) familiar forms of Kaila. Forms of Kaylee.
Kaile, Kaileh, Kaileigh, Kaili, Kailia, Kailie, Kailli, Kaillie, Kaily, Kailya

Kailyn, Kailynn (American) forms of Kaitlin.
Kailan, Kaileen, Kaileena, Kailen, Kailena, Kailene, Kaileyne, Kailin, Kailina, Kailon, Kailynne

Kairos (Greek) last, final, complete. Mythology: the last goddess born to Jupiter.
Kaira, Kairra

Kaishawn (American) a combination of Kai + Shawna.
Kaeshun, Kaisha, Kaishala, Kaishon

Kaitlin (Irish) pure. See also Katelin.
Kaetlyn, Kailyn, Kailynn, Kaitlan, Kaitland, Kaitleen, Kaitlen, Kaitlind, Kaitlinn, Kaitlinne, Kaitlon, Kaytlin

Kaitlyn, Kaitlynn (Irish) forms of Caitlyn.
Kaitelynne, Kaitlynne

Kaiya (Japanese) forgiveness.
Kaiyah, Kaiyia

Kala (Arabic) a short form of Kalila. A form of Cala.
Kalah, Kalla, Kallah

Kalama (Hawaiian) torch.

Kalani (Hawaiian) chieftain; sky.
Kailani, Kalanie, Kaloni

Kalare (Latin, Basque) bright; clear.

Kalea (Hawaiian) bright; clear.
Kahlea, Kahleah, Kailea, Kaileah, Kaleah, Kaleeia, Kaleia, Kalia, Kallea, Kalleah, Kaylea, Kayleah, Khalea, Khaleah

Kalee, Kaleigh, Kaley, Kalie
(American) forms of Caley,
Kaylee.
*Kalei, Kalleigh, Kalley, Kally,
Kaly*

Kalei (Hawaiian) flower
wreath.
*Kahlei, Kailei, Kallei, Kaylei,
Khalei*

Kalena (Hawaiian) pure. See
also Kalina.
*Kaleen, Kaleena, Kalene,
Kalenea, Kalenna*

Kalere (Swahili) short woman.
Kaleer

Kali (Hindi) the black one.
(Hawaiian) hesitating.
Religion: a form of the
Hindu goddess Devi. See
also Cali.
*Kalee, Kaleigh, Kaley, Kalie,
Kallee, Kalley, Kalli, Kallie,
Kally, Kallye, Kaly*

Kalia (Hawaiian) a form of
Kalea.
Kaliah, Kaliea, Kalieya

Kalifa (Somali) chaste; holy.

Kalila (Arabic) beloved, sweet-
heart. See also Kaela.
*Kahlila, Kala, Kaleela, Kalilla,
Kaylil, Kaylila, Kelila, Khalila,
Khalilah, Khalillah, Kylila,
Kylilah, Kylillah*

Kalina (Slavic) flower.
(Hawaiian) a form of Karen.
See also Kalena.
*Kalin, Kalinna, Kalyna,
Kalynah, Kalynna*

Kalinda (Hindi) sun.
*Kaleenda, Kalindi, Kalynda,
Kalyndi*

Kalisa (American) a combination of Kate + Lisa.
Kalise, Kalissa, Kalysa, Kalyssa

Kalisha (American) a combination of Kate + Aisha.
Kaleesha, Kaleisha, Kalishia

Kaliska (Moquelumnan) coyote chasing deer.

Kallan (Slavic) stream, river.
*Kalahn, Kalan, Kalen, Kallen,
Kallon, Kalon*

Kalle (Finnish) a form of
Carol.
Kaille, Kaylle

Kalli, Kallie (Greek) forms of
Callie. Familiar forms of
Kalliope, Kallista, Kalliyan.
*Kalle, Kallee, Kalley, Kallita,
Kally*

Kalliope (Greek) a form of
Calliope.
Kalli, Kallie, Kallyope

Kallista (Greek) a form of
Callista.
*Kalesta, Kalista, Kallesta, Kalli,
Kallie, Kallysta, Kaysta*

Kalliyan (Cambodian) best.
Kalli, Kallie

Kaltha (English) marigold,
yellow flower.

Kaluwa (Swahili) forgotten
one.
Kalua

Kalyca (Greek) rosebud.
Kalica, Kalika, Kaly

Kalyn, Kalynn (American)
forms of Kaylyn.
*Kalin, Kallen, Kallin, Kallon,
Kallyn, Kalyne, Kalynne*

Kama (Sanskrit) loved one.
Religion: the Hindu god of
love.

Kamala (Hindi) lotus.
Kamalah, Kammala

Kamali (Mahona) spirit guide;
protector.
Kamalie

Kamaria (Swahili) moonlight.
*Kamar, Kamara, Kamarae,
Kamaree, Kamari, Kamariah,
Kamarie, Kamariya,
Kamariyah, Kamarya*

Kamata (Moquelumnan)
gambler.

Kambria (Latin) a form of
Cambria.
*Kambra, Kambrie, Kambriea,
Kambry*

Kamea (Hawaiian) one and
only; precious.
Kameah, Kameo, Kamiya

Kameke (Swahili) blind.

Kameko (Japanese) turtle
child. Mythology: the turtle
symbolizes longevity.

Kameron (American) a form
of Cameron.
Kameran, Kamri

Kami (Japanese) divine aura.
(Italian, North African) a
short form of Kamila,
Kamilah. See also Cami.
*Kamie, Kammi, Kammie,
Kammy, Kammye, Kamy*

Kamila (Slavic) a form of
Camila. See also Millie.
*Kameela, Kamela, Kamelia,
Kamella, Kami, Kamilah,
Kamilia, Kamilka, Kamilla,
Kamille, Kamma, Kammilla,
Kamyla*

Kamilah (North African)
perfect.
*Kameela, Kameelah, Kami,
Kamillah, Kammilah*

Kamiya (Hawaiian) a form of
Kamea.
Kamia, Kamiah, Kamiyah

Kamri (American) a short
form of Kameron. See also
Camri.
*Kamree, Kamrey, Kamrie,
Kamry, Kamrye*

Kamryn (American) a short form of Kameron. See also Camryn.
Kameryn, Kamren, Kamrin, Kamron, Kamrynn

Kanani (Hawaiian) beautiful.
Kana, Kanae, Kanan

Kanda (Native American) magical power.

Kandace, Kandice (Greek) glittering white; glowing. (American) forms of Candace, Candice.
Kandas, Kandess, Kandi, Kandis, Kandise, Kandiss, Kandus, Kandyce, Kandys, Kandyse

Kandi (American) a familiar form of Kandace, Kandice. See also Candi.
Kandhi, Kandia, Kandie, Kandy, Kendi, Kendie, Kendy, Kenndi, Kenndie, Kenndy

Kandra (American) a form of Kendra. See also Candra.
Kandrea, Kandree, Kandria

Kane (Japanese) two right hands.

Kaneisha, Kanisha (American) forms of Keneisha.
Kaneasha, Kanecia, Kaneesha, Kanesah, Kanesha, Kaneshea, Kaneshia, Kanessa, Kaneysha, Kaniece, Kanishia

Kanene (Swahili) a little important thing.

Kani (Hawaiian) sound.

Kanika (Mwera) black cloth.
Kanica, Kanicka

Kannitha (Cambodian) angel.

Kanoa (Hawaiian) free.

Kanya (Hindi) virgin. (Tai) young lady. Religion: a form of the Hindu goddess Devi.
Kanea, Kania, Kaniya, Kanyia

Kapri (American) a form of Capri.
Kapre, Kapree, Kapria, Kaprice, Kapricia, Kaprisha, Kaprisia

Kapua (Hawaiian) blossom.

Kapuki (Swahili) first-born daughter.

Kara (Greek, Danish) pure.
Kaira, Kairah, Karah, Karalea, Karaleah, Karalee, Karalie, Kari, Karra

Karah (Greek, Danish) a form of Kara. (Irish, Italian) a form of Cara.
Karrah

Karalynn (English) a combination of Kara + Lynn.
Karalin, Karaline, Karalyn, Karalyne, Karalynne

Karelle (American) a form of Carol.
Karel, Kareli, Karell, Karely

Karen (Greek) pure. See also
Carey, Carina, Caryn.
*Kaaren, Kalina, Karaina,
Karan, Karena, Karin, Karina,
Karine, Karna, Karon, Karren,
Karron, Karyn, Kerron, Koren*

Karena (Scandinavian) a form
of Karen.
*Kareen, Kareena, Kareina,
Karenah, Karene, Karreen,
Karreena, Karrena, Karrene*

Karessa (French) a form of
Caressa.

Kari (Greek) pure. (Danish) a
form of Caroline, Katherine.
See also Carey, Cari, Carrie.
*Karee, Karey, Karia, Kariah,
Karie, Karrey, Karri, Karrie,
Karry, Kary*

Kariane, Karianne
(American) combinations of
Kari + Ann.
*Karian, Kariana, Kariann,
Karianna*

Karida (Arabic) untouched,
pure.
Kareeda, Karita

Karilynn (American) a combi-
nation of Kari + Lynn.
*Kareelin, Kareeline, Kareelinn,
Kareelyn, Kareelyne, Kareelynn,
Kareelynne, Karilin, Kariline,
Karilinn, Karilyn, Karilyne,
Karilynne, Karylin, Karyline,
Karylinn, Karylyn, Karylyne,
Karylynn, Karylynne*

Karimah (Arabic) generous.
*Kareema, Kareemah, Karima,
Karime*

Karin (Scandinavian) a form
of Karen.
*Kaarin, Kareen, Karina,
Karine, Karinne, Karrin, Kerrin*

Karina (Russian) a form of
Karen.
*Kaarina, Karinna, Karrina,
Karryna, Karyna, Karynna*

Karine (Russian) a form of
Karen.
Karrine, Karryne, Karyne

Karis (Greek) graceful.
*Karess, Karice, Karise, Karisse,
Karris, Karys, Karyss*

Karissa (Greek) a form of
Carissa.
*Karese, Karesse, Karisa,
Karisha, Karishma, Karisma,
Karissimia, Kariza, Karrisa,
Karrissa, Karysa, Karyssa,
Kerisa*

Karla (German) a form of
Carla. (Slavic) a short form
of Karoline.
*Karila, Karilla, Karle, Karlene,
Karlicka, Karlinka, Karlisha,
Karlisia, Karlitha, Karlla,
Karlon, Karlyn*

Karlee, Karleigh (American)
forms of Karley, Karly. See
also Carlee.
Karlea, Karleah, Karlei

Karlene, Karlyn (American)
forms of Karla. See also
Carleen.
*Karleen, Karlen, Karlena,
Karlign, Karlin, Karlina,
Karlinna, Karlyan, Karlynn,
Karlynne*

Karley, Karly (Latin) little and
strong. (American) forms of
Carly.
*Karlee, Karley, Karlie, Karlyan,
Karlye*

Karli, Karlie (American)
forms of Karley, Karly. See
also Carli.

Karlotte (American) a form of
Charlotte.
*Karlita, Karletta, Karlette,
Karlotta*

Karma (Hindi) fate, destiny;
action.

Karmel (Hebrew) a form of
Carmela.
*Karmeita, Karmela, Karmelina,
Karmella, Karmelle, Karmiella,
Karmielle, Karmyla*

Karmen (Latin) song.
*Karman, Karmencita, Karmin,
Karmina, Karmine, Karmita,
Karmon, Karmyn, Karmyne*

Karolane (American) a com-
bination of Karoll + Anne.
*Karolan, Karolann, Karolanne,
Karol-Anne*

Karolina, Karoline (Slavic)
forms of Caroline. See also
Carolina.
*Karaleen, Karalena, Karalene,
Karalin, Karaline, Karileen,
Karilena, Karilene, Karilin,
Karilina, Kariline, Karleen,
Karlen, Karlena, Karlene,
Karling, Karoleena, Karolena,
Karolinka, Karroleen,
Karrolena, Karrolene, Karrolin,
Karroline*

Karoll (Slavic) a form of
Carol.
*Karel, Karilla, Karily, Karol,
Karola, Karole, Karoly, Karrol,
Karyl, Kerril*

Karolyn (American) a form of
Carolyn.
*Karalyn, Karalyna, Karalynn,
Karalynne, Karilyn, Karilyna,
Karilynn, Karilynne, Karlyn,
Karlynn, Karlynne, Karolyna,
Karolynn, Karolynne, Karrolyn,
Karrolyna, Karrolynn,
Karrolynne*

Karri, Karrie (American)
forms of Carrie.
Kari, Karie, Karry, Kary

Karsen, Karsyn (English) child
of Kar. Forms of Carson.
Karson

Karuna (Hindi) merciful.

Karyn (American) a form of
Karen.
*Karyne, Karynn, Karynna,
Kerrynn, Kerrynne*

Kasa (Hopi) fur robe.

Kasandra (Greek) a form of Kassandra.
Kasander, Kasandria, Kasandra, Kasaundra, Kasondra, Kasoundra

Kasey, Kasie (Irish) brave. (American) forms of Casey, Kacey.
Kaisee, Kaisie, Kasci, Kascy, Kasee, Kasi, Kassee, Kassey, Kasy, Kasya, Kaysci, Kaysea, Kaysee, Kaysey, Kaysi, Kaysie, Kaysy

Kashawna (American) a com-bination of Kate + Shawna.
Kasha, Kashae, Kashana, Kashanna, Kashauna, Kashawn, Kasheana, Kasheanna, Kasheena, Kashena, Kashonda, Kashonna

Kashmir (Sanskrit) Geography: a region located between India and Pakistan.
Cashmere, Kashmear, Kashmere, Kashmia, Kashmira, Kasmir, Kasmira, Kazmir, Kazmira

Kasi (Hindi) from the holy city.

Kasia (Polish) a form of Katherine. See also Cassia.
Kashia, Kasiah, Kasian, Kasienka, Kasja, Kaska, Kassa, Kassia, Kassya, Kasya

Kasinda (Umbundu) our last baby.

Kassandra (Greek) a form of Cassandra.
Kassandr, Kassandre, Kassandré, Kassaundra, Kassi, Kassondra, Kassondria, Kassundra, Kazandra, Khrisandra, Krisandra, Krissandra

Kassi, Kassie (American) familiar forms of Kassandra, Kassidy. See also Cassie.
Kassey, Kassia, Kassy

Kassidy (Irish) clever. (American) a form of Cassidy.
Kassadee, Kassadi, Kassadie, Kassadina, Kassady, Kasseday, Kassedee, Kassi, Kassiddy, Kassidee, Kassidi, Kassidie, Kassity, Kassydi

Katalina (Irish) a form of Caitlin. See also Catalina.
Kataleen, Kataleena, Katalena, Katalin, Katalyn, Katalynn

Katarina (Czech) a form of Katherine.
Kata, Katareena, Katarena, Katarin, Katarine, Katarinna, Katarinne, Katarrina, Kataryna, Katarzyna, Katinka, Katrika, Katrinka

Kate (Greek) pure. (English) a short form of Katherine.
Kait, Kata, Katee, Kati, Katica, Katie, Katka, Katy, Katya

Katee, Katey (English) famil-iar forms of Kate, Katherine.

Katelin (Irish) a form of
Caitlin. See also Kaitlin.
Kaetlin, Katalin, Katelan,
Kateland, Kateleen, Katelen,
Katelene, Katelind, Kateline,
Katelinn, Katelun, Kaytlin

Katelyn, Katelynn (Irish)
forms of Caitlin.
Kaetlyn, Kaetlynn, Kaetlynne,
Katelyne, Katelynne, Kaytlyn,
Kaytlynn, Kaytlynne

Katerina (Slavic) a form of
Katherine.
Katenka, Katerine, Katerini,
Katerinka

Katharine (Greek) a form of
Katherine.
Katharaine, Katharin,
Katharina, Katharyn

Katherine (Greek) pure. See
also Carey, Catherine,
Ekaterina, Kara, Karen, Kari,
Kasia, Katerina,Yekaterina.
Ekaterina, Ekatrinna, Kasienka,
Kasin, Kat, Katarina, Katchen,
Kate, Katee, Kathann,
Kathanne, Katharine,
Kathereen, Katheren, Katherene,
Katherenne, Katherin,
Katherina, Katheryn,
Katheryne, Kathi, Kathleen,
Kathrine, Kathryn, Kathy,
Kathyrine, Katia, Katina,
Katlaina, Katoka, Katreeka,
Katrina, Kay, Kitty

Kathi, Kathy (English) familiar forms of Katherine,

Kathleen. See also Cathi.
Kaethe, Katha, Kathe, Kathee,
Kathey, Kathi, Kathie, Katka,
Katla, Kató

Kathleen (Irish) a form of
Katherine. See also Cathleen.
Katheleen, Kathelene, Kathi,
Kathileen, Kathlean, Kathleena,
Kathleene, Kathlene, Kathlin,
Kathlina, Kathlyn, Kathlyne,
Kathlynn, Kathy, Katleen

Kathrine (Greek) a form of
Katherine.
Kathreen, Kathreena, Kathrene,
Kathrin, Kathrina

Kathryn (English) a form of
Katherine.
Kathren, Kathryne, Kathrynn,
Kathrynne

Kati (Estonian) a familiar form
of Kate.
Katja, Katya, Katye

Katia, Katya (Russian) forms
of Katherine.
Cattiah, Katiya, Kattia,
Kattiah, Katyah

Katie (English) a familiar form
of Kate.
Katee, Kati, Kãtia, Katti,
Kattie, Katy, Kayte, Kaytee,
Kaytie

Katilyn (Irish) a form of
Katlyn.
Katilin, Katilynn

Katlin (Irish) a form of Katlyn.
Katlina, Katline

Katlyn (Greek) pure. (Irish) a
form of Katelin.
*Kaatlain, Katilyn, Katland,
Katlin, Katlynd, Katlyne,
Katlynn, Katlynne*

Katriel (Hebrew) God is my
crown.
*Katrelle, Katri, Katrie, Katry,
Katryel*

Katrina (German) a form of
Katherine. See also Catrina,
Trina.
*Katreen, Katreena, Katrene,
Katri, Katrice, Katricia, Katrien,
Katrin, Katrine, Katrinia,
Katriona, Katryn, Katryna,
Kattrina, Kattryna, Katus,
Katuska*

Katy (English) a familiar form
of Kate. See also Cady.
Kady, Katey, Katty, Kayte

Kaulana (Hawaiian) famous.
Kaula, Kauna, Kahuna

Kaveri (Hindi) Geography: a
sacred river in India.

Kavindra (Hindi) poet.

Kawena (Hawaiian) glow.
Kawana, Kawona

Kay (Greek) rejoicer.
(Teutonic) a fortified place.
(Latin) merry. A short form
of Katherine.
Caye, Kae, Kai, Kaye, Kayla

Kaya (Hopi) wise child.
(Japanese) resting place.
Kaja, Kayah, Kayia

Kaycee (American) a combi-
nation of the initials K. + C.
*Kayce, Kaysee, Kaysey, Kaysi,
Kaysie, Kaysii*

Kaydee (American) a combi-
nation of the initials K. + D.
*Kayda, Kayde, Kayden, Kaydi,
Kaydie*

Kayla (Arabic, Hebrew) laurel;
crown. A form of Kaela,
Kaila. See also Cayla.
*Kaylah, Kaylea, Kaylee,
Kayleen, Kaylene, Kaylia,
Keila, Keyla*

Kaylah (Arabic, Hebrew) a
form of Kayla.
Kayleah, Kaylia, Keylah

Kaylan, Kaylen (Hebrew)
forms of Kayleen.
*Kaylana, Kayland, Kaylani,
Kaylann, Kaylean, Kayleana,
Kayleanna, Kaylenn*

Kaylee (American) a form of
Kayla. See also Caeley, Kalee.
*Kailee, Kayle, Kayleigh, Kayley,
Kayli, Kaylie*

Kayleen, Kaylene (Hebrew)
beloved, sweetheart. Forms of
Kayla.
*Kaylan, Kayleena, Kayleene,
Kaylen, Kaylena*

Kayleigh (American) a form of Kaylee.
Kaylei

Kayley, Kayli, Kaylie (American) forms of Kaylee.

Kaylin (American) a form of Kaylyn.
Kaylon

Kaylyn, Kaylynn (American) combinations of Kay + Lynn. See also Kaelyn.
Kalyn, Kalynn, Kayleen, Kaylene, Kaylin, Kaylyna, Kaylyne, Kaylynne

Kaytlin, Kaytlyn (Irish) forms of Kaitlin.
Kaytlan, Kaytlann, Kaytlen, Kaytlyne, Kaytlynn, Kaytlynne

Keaira (Irish) a form of Keara.
Keair, Keairah, Keairra, Keairre, Keairrea

Keala (Hawaiian) path.

Keana, Keanna (German) bold; sharp. (Irish) beautiful.
Keanah, Keanne, Keanu, Keenan, Keeyana, Keeyanah, Keeyanna, Keeyona. Keeyonna, Keiana, Keianna, Keona, Keonna

Keandra, Keondra (American) forms of Kenda.
Keandrah, Keandre, Keandrea, Keandria, Kedeana, Kedia, Keonda, Keondre, Keondria

Keara (Irish) dark; black. Religion: an Irish saint.
Keaira, Kearah, Kearia, Kearra, Keera, Keerra, Keiara, Keiarah, Keiarra, Keira, Kera

Kearsten, Keirsten (Greek) forms of Kirstin.
Kearstin, Kearston, Kearstyn, Keirstan, Keirstein, Keirstin, Keirston, Keirstyn, Keirstynne

Keeley, Keely (Irish) forms of Kelly.
Kealee, Kealey, Keali, Kealie, Keallie, Kealy, Keela, Keelan, Keele, Keelee, Keeleigh, Keeli, Keelia, Keelie, Keellie, Keelye, Keighla, Keilee, Keileigh, Keiley, Keilly, Kiela, Kiele, Kieley, Kielly, Kiely

Keelyn (Irish) a form of Kellyn.
Kealyn, Keelin, Keilan, Kielyn

Keena (Irish) brave.
Keenya, Kina

Keesha (American) a form of Keisha.
Keesa, Keeshae, Keeshana, Keeshanne, Keeshawna, Keeshonna, Keeshya, Keiosha

Kei (Japanese) reverent.

Keiana, Keianna (Irish) forms of Keana. (American) forms of Kiana.
Keiann, Keiannah, Keionna

Keiki (Hawaiian) child.
Keikana, Keikann, Keikanna, Keikanne

Keiko (Japanese) happy child.

Keila (Arabic, Hebrew) a form of Kayla.
Keilah, Kela, Kelah

Keilani (Hawaiian) glorious chief.
Kaylani, Keilan, Keilana, Keilany, Kelana, Kelanah, Kelane, Kelani, Kelanie

Keira (Irish) a form of Keara.
Keiara, Keiarra, Keirra, Keirrah, Kera, Keyeira

Keisha (American) a short form of Keneisha.
Keasha, Keashia, Keesha, Keishaun, Keishauna, Keishawn, Kesha, Keysha, Kiesha, Kisha, Kishanda

Keita (Scottish) woods; enclosed place.
Keiti

Kekona (Hawaiian) second-born child.

Kelcey, Kelci, Kelcie (Scottish) forms of Kelsey.
Kelse, Kelcee, Kelcy

Kelila (Hebrew) crown, laurel. See also Kaela, Kayla, Kalila.
Kelilah, Kelula

Kelley (Irish) a form of Kelly.

Kelli, Kellie (Irish) familiar forms of Kelly.
Keleigh, Keli, Kelia, Keliah, Kelie, Kellee, Kelleigh, Kellia, Kellisa

Kelly (Irish) brave warrior. See also Caeley.
Keeley, Keely, Kelley, Kelley, Kelli, Kellie, Kellye

Kellyanne (Irish) a combination of Kelly + Anne.
Kelliann, Kellianne, Kellyann

Kellyn (Irish) a combination of Kelly + Lyn.
Keelyn, Kelleen, Kellen, Kellene, Kellina, Kelline, Kellynn, Kellynne

Kelsea (Scottish) a form of Kelsey.
Kelcea, Kelcia, Kelsa, Kelsae, Kelsay, Kelse

Kelsey (Scandinavian, Scottish) ship island. (English) a form of Chelsea.
Kelcey, Kelda, Kellsee, Kellsei, Kellsey, Kellsie, Kellsy, Kelsea, Kelsei, Kelsey, Kelsi, Kelsie, Kelsy, Kelsye

Kelsi, Kelsie, Kelsy (Scottish) forms of Chelsea.
Kalsie, Kelci, Kelcie, Kellsi

Kenda (English) water baby. (Dakota) magical power.
Keandra, Kendra, Kennda

Kendal (English) a form of Kendall.
Kendahl, Kendale, Kendalie, Kendalin, Kendalyn, Kendalynn, Kendel, Kendele, Kendil, Kindal

Kendall (English) ruler of the valley.
Kendal, Kendalla, Kendalle, Kendell, Kendelle, Kendera, Kendia, Kendyl, Kinda, Kindall, Kindi, Kindle, Kynda, Kyndal, Kyndall, Kyndel

Kendra (English) a form of Kenda.
Kandra, Kendrah, Kendre, Kendrea, Kendreah, Kendria, Kenndra, Kentra, Kentrae, Kindra, Kyndra

Kendyl (English) a form of Kendall.
Kendyle, Kendyll

Keneisha (American) a combination of the prefix Ken + Aisha.
Kaneisha, Keisha, Keneesha, Kenesha, Keneshia, Kenisha, Kenneisha, Kennesha, Kenneshia, Keosha, Kineisha

Kenenza (English) a form of Kennice.
Kenza

Kenia (Hebrew) a form of Kenya.
Keniya, Kennia

Kenisha (American) a form of Keneisha.
Kenisa, Kenise, Kenishia, Kenissa, Kennisa, Kennisha, Kennysha

Kenna (Irish) a short form of Kennice.

Kennedy (Irish) helmeted chief. History: John F. Kennedy was the thirty-fifth U. S. president.
Kenedee, Kenedey, Kenedi, Kenedie, Kenedy, Kenidee, Kenidi, Kenidie, Kenidy, Kennadee, Kennadi, Kennadie, Kennady, Kennedee, Kennedey, Kennedi, Kennedie, Kennidee, Kennidi, Kennidy, Kynnedi

Kennice (English) beautiful.
Kanice, Keneese, Kenenza, Kenese, Kennise

Kenya (Hebrew) animal horn. Geography: a country in Africa.
Keenya, Kenia, Kenja, Kenyah, Kenyana, Kenyatta, Kenyia

Kenyatta (American) a form of Kenya.
Kenyata, Kenyatah, Kenyatte, Kenyattia, Kenyatta, Kenyette

Kenzie (Scottish) light skinned. (Irish) a short form of Mackenzie.
Kenzea, Kenzee, Kenzey, Kenzi, Kenzia, Kenzy, Kinzie

Keona, Keonna (Irish) forms of Keana.
Keiona, Keionna, Keoana, Keoni, Keonia, Keonnah, Keonni, Keonnia

Keosha (American) a short form of Keneisha.
Keoshae, Keoshi, Keoshia, Keosia

Kerani (Hindi) sacred bells. See also Rani.
Kera, Kerah, Keran, Kerana

Keren (Hebrew) animal's horn.
Kerrin, Keryn

Kerensa (Cornish) a form of Karenza.
Karensa, Karenza, Kerenza

Keri, Kerri, Kerrie (Irish) forms of Kerry.
Keriann, Kerianne, Kerriann, Kerrianne

Kerry (Irish) dark haired. Geography: a county in Ireland.
Keary, Keiry, Keree, Kerey, Keri, Kerri, Kerrie, Kerryann, Kerryanne, Kery, Kiera, Kierra

Kerstin (Scandinavian) a form of Kirsten.
Kerstan, Kerste, Kerstein, Kersten, Kerstie, Kerstien, Kerston, Kerstyn, Kerstynn

Kesare (Latin) long haired. (Russian) a form of Caesar (see Boys' Names).

Kesha (American) a form of Keisha.
Keshah, Keshal, Keshala, Keshan, Keshana, Keshara, Keshawn, Keshawna, Keshawnna

Keshia (American) a form of Keisha. A short form of Keneisha.
Kecia, Keishia, Keschia, Keshea, Kesia, Kesiah, Kessia, Kessiah

Kesi (Swahili) born during difficult times.

Kessie (Ashanti) chubby baby.
Kess, Kessa, Kesse, Kessey, Kessi

Kevyn (Irish) beautiful.
Keva, Kevan, Keven, Kevia, Keviana, Kevinna, Kevina, Kevion, Kevionna, Kevon, Kevona, Kevone, Kevonia, Kevonna, Kevonne, Kevonya, Kevynn

Keyana, Keyanna (American) forms of Kiana.
Keya, Keyanah, Keyanda, Keyandra, Keyannah

Keyara (Irish) a form of Kiara.
Keyarah, Keyari, Keyarra, Keyera, Keyerah, Keyerra

Keyona, Keyonna (American) forms of Kiana.
Keyonda, Keyondra, Keyonnia, Keyonnie

Keysha (American) a form of Keisha.
Keyosha, Keyoshia, Keyshana, Keyshanna, Keyshawn, Keyshawna, Keyshia, Keyshla, Keyshona, Keyshonna

Keziah (Hebrew) cinnamon-like spice. Bible: one of the daughters of Job.
Kazia, Kaziah, Ketzi, Ketzia, Ketziah, Kezi, Kezia, Kizzy

Khadijah (Arabic) trustworthy. History: Muhammed's first wife.
Khadaja, Khadajah, Khadeeja, Khadeejah, Khadeja, Khadejah, Khadejha, Khadija, Khadije, Khadijia, Khadijiah

Khalida (Arabic) immortal, everlasting.
Khali, Khalia, Khaliah, Khalidda, Khalita

Khrissa (American) a form of Chrissa. (Czech) a form of Krista.
Khrishia, Khryssa, Krisha, Krisia, Krissa, Krysha, Kryssa

Khristina (Russian, Scandinavian) a form of Kristina, Christina.
Khristeen, Khristen, Khristin, Khristine, Khyristya, Khristyana, Khristyna, Khrystyne

Ki (Korean) arisen.

Kia (African) season's beginning. (American) a short form of Kiana.
Kiah

Kiana (American) a combination of the prefix Ki + Ana.
Keanna, Keiana, Keyana, Keyona, Khiana, Khianah, Khianna, Ki, Kiahna, Kiane, Kiani, Kiania, Kianna, Kiauna, Kiandra, Kiandria, Kiauna, Kiaundra, Kiyana, Kyana

Kianna (American) a form of Kiana.
Kiannah, Kianne, Kianni

Kiara (Irish) little and dark.
Keyara, Kiarra, Kieara, Kiearah, Kiearra, Kyara

Kiaria, Kiarra, Kichi (Japanese) fortunate.

Kiele (Hawaiian) gardenia; fragrant blossom.
Kiela, Kieley, Kieli, Kielli, Kielly

Kiera, Kierra (Irish) forms of Kerry.
Kierana, Kieranna, Kierea

Kiersten, Kierstin (Scandanavian) forms of Kirsten.
Keirstan, Kerstin, Kierstan, Kierston, Kierstyn, Kierstynn

Kiki (Spanish) a familiar form of names ending in "queta."

Kiku (Japanese) chrysanthemum.
Kiko

Kiley (Irish) attractive; from
the straits.
*Kilea, Kilee, Kileigh, Kili, Kilie,
Kylee, Kyli, Kylie*

Kim (Vietnamese) needle.
(English) a short form of
Kimberly.
Kima, Kimette, Kym

Kimana (Shoshone) butterfly.
Kiman, Kimani

Kimber (English) a short form
of Kimberly.
Kimbra

Kimberlee, Kimberley
(English) forms of Kimberly.
*Kimbalee, Kimberlea, Kimberlei,
Kimberleigh, Kimbley*

Kimberly (English) chief,
ruler.
*Cymberly, Cymbre, Kim,
Kimba, Kimbely, Kimber,
Kimbereley, Kimberely,
Kimberlee, Kimberli, Kimberlie,
Kimberlyn, Kimbery, Kimbria,
Kimbrie, Kimbry, Kimmie,
Kymberly*

Kimberlyn (English) a form of
Kimberly.
Kimberlin, Kimberlynn

Kimi (Japanese) righteous.
*Kimia, Kimika, Kimiko,
Kimiyo, Kimmi, Kimmie,
Kimmy*

Kimmie (English) a familiar
form of Kimberly.
*Kimee, Kimme, Kimmee,
Kimmi, Kimmy, Kimy*

Kina (Hawaiian) from China.

Kineisha (American) a form
of Keneisha.
*Kineesha, Kinesha, Kineshia,
Kinisha, Kinishia*

Kineta (Greek) energetic.
Kinetta

Kini (Hawaiian) a form of Jean.
Kina

Kinsey (English) offspring;
relative.
*Kinsee, Kinsley, Kinza, Kinze,
Kinzee, Kinzey, Kinzi, Kinzie,
Kinzy*

Kinsley (American) a form of
Kinsey.
Kinslee, Kinslie, Kinslyn

Kioko (Japanese) happy child.
Kiyo, Kiyoko

Kiona (Native American)
brown hills.
Kionah, Kioni, Kionna

Kira (Persian) sun. (Latin) light.
*Kirah, Kiri, Kiria, Kiro, Kirra,
Kirrah, Kirri*

Kiran (Hindi) ray of light.

Kirby (Scandinavian) church
village. (English) cottage by
the water.
Kirbee, Kirbi

Kirima (Eskimo) hill.

Kirsi (Hindi) amaranth blossoms.
Kirsie

Kirsta (Scandinavian) a form of Kirsten.

Kirsten (Greek) Christian; annointed. (Scandinavian) a form of Christine.
Karsten, Kearsten, Keirstan, Kerstin, Kiersten, Kirsteni, Kirsta, Kirstan, Kirstene, Kirstie, Kirstin, Kirston, Kirsty, Kirstyn, Kjersten, Kursten, Kyersten, Kyrsten, Kyrstin

Kirstin (Scandinavian) a form of Kirsten.
Karstin, Kirsteen, Kirstien, Kirstine

Kirstie, Kirsty (Scandinavian) familiar forms of Kirsten.
Kerstie, Kirsta, Kirste, Kirstee, Kirstey, Kirsti, Kjersti, Kyrsty

Kirstyn (Greek) a form of Kirsten.
Kirstynn

Kisa (Russian) kitten.
Kisha, Kiska, Kissa, Kiza

Kishi (Japanese) long and happy life.

Kissa (Ugandan) born after twins.

Kita (Japanese) north.

Kitra (Hebrew) crowned.

Kitty (Greek) a familiar form of Katherine.
Ketter, Ketti, Ketty, Kit, Kittee, Kitteen, Kittey, Kitti, Kittie

Kiwa (Japanese) borderline.

Kiyana (American) a form of Kiana.
Kiya, Kiyah, Kiyan, Kiyani, Kiyanna, Kiyenna

Kizzy (American) a familiar form of Keziah.
Kezi, Kissie, Kizzi, Kizzie

Klara (Hungarian) a form of Clara.
Klára, Klari, Klarika

Klarise (German) a form of Klarissa.
Klarice, Kláris, Klaryce

Klarissa (German) clear, bright. (Italian) a form of Clarissa.
Klarisa, Klarise, Klarrisa, Klarrissa, Klarrissia, Klarisza, Klarysa, Klaryssa, Kleresa

Klaudia (American) a form of Claudia.
Klaudija

Kloe (American) a form of Chloe.
Khloe, Kloee, Kloey, Klohe, Kloie

Kodi (American) a form of Codi.
Kodee, Kodey, Kodie, Kody, Kodye, Koedi

Koffi (Swahili) born on Friday.
Kaffe, Kaffi, Koffe, Koffie

Koko (Japanese) stork. See also
Coco.

Kolby (American) a form of
Colby.
*Kobie, Koby, Kolbee, Kolbey,
Kolbi, Kolbie*

Kolina (Swedish) a form of
Katherine. See also Colleen.
*Koleen, Koleena, Kolena,
Kolene, Koli, Kolleen, Kollena,
Kollene, Kolyn, Kolyna*

Kona (Hawaiian) lady. (Hindi)
angular.
Koni, Konia

Konstance (Latin) a form of
Constance.
*Konstantina, Konstantine,
Konstanza, Konstanze*

Kora (Greek) a form of Cora.
*Korah, Kore, Koren, Koressa,
Koretta, Korra*

Koral (American) a form of
Coral.
*Korel, Korele, Korella, Korilla,
Korral, Korrel, Korrell, Korrelle*

Kori (American) a short form
of Korina. See also Corey,
Cori.
*Koree, Korey, Koria, Korie,
Korri, Korrie, Korry, Kory*

Korina (Greek) a form of
Corina.
*Koreena, Korena, Koriana,
Korianna, Korine, Korinna,
Korreena, Korrina, Korrinna,
Koryna, Korynna*

Korine (Greek) a form of
Korina.
*Koreen, Korene, Koriane,
Korianne, Korin, Korinn,
Korinne, Korrin, Korrine,
Korrinne, Korryn, Korrynne,
Koryn, Koryne, Korynn*

Kornelia (Latin) a form of
Cornelia.
*Karniela, Karniella, Karnis,
Kornelija, Kornelis, Kornelya,
Korny*

Kortney (English) a form of
Courtney.
*Kortnay, Kortnee, Kortni,
Kortnie, Kortny*

Kosma (Greek) order;
universe.
Cosma

Kosta (Latin) a short form of
Constance.
Kostia, Kostusha, Kostya

Koto (Japanese) harp.

Kourtney (American) a form
of Courtney.
*Kourtnay, Kourtne, Kourtnee,
Kourtnei, Kourtneigh, Kourtni,
Kourtny, Kourtynie*

Kris (American) a short form
of Kristine. A form of Chris.
Khris, Krissy

Krissy (American) a familiar form of Kris.
Krissey, Krissi, Krissie

Krista (Czech) a form of ~Christina. See also Christa.
Khrissa, Khrista, Khryssa, Khrysta, Krissa, Kryssa, Krysta

Kristal (Latin) a form of Crystal.
Kristale, Kristall, Kristill, Kristl, Kristle, Kristy

Kristan (Greek) a form of Kristen.
Kristana, Kristanna, Kristanne, Kriston, Krystan, Krystane

Kristen (Greek) Christian; annointed. (Scandinavian) a form of Christine.
Christen, Kristan, Kristene, Kristien, Kristin, Kristyn, Krysten

Kristi, Kristie (Scandinavian) short forms of Kristine.
Christi

Kristian, Kristiana (Greek) Christian; anointed. Forms of Christian.
Khristian, Kristian, Kristiane, Kristiann, Kristi-Ann, Kristianna, Kristianne, Kristi-Anne, Kristienne, Kristyan, Kristyana, Kristy-Ann, Kristy-Anne

Kristin (Scandinavian) a form of Kristen. See also Cristen.
Kristiin, Krystin

Kristina (Greek) Christian; annointed. (Scandinavian) a form of Christina. See also Cristina.
Khristina, Kristena, Kristina, Kristeena, Kristena, Kristinka, Krystina

Kristine (Scandinavian) a form of Christine.
Kris, Kristeen, Kristene, Kristi, Kristie, Kristy, Krystine, Krystyne

Kristy (American) a familiar form of Kristine, Krystal. See also Cristy.
Kristi, Kristia, Kristie, Krysia, Krysti

Kristyn (Greek) a form of Kristen.
Kristyne, Kristynn

Krysta (Polish) a form of Krista.
Krystah, Krystka

Krystal (American) clear, brilliant glass.
Kristabel, Kristal, Krystalann, Krystalanne, Krystale, Krystall, Krystalle, Krystel, Krystil, Krystle, Krystol

Krystalee (American) a combination of Krystal + Lee.
Kristalea, Kristaleah, Kristalee, Krystalea, Krystaleah, Krystlea, Krystleah, Krystlee, Krystlelea, Krystleleah, Krystlelee

Krystalynn (American) a
combination of Krystal +
Lynn.
*Kristaline, Kristalyn,
Kristalynn, Kristilyn,
Kristilynn, Kristlyn, Krystaleen,
Krystalene, Krystalin,
Krystalina, Krystallyn,
Krystalyn, Krystalynne*

Krystel (Latin) a form of
Krystal.
*Kristel, Kristell, Kristelle,
Krystelle*

Krysten (Greek) a form of
Kristen.
Krystene, Krystyn, Krystyne

Krystian, Krystiana (Greek)
forms of Christian.
*Krystiana, Krystianna,
Krystianne, Krysty-Ann,
Krystyan, Kristyana,
Krystyanna, Krystyanne,
Krysty-Anne, Krystyen*

Krystin (Czech) a form of
Kristin.

Krystina (Greek) a form of
Kristina.
*Krysteena, Krystena, Krystyna,
Krystynka*

Krystle (American) a form of
Krystal.
Krystl, Krystyl

Kudio (Swahili) born on
Monday.

Kuma (Japanese) bear.
(Tongan) mouse.

Kumiko (Japanese) girl with
braids.
Kumi

Kumuda (Sanskrit) lotus
flower.

Kuniko (Japanese) child from
the country.

Kunto (Twi) third-born.

Kuri (Japanese) chestnut.

Kusa (Hindi) God's grass.

Kwanita (Zuni) a form of
Juanita.

Kwashi (Swahili) born on
Sunday.

Kwau (Swahili) born on
Thursday.

Kyana (American) a form of
Kiana.
*Kyanah, Kyani, Kyann,
Kyanna, Kyanne, Kyanni,
Kyeana, Kyeanna*

Kyara (Irish) a form of Kiara.
*Kiyara, Kiyera, Kiyerra,
Kyarah, Kyaria, Kyarie, Kyarra,
Kyera, Kyerra*

Kyla (Irish) attractive.
(Yiddish) crown; laurel.
*Khyla, Kylah, Kylea, Kyleah,
Kylia*

Kyle (Irish) attractive.
*Kial, Kiele, Kylee, Kyleigh,
Kylene, Kylie*

Kylee (Irish) a familiar form of Kyle.
Kylea, Kyleah, Kylie, Kyliee

Kyleigh (Irish) a form of Kyle.
Kyliegh

Kylene (Irish) a form of Kyle.
Kyleen, Kylen, Kylyn, Kylynn

Kylie (West Australian Aboriginal) curled stick; boomerang. (Irish) a familiar form of Kyle.
Keiley, Keilley, Keilly, Keily, Kiley, Kye, Kylee, Kyley, Kyli, Kyllie

Kymberly (English) a form of Kimberly.
Kymber, Kymberlee, Kymberleigh, Kymberley, Kymberli, Kymberlie, Kymberlyn, Kymberlynn, Kymberlynne

Kyndal, Kyndall (English) forms of Kendall.
Kyndahl, Kyndalle, Kyndel, Kyndell, Kyndelle, Kyndle, Kyndol

Kynthia (Greek) a form of Cynthia.
Kyndi

Kyoko (Japanese) mirror.

Kyra (Greek) ladylike. A form of Cyrilla.
Keera, Keira, Kira, Kyrah, Kyrene, Kyria, Kyriah, Kyriann, Kyrie

L

Lacey, Lacy (Latin) cheerful. (Greek) familiar forms of Larissa.
Lacee, Laci, Lacie, Lacye

Lachandra (American) a combination of the prefix La + Chandra.
Lachanda, Lachandice

Laci, Lacie (Latin) forms of Lacey.
Lacia, Laciann, Lacianne

Lacrecia (Latin) a form of Lucretia.
Lacrasha, Lacreash, Lacreasha, Lacreashia, Lacreisha, Lacresha, Lacreshia, Lacresia, Lacretia, Lacricia, Lacriesha, Lacrisah, Lacrisha, Lacrishia, Lacrissa

Lada (Russian) Mythology: the Slavic goddess of beauty.

Ladasha (American) a combination of the prefix La + Dasha.
Ladaesha, Ladaisa, Ladaisha, Ladaishea, Ladaishia, Ladashiah, Ladaseha, Ladashia, Ladasia, Ladassa, Ladaysha, Ladesha, Ladisha, Ladosha

Ladeidra (American) acombinatione of the prefix La + Deidra.
Ladedra, Ladiedra

Ladonna (American) a combination of the prefix La + Donna.
Ladan, Ladana, Ladon, Ladona, Ladonne, Ladonya

Laela (Arabic, Hebrew) a form of Leila.
Lael, Laelle

Lahela (Hawaiian) a form of Rachel.

Laila (Arabic) a form of Leila.
Lailah, Laili, Lailie

Laine, Layne (French) short forms of Elaine.
Lain, Laina, Lainah, Lainee, Lainna, Layna

Lainey, Layney (French) familiar forms of Elaine.
Laini, Lainie, Laynee, Layni, Laynie

Lajila (Hindi) shy, coy.

Lajuana (American) a combination of the prefix La + Juana.
Lajuanna, Lawana, Lawanna, Lawanza, Lawanze, Laweania

Laka (Hawaiian) attractive; seductive; tame. Mythology: the goddess of the hula.

Lakayla (American) a combination of the prefix La + Kayla.
Lakala, Lakaya, Lakeila, Lakela, Lakella

Lakeisha (American) a combination of the prefix La + Keisha. See also Lekasha.
Lakaiesha, Lakaisha, Lakasha, Lakashia, Lakaysha, Lakaysia, Lakeasha, Lakecia, Lakeesh, Lakeesha, Lakeeshia, Lakesha, Lakeshia, Lakeysha, Lakezia, Lakicia, Lakieshia, Lakisha

Laken, Lakin, Lakyn (American) short forms of Lakendra.
Lakena, Lakyna, Lakynn

Lakendra (American) a combination of the prefix La + Kendra.
Lakanda, Lakedra, Laken, Lakenda

Lakenya (American) a combination of the prefix La + Kenya.
Lakeena, Lakeenna, Lakeenya, Lakena, Lakenia, Lakinja, Lakinya, Lakwanya, Lekenia, Lekenya

Lakesha, Lakeshia, Lakisha (American) forms of Lakeisha.
Lakecia, Lakeesha, Lakesa, Lakese, Lakeseia, Lakeshya, Lakesi, Lakesia, Lakeyshia, Lakiesha

Laketa (American) a combination of the prefix La + Keita.
Lakeeta, Lakeetah, Lakeita, Lakeitha, Lakeithia, Laketha, Laketia, Laketta, Lakieta, Lakietha, Lakita, Lakitia, Lakitra, Lakitri, Lakitta

Lakia (Arabic) found treasure.
Lakiea, Lakkia

Lakota (Dakota) a tribal name.
Lakoda, Lakohta, Lakotah

Lakresha (American) a form
of Lucretia.
*Lacresha, Lacreshia, Lacresia,
Lacretia, Lacrisha, Lakreshia,
Lakrisha, Lekresha, Lekresia*

Lakya (Hindi) born on
Thursday.
*Lakeya, Lakeyah, Lakieya,
Lakiya, Lakyia*

Lala (Slavic) tulip.
Lalah, Lalla

Lalasa (Hindi) love.

Laleh (Persian) tulip.
Lalah

Lali (Spanish) a form of
Lulani.
Lalia, Lalli, Lally

Lalita (Greek) talkative.
(Sanskrit) charming; candid.

Lallie (English) babbler.
Lalli, Lally

Lamesha (American) a com-
bination of the prefix La +
Mesha.
*Lamees, Lameesha, Lameise,
Lameisha, Lameshia, Lamisha,
Lamishia, Lemisha*

Lamia (German) bright land.
Lama, Lamiah

Lamis (Arabic) soft to the touch.
Lamese, Lamise

Lamonica (American) a com-
bination of the prefix La +
Monica.
Lamoni, Lamonika

Lamya (Arabic) dark lipped.
Lama

Lan (Vietnamese) flower.

Lana (Latin) woolly. (Irish)
attractive, peaceful. A short
form of Alana, Elana.
(Hawaiian) floating; bouyant.
*Lanae, Lanai, Lanata, Lanay,
Laneah, Laneetra, Lanette,
Lanna, Lannah*

Landa (Basque) another name
for the Virgin Mary.

Landon (English) open, grassy
meadow.
*Landan, Landen, Landin,
Landyn, Landynne*

Landra (German, Spanish)
counselor.
Landrea

Lane (English) narrow road.
Laina, Laney, Layne

Laneisha (American) a com-
bination of the prefix La +
Keneisha.
*Laneasha, Lanecia, Laneesha,
Laneise, Laneishia, Lanesha,
Laneshe, Laneshea, Laneshia,
Lanesia, Lanessa, Lanesse,
Lanisha, Lanishia*

Laney (English) a familiar
form of Lane.
Lanie, Lanni, Lanny, Lany

Lani (Hawaiian) sky; heaven. A
short form of Atalanta,
'Aulani, Leilani.
*Lanee, Lanei, Lania, Lanie,
Lanita, Lanney, Lanni, Lannie*

Laporsha (American) a com-
bination of the prefix La +
Porsha.
*Laporcha, Laporche, Laporscha,
Laporsche, Laporschia, Laporshe,
Laporshia, Laportia*

Laqueena (American) a com-
bination of the prefix La +
Queenie.
*Laqueen, Laquena, Laquenetta,
Laquinna*

Laquinta (American) a com-
bination of the prefix La +
Quintana.
*Laquanta, Laqueinta,
Laquenda, Laquenta, Laquinda*

Laquisha (American) a com-
bination of the prefix La +
Queisha.
*Laquasha, Laquaysha,
Laqueisha, Laquesha, Laquiesha*

Laquita (American) a combi-
nation of the prefix La +
Queta.
*Laqeita, Laqueta, Laquetta,
Laquia, Laquiata, Laquieta,
Laquitta, Lequita*

Lara (Greek) cheerful. (Latin)
shining; famous. Mythology:
a Roman nymph. A short
form of Laraine, Larissa,
Laura.
Larae, Larah, Laretta, Larette

Laraine (Latin) a form of
Lorraine.
*Lara, Laraene, Larain, Larane,
Larayn, Larayne, Laraynna,
Larein, Lareina, Lareine, Laren,
Larenn, Larenya, Lauraine,
Laurraine*

Larina (Greek) seagull.
Larena, Larine

Larisa (Greek) a form of
Larissa.
*Lareesa, Lareese, Laresa, Laris,
Larise, Larisha, Larrisa, Larysa,
Laurisa*

Larissa (Greek) cheerful. See
also Lacey.
*Lara, Laressa, Larisa, Larissah,
Larrissa, Larryssa, Laryssa,
Laurissa, Laurissah*

Lark (English) skylark.

Lashae, Lashay (American)
combinations of the prefix
La + Shay.
*Lasha, Lashai, Lashaia,
Lashaya, Lashaye, Lashea*

Lashana (American) a combi-
nation of the prefix La +
Shana.
*Lashanay, Lashane, Lashanna,
Lashannon, Lashona, Lashonna*

Lashanda (American) a combination of the prefix La + Shanda.
Lashandra, Lashanta, Lashante

Lashawna (American) a combination of the prefix La + Shawna.
Lashaun, Lashauna, Lashaune, Lashaunna, Lashaunta, Lashawn, Lashawnd, Lashawnda, Lashawndra, Lashawne, Lashawnia, Leshawn, Leshawna

Lashonda (American) a combination of the prefix La + Shonda.
Lachonda, Lashaunda, Lashaundra, Lashon, Lashond, Lashonde, Lashondia, Lashondra, Lashonta, Lashunda, Lashundra, Lashunta, Lashunte, Leshande, Leshandra, Leshondra, Leshundra

Latanya (American) a combination of the prefix La + Tanya.
Latana, Latandra, Latania, Latanja, Latanna, Latanua, Latonshia

Latara (American) a combination of the prefix La + Tara.

Latasha (American) a combination of the prefix La + Tasha.
Latacha, Latacia, Latai, Lataisha, Latashia, Latasia, Lataysha, Letasha, Letashia, Letasiah

Latavia (American) a combination of the prefix La + Tavia.

Lateefah (Arabic) pleasant. (Hebrew) pat, caress.
Lateefa, Latifa, Latifah, Latipha

Latesha (American) a form of Leticia.
Lataeasha, Lateasha, Lateashia, Latecia, Lateicia, Lateisha, Latesa, Lateshia, Latessa, Lateysha, Latisa, Latissa, Leteisha, Leteshia

Latia (American) a combination of the prefix La + Tia.
Latea, Lateia, Lateka

Latika (Hindi) elegant.
Lateeka, Lateka

Latisha (Latin) joy. (American) a combination of the prefix La + Tisha.
Laetitia, Laetizia, Latashia, Lateasha, Lateashia, Latecia, Lateesha, Lateicia, Lateisha, Latice, Laticia, Latiesha, Latishia, Latishya, Latissha, Latitia, Latysha

Latona (Latin) Mythology: the powerful goddess who bore Apollo and Diana.
Latonna, Latonnah

Latonya (American) a combination of the prefix La + Tonya. (Latin) a form of Latona.
Latoni, Latonia

Latoria (American) a combi-
nation of the prefix La +
Tori.
Latoira, Latorio, Latorja,
Latorray, Latorreia, Latory,
Latorya, Latoyra, Latoyria

Latosha (American) a combi-
nation of the prefix La +
Tosha.
Latoshia, Latoshya, Latosia

Latoya (American) a combi-
nation of the prefix La +
Toya.
Latoia, Latoiya, LaToya,
Latoyia, Latoye, Latoyia,
Latoyita, Latoyo

Latrice (American) a combi-
nation of the prefix La +
Trice.
Latrece, Latreece, Latreese,
Latresa, Latrese, Latressa,
Letreece, Letrice

Latricia (American) a combi-
nation of the prefix La +
Tricia.
Latrecia, Latresh, Latresha,
Latreshia, Latrica, Latrisha,
Latrishia

Laura (Latin) crowned with
laurel.
Lara, Laurah, Lauralee,
Laurelen, Laurella, Lauren,
Lauricia, Laurie, Laurka, Laury,
Lauryn, Lavra, Lolly, Lora,
Loretta, Lori, Lorinda, Lorna,
Loura

Laurel (Latin) laurel tree.
Laural, Laurell, Laurelle, Lorel,
Lorelle

Lauren (English) a form of
Laura.
Lauran, Laureen, Laurena,
Laurene, Laurien, Laurin,
Laurine, Lawren, Loren, Lorena

Laurence (Latin) crowned
with laurel.
Laurencia, Laurens, Laurent,
Laurentana, Laurentina,
Lawrencia

Laurianna (English) a combi-
nation of Laurie + Anna.
Laurana, Laurann, Laureana,
Laureanne, Laureen, Laureena,
Laurian, Lauriana, Lauriane,
Laurianna, Laurie Ann, Laurie
Anne, Laurina

Laurie (English) a familiar
form of Laura.
Lari, Larilia, Laure, Lauré,
Lauri, Lawrie

Laury (English) a familiar
form of Laura.

Lauryn (English) a familiar
form of Laura.
Laurynn

Laveda (Latin) cleansed, purified.
Lavare, Lavetta, Lavette

Lavelle (Latin) cleansing.
Lavella

Lavena (Irish, French) joy. (Latin) a form of Lavina.

Laverne (Latin) springtime. (French) grove of alder trees. See also Verna.
Laverine, Lavern, Laverna, La Verne

Lavina (Latin) purified; woman of Rome. See also Vina.
Lavena, Lavenia, Lavinia, Lavinie, Levenia, Levinia, Livinia, Louvinia, Lovina, Lovinia

Lavonna (American) a combination of the prefix La + Yvonne.
Lavon, Lavonda, Lavonder, Lavondria, Lavone, Lavonia, Lavonica, Lavonn, Lavonne, Lavonnie, Lavonya

Lawan (Tai) pretty.
Lawanne

Lawanda (American) a combination of the prefix La + Wanda.
Lawonda, Lawynda

Layce (American) a form of Lacey.
Laycee, Layci, Laycia, Laycie, Laysa, Laysea, Laysie

Layla (Hebrew, Arabic) a form of Leila.
Laylah, Layli, Laylie

Le (Vietnamese) pearl.

Lea (Hawaiian) Mythology: the goddess of canoe makers. (Hebrew) a form of Leah.

Leah (Hebrew) weary. Bible: the first wife of Jacob. See also Lia.
Lea, Léa, Lee, Leea, Leeah, Leia

Leala (French) faithful, loyal.
Lealia, Lealie, Leial

Lean, Leann, Leanne (English) forms of Leeann, Lian.
Leana, Leane, Leanna

Leandra (Latin) like a lioness.
Leanda, Leandre, Leandrea, Leandria, Leeanda, Leeandra

Leanna, Leeanna (English) forms of Liana.
Leana, Leeana, Leianna

Leanore (Greek) a form of Eleanor. (English) a form of Helen.
Leanora, Lanore

Lecia (Latin) a short form of Felecia.
Leasia, Leecia, Leesha, Leesia, Lesha, Leshia, Lesia

Leda (Greek) lady. Mythology: the queen of Sparta and the mother of Helen of Troy.
Ledah, Lyda, Lydah

Lee (Chinese) plum. (Irish) poetic. (English) meadow. A short form of Ashley, Leah.
Lea, Leigh

Leeann, Leeanne (English) combinations of Lee + Ann. Forms of Lian.
Leane, Leean, Leian, Leiann, Leianne

Leena (Estonian) a form of Helen. (Greek, Latin, Arabic) a form of Lina.

Leeza (Hebrew) a short form of Aleeza. (English) a form of Lisa, Liza.
Leesa

Lei (Hawaiian) a familiar form of Leilani.

Leigh, Leigha (English) forms of Leah.
Leighann, Leighanna, Leighanne

Leiko (Japanese) arrogant.

Leila (Hebrew) dark beauty; night. (Arabic) born at night. See also Laela, Layla, Lila.
Laila, Leela, Leelah, Leilah, Leilia, Lela, Lelah, Leland, Lelia, Leyla

Leilani (Hawaiian) heavenly flower; heavenly child.
Lailanee, Lailani, Lailanie, Lailany, Lailoni, Lani, Lei, Leilany, Leiloni, Leilony, Lelani, Lelania

Lekasha (American) a form of Lakeisha.
Lekeesha, Lekeisha, Lekesha, Lekeshia, Lekesia, Lekicia, Lekisha

Leli (Swiss) a form of Magdalen.
Lelie

Lelia (Greek) fair speech. (Hebrew, Arabic) a form of Leila.
Leliah, Lelika, Lelita, Lellia

Lelya (Russian) a form of Helen.

Lena (Hebrew) dwelling or lodging. (Latin) temptress. (Norwegian) illustrious. (Greek) a short form of Eleanor. Music: Lena Horne, a well-known African American singer and actress.
Lenah, Lene, Lenee, Leni, Lenka, Lenna, Lennah, Lina, Linah

Lenci (Hungarian) a form of Helen.
Lency

Lene (German) a form of Helen.
Leni, Line

Leneisha (American) a combination of the prefix Le + Keneisha.
Lenece, Lenesha, Leniesha, Lenieshia, Leniesia, Leniessia, Lenisa, Lenise, Lenisha, Lennise, Lennisha, Lynesha

Lenia (German) a form of Leona.
Lenayah, Lenda, Lenea, Leneen, Lenna, Lennah, Lennea, Leny

Lenita (Latin) gentle.
Leneta, Lenette, Lennette

Lenore (Greek, Russian) a form of Eleanor.
Lenni, Lenor, Lenora, Lenorah

Leona (German) brave as a lioness. See also Lona.
Lenia, Leoine, Leola, Leolah, Leonae, Leonah, Leondra, Leone, Leonelle, Leonia, Leonice, Leonicia, Leonie, Leonissa, Leonna, Leonne, Liona

Leonie (German) a familiar form of Leona.
Leoni, Léonie, Leony

Leonore (Greek) a form of Eleanor. See also Nora.
Leonor, Leonora, Leonorah, Léonore

Leontine (Latin) like a lioness.
Leona, Leonine, Leontyne, Léontyne

Leora (Hebrew) light. (Greek) a familiar form of Eleanor. See also Liora.
Leorah, Leorit

Leotie (Native American) prairie flower.

Lera (Russian) a short form of Valera.
Lerka

Lesley (Scottish) gray fortress.
Leslea, Leslee, Leslie, Lesly, Lezlee, Lezley

Leslie (Scottish) a form of Lesley.
Leslei, Lesleigh, Lesli, Lesslie, Lezli

Lesly (Scottish) a form of Lesley.
Leslye, Lessly, Lezly

Leta (Latin) glad. (Swahili) bringer. (Greek) a short form of Aleta.
Lita, Lyta

Leticia (Latin) joy. See also Latisha, Tisha.
Laticia, Leisha, Leshia, Let, Leta, Letesa, Letesha, Leteshia, Letha, Lethia, Letice, Letichia, Letisha, Letishia, Letisia, Letissa, Letita, Letitia, Letiticia, Letiza, Letizia, Letty, Letycia, Loutitia

Letty (English) a familiar form of Leticia.
Letta, Letti, Lettie

Levana (Hebrew) moon; white. (Latin) risen. Mythology: the goddess of newborn babies.
Lévana, Levania, Levanna, Levenia, Lewana, Livana

Levani (Fijian) anointed with oil.

Levia (Hebrew) joined, attached.
Leevya, Levi, Levie

Levina (Latin) flash of lightning.
Levene

Levona (Hebrew) spice; incense.
Leavonia, Levonat, Levonna, Levonne, Livona

Lewana (Hebrew) a form of Levana.
Lebhanah, Lewanna

Lexandra (Greek) a short form of Alexandra.
Lisandra

Lexi, Lexie (Greek) familiar forms of Alexandra.
Leksi, Lexey, Lexy

Lexia (Greek) a familiar form of Alexandra.
Leska, Lesya, Lexa, Lexane, Lexina, Lexine

Lexis (Greek) a short form of Alexius, Alexus.
Laexis, Lexius, Lexsis, Lexxis

Lexus (Greek) a short form of Alexis.
Lexuss, Lexxus, Lexyss

Leya (Spanish) loyal. (Tamil) the constellation Leo.
Leyah, Leyla

Lia (Greek) bringer of good news. (Hebrew, Dutch, Italian) dependent. See also Leah.
Liah

Lian (Chinese) graceful willow. (Latin) a short form of Gillian, Lillian.
Lean, Leeann, Liane, Liann, Lianne

Liana, Lianna (Latin) youth. (French) bound, wrapped up; tree covered with vines. (English) meadow. (Hebrew) short forms of Eliana.
Leanna

Liane, Lianne (Hebrew) short forms of Eliane. (English) forms of Lian.
Leeanne

Libby (Hebrew) a familiar form of Elizabeth.
Ibby, Lib, Libbee, Libbey, Libbie

Liberty (Latin) free.
Liberti, Libertie

Licia (Greek) a short form of Alicia.
Licha, Lishia, Lisia, Lycia

Lida (Greek) happy. (Slavic) loved by people. (Latin) a short form of Alida, Elita.
Leeda, Lidah, Lidochka, Lyda

Lide (Latin, Basque) life.

Lidia (Greek) a form of Lydia.
Lidea, Lidi, Lidija, Lidiya, Lidka, Lidya

Lien (Chinese) lotus.
Lienne

Liesabet (German) a short form of Elizabeth.
Liesbeth, Lisbete

Liese (German) a familiar form of Elise, Elizabeth.
Liesa, Lieschen, Lise

Liesel (German) a familiar form of Elizabeth.
Leesel, Leesl, Leezel, Leezl, Liesl, Liezel, Liezl, Lisel

Lila (Arabic) night. (Hindi) free will of God. (Persian) lilac. A short form of Dalila, Delilah, Lillian.
Lilah, Lilia, Lyla, Lylah

Lilac (Sanskrit) lilac; blue purple.

Lilia (Persian) a form of Lila.
Lili

Lilian (Latin) a form of Lillian.
Liliane, Liliann, Lilianne

Liliana (Latin) a form of Lillian.
Lileana, Lilliana, Lilianna, Lilliana, Lillianna

Lilibeth (English) a combination of Lilly + Beth.
Lilibet, Lillibeth, Lillybeth, Lilybet, Lilybeth

Lilith (Arabic) of the night; night demon. Mythology: the first wife of Adam, according to ancient Jewish legends.
Lillis, Lily

Lillian (Latin) lily flower.
Lian, Lil, Lila, Lilas, Lileane, Lilia, Lilian, Liliana, Lilias,

Liliha, Lilja, Lilla, Lilli, Lillia, Lilliane, Lilliann, Lillianne, Lillyann, Lis, Liuka

Lillyann (English) a combination of Lilly + Ann. (Latin) a form of Lillian.
Lillyan, Lillyanne, Lily, Lilyan, Lilyana, Lilyann, Lilyanna, Lilyanne

Lily (Latin, Arabic) a familiar form of Lilith, Lillian, Lillyann.
Lil, Líle, Lili, Lilie, Lilijana, Lilika, Lilike, Liliosa, Lilium, Lilka, Lille, Lilli, Lillie, Lilly

Limber (Tiv) joyful.

Lin (Chinese) beautiful jade. (English) a form of Lynn.
Linh, Linn

Lina (Greek) light. (Arabic) tender. (Latin) a form of Lena.

Linda (Spanish) pretty.
Lind, Lindy, Linita, Lynda

Lindsay (English) a form of Lindsey.
Lindsi, Linsay, Lyndsay

Lindsey (English) linden tree island; camp near the stream.
Lind, Lindsea, Lindsee, Lindsi, Linsey, Lyndsey, Lynsey

Lindsi (American) a familiar form of Lindsay, Lindsey.
Lindsie, Lindsy, Lindze, Lindzee, Lindzey, Lindzy

Lindy (Spanish) a familiar
form of Linda.
Linde, Lindee, Lindey, Lindi,
Lindie

Linette (Welsh) idol. (French)
bird.
Lanette, Linet, Linnet, Linnetta,
Linnette, Lyannette, Lynette

Ling (Chinese) delicate, dainty.

Linnea (Scandinavian) lime
tree. Botany: the national
flower of Sweden.
Lin, Linae, Linea, Linnae,
Linnaea, Linneah, Lynea,
Lynnea

Linsey (English) a form of
Lindsey.
Linsea, Linsee, Linsi, Linsie,
Linsy, Linzee, Linzey, Linzi,
Linzie, Linzy, Linzzi, Lynsey

Liolya (Russian) a form of
Helen.

Liora (Hebrew) light. See also
Leora.

Lirit (Hebrew) poetic; lyrical,
musical.

Liron (Hebrew) my song.
Leron, Lerone, Lirone

Lisa (Hebrew) consecrated to
God. (English) a short form
of Elizabeth.
Leeza, Liesa, Liisa, Lise,
Lisenka, Lisette, Liszka, Litsa,
Lysa

Lisbeth (English) a short form
of Elizabeth.
Lisbet

Lise (German) a form of Lisa.

Lisette, Lissette (French)
forms of Lisa. (English)
familiar forms of Elise,
Elizabeth.
Liset, Liseta, Lisete, Liseth,
Lisett, Lisetta, Lisettina, Lisset,
Lissete, Lissett, Lizet, Lizette,
Lysette

Lisha (Arabic) darkness before
midnight. (Hebrew) a short
form of Alisha, Elisha, Ilisha.
Lishe

Lissa (Greek) honey bee. A
short form of Elissa,
Elizabeth, Melissa, Millicent.
Lyssa

Lissie (American) a familiar
form of Allison, Elise,
Elizabeth.
Lissee, Lissey, Lissi, Lissy, Lissye

Lita (Latin) a familiar form of
names ending in "lita."
Leta, Litah, Litta

Litonya (Moquelumnan) dart-
ing hummingbird.

Liv (Latin) a short form of
Livia, Olivia.

Livana (Hebrew) a form of
Levana.
Livna, Livnat

Livia (Hebrew) crown. A
familiar form of Olivia.
(Latin) olive.
*Levia, Liv, Livie, Livy, Livya,
Livye*

Liviya (Hebrew) brave lioness;
royal crown.
Leviya, Levya, Livya

Livona (Hebrew) a form of
Levona.

Liz (English) a short form of
Elizabeth.

Liza (American) a short form
of Elizabeth.
Leeza, Lizela, Lizka, Lyza

Lizabeta (Russian) a form of
Elizabeth.
Lizabetah, Lizaveta, Lizonka

Lizabeth (English) a short
form of Elizabeth.
*Lisabet, Lisabeth, Lisabette,
Lizabette*

Lizbeth (English) a short form
of Elizabeth.
Lizbet, Lizbett

Lizet, Lizette (French) forms
of Lisette.
*Lizet, Lizete, Lizeth, Lizett,
Lizzet, Lizzeth, Lizzette*

Lizina (Latvian) a familiar
form of Elizabeth.

Lizzy (American) a familiar
form of Elizabeth.
Lizzie, Lizy

Logan (Irish) meadow.
*Logann, Loganne, Logen,
Loghan, Logun, Logyn, Logynn*

Lois (German) famous warrior.

Lola (Spanish) a familiar form
of Carlota, Dolores, Louise.
Lolah, Lolita

Lolita (Spanish) sorrowful. A
familiar form of Lola.
Lita, Lulita

Lolly (English) sweet; candy. A
familiar form of Laura.

Lolotea (Zuni) a form of
Dorothy.

Lomasi (Native American)
pretty flower.

Lona (Latin) lioness. (English)
solitary. (German) a short
form of Leona.
Loni, Lonna

London (English) fortress of
the moon. Geography: the
capital of the United
Kingdom.
*Landyn, Londen, Londun,
Londyn*

Loni (American) a form of
Lona.
Lonee, Lonie, Lonni, Lonnie

Lora (Latin) crowned with
laurel. (American) a form of
Laura.
*Lorah, Lorane, Lorann, Lorra,
Lorrah, Lorrane*

Lore (Basque) flower. (Latin) a short form of Flora.
Lor

Lorelei (German) alluring. Mythology: the siren of the Rhine River who lured sailors to their deaths. See also Lurleen.
Loralee, Loralei, Lorali, Loralie, Loralyn, Loreal, Lorelea, Loreli, Lorilee, Lorilyn

Lorelle (American) a form of Laurel.

Loren (American) a form of Lauren.
Loreen, Lorena, Lorin, Lorne, Lorren, Lorrin, Lorryn, Loryn, Lorynn, Lorynne

Lorena (English) a form of Lauren.
Lorene, Lorenea, Lorenia, Lorenna, Lorina, Lorrina, Lorrine, Lurana

Lorenza (Latin) a form of Laura.
Laurencia, Laurentia, Laurentina

Loretta (English) a familiar form of Laura.
Larretta, Lauretta, Laurette, Loretah, Lorette, Lorita, Lorretta, Lorrette

Lori (Latin) crowned with laurel. (French) a short form of Lorraine. (American) a familiar form of Laura.
Loree, Lorey, Loria, Lorianna,
Lorianne, Lorie, Lorree, Lorri, Lorrie, Lory

Lorin (American) a form of Loren.
Lorine

Lorinda (Spanish) a form of Laura.

Loris (Latin) thong. (Dutch) clown. (Greek) a short form of Chloris.
Laurice, Laurys, Lorice

Lorna (Latin) crowned with laurel. Literature: probably coined by Richard Blackmore in his novel *Lorna Doone*.
Lorrna

Lorraine (Latin) sorrowful. (French) from Lorraine, a former province of France. See also Rayna.
Laraine, Lorain, Loraine, Lorayne, Lorein, Loreine, Lori, Lorine, Lorrain, Lorraina, Lorrayne, Lorreine

Lotte (German) a short form of Charlotte.
Lotie, Lotta, Lottchen, Lottey, Lottie, Lotty, Loty

Lotus (Greek) lotus.

Lou (American) a short form of Louise, Luella.
Lu

Louam (Ethiopian) sleep well.

Louisa (English) a familiar form of Louise. Literature: Louisa May Alcott was an American writer and reformer best known for her novel *Little Women*.
Aloisa, Eloisa, Heloisa, Lou, Louisian, Louisane, Louisina, Louiza, Lovisa, Luisa, Luiza, Lujza, Lujzika

Louise (German) famous warrior. See also Alison, Eloise, Heloise, Lois, Lola, Ludovica, Luella, Lulu.
Loise, Lou, Louisa, Louisette, Louisiane, Louisine, Lowise, Loyce, Loyise, Luise

Lourdes (French) from Lourdes, France. Religion: a place where the Virgin Mary was said to have appeared.

Love (English) love, kindness, charity.
Lovely, Lovewell, Lovey, Lovie, Lovy, Luv, Luvvy

Lovisa (German) a form of Louisa.

Luann (Hebrew, German) graceful woman warrior. (Hawaiian) happy; relaxed. (American) a combination of Louise + Ann.
Louann, Louanne, Lu, Lua, Luan, Luane, Luanna, Luanne, Luanni, Luannie

Luanna (German) a form of Luann.
Lewanna, Louanna, Luana, Luwana

Lubov (Russian) love.
Luba, Lubna, Lubochka, Lyuba, Lyubov

Lucerne (Latin) lamp; circle of light. Geography: the Lake of Lucerne is in Switzerland.
Lucerna, Lucero

Lucero (Latin) a form of Lucerne.

Lucetta (English) a familiar form of Lucy.
Lucette

Lucia (Italian, Spanish) a form of Lucy.
Luciana, Lucianna

Lucie (French) a familiar form of Lucy.

Lucille (English) a familiar form of Lucy.
Lucila, Lucile, Lucilla

Lucinda (Latin) a form of Lucy. See also Cindy.

Lucine (Arabic) moon. (Basque) a form of Lucy.
Lucienne, Lucina, Lucyna, Lukene, Lusine, Luzine

Lucita (Spanish) a form of Lucy.
Lusita

Lucretia (Latin) rich; rewarded.
Lacrecia, Lucrece, Lucréce, Lucrecia,
Lucreecia, Lucresha, Lucreshia,
Lucrezia, Lucrisha, Lucrishia

Lucrezia (Italian) a form of
Lucretia. History: Lucrezia
Borgia was the Duchess of
Ferrara and a patron of
learning and the arts.

Lucy (Latin) light; bringer of
light.
Luca, Luce, Lucetta, Luci, Lucia,
Lucida, Lucie, Lucija, Lucika,
Lucille, Lucinda, Lucine, Lucita,
Luciya, Lucya, Luzca, Luzi

Ludmilla (Slavic) loved by the
people. See also Mila.
Ludie, Ludka, Ludmila, Lyuba,
Lyudmila

Ludovica (German) a form of
Louise.
Ludovika, Ludwiga

Luella (English) elf. (German)
a familiar form of Louise.
Loella, Lou, Louella, Ludella,
Luelle, Lula, Lulu

Luisa (Spanish) a form of Louisa.

Lulani (Polynesian) highest
point of heaven.

Lulu (Arabic) pearl. (English)
soothing, comforting. (Native
American) hare. (German) a
familiar form of Louise,
Luella.
Loulou, Lula, Lulie

Luna (Latin) moon.
Lunetta, Lunette, Lunneta,
Lunnete

Lupe (Latin) wolf. (Spanish) a
short form of Guadalupe.
Lupi, Lupita, Luppi

Lupita (Latin) a form of Lupe.

Lurleen, Lurlene
(Scandinavian) war horn.
(German) forms of Lorelei.
Lura, Lurette, Lurline

Lusa (Finnish) a form of
Elizabeth.

Lusela (Moquelumnan) like a
bear swinging its foot when
licking it.

Luvena (Latin, English) little;
beloved.
Lovena, Lovina, Luvenia, Luvina

Luyu (Moquelumnan) like a
pecking bird.

Luz (Spanish) light. Religion:
Nuestra Señora de Luz—Our
Lady of the Light—is another
name for the Virgin Mary.
Luzi, Luzija

Lycoris (Greek) twilight.

Lyda (Greek) a short form of
Lidia, Lydia.

Lydia (Greek) from Lydia, an
ancient land in Asia. (Arabic)
strife.
Lidia, Lidija, Lidiya, Lyda,
Lydie, Lydië

Lyla (French) island. (English) a form of Lyle (see Boys' Names). (Arabic, Hindi, Persian) a form of Lila.
Lila, Lilah

Lynda (Spanish) pretty. (American) a form of Linda.
Lyndah, Lynde, Lyndi, Lynnda

Lyndell (English) a form of Lynelle.
Lyndall, Lyndel, Lyndella

Lyndi (Spanish) a familiar form of Lynda.
Lyndee, Lindie, Lyndy, Lynndie, Lynndy

Lyndsay (American) a form of Lindsay.
Lyndsaye

Lyndsey (English) linden tree island; camp near the stream. (American) a form of Lindsey.
Lyndsea, Lyndsee, Lyndsi, Lyndsie, Lyndsy, Lyndzee, Lyndzey, Lyndzi, Lyndzie, Lynndsie

Lynelle (English) pretty.
Linel, Linell, Linnell, Lyndell, Lynel, Lynell, Lynella, Lynnell

Lynette (Welsh) idol. (English) a form of Linette.
Lynett, Lynetta, Lynnet, Lynnette

Lynn, Lynne (English) waterfall; pool below a waterfall.
Lin, Lina, Linley, Linn, Lyn,
Lynlee, Lynley, Lynna, Lynnae, Lynnea

Lynnell (English) a form of Lynelle.
Linnell, Lynnelle

Lynsey (American) a form of Lyndsey.
Lynnsey, Lynnzey, Lynsie, Lynsy, Lynzee, Lynzey, Lynzi, Lynzie, Lynzy

Lyra (Greek) lyre player.
Lyre, Lyric, Lyrica, Lyrie, Lyris

Lysandra (Greek) liberator.
Lisandra, Lysandre, Lytle

Lysanne (American) a combination of Lysandra + Anne.
Lisanne, Lizanne

M

Mab (Irish) joyous. (Welsh) baby. Literature: queen of the fairies.
Mabry

Mabel (Latin) lovable. A short form of Amabel.
Mabelle, Mable, Mabyn, Maible, Maybel, Maybeline, Maybelle, Maybull

Macawi (Dakota) generous; motherly.

Macayla (American) a form of
Michaela.
Macaela, Macaila, Macala,
Macalah, Macaylah, Macayle,
Macayli, Mackayla

Macey, Macie, Macy (Polish)
familiar forms of Macia.
Macee, Maci, Macye

Machaela (Hebrew) a form of
Michaela.
Machael, Machaelah, Machaelie,
Machaila, Machala, Macheala

Machiko (Japanese) fortunate
child.
Machi

Macia (Polish) a form of
Miriam.
Macelia, Macey, Machia, Macie,
Macy, Masha, Mashia

Mackenna (American) a form
of Mackenzie.
Mackena, Makenna, Mckenna

Mackenzie (Irish) child of the
wise leader. See also Kenzie.
Macenzie, Mackenna, Mackensi,
Mackensie, Mackenze,
Mackenzee, Mackenzey,
Mackenzi, Mackenzia,
Mackenzy, Mackenzye,
Mackinsey, Mackynze,
Makenzie, McKenzie,
Mckinzie, Mekenzie, Mykenzie

Mackinsey (Irish) a form of
Mackenzie.
Mackinsie, Mackinze, Mackinzee,
Mackinzey, Mackinzi, Mackinzie

Mada (English) a short form
of Madaline, Magdalen.
Madda, Mahda

Madaline (English) a form of
Madeline.
Mada, Madailéin, Madaleen,
Madaleine, Madalene, Madalin,
Madaline

Madalyn (Greek) a form of
Madeline.
Madalyne, Madalynn,
Madalynne

Maddie (English) a familiar
form of Madeline.
Maddi, Maddy, Mady, Maidie,
Maydey

Maddison (English) a form of
Madison.
Maddisan, Maddisen,
Maddisson, Maddisyn,
Maddyson

Madelaine (French) a form of
Madeline.
Madelane, Madelayne

Madeleine (French) a form of
Madeline.
Madalaine, Madalayne,
Madelaine, Madelein, Madeliene

Madelena (English) a form of
Madeline.
Madalaina, Madalena,
Madalina, Maddalena,
Madelaina, Madeleina,
Madelina, Madelyna

Madeline (Greek) high tower.
See also Lena, Lina, Maud.
*Madaline, Madalyn, Maddie,
Madel, Madelaine, Madeleine,
Madelena, Madelene, Madelia,
Madella, Madelle, Madelon,
Madelyn, Madge, Madilyn,
Madlen, Madlin, Madline,
Madlyn, Madolyn, Maida*

Madelyn (Greek) a form of
Madeline.
*Madelyne, Madelynn, Madelynne,
Madilyn, Madlyn, Madolyn*

Madge (Greek) a familiar
form of Madeline, Margaret.
Madgi, Madgie, Mady

Madilyn (Greek) a form of
Madeline.
*Madilen, Madiline, Madilyne,
Madilynn*

Madisen (English) a form of
Madison.
*Madisan, Madisin, Madissen,
Madisun*

Madison (English) good; child
of Maud.
*Maddison, Madisen, Madisson,
Madisyn, Madyson, Mattison*

Madisyn (English) a form of
Madison.
*Madissyn, Madisynn,
Madisynne*

Madolyn (Greek) a form of
Madeline.
*Madoline, Madolyne,
Madolynn, Madolynne*

Madonna (Latin) my lady.
Madona

Madrona (Spanish) mother.
Madre, Madrena

Madyson (English) a form of
Madison.
Madysen, Madysun

Mae (English) a form of May.
History: Mae Jemison was
the first African American
woman in space.
*Maelea, Maeleah, Maelen,
Maelle, Maeona*

Maegan (Irish) a form of
Megan.
Maegen, Maeghan, Maegin

Maeko (Japanese) honest
child.
Mae, Maemi

Maeve (Irish) joyous.
Mythology: a legendary
Celtic queen. See also Mavis.
Maevi, Maevy, Maive, Mayve

Magali, Magaly (Hebrew)
from the high tower.
Magalie, Magally

Magan, Magen (Greek) forms
of Megan.
Maggen, Maggin

Magda (Czech, Polish, Russian)
a form of Magdalen.
Mahda, Makda

Magdalen (Greek) high tower.
Bible: Magdala was the home
of Saint Mary Magdalen. See

also Madeline, Malena,
Marlene.
Mada, Magda, Magdala,
Magdaleen, Magdalena,
Magdalene, Magdaline,
Magdalyn, Magdalynn,
Magdelane, Magdelene,
Magdeline, Magdelyn, Magdlen,
Magdolna, Maggie, Magola,
Maighdlin, Mala, Malaine

Magdalena (Greek) a form of
Magdalen.
Magdalina, Magdelana,
Magdelena, Magdelina

Magena (Native American)
coming moon.

Maggie (Greek) pearl.
(English) a familiar form of
Magdalen, Margaret.
Mag, Magge, Maggee, Maggi,
Maggia, Maggie, Maggiemae,
Maggy, Magi, Magie, Mags

Maggy, Meggy (English)
forms of Maggie.
Maggey, Magy

Magnolia (Latin) flowering
tree. See also Nollie.
Nola

Mahal (Filipino) love.

Mahala (Arabic) fat, marrow;
tender. (Native American)
powerful woman.
Mahalah, Mahalar, Mahalla,
Mahela, Mahila, Mahlah,
Mahlaha, Mehala, Mehalah

Mahalia (American) a form of
Mahala.
Mahaley, Mahaliah, Mahalie,
Mahayla, Mahaylah, Mahaylia,
Mahelea, Maheleah, Mahelia,
Mahilia, Mehalia

Maharene (Ethiopian) forgive
us.

Mahesa (Hindi) great lord.
Religion: a name for the
Hindu god Shiva.
Maheesa, Mahisa

Mahila (Sanskrit) woman.

Mahina (Hawaiian) moon
glow.

Mahira (Hebrew) energetic.
Mahri

Mahogony (Spanish) rich;
strong.
Mahagony, Mahoganey,
Mahogani, Mahoganie,
Mahogany, Mahogney,
Mahogny, Mohogany, Mohogony

Mai (Japanese) brightness.
(Vietnamese) flower.
(Navajo) coyote.

Maia (Greek) mother; nurse.
(English) kinswoman;
maiden. Mythology: the
loveliest of the Pleiades, the
seven daughters of Atlas, and
the mother of Hermes. See
also Maya.
Maiah, Maie, Maiya

Maida (English) maiden.
(Greek) a short form of
Madeline.
Maidel, Mayda, Maydena

Maija (Finnish) a form of
Mary.
Maiji, Maikki

Maika (Hebrew) a familiar
form of Michaela.
Maikala, Maikka, Maiko

Maira, Maire (Irish) forms of
Mary.
*Maairah, Mair, Mairi, Mairim,
Mairin, Mairona, Mairwen*

Maisie (Scottish) familiar
forms of Margaret.
*Maisa, Maise, Maisey, Maisi,
Maisy, Maizie, Maycee, Maysie,
Mayzie, Mazey, Mazie, Mazy,
Mazzy, Mysie, Myzie*

Maita (Spanish) a form of
Martha.
Maite, Maitia

Maitlyn (American) a combi-
nation of Maita + Lynn.
*Maitlan, Maitland, Maitlynn,
Mattilyn*

Maiya (Greek) a form of
Maia.
Maiyah

Maja (Arabic) a short form of
Majidah.
*Majal, Majalisa, Majalyn,
Majalynn*

Majidah (Arabic) splendid.
Maja, Majida

Makaela, Makaila (American)
forms of Michaela.
*Makaelah, Makaelee, Makaella,
Makaely, Makail, Makailah,
Makailee, Makailla, Makaillah,
Makealah, Makell*

Makala (Hawaiian) myrtle.
(Hebrew) a form of
Michaela.
*Makalae, Makalah, Makalai,
Makalea, Makalee, Makaleh,
Makaleigh, Makaley, Makalia,
Makalie, Makalya, Makela,
Makelah, Makell, Makella*

Makana (Hawaiian) gift, present.

Makani (Hawaiian) wind.

Makara (Hindi) Astrology:
another name for the zodiac
sign Capricorn.

Makayla (American) a form of
Michaela.
*Macayla, Makaylah, Makaylee,
Makayleigh, Makayli,
Makaylia, Makaylla, Makell,
Makyla, Makylah, Mckayla,
Mekayla, Mikayla*

Makell (American) a short
form of Makaela, Makala,
Makayla.
Makele, Makelle, Mckell, Mekel

Makenna (American) a form
of Mackenna.
Makena, Makennah, Mikenna

Makenzie (Irish) a form of
Mackenzie.
*Makense, Makensey, Makensie,
Makenze, Makenzee,
Makenzey, Makenzi, Makenzy,
Makenzye, Makinzey,
Makynzey, Mekenzie,
Mykenzie*

Mala (Greek) a short form of
Magdalen.
Malana, Malee, Mali

Malana (Hawaiian) bouyant,
light.

Malaya (Filipino) free.
*Malayaa, Malayah, Malayna,
Malea, Maleah*

Malena (Swedish) a familiar
form of Magdalen.
*Malen, Malenna, Malin,
Malina, Maline, Malini,
Malinna*

Malha (Hebrew) queen.
*Maliah, Malkah, Malkia,
Malkiah, Malkie, Malkiya,
Malkiyah, Miliah*

Mali (Tai) jasmine flower.
(Tongan) sweet. (Hungarian)
a short form of Malika.
Malea, Malee, Maley

Malia (Hawaiian, Zuni) a form
of Mary. (Spanish) a form of
Maria.
*Malea, Maleah, Maleeya,
Maleeyah, Maleia, Maliah,
Maliasha, Malie, Maliea,
Maliya, Maliyah, Malli, Mally*

Malika (Hungarian) industri-
ous. (Arabic) queen.
*Malak, Maleeka, Maleka, Mali,
Maliaka, Malik, Malikah,
Malikee, Maliki, Malikia,
Malky*

Malina (Hebrew) tower.
(Native American) soothing.
(Russian) raspberry.
*Malin, Maline, Malina,
Malinna, Mallie*

Malinda (Greek) a form of
Melinda.
Malinde, Malinna, Malynda

Malini (Hindi) gardener.
Maliny

Malissa (Greek) a form of
Melissa.
Malisa, Malisah, Malyssa

Mallalai (Pashto) beautiful.

Malley (American) a familiar
form of Mallory.
*Mallee, Malli, Mallie, Mally,
Maly*

Mallorie (French) a form of
Mallory.
*Malerie, Mallari, Mallerie,
Malloreigh, Mallori*

Mallory (German) army
counselor. (French) unlucky.
*Maliri, Mallary, Mallauri,
Mallery, Malley, Malloree,
Mallorey, Mallorie, Malorie,
Malory, Malorym, Malree,
Malrie, Mellory*

Malorie, Malory (German) forms of Mallory.
Malarie, Maloree, Malori, Melorie, Melory

Malva (English) a form of Melba.
Malvi, Malvy

Malvina (Scottish) a form of Melvina. Literature: a name created by the eighteenth-century romantic poet James Macpherson.
Malvane, Malvi

Mamie (American) a familiar form of Margaret.
Mame, Mamee, Mami, Mammie, Mamy, Mamye

Mamo (Hawaiian) saffron flower; yellow bird.

Mana (Hawaiian) psychic; sensitive.
Manal, Manali, Manna, Mannah

Manar (Arabic) guiding light.
Manayra

Manda (Spanish) woman warrior. (Latin) a short form of Amanda.
Mandy

Mandara (Hindi) calm.

Mandeep (Punjabi) enlightened.

Mandisa (Xhosa) sweet.

Mandy (Latin) lovable. A familiar form of Amanda, Manda, Melinda.
Mandee, Mandi, Mandie

Manette (French) a form of Mary.

Mangena (Hebrew) song, melody.
Mangina

Mani (Chinese) a mantra repeated in Tibetan Buddhist prayer to impart understanding.
Manee

Manka (Polish, Russian) a form of Mary.

Manon (French) a familiar form of Marie.
Mannon

Manpreet (Punjabi) mind full of love.
Manprit

Mansi (Hopi) plucked flower.
Mancey, Manci, Mancie, Mansey, Mansie, Mansy

Manuela (Spanish) a form of Emmanuelle.
Manuala, Manuelita, Manuella, Manuelle

Manya (Russian) a form of Mary.

Mara (Hebrew) melody. (Greek) a short form of Amara. (Slavic) a form of Mary.
Mahra, Marae, Marah, Maralina, Maraline, Marra

Marabel (English) a form of Mirabel.
Marabella, Marabelle

Maranda (Latin) a form of Miranda.

Maraya (Hebrew) a form of Mariah.
Mareya

Marcela (Latin) a form of Marcella.
Marcele, Marcelen, Marcelia, Marcelina, Marceline, Maricela

Marcelen (English) a form of Marcella.
Marcelen, Marcelin, Marcelina, Marceline, Marcellin, Marcellina, Marcelline, Marcelyn, Marcilen

Marcella (Latin) martial, warlike. Mythology: Mars was the god of war.
Mairsil, Marca, Marce, Marceil, Marcela, Marcelen, Marcell, Marcelle, Marcello, Marcena, Marchella, Marchelle, Marci, Marcia, Marcie, Marciella, Marcile, Marcilla, Marcille, Marella, Marsella, Marselle, Marsiella

Marcena (Latin) a form of Marcella, Marcia.
Maracena, Marceen, Marcene, Marcenia, Marceyne, Marcina

Marci, Marcie (English) familiar forms of Marcella, Marcia.
Marca, Marcee, Marcita, Marcy, Marsi, Marsie

Marcia (Latin) martial, warlike. See also Marquita.
Marcena, Marchia, Marci, Marciale, Marcie, Marcsa, Marsha, Martia

Marciann (American) a combination of Marci + Ann.
Marciane, Marcianna, Marcianne, Marcyane, Marcyanna, Marcyanne

Marcilynn (American) a combination of Marci + Lynn.
Marcilen, Marcilin, Marciline, Marcilyn, Marcilyne, Marcilynne, Marcylen, Marcylin, Marcyline, Marcylyn, Marcylyne, Marcylynn, Marcylynne

Marcy (English) a form of Marci.
Marsey, Marsy

Mardi (French) born on Tuesday. (Aramaic) a familiar form of Martha.

Mare (Irish) a form of Mary.
Mair, Maire

Marelda (German) renowned warrior.
Marella, Marilda

Maren (Latin) sea. (Aramaic) a form of Mary. See also Marina.
Marin, Marine, Marinn, Miren

Maresa, Maressa (Latin)
forms of Marisa.
Maresha, Meresa

Maretta (English) a familiar
form of Margaret.
Maret, Marette

Margaret (Greek) pearl.
History: Margaret Hilda
Thatcher served as British
prime minister. See also Gita,
Greta, Gretchen, Marjorie,
Markita, Meg, Megan, Peggy,
Reet, Rita.
*Madge, Maergrethe, Maggie,
Maisie, Mamie, Maretta, Marga,
Margalo, Marganit, Margara,
Maretha, Margarett, Margarette,
Margarida, Margarit, Margarita,
Margaro, Margaux, Marge,
Margeret, Margeretta,
Margerette, Margery, Margetta,
Margiad, Margie, Margisia,
Margit, Margo, Margot, Margret,
Marguerite, Meta*

Margarit (Greek) a form of
Margaret.
*Margalide, Margalit, Margalith,
Margarid, Margaritt, Margerit*

Margarita (Italian, Spanish) a
form of Margaret.
*Margareta, Margaretta,
Margarida, Margaritis,
Margaritta, Margeretta,
Margharita, Margherita,
Margrieta, Margrita,
Marguarita, Marguerita,
Margurita*

Margaux (French) a form of
Margaret.
Margeaux

Marge (English) a short form
of Margaret, Marjorie.
Margie

Margery (English) a form of
Margaret.
Margerie, Margorie

Margie (English) a familiar
form of Marge, Margaret.
Margey, Margi, Margy

Margit (Hungarian) a form of
Margaret.
Marget, Margette, Margita

Margo, Margot (French)
forms of Margaret.
Mago, Margaro

Margret (German) a form of
Margaret.
*Margreta, Margrete, Margreth,
Margrett, Margretta, Margrette,
Margrieta, Margrita*

Marguerite (French) a form
of Margaret.
*Margarete, Margaretha,
Margarethe, Margarite,
Margerite, Marguaretta,
Marguarette, Marguarite,
Marguerette, Margurite*

Mari (Japanese) ball. (Spanish)
a form of Mary.

Maria (Hebrew) bitter; sea of
bitterness. (Italian, Spanish) a
form of Mary.
*Maie, Malia, Marea, Mareah,
Mariabella, Mariae, Mariesa,
Mariessa, Mariha, Marija,
Mariya, Mariyah, Marja, Marya*

Mariah (Hebrew) a form of
Mary. See also Moriah.
*Maraia, Maraya, Mariyah,
Marriah, Meriah*

Mariam (Hebrew) a form of
Miriam.
*Mariama, Mariame, Mariem,
Meryam*

Marian (English) a form of
Maryann.
*Mariana, Mariane, Mariann,
Marianne, Mariene, Marion,
Marrian, Marriann*

Mariana, Marianna (Spanish)
forms of Marian.
*Marriana, Marrianna, Maryana,
Maryanna*

Mariane, Marianne (English)
forms of Marian.
Marrianne, Maryanne

Maribel (French) beautiful.
(English) a combination of
Maria + Bell.
*Marabel, Marbelle, Mariabella,
Maribella, Maribelle, Maridel,
Marybel, Marybella, Marybelle*

Marice (Italian) a form of
Mary. See also Maris.
Marica, Marise, Marisse

Maricela (Latin) a form of
Marcella.
*Maricel, Mariceli, Maricelia,
Maricella, Maricely*

Maridel (English) a form of
Maribel.

Marie (French) a form of
Mary.
Maree, Marietta, Marrie

Mariel, Marielle (German,
Dutch) forms of Mary.
*Marial, Marieke, Marielana,
Mariele, Marieli, Marielie,
Marieline, Mariell, Mariellen,
Marielsie, Mariely, Marielys*

Mariela, Mariella (German,
Dutch) forms of Mary.

Marietta (Italian) a familiar
form of Marie.
*Maretta, Marette, Mariet,
Mariette, Marrietta*

Marieve (American) a combination of Mary + Eve.

Marigold (English) Mary's
gold. Botany: a plant with
yellow or orange flowers.
Marygold

Marika (Dutch, Slavic) a form
of Mary.
*Marica, Marieke, Marija,
Marijke, Marikah, Marike,
Marikia, Marikka, Mariska,
Mariske, Marrika, Maryk,
Maryka, Merica, Merika*

Mariko (Japanese) circle.

Marilee (American) a combi-
nation of Mary + Lee.
*Marili, Marilie, Marily,
Marrilee, Marylea, Marylee,
Merrilee, Merrili, Merrily*

Marilla (Hebrew, German) a
form of Mary.
Marella, Marelle

Marilou (American) a form of
Marylou.
Marilu, Mariluz

Marilyn (Hebrew) Mary's line
of descendants. See also
Merilyn.
*Maralin, Maralyn, Maralyne,
Maralynn, Maralynne, Marelyn,
Marilin, Marillyn, Marilyne,
Marilynn, Marilynne, Marlyn,
Marolyn, Marralynn, Marrilin,
Marrilyn, Marrilynn,
Marrilynne, Marylin, Marylinn,
Marylyn, Marylyne, Marylynn,
Marylynne*

Marina (Latin) sea. See also
Maren.
*Mareena, Marena, Marenka,
Marinae, Marinah, Marinda,
Marindi, Marinka, Marinna,
Marrina, Maryna, Merina,
Mirena*

Marini (Swahili) healthy;
pretty.

Marion (French) a form of
Mary.
*Marrian, Marrion, Maryon,
Maryonn*

Maris (Latin) sea. (Greek) a
short form of Amaris,
Damaris. See also Marice.
*Maries, Marise, Marris, Marys,
Maryse, Meris*

Marisa (Latin) sea.
*Maresa, Mariesa, Mariessa,
Marisela, Marissa, Marita,
Mariza, Marrisa, Marrissa,
Marysa, Maryse, Maryssa,
Merisa*

Marisela (Latin) a form of
Marisa.
*Mariseli, Marisella, Marishelle,
Marissela*

Marisha (Russian) a familiar
form of Mary.
*Mareshah, Marishenka,
Marishka, Mariska*

Marisol (Spanish) sunny sea.
Marise, Marizol, Marysol

Marissa (Latin) a form of
Maris, Marisa.
*Maressa, Marisa, Marisha,
Marissah, Marisse, Marizza,
Marrissa, Marrissia, Maryssa,
Merissa, Morissa*

Marit (Aramaic) lady.
Marita, Marite

Marita (Spanish) a form of
Marisa. (Aramaic) a form of
Marit.
Marité, Maritha

Maritza (Arabic) blessed.
Maritsa, Maritssa

Mariyan (Arabic) purity.
*Mariya, Mariyah, Mariyana,
Mariyanna*

Marja (Finnish) a form of
Mary.
Marjae, Marjatta, Marjie

Marjan (Persian) coral. (Polish)
a form of Mary.
Marjaneh, Marjanna

Marjie (Scottish) a familiar
form of Marjorie.
Marje, Marjey, Marji, Marjy

Marjolaine (French) marjo-
ram.

Marjorie (Greek) a familiar
form of Margaret. (Scottish)
a form of Mary.
*Majorie, Marge, Margeree,
Margerey, Margerie, Margery,
Margorie, Margory, Marjarie,
Marjary, Marjerie, Marjery,
Marjie, Marjorey, Marjori,
Marjory*

Markayla (American) a com-
bination or Mary + Kayla.
*Marka, Markaiah, Markaya,
Markayel, Markeela, Markel*

Markeisha (English) a combi-
nation of Mary + Keisha.
*Markasha, Markeisa, Markeisia,
Markesha, Markeshia,
Markesia, Markiesha, Markisha,
Markishia, Marquesha*

Markita (Czech) a form of
Margaret.
Marka, Markeah, Markeda,

*Markee, Markeeta, Marketa,
Marketta, Marki, Markia,
Markie, Markieta, Markita,
Markitha, Markketta, Merkate*

Marla (English) a short form
of Marlena, Marlene.
Marlah, Marlea, Marleah

Marlana (English) a form of
Marlena.
*Marlaena, Marlaina, Marlainna,
Marlania, Marlanna, Marlayna,
Marleana*

Marlee (English) a form of
Marlene.
Marlea, Marleah, Marleigh

Marlena (German) a form of
Marlene.
*Marla, Marlaina, Marlana,
Marlanna, Marleena, Marlina,
Marlinda, Marlyna, Marna*

Marlene (Greek) high tower.
(Slavic) a form of Magdalen.
*Marla, Marlaine, Marlane,
Marlayne, Marlee, Marleen,
Marleene, Marlen, Marlena,
Marlenne, Marley, Marlin,
Marline, Marlyne*

Marley (English) a familiar
form of Marlene.
Marlee, Marli, Marlie, Marly

Marlis (English) a combina-
tion of Maria + Lisa.
*Marles, Marlisa, Marlise,
Marlys, Marlyse, Marlyssa*

Marlo (English) a form of Mary.
Marlon, Marlow, Marlowe

Marlyn (Hebrew) a short form of Marilyn. (Greek, Slavic) a form of Marlene.
Marlynn, Marlynne

Marmara (Greek) sparkling, shining.
Marmee

Marni (Hebrew) a form of Marnie.
Marnia, Marnique

Marnie (Hebrew) a short form of Marnina.
Marna, Marnay, Marne, Marnee, Marney, Marni, Marnisha, Marnja, Marny, Marnya, Marnye

Marnina (Hebrew) rejoice.

Maroula (Greek) a form of Mary.

Marquise (French) noblewoman.
Markese, Marquees, Marquese, Marquice, Marquies, Marquiese, Marquis, Marquisa, Marquisee, Marquisha, Marquisse, Marquiste

Marquisha (American) a form of Marquise.
Marquiesha, Marquisia

Marquita (Spanish) a form of Marcia.
Marquatte, Marqueda,

Marquedia, Marquee, Marqueita, Marquet, Marqueta, Marquetta, Marquette, Marquia, Marquida, Marquietta, Marquitra, Marquitia, Marquitta

Marrim (Chinese) tribal name in Manpur state.

Marsala (Italian) from Marseilles, France.
Marsali, Marseilles

Marsha (English) a form of Marcia.
Marcha, Marshae, Marshay, Marshel, Marshele, Marshell, Marshia, Marshiela

Marta (English) a short form of Martha, Martina.
Martá, Martä, Marte, Martia, Marttaha, Merta

Martha (Aramaic) lady; sorrowful. Bible: a friend of Jesus. See also Mardi.
Maita, Marta, Martaha, Marth, Marthan, Marthe, Marthy, Marti, Marticka, Martita, Mattie, Matty, Martus, Martuska, Masia

Marti (English) a familiar form of Martha, Martina.
Martie, Marty

Martina (Latin) martial, warlike. See also Tina.
Marta, Martel, Martella, Martelle, Martene, Marthena, Marthina, Marthine, Marti, Martine, Martinia, Martino,

Martisha, Martosia, Martoya,
Martricia, Martrina, Martyna,
Martyne, Martynne

Martiza (Arabic) blessed.

Maru (Japanese) round.

Maruca (Spanish) a form of
Mary.
Maruja, Maruska

Marvella (French) marvelous.
Marva, Marvel, Marvela,
Marvele, Marvelle, Marvely,
Marvetta, Marvette, Marvia,
Marvina

Mary (Hebrew) bitter; sea of
bitterness. Bible: the mother
of Jesus. See also Maija,
Malia, Maren, Mariah,
Marjorie, Maura, Maureen,
Miriam, Mitzi, Moira,
Mollie, Muriel.
Maira, Maire, Manette, Manka,
Manon, Manya, Mara, Mare,
Maree, Maren, Marella, Marelle,
Mari, Maria, Maricara, Marice,
Marie, Mariel, Mariela, Marika,
Marilla, Marilyn, Marion,
Mariquilla, Mariquita, Marisha,
Marja, Marjan, Marlo, Maroula,
Maruca, Marye, Maryla,
Marynia, Masha, Mavra,
Mendi, Mérane, Meridel,
Mhairie, Mirja, Molara, Morag,
Moya

Marya (Arabic) purity; bright
whiteness.
Maryah

Maryam (Hebrew) a form of
Miriam.
Maryama

Maryann, Maryanne (English)
combinations of Mary +
Ann.
Marian, Marryann, Maryan,
Meryem

Marybeth (American) a combination of Mary + Beth.
Maribeth, Maribette

Maryellen (American) a combination of Mary + Ellen.
Mariellen

Maryjane (American) a combination of Mary + Jane.

Maryjo (American) a combination of Mary + Jo.
Marijo, Maryjoe

Marykate (American) a combination of Mary + Kate.
Mary-Kate

Marylou (American) a combination of Mary + Lou.
Marilou, Marylu

Maryssa (Latin) a form of
Marissa.
Maryse, Marysia

Masago (Japanese) sands of
time.

Masani (Luganda) gap
toothed.

Masha (Russian) a form of
Mary.
Mashka, Mashenka

Mashika (Swahili) born during the rainy season.
Masika

Matana (Hebrew) gift.
Matat

Mathena (Hebrew) gift of
God.

Mathilde (German) a form of
Matilda.
Mathilda

Matilda (German) powerful
battler. See also Maud, Tilda,
Tillie.
*Máda, Mahaut, Maitilde,
Malkin, Mat, Matelda,
Mathilde, Matilde, Mattie,
Matty, Matusha, Matylda*

Matrika (Hindi) mother.
Religion: a name for the
Hindu goddess Shakti in the
form of the letters of the
alphabet.
Matrica

Matsuko (Japanese) pine tree.

Mattea (Hebrew) gift of God.
*Matea, Mathea, Mathia, Matia,
Matte, Matthea, Matthia,
Mattia, Matya*

Mattie, Matty (English) familiar forms of Martha, Matilda.
Matte, Mattey, Matti, Mattye

Matusha (Spanish) a form of
Matilda.
Matuja, Matuxa

Maud, Maude (English) short
forms of Madeline, Matilda.
See also Madison.
Maudie, Maudine, Maudlin

Maura (Irish) dark. A form of
Mary, Maureen. See also
Moira.
*Maurah, Maure, Maurette,
Mauricette, Maurita*

Maureen (French) dark. (Irish)
a form of Mary.
*Maura, Maurene, Maurine, Mo,
Moreen, Morena, Morene,
Morine, Morreen, Moureen*

Maurelle (French) dark; elfin.
Mauriel, Mauriell, Maurielle

Maurise (French) dark
skinned; moor; marshland.
*Maurisa, Maurissa, Maurita,
Maurizia*

Mausi (Native American)
plucked flower.

Mauve (French) violet
colored.

Mavis (French) thrush, song-
bird. See also Maeve.
*Mavies, Mavin, Mavine,
Mavon, Mavra*

Maxie (English) a familiar
form of Maxine.
Maxi, Maxy

Maxine (Latin) greatest.
Max, Maxa, Maxeen, Maxena,
Maxene, Maxie, Maxima,
Maxime, Maximiliane, Maxina,
Maxna, Maxyne

May (Latin) great. (Arabic)
discerning. (English) flower;
month of May. See also Mae,
Maia.
Maj, Mayberry, Maybeth,
Mayday, Maydee, Maydena,
Maye, Mayela, Mayella,
Mayetta, Mayrene

Maya (Hindi) God's creative
power. (Greek) mother;
grandmother. (Latin) great. A
form of Maia.
Mayam, Mya

Maybeline (Latin) a familiar
form of Mabel.

Maygan, Maygen (Irish) forms
of Megan.
Mayghan, Maygon

Maylyn (American) a combi-
nation of May + Lynn.
Mayelene, Mayleen, Maylen,
Maylene, Maylin, Maylon,
Maylynn, Maylynne

Mayoree (Tai) beautiful.
Mayra, Mayree, Mayariya

Mayra (Tai) a form of
Mayoree.

Maysa (Arabic) walks with a
proud stride.

Maysun (Arabic) beautiful.

Mazel (Hebrew) lucky.
Mazal, Mazala, Mazella

Mckayla (American) a form of
Makayla.
Mckaela, Mckaila, Mckala,
Mckaylah, Mckayle, Mckaylee,
Mckayleh, Mckayleigh, Mckayli,
Mckaylia, Mckaylie

Mckell (American) a form of
Makell.
Mckelle

Mckenna (American) a form
of Mackenna.
Mckena, Mckennah, Mckinna,
Mckinnah

Mckenzie (Scottish) a form of
Mackenzie.
Mckennzie, Mckensee,
Mckensey, McKensi, Mckensi,
Mckensie, Mckensy, Mckenze,
Mckenzee, Mckenzey, Mckenzi,
Mckenzy, Mckenzye, Mekensie,
Mekenzi, Mekenzie

Mckinley (Irish) daughter of
the learned ruler.
Mckinlee, Mckinleigh, Mckinlie,
Mckinnley

Mckinzie (American) a form
of Mackenzie.
Mckinsey, Mckinze, Mckinzea,
Mckinzee, Mckinzi, Mckinzy,
Mckynze, Mckynzie

Mead, Meade (Greek) honey
wine.

Meagan (Irish) a form of
Megan.
*Maegan, Meagain, Meagann,
Meagen, Meagin, Meagnah,
Meagon*

Meaghan (Welsh) a form of
Megan.
*Maeghan, Meaghann, Meaghen,
Meahgan*

Meara (Irish) mirthful.

Meda (Native American)
prophet; priestess.

Medea (Greek) ruling. (Latin)
middle. Mythology: a sorcer-
ess who helped Jason get the
Golden Fleece.
Medeia

Medina (Arabic) History: the
site of Muhammed's tomb.
Medinah

Medora (Greek) mother's gift.
Literature: a character in
Lord Byron's poem *The
Corsair.*

Meena (Hindi) blue
semiprecious stone; bird.
(Greek, German, Dutch) a
form of Mena.

Meg (English) a short form of
Margaret, Megan.

Megan (Greek) pearl; great.
(Irish) a form of Margaret.
*Maegan, Magan, Magen,
⸤aegan, Meaghan, Magen,
⸤ ⸥gan, Maygen, Meg, Megane,*

*Megann, Megean, Megen,
Meggan, Meggen, Meggie,
Meghan, Megyn, Meygan*

Megane (Irish) a form of
Megan.
Magana, Meganna, Meganne

Megara (Greek) first.
Mythology: Heracles's first
wife.

Meggie (English) a familiar
form of Margaret, Megan.
Meggi, Meggy

Meghan (Welsh) a form of
Megan.
*Meeghan, Meehan, Megha,
Meghana, Meghane, Meghann,
Meghanne, Meghean, Meghen,
Mehgan, Mehgen*

Mehadi (Hindi) flower.

Mehira (Hebrew) speedy;
energetic.
Mahira

Mehitabel (Hebrew) benefited
by trusting God.
*Mehetabel, Mehitabelle, Hetty,
Hitty*

Mehri (Persian) kind; lovable;
sunny.

Mei (Hawaiian) great. (Chinese)
a short form of Meiying.
Meiko

Meira (Hebrew) light.
Meera

Meit (Burmese) affectionate.

Meiying (Chinese) beautiful flower.
Mei

Meka (Hebrew) a familiar form of Michaela.

Mekayla (American) a form of Michaela.
Mekaela, Mekaila, Mekayela, Mekaylia

Mel (Portuguese, Spanish) sweet as honey.

Mela (Hindi) religious service. (Polish) a form of Melanie.

Melana (Russian) a form of Melanie.
Melanna, Melashka, Melenka, Milana

Melanie (Greek) dark skinned.
Malania, Malanie, Meila, Meilani, Meilin, Melaine, Melainie, Melana, Melane, Melanee, Melaney, Melani, Melania, Mélanie, Melanka, Melanney, Melannie, Melany, Melanya, Melasya, Melayne, Melenia, Mella, Mellanie, Melonie, Melya, Milena, Milya

Melantha (Greek) dark flower.

Melba (Greek) soft; slender. (Latin) mallow flower.
Malva, Melva

Mele (Hawaiian) song; poem.

Melesse (Ethiopian) eternal.
Mellesse

Melia (German) a short form of Amelia.
Melcia, Melea, Meleah, Meleia, Meleisha, Meli, Meliah, Melida, Melika, Mema

Melina (Latin) canary yellow. (Greek) a short form of Melinda.
Melaina, Meleana, Meleena, Melena, Meline, Melinia, Melinna, Melynna

Melinda (Greek) honey. See also Linda, Melina, Mindy.
Maillie, Malinda, Melinde, Melinder, Mellinda, Melynda, Melyne, Milinda, Milynda, Mylenda, Mylinda, Mylynda

Meliora (Latin) better.
Melior, Meliori, Mellear, Melyor, Melyora

Melisa (Greek) a form of Melissa.
Melesa, Mélisa, Melise, Melisha, Melishia, Melisia, Meliza, Melizah, Mellisa, Melosa, Milisa, Mylisa, Mylisia

Melisande (French) a form of Melissa, Millicent.
Lisandra, Malisande, Malissande, Malyssandre, Melesande, Melisandra, Melisandre, Mélisandré, Melisenda, Melissande, Melissandre, Mellisande, Melond, Melysande, Melyssandre

Melissa (Greek) honey bee.
See also Elissa, Lissa,
Melisande, Millicent.
*Malissa, Mallissa, Melessa,
Meleta, Melisa, Mélissa,
Melisse, Melissia, Mellie,
Mellissa, Melly, Melyssa,
Milissa, Millie, Milly, Missy,
Molissia, Mollissa, Mylissa,
Mylissia*

Melita (Greek) a form of
Melissa. (Spanish) a short
form of Carmelita.
*Malita, Meleeta, Melitta,
Melitza, Melletta, Molita*

Melly (American) a familiar
form of names beginning
with "Mel." See also Millie.
Meli, Melie, Melli, Mellie

Melody (Greek) melody. See
also Elodie.
*Meladia, Melodee, Melodey,
Melodi, Melodia, Melodie,
Melodyann, Melodye*

Melonie (American) a form of
Melanie.
*Melloney, Mellonie, Mellony,
Melonee, Meloney, Meloni,
Melonie, Melonnie, Melony*

Melosa (Spanish) sweet; tender.

Melvina (Irish) armored chief.
See also Malvina.
*Melevine, Melva, Melveen,
Melvena, Melvene, Melvonna*

Melyne (Greek) a short form
of Melinda.
Melyn, Melynn, Melynne

Melyssa (Greek) a form of
Melissa.

Mena (German, Dutch)
strong. (Greek) a short form
of Philomena. History:
Menes is believed to be the
first king of Egypt.
Menah

Mendi (Basque) a form of
Mary.
Menda, Mendy

Meranda (Latin) a form of
Miranda.
*Merana, Merandah, Merandia,
Merannda*

Mérane (French) a form of
Mary.
Meraine, Merrane

Mercedes (Latin) reward, pay-
ment. (Spanish) merciful.
*Mercades, Mercadez, Mercadie,
Meceades, Merced, Mercede,
Mercedees, Mercedeez,
Mercedez, Mercedies, Mercedis,
Mersade, Mersades*

Mercia (English) a form of
Marcia. History: an ancient
British kingdom.

Mercy (English) compassion-
ate, merciful. See also Merry.
*Mercey, Merci, Mercie, Mercille,
Mersey*

Meredith (Welsh) protector of the sea.
Meredeth, Meredithe, Meredy, Meredyth, Meredythe, Meridath, Merideth, Meridie, Meridith, Merridie, Merridith, Merry

Meri (Finnish) sea. (Irish) a short form of Meriel.

Meriel (Irish) shining sea.
Meri, Merial, Meriol, Meryl

Merilyn (English) a combination of Merry + Lynn. See also Marilyn.
Merelyn, Merlyn, Merralyn, Merrelyn, Merrilyn

Merissa (Latin) a form of Marissa.
Merisa, Merisha

Merle (Latin, French) blackbird.
Merl, Merla, Merlina, Merline, Merola, Murle, Myrle, Myrleen, Myrlene, Myrline

Merry (English) cheerful, happy. A familiar form of Mercy, Meredith.
Merie, Merree, Merri, Merrie, Merrielle, Merrilee, Merrili, Merrilyn, Merris, Merrita

Meryl (German) famous. (Irish) shining sea. A form of Meriel, Muriel.
Meral, Merel, Merrall, Merrell, Merril, Merrile, Merrill, Merryl, Meryle, Meryll

Mesha (Hindi) another name for the zodiac sign Aries.
Meshal

Meta (German) a short form of Margaret.
Metta, Mette, Metti

Mhairie (Scottish) a form of Mary.
Mhaire, Mhairi, Mhari, Mhary

Mia (Italian) mine. A familiar form of Michaela, Michelle.
Mea, Meah, Miah

Micaela (Hebrew) a form of Michaela.
Macaela, Micaella, Micaila, Micala, Miceala

Micah (Hebrew) a short form of Michaela. Bible: one of the Old Testament prophets.
Meecah, Mica, Micha, Mika, Myca, Mycah

Micayla, Michayla (Hebrew) forms of Michaela.
Micayle, Micaylee, Michaylah

Michaela (Hebrew) who is like God?
Machaela, Maika, Makaela, Makaila, Makala, Makayla, Mia, Micaela, Micayla, Michael, Michaelann, Michala, Michayla, Michealia, Michaelina, Michaeline, Michaell, Michaella, Michaelyn, Michaila, Michal, Michala, Micheal, Micheala, Michelia, Michelina, Michelle, Michely, Michelyn, Micheyla,

Michaela (cont.)
Micheline, Micki, Miguela,
Mikaela, Mikala, Misha,
Mycala, Mychael, Mychal

Michala (Hebrew) a form of
Michaela.
Michalann, Michale, Michalene,
Michalin, Mchalina, Michalisha,
Michalla, Michalle, Michayla,
Michayle, Michela

Michele (Italian) a form of
Michaela.
Michaelle, Michal, Michela

Michelle (French) who is like
God? See also Shelley.
Machealle, Machele, Machell,
Machella, Machelle, Mechelle,
Meichelle, Meschell, Meshell,
Meshelle, Mia, Michel, Michéle,
Michell, Michella, Michellene,
Michellyn, Mischel, Mischelle,
Mishael, Mishaela, Mishayla,
Mishell, Mishelle, Mitchele,
Mitchelle

Michi (Japanese) righteous
way.
Miche, Michee, Michiko

Micki (American) a familiar
form of Michaela.
Mickee, Mickeeya, Mickia,
Mickie, Micky, Mickya, Miquia

Midori (Japanese) green.

Mieko (Japanese) prosperous.
Mieke

Mielikki (Finnish) pleasing.

Miette (French) small; sweet.

Migina (Omaha) new moon.

Mignon (French) dainty,
petite; graceful.
Mignonette, Minnionette,
Minnonette, Minyonette,
Minyonne

Miguela (Spanish) a form of
Michaela.
Micquel, Miguelina, Miguelita,
Miquel, Miquela, Miquella

Mika (Japanese) new moon.
(Russian) God's child.
(Native American) wise
racoon. (Hebrew) a form of
Micah. (Latin) a form of
Dominica.
Mikah, Mikka

Mikaela (Hebrew) a form of
Michaela.
Mekaela, Mekala, Mickael,
Mickaela, Mickala, Mickalla,
Mickeel, Mickell, Mickelle,
Mikael, Mikail, Mikaila, Mikal,
Mikalene, Mikalovna, Mikalyn,
Mikayla, Mikea, Mikeisha,
Mikeita, Mikel, Mikela, Mikele,
Mikell, Mikella, Mikesha,
Mikeya, Mikhaela, Mikie,
Mikiela, Mikkel, Mikyla,
Mykaela

Mikala (Hebrew) a form of
Michaela.
Mickala, Mikalah, Mikale,
Mikalea, Mikalee, Mikaleh

Mikayla (American) a form of Mikaela.
Mekayla, Mickayla, Mikala, Mikayle, Mikyla

Mikhaela (American) a form of Mikaela.
Mikhail, Mikhaila, Mikhala, Mikhalea, Mikhayla, Mikhelle

Miki (Japanese) flower stem.
Mikia, Mikiala, Mikie, Mikita, Mikiyo, Mikki, Mikkie, Mikkiya, Mikko, Miko

Mila (Russian) dear one. (Italian, Slavic) a short form of Camila, Ludmilla.
Milah, Milla

Milada (Czech) my love.
Mila, Milady

Milagros (Spanish) miracle.
Mila, Milagritos, Milagro, Milagrosa, Mirari

Milana (Italian) from Milan, Italy. (Russian) a form of Melana.
Milan, Milane, Milani, Milanka, Milanna, Milanne

Mildred (English) gentle counselor.
Mil, Mila, Mildrene, Mildrid, Millie, Milly

Milena (Greek, Hebrew, Russian) a form of Ludmilla, Magdalen, Melanie.
Mila, Milène, Milenia, Milenny, Milini, Millini

Mileta (German) generous, merciful.

Milia (German) industrious. A short form of Amelia, Emily.
Mila, Milka, Milla, Milya

Miliani (Hawaiian) caress.
Milanni, Miliany

Mililani (Hawaiian) heavenly caress.
Milliani

Milissa (Greek) a form of Melissa.
Milessa, Milisa, Millisa, Millissa

Milka (Czech) a form of Amelia.
Milica, Milika

Millicent (English) industrious. (Greek) a form of Melissa. See also Lissa, Melisande.
Melicent, Meliscent, Mellicent, Mellisent, Melly, Milicent, Milisent, Millie, Milliestone, Millisent, Milly, Milzie, Missy

Millie, Milly (English) familiar forms of Amelia, Camille, Emily, Kamila, Melissa, Mildred, Millicent.
Mili, Milla, Millee, Milley, Millie, Mylie

Mima (Burmese) woman.
Mimma

Mimi (French) a familiar form of Miriam.

Mina (German) love. (Persian) blue sky. (Arabic) harbor. (Japanese) south. A short form of names ending in "mina."
Meena, Mena, Min

Minal (Native American) fruit.

Minda (Hindi) knowledge.

Mindy (Greek) a familiar form of Melinda.
Mindee, Mindi, Mindie, Mindyanne, Mindylee, Myndy

Mine (Japanese) peak; mountain range.
Mineko

Minerva (Latin) wise. Mythology: the goddess of wisdom.
Merva, Minivera, Minnie, Myna

Minette (French) faithful defender
Minnette, Minnita

Minka (Polish) a short form of Wilhelmina.

Minna (German) a short form of Wilhelmina.
Mina, Minka, Minnie, Minta

Minnie (American) a familiar form of Mina, Minerva, Minna, Wilhelmina.
Mini, Minie, Minne, Minni, Minny

Minowa (Native American) singer.
Minowah

Minta (English) Literature: originally coined by playwright Sir John Vanbrugh in his comedy *The Confederacy.*
Minty

Minya (Osage) older sister.

Mio (Japanese) three times as strong.

Mira (Latin) wonderful. (Spanish) look, gaze. A short form of Almira, Amira, Marabel, Mirabel, Miranda.
Mirae, Mirra, Mirah

Mirabel (Latin) beautiful.
Mira, Mirabell, Mirabella, Mirabelle, Mirable

Miracle (Latin) wonder, marvel.

Miranda (Latin) strange; wonderful; admirable. Literature: the heroine of Shakespeare's *The Tempest.* See also Randi.
Maranda, Marenda, Meranda, Mira, Miran, Miranada, Mirandia, Mirinda, Mirindé, Mironda, Mirranda, Muranda, Myranda

Mireille (Hebrew) God spoke. (Latin) wonderful.
Mireil, Mirel, Mirella, Mirelle, Mirelys, Mireya, Mireyda, Mirielle, Mirilla, Myrella, Myrilla

Mireya (Hebrew) a form of
Mireille.
Mireea, Miriah, Miryah

Miri (Gypsy) a short form of
Miriam.
Miria, Miriah

Miriam (Hebrew) bitter; sea of
bitterness. Bible: the original
form of Mary. See also
Macia, Mimi, Mitzi.
*Mairwen, Mariam, Maryam,
Miram, Mirham, Miri, Miriain,
Miriama, Miriame, Mirian,
Mirit, Mirjam, Mirjana,
Mirriam, Mirrian, Miryam,
Miryan, Myriam*

Misha (Russian) a form of
Michaela.
Mischa, Mishae

Missy (English) a familiar form
of Melissa, Millicent.
Missi, Missie

Misty (English) shrouded by
mist.
*Missty, Mistee, Mistey, Misti,
Mistie, Mistin, Mistina, Mistral,
Mistylynn, Mystee, Mysti,
Mystie*

Mitra (Hindi) Religion: god
of daylight. (Persian) angel.
Mita

Mituna (Moquelumnan) like a
fish wrapped up in leaves.

Mitzi (German) a form of
Mary, Miriam.
Mieze, Mitzee, Mitzie, Mitzy

Miwa (Japanese) wise eyes.
Miwako

Miya (Japanese) temple.
Miyah, Miyana, Miyanna

Miyo (Japanese) beautiful
generation.
Miyoko, Miyuko

Miyuki (Japanese) snow.

Moana (Hawaiian) ocean; fragrance.

Mocha (Arabic) chocolate-
flavored coffee.
Moka

Modesty (Latin) modest.
*Modesta, Modeste, Modestia,
Modestie, Modestina, Modestine,
Modestus*

Moesha (American) a short
form of Monisha.
Myesha

Mohala (Hawaiian) flowers in
bloom.
Moala

Moira (Irish) great. A form of
Mary. See also Maura.
*Moirae, Moirah, Moire, Moya,
Moyra, Moyrah*

Molara (Basque) a form of
Mary.

Mollie, Molly (Irish) familiar
forms of Mary.
*Moli, Molie, Moll, Mollee,
Molley, Molli, Mollissa*

Mona (Irish) noble. (Greek) a
short form of Monica,
Ramona, Rimona.
*Moina, Monah, Mone, Monea,
Monna, Moyna*

Monet (French) Art: Claude
Monet was a leading French
impressionist remembered
for his paintings of water
lilies.
Monae, Monay, Monee

Monica (Greek) solitary.
(Latin) advisor.
*Mona, Monca, Monee, Monia,
Monic, Monice, Monicia,
Monicka, Monika, Monique,
Monise, Monn, Monnica,
Monnie, Monya*

Monifa (Yoruba) I have my
luck.

Monika (German) a form of
Monica.
*Moneka, Monieka, Monike,
Monnika*

Monique (French) a form of
Monica.
*Moneeke, Moneik, Moniqua,
Moniquea, Moniquie, Munique*

Monisha (American) a combination of Monica + Aisha.
Moesha, Moneisha, Monishia

Montana (Spanish) mountain.
Geography: a U. S. state.
Montanna

Mora (Spanish) blueberry.
Morae, Morea, Moria, Morita

Morela (Polish) apricot.
Morelia, Morelle

Morena (Irish) a form of
Maureen.

Morgan (Welsh) seashore.
Literature: Morgan le Fay
was the half-sister of King
Arthur.
*Morgana, Morgance, Morgane,
Morganetta, Morganette,
Morganica, Morgann,
Morganna, Morganne, Morgen,
Morghan, Morgyn, Morrigan*

Morghan (Welsh) a form of
Morgan.
Morghen, Morghin, Morghyn

Moriah (Hebrew) God is my
teacher. (French) dark
skinned. Bible: the mountain
on which the Temple of
Solomon was built. See also
Mariah.
*Moria, Moriel, Morit, Morria,
Morriah*

Morie (Japanese) bay.

Morowa (Akan) queen.

Morrisa (Latin) dark skinned;
moor; marshland.
Morisa, Morissa, Morrissa

Moselle (Hebrew) drawn
from the water. (French) a
white wine.
Mozelle

Mosi (Swahili) first-born.

Moswen (Tswana) white.

Mouna (Arabic) wish, desire.
*Moona, Moonia, Mounia,
Muna, Munia*

Mrena (Slavic) white eyes.
Mren

Mumtaz (Arabic)
distinguished.

Mura (Japanese) village.

Muriel (Arabic) myrrh. (Irish)
shining sea. A form of Mary.
See also Meryl.
*Merial, Meriel, Meriol, Merrial,
Merriel, Muire, Murial, Muriell,
Murielle*

Musetta (French) little bag-
pipe.
Musette

Muslimah (Arabic) devout
believer.

Mya (Burmese) emerald.
(Italian) a form of Mia.
My, Myah, Myia, Myiah

Myesha (American) a form of
Moesha.
*Myeisha, Myeshia, Myiesha,
Myisha*

Mykaela, Mykayla (American)
forms of Mikaela.
*Mykael, Mykaila, Mykal,
Mykala, Mykaleen, Mykel,
Mykela, Mykyla*

Myla (English) merciful.

Mylene (Greek) dark.
*Mylaine, Mylana, Mylee,
Myleen*

Myra (Latin) fragrant
ointment.
Mayra, Myrena, Myria

Myranda (Latin) a form of
Miranda.
*Myrandah, Myrandia,
Myrannda*

Myriam (American) a form of
Miriam.
Myriame, Myryam

Myrna (Irish) beloved.
Merna, Mirna, Morna, Muirna

Myrtle (Greek) dark green
shrub.
*Mertis, Mertle, Mirtle, Myrta,
Myrtia, Myrtias, Myrtice,
Myrtie, Myrtilla, Myrtis*

N

Nabila (Arabic) born to nobility.
Nabeela, Nabiha, Nabilah

Nadda (Arabic) generous;
dewy.
Nada

Nadette (French) a short form
of Bernadette.

Nadia (French, Slavic) hopeful.
Nadea, Nadenka, Nadezhda, Nadiah, Nadie, Nadija, Nadijah, Nadine, Nadiya, Nadiyah, Nadja, Nadjae, Nadjah, Nadka, Nadusha, Nady, Nadya

Nadine (French, Slavic) a form of Nadia.
Nadean, Nadeana, Nadeen, Nadena, Nadene, Nadien, Nadin, Nadina, Nadyne, Naidene, Naidine

Nadira (Arabic) rare, precious.
Naadirah, Nadirah

Naeva (French) a form of Eve.
Nahvon

Nafuna (Luganda) born feet first.

Nagida (Hebrew) noble; prosperous.
Nagda, Nageeda

Nahid (Persian) Mythology: another name for Venus, the goddess of love and beauty.

Nahimana (Dakota) mystic.

Naida (Greek) water nymph.
Naiad, Naiya, Nayad, Nyad

Naila (Arabic) successful.
Nailah

Nairi (Armenian) land of rivers. History: a name for ancient Armenia.
Naira, Naire, Nayra

Naiya (Greek) a form of Naida.
Naia, Naiyana, Naja, Najah, Naya

Najam (Arabic) star.
Naja, Najma

Najila (Arabic) brilliant eyes.
Naja, Najah, Najia, Najja, Najla

Nakeisha (American) a combination of the prefix Na + Keisha.
Nakeesha, Nakesha, Nakeshea, Nakeshia, Nakeysha, Nakiesha, Nakisha, Nekeisha

Nakeita (American) a form of Nikita.
Nakeeta, Nakeitha, Nakeithra, Nakeitra, Nakeitress, Nakeitta, Nakeittia, Naketta, Nakieta, Nakitha, Nakitia, Nakitta, Nakyta

Nakia (Arabic) pure.
Nakea, Nakeia, Nakeya, Nakeyah, Nakeyia, Nakiah, Nakiaya, Nakiea, Nakiya, Nakiyah, Nekia

Nakita (American) a form of Nikita.
Nakkita, Naquita

Nalani (Hawaiian) calm as the heavens.
Nalanie, Nalany

Nami (Japanese) wave.
Namika, Namiko

`Girls` 185

Nan (German) a short form of
Fernanda. (English) a form of
Ann.
*Nana, Nanice, Nanine, Nanna,
Nanon*

Nana (Hawaiian) spring.

Nanci (English) a form of
Nancy.
Nancie, Nancsi, Nansi

Nancy (English) gracious. A
familiar form of Nan.
*Nainsi, Nance, Nancee, Nancey,
Nanci, Nancine, Nancye,
Nanette, Nanice, Nanncey,
Nanncy, Nanouk, Nansee,
Nansey, Nanuk*

Nanette (French) a form of
Nancy.
*Nan, Nanete, Nannette, Nettie,
Nineta, Ninete, Ninetta,
Ninette, Nini, Ninita, Ninnetta,
Ninnette, Nynette*

Nani (Greek) charming.
(Hawaiian) beautiful.
Nanni, Nannie, Nanny

Naomi (Hebrew) pleasant,
beautiful. Bible: Ruth's
mother-in-law.
*Naoma, Naomia, Naomie,
Naomy, Navit, Neoma, Neomi,
Noami, Noemi, Noma, Nomi,
Nyomi*

Naomie (Hebrew) a form of
Naomi.
Naome, Naomee, Noemie

Nara (Greek) happy. (English)
north. (Japanese) oak.
Narah

Narcissa (Greek) daffodil.
Mythology: Narcissus was
the youth who fell in love
with his own reflection.
*Narcessa, Narcisa, Narcisse,
Narcyssa, Narissa, Narkissa*

Narelle (Australian) woman
from the sea.
Narel

Nari (Japanese) thunder.
Narie, Nariko

Narmada (Hindi) pleasure
giver.

Nashawna (American) a com-
bination of the prefix Na +
Shawna.
*Nashan, Nashana, Nashanda,
Nashaun, Nashauna,
Nashaunda, Nashauwna,
Nashawn, Nasheena,
Nashounda, Nashuana*

Nashota (Native American)
double; second-born twin.

Nastasia (Greek) a form of
Anastasia.
*Nastasha, Nastashia, Nastasja,
Nastassa, Nastassia, Nastassiya,
Nastassja, Nastassya, Nastasya,
Nastazia, Nastisija, Nastka,
Nastusya, Nastya*

Nasya (Hebrew) miracle.
Nasia, Nasyah

Nata (Sanskrit) dancer. (Latin)
swimmer. (Native American)
speaker; creator. (Polish,
Russian) a form of Natalie.
See also Nadia.
Natia, Natka, Natya

Natacha (Russian) a form of
Natasha.
Natachia, Natacia, Naticha

Natalee, Natali (Latin) forms
of Natalie.
*Natale, Nataleh, Nataleigh,
Nattlee*

Natalia (Russian) a form of
Natalie. See also Talia.
*Nacia, Natala, Natalea,
Nataliia, Natalija, Natalina,
Nataliya, Nataliyah, Natalja,
Natalka, Natallea, Natallia,
Natalya, Nathalia, Natka*

Natalie (Latin) born on
Christmas day. See also Nata,
Natasha, Noel, Talia.
*Nat, Natalee, Natali, Natalia,
Nataliee, Nataline, Natalle,
Natallie, Nataly, Natelie,
Nathalie, Nathaly, Natie,
Natilie, Natlie, Nattalie, Nattilie*

Nataline (Latin) a form of
Natalie.
Natalene, Nataléne, Natalyn

Natalle (French) a form of
Natalie.
Natale

Nataly (Latin) a form of
Natalie.
Nathaly, Natally, Natallye

Natane (Arapaho) daughter.
Natanne

Natania (Hebrew) gift of
God.
*Natanya, Natée, Nathania,
Nathenia, Netania, Nethania*

Natara (Arabic) sacrifice.
Natori, Natoria

Natasha (Russian) a form of
Natalie. See also Stacey,
Tasha.
*Nahtasha, Natacha, Natasa,
Natascha, Natashah, Natashea,
Natashenka, Natashia,
Natashiea, Natashja, Natashka,
Natasia, Natassia, Natassija,
Natassja, Natasza, Natausha,
Natawsha, Natesha, Nateshia,
Nathasha, Nathassha, Natisha,
Natishia, Natosha, Netasha,
Notosha*

Natesa (Hindi) cosmic dancer.
Religion: another name for
the Hindu god Shiva.
Natisa, Natissa

Nathalie, Nathaly (Latin)
forms of Natalie.
*Nathalee, Nathali, Nathalia,
Nathalya*

Natie (English) a familiar
form of Natalie.
Nati, Natti, Nattie, Natty

Natosha (Russian) a form of Natasha.
Natoshia, Natoshya, Netosha, Notosha

Nava (Hebrew) beautiful; pleasant.
Navah, Naveh, Navit

Nayely (Irish) a form of Neila.
Naeyli, Nayelia, Nayelli, Nayelly, Nayla

Neala (Irish) a form of Neila.
Nayela, Naylea, Naylia, Nealia, Neela, Neelia, Neila

Necha (Spanish) a form of Agnes.
Necho

Neci (Hungarian) fiery, intense.
Necia, Necie

Neda (Slavic) born on Sunday.
Nedah, Nedi, Nedia, Neida

Nedda (English) prosperous guardian.
Neddi, Neddie, Neddy

Neely (Irish) a familiar form of Neila, Nelia.
Nealee, Nealie, Nealy, Neelee, Neeley, Neeli, Neelie, Neili, Neilie

Neema (Swahili) born during prosperous times.

Neena (Spanish) a form of Nina.
Neenah, Nena

Neila (Irish) champion. See also Neala, Neely.
Nayely, Neilah, Neile, Neilia, Neilla, Neille

Nekeisha (American) a form of Nakeisha.
Nechesa, Neikeishia, Nekesha, Nekeshia, Nekiesha, Nekisha, Nekysha

Nekia (Arabic) a form of Nakia.
Nekeya, Nekiya, Nekiyah, Nekya, Nekiya

Nelia (Spanish) yellow. (Latin) a familiar form of Cornelia.
Neelia, Neely, Neelya, Nela, Neli, Nelka, Nila

Nelle (Greek) stone.

Nellie, Nelly (English) familiar forms of Cornelia, Eleanor, Helen, Prunella.
Nel, Neli, Nell, Nella, Nelley, Nelli, Nellianne, Nellice, Nellis, Nelma

Nenet (Egyptian) born near the sea. Mythology: Nunet was the goddess of the sea.

Neola (Greek) youthful.
Neolla

Neona (Greek) new moon.

Nereida (Greek) a form of Nerine.
Nereyda, Nereyida, Nerida

Nerine (Greek) sea nymph.
Nereida, Nerina, Nerita,
Nerline

Nerissa (Greek) sea nymph.
See also Rissa.
Narice, Narissa, Nerice, Nerisa,
Nerisse, Nerrisa, Nerys, Neryssa

Nessa (Scandinavian) promon-
tory. (Greek) a short form of
Agnes. See also Nessie.
Nesa, Nesha, Neshia, Nesiah,
Nessia, Nesta, Nevsa, Neysa,
Neysha, Neyshia

Nessie (Greek) a familiar form
of Agnes, Nessa, Vanessa.
Nese, Neshie, Nesho, Nesi,
Ness, Nessi, Nessy, Nest, Neys

Neta (Hebrew) plant, shrub.
See also Nettie.
Netia, Netta, Nettia

Netis (Native American) trustworthy.

Nettie (French) a familiar
form of Annette, Nanette,
Antoinette.
Neti, Netie, Netta, Netti, Netty,
Nety

Neva (Spanish) snow. (English)
new. Geography: a river in
Russia.
Neiva, Neve, Nevia, Neyva,
Nieve, Niva, Nivea, Nivia

Nevada (Spanish) snow.
Geography: a western U. S.
state.
Neiva, Neva

Nevina (Irish) worshipper of
the saint.
Neveen, Nevein, Nevena,
Neveyan, Nevin, Nivena

Neylan (Turkish) fulfilled
wish.
Neya, Neyla

Neza (Slavic) a form of Agnes.

Nia (Irish) a familiar form of
Neila. Mythology: Nia Ben
Aur was a legendary Welsh
woman.
Neya, Niah, Niajia, Niya, Nya

Niabi (Osage) fawn.

Nichelle (American) a combination of Nicole + Michelle.
Culture: Nichelle Nichols was
the first African American
woman featured in a television
drama (*Star Trek*).
Nichele, Nichell, Nishelle

Nichole (French) a form of
Nicole.
Nichol, Nichola, Nicholas,
Nicholle

Nicki (French) a familiar form
of Nicole.
Nicci, Nickey, Nickeya, Nickia,
Nickie, Nickiya, Nicky, Niki

Nickole (French) a form of
Nicole.
Nickol

Nicola (Italian) a form of
Nicole.
Nacola, Necola, Nichola,

Nickola, Nicolea, Nicolla,
Nikkola, Nikola, Nikolia,
Nykola

Nicole (French) a form of
Nicholas. See also Colette,
Cosette, Nikita.
Nacole, Necole, Nica, Nichole,
Nicia, Nicki, Nickole, Nicol,
Nicola, Nicolette, Nicoli, Nicolie,
Nicoline, Nicolle, Nikayla,
Nikelle, Nikki, Niquole, Nocole,
Nycole

Nicolette (French) a form of
Nicole.
Nicholette, Nicoletta, Nicollete,
Nicollette, Nikkolette, Nikoleta,
Nikoletta, Nikolette

Nicoline (French) a familiar
form of Nicole.
Nicholine, Nicholyn, Nicoleen,
Nicolene, Nicolina, Nicolyn,
Nicolyne, Nicolynn, Nicolynne,
Nikolene, Nikolina, Nikoline

Nicolle (French) a form of
Nicole.
Nicholle

Nida (Omaha) Mythology: an
elflike creature.
Nidda

Nidia (Latin) nest.
Nidi, Nidya

Niesha (American) pure.
(Scandinavian) a form of
Nissa.
Neisha, Neishia, Neissia,

Nesha, Neshia, Nesia, Nessia,
Niessia, Nisha, Nyesha

Nige (Latin) dark night.
Nigea, Nigela, Nija, Nijae,
Nijah

Nika (Russian) belonging to
God.
Nikka

Nikayla, Nikelle (American)
forms of Nicole.
Nikeille, Nikel, Nikela, Nikelie

Nike (Greek) victorious.
Mythology: the goddess of
victory.

Niki (Russian) a short form of
Nikita. (American) a familiar
form of Nicole.
Nikia, Nikiah

Nikita (Russian) victorious
people.
Nakeita, Nakita, Niki, Nikitah,
Nikitia, Nikitta, Nikki,
Nikkita, Niquita, Niquitta

Nikki (American) a familiar
form of Nicole, Nikita.
Nicki, Nikia, Nikkea, Nikkey,
Nikkia, Nikkiah, Nikkie,
Nikko, Nikky

Nikole (French) a form of
Nicole.
Nikkole, Nikkolie, Nikola,
Nikole, Nikolena, Nicolia,
Nikolina, Nikolle

Nila (Latin) Geography: the Nile River is in Africa. (Irish) a form of Neila.
Nilah, Nilesia, Nyla

Nili (Hebrew) Botany: a pea plant that yields indigo.

Nima (Hebrew) thread. (Arabic) blessing.
Nema, Niama, Nimali

Nina (Hebrew) a familiar form of Hannah.(Spanish) girl. (Native American) mighty. (Hebrew) a familiar form of Hannah.
Neena, Ninah, Ninacska, Ninja, Ninna, Ninon, Ninosca, Ninoshka

Ninon (French) a form of Nina.

Nirel (Hebrew) light of God.
Nirali, Nirelle

Nirveli (Hindi) water child.

Nisa (Arabic) woman.

Nisha (American) a form of Niesha, Nissa.
Niasha, Nishay

Nishi (Japanese) west.

Nissa (Hebrew) sign, emblem. (Scandinavian) friendly elf; brownie. See also Nyssa.
Nisha, Nisse, Nissie, Nissy

Nita (Hebrew) planter. (Choctaw) bear. (Spanish) a short form of Anita, Juanita.
Nitai, Nitha, Nithai, Nitika

Nitara (Hindi) deeply rooted.

Nitasha (American) a form of Natasha.
Nitasia, Niteisha, Nitisha, Nitishia

Nitsa (Greek) a form of Helen.

Nituna (Native American) daughter.

Nitza (Hebrew) flower bud.
Nitzah, Nitzana, Nitzanit, Niza, Nizah

Nixie (German) water sprite.

Niya (Irish) a form of Nia.
Niyah, Niyana, Niyia, Nyia

Nizana (Hebrew) a form of Nitza.
Nitzana, Nitzania, Zana

Noel (Latin) Christmas. See also Natalie.
Noël, Noela, Noelani, Noele, Noeleen, Noelene, Noelia, Noeline, Noelle, Noelyn, Noelynn, Nohely, Noleen, Novelenn, Novelia, Nowel, Noweleen, Nowell

Noelani (Hawaiian) beautiful one from heaven.
Noela

Noelle (French) Christmas.
Noell, Noella, Noelleen, Noelly, Noellyn

Noemi (Hebrew) a form of
Naomi.
Noam, Noemie, Noemy,
Nohemi, Nomi

Noemie (Hebrew) a form of
Noemi.

Noemy (Hebrew) a form of
Noemi.
Noamy

Noga (Hebrew) morning
light.

Nohely (Latin) a form of
Noel.
Noeli, Noelie, Noely, Nohal,
Noheli

Nokomis (Dakota) moon
daughter.

Nola (Latin) small bell. (Irish)
famous; noble. A short form
of Fionnula.
Nuala

Noleta (Latin) unwilling.
Nolita

Nollie (English) a familiar
form of Magnolia.
Nolia, Nolle, Nolley, Nolli,
Nolly

Noma (Hawaiian) a form of
Norma.

Nona (Latin) ninth.
Nonah, Noni, Nonia, Nonie,
Nonna, Nonnah, Nonya

Noor (Aramaic) a form of
Nura.
Noorie, Nour, Nur

Nora (Greek) light. A familiar
form of Eleanor, Honora,
Leonore.
Norah, Noreen

Noreen (Irish) a form of
Eleanor, Nora. (Latin) a
familiar form of Norma.
Noorin, Noreena, Noreene,
Noren, Norena, Norene,
Norina, Norine, Nureen

Norell (Scandinavian) from
the north.
Narell, Narelle, Norela, Norelle,
Norely

Nori (Japanese) law, tradition.
Noria, Norico, Noriko, Norita

Norma (Latin) rule, precept.
Noma, Noreen, Normi, Normie

Nova (Latin) new. A short
form of Novella, Novia.
(Hopi) butterfly chaser.
Astronomy: a star that
releases bright bursts of
energy.

Novella (Latin) newcomer.
Nova, Novela

Novia (Spanish) sweetheart.
Nova, Novka, Nuvia

Nu (Burmese) tender.
(Vietnamese) girl.
Nue

Nuala (Irish) a short form of
Fionnula.
Nola, Nula

Nuela (Spanish) a form of
Amelia.

Nuna (Native American) land.

Nunciata (Latin) messenger.
Nunzia

Nura (Aramaic) light.
Noor, Noora, Noorah, Noura,
Nurah

Nuria (Aramaic) the Lord's
light.
Nuri, Nuriel, Nurin

Nurita (Hebrew) Botany: a
flower with red and yellow
blossoms.
Nurit

Nuru (Swahili) daylight.

Nusi (Hungarian) a form of
Hannah.

Nuwa (Chinese) mother goddess. Mythology: another
name for Nü-gua, the creator
of mankind.

Nya (Irish) a form of Nia.
Nyaa, Nyah, Nyia

Nycole (French) a form of
Nicole.
Nychelle, Nycolette, Nycolle

Nydia (Latin) nest.
Nyda

Nyesha (American) a form of
Niesha.
Nyeisha, Nyeshia

Nyla (Latin, Irish) a form of
Nila.
Nylah

Nyoko (Japanese) gem, treasure.

Nyomi (Hebrew) a form of
Naomi.
Nyome, Nyomee, Nyomie

Nyree (Maori) sea.
Nyra, Nyrie

Nyssa (Greek) beginning. See
also Nissa.
Nisha, Nissi, Nissy, Nyasia,
Nysa

Nyusha (Russian) a form of
Agnes.
Nyushenka, Nyushka

Oba (Yoruba) chief, ruler.

Obelia (Greek) needle.

Oceana (Greek) ocean.
Mythology: Oceanus was the
god of the ocean.
Ocean, Oceananna, Oceane,
Oceania, Oceanna, Oceanne,
Oceaonna, Oceon

Octavia (Latin) eighth. See also Tavia.
Octabia, Octaviah, Octaviais, Octavice, Octavie, Octavienne, Octavio, Octavious, Octavise, Octavya, Octivia, Otavia, Ottavia

Odeda (Hebrew) strong; courageous.

Odele (Greek) melody, song.
Odelet, Odelette, Odell, Odelle

Odelia (Greek) ode; melodic. (Hebrew) I will praise God. (French) wealthy. See also Odetta.
Oda, Odeelia, Odeleya, Odelina, Odelinda, Odelyn, Odila, Odile, Odilia

Odella (English) wood hill.
Odela, Odelle, Odelyn

Odera (Hebrew) plough.

Odessa (Greek) odyssey, long voyage.
Adesha, Adeshia, Adessa, Adessia, Odessia

Odetta (German, French) a form of Odelia.
Oddetta, Odette

Odina (Algonquin) mountain.

Ofelia (Greek) a form of Ophelia.
Ofeelia, Ofilia

Ofira (Hebrew) gold.
Ofarrah, Ophira

Ofra (Hebrew) a form of Aphra.
Ofrat

Ogin (Native American) wild rose.

Ohanna (Hebrew) God's gracious gift.

Okalani (Hawaiian) heaven.
Okilani

Oki (Japanese) middle of the ocean.
Okie

Oksana (Latin) a form of Osanna.
Oksanna

Ola (Greek) a short form of Olesia.(Scandinavian) ancestor.

Olathe (Native American) beautiful.
Olathia

Oleda (Spanish) a form of Alida. See also Leda.
Oleta, Olida, Olita

Olena (Russian) a form of Helen.
Oleena, Olenka, Olenna, Olenya, Olya

Olesia (Greek) a form of Alexandra.
Cesya, Ola, Olecia, Oleesha, Oleishia, Olesha, Olesya, Olexa, Olice, Olicia, Olisha, Olishia, Ollicia

Oletha (Scandinavian) nimble.
Oleta, Yaletha

Olethea (Latin) truthful. See
also Alethea.
Oleta

Olga (Scandinavian) holy. See
also Helga, Olivia.
*Olenka, Olia, Olja, Ollya,
Olva, Olya*

Oliana (Polynesian) oleander.

Olina (Hawaiian) filled with
happiness.

Olinda (Latin) scented.
(Spanish) protector of prop-
erty. (Greek) a form of
Yolanda.

Olisa (Ibo) God.

Olive (Latin) olive tree.
Oliff, Oliffe, Olivet, Olivette

Olivia (Latin) a form of Olive.
(English) a form of Olga. See
also Liv, Livia.
*Alivia, Alyvia, Olevia, Oliva,
Olivea, Oliveia, Olivetta, Olivi,
Olivianne, Olivya, Oliwia,
Ollie, Olva, Olyvia*

Ollie (English) a familiar form
of Olivia.
Olla, Olly, Ollye

Olwen (Welsh) white
footprint.
*Olwenn, Olwin, Olwyn,
Olwyne, Olwynne*

Olympia (Greek) heavenly.
Olimpia, Olympe, Olympie

Olyvia (Latin) a form of
Olivia.

Oma (Hebrew) reverent.
(German) grandmother.
(Arabic) highest.

Omaira (Arabic) red.
*Omar, Omara, Omarah,
Omari, Omaria, Omarra*

Omega (Greek) last, final, end.
Linguistics: the last letter in
the Greek alphabet.

Ona (Latin, Irish) a form of
Oona, Una. (English) river.

Onatah (Iroquois) daughter of
the earth and the corn spirit.

Onawa (Native American)
wide awake.
Onaja, Onajah

Ondine (Latin) a form of
Undine.
Ondene, Ondina, Ondyne

Ondrea (Czech) a form of
Andrea.
*Ohndrea, Ohndreea, Ohndreya,
Ohndria, Ondraya, Ondreana,
Ondreea, Ondreya, Ondria,
Ondrianna, Ondriea*

Oneida (Native American)
eagerly awaited.
Onida, Onyda

Onella (Hungarian) a form of
Helen.

Onesha (American) a combination of Ondrea + Aisha.
Oneshia, Onesia, Onessa, Onessia, Onethia, Oniesha, Onisha

Oni (Yoruba) born on holy ground.
Onnie

Onora (Latin) a form of Honora.
Onoria, Onorine, Ornora

Oona (Latin, Irish) a form of Una.
Ona, Onna, Onnie, Oonagh, Oonie

Opa (Choctaw) owl. (German) grand-father.

Opal (Hindi) precious stone.
Opale, Opalina, Opaline

Ophelia (Greek) helper. Literature: Hamlet's love interest in the Shakespearean play *Hamlet*.
Filia, Ofelia, Ophélie, Ophilia, Phelia

Oprah (Hebrew) a form of Orpah.
Ophra, Ophrah, Opra

Ora (Latin) prayer. (Spanish) gold. (English) seacoast. (Greek) a form of Aura.
Orah, Orlice, Orra

Orabella (Latin) a form of Arabella.
Orabel, Orabela, Orabelle

Oralee (Hebrew) the Lord is my light. See also Yareli.
Areli, Orali, Oralit, Orelie, Orlee, Orli, Orly

Oralia (French) a form of Aurelia. See also Oriana.
Oralis, Oriel, Orielda, Orielle, Oriena, Orlena, Orlene

Orea (Greek) mountains.
Oreal, Oria, Oriah

Orela (Latin) announcement from the gods; oracle.
Oreal, Orella, Orelle, Oriel, Orielle

Orenda (Iroquois) magical power.

Oretha (Greek) a form of Aretha.
Oreta, Oretta, Orette

Oriana (Latin) dawn, sunrise. (Irish) golden.
Orane, Orania, Orelda, Orelle, Ori, Oria, Orian, Oriane, Orianna, Orieana, Oryan

Orina (Russian) a form of Irene.
Orya, Oryna

Orinda (Hebrew) pine tree. (Irish) light skinned, white.
Orenda

Orino (Japanese) worker's field.
Ori

Oriole (Latin) golden; black-and-orange bird.
Auriel, Oriel, Oriell, Oriella, Oriola

Orla (Irish) golden woman.
Orlagh, Orlie, Orly

Orlanda (German) famous
throughout the land.
*Orlandia, Orlantha, Orlenda,
Orlinda*

Orlenda (Russian) eagle.

Orli (Hebrew) light.
Orlice, Orlie, Orly

Ormanda (Latin) noble.
(German) mariner.
Orma

Ornice (Hebrew) cedar tree.
(Irish) pale; olive colored.
*Orna, Ornah, Ornat, Ornette,
Ornit*

Orpah (Hebrew) runaway. See
also Oprah.
Orpa, Orpha, Orphie

Orquidea (Spanish) orchid.
Orquidia

Orsa (Latin) a short form of
Orseline. See also Ursa.
*Orsaline, Orse, Orsel, Orselina,
Orseline, Orsola*

Ortensia (Italian) a form of
Hortense.

Orva (French) golden; worthy.
(English) brave friend.

Osanna (Latin) praise the
Lord.
Oksana, Osana

Osen (Japanese) one thousand.

Oseye (Benin) merry.

Osma (English) divine protector.
Ozma

Otilie (Czech) lucky heroine.
*Otila, Otilia, Otka, Ottili,
Otylia*

Ovia (Latin, Danish) egg.

Owena (Welsh) born to nobility; young warrior.

Oya (Moquelumnan) called
forth.

Oz (Hebrew) strength.

Ozara (Hebrew) treasure,
wealth.

P

Paca (Spanish) a short form of
Pancha. See also Paka.

Padget (French) a form of Page.
Padgett, Paget, Pagett

Padma (Hindi) lotus.

Page (French) young assistant.
Padget, Pagen, Pagi, Payge

Paige (English) young child.
Payge

Paisley (Scottish) patterned
fabric first made in Paisley,
Scotland.
Paislay, Paislee, Paisleyann,

Paisleyanne, Paizlei, Paizleigh, Paizley, Pasley, Pazley

Paiton (English) warrior's town.
Paiten, Paityn, Paityne, Paiyton, Paten, Patton

Paka (Swahili) kitten. See also Paca.

Pakuna (Moquelumnan) deer bounding while running downhill.

Palila (Polynesian) bird.

Pallas (Greek) wise. Mythology: another name for Athena, the goddess of wisdom.

Palma (Latin) palm tree.
Pallma, Palmira

Palmira (Spanish) a form of Palma.
Pallmirah, Pallmyra, Palmer, Palmyra

Paloma (Spanish) dove. See also Aloma.
Palloma, Palometa, Palomita, Paluma, Peloma

Pamela (Greek) honey.
Pam, Pama, Pamala, Pamalla, Pamelia, Pamelina, Pamella, Pamila, Pamilla, Pammela, Pammi, Pammie, Pammy, Pamula

Pancha (Spanish) free; from France.
Paca, Panchita

Pandita (Hindi) scholar.

Pandora (Greek) all-gifted. Mythology: a woman who opened a box out of curiosity and released evil into the world. See also Dora.
Pandi, Pandorah, Pandorra, Pandorrah, Pandy, Panndora, Panndorah, Panndorra, Panndorrah

Pansy (Greek) flower; fragrant. (French) thoughtful.
Pansey, Pansie

Panthea (Greek) all the gods.
Pantheia, Pantheya

Panya (Swahili) mouse; tiny baby. (Russian) a familiar form of Stephanie.
Panyia

Panyin (Fante) older twin.

Paola (Italian) a form of Paula.
Paoli, Paolina

Papina (Moquelumnan) vine growing on an oak tree.

Paquita (Spanish) a form of Frances.
Paqua

Pari (Persian) fairy eagle.

Paris (French) Geography: the capital of France. Mythology: the Trojan prince who started the Trojan War by abducting Helen.
Parice, Paries, Parisa, Parise, Parish, Parisha, Pariss, Parissa, Parisse, Parris, Parys, Parysse

Parker (English) park keeper.
Park, Parke

Parris (French) a form of Paris.
Parrise, Parrish, Parrisha, Parrys, Parrysh

Parthenia (Greek) virginal.
Partheenia, Parthenie, Parthinia, Pathina

Parveneh (Persian) butterfly.

Pascale (French) born on Easter or Passover.
Pascalette, Pascaline, Pascalle, Paschale, Paskel

Pasha (Greek) sea.
Palasha, Pascha, Pasche, Pashae, Pashe, Pashel, Pashka, Pasia, Passia

Passion (Latin) passion.
Pashion, Pashonne, Pasion, Passionaé, Passionate, Passionette

Pasua (Swahili) born by cesarean section.

Pat (Latin) a short form of Patricia, Patsy.

Pati (Moquelumnan) fish baskets made of willow branches.

Patia (Gypsy, Spanish) leaf. (Latin, English) a familiar form of Patience, Patricia.

Patience (English) patient.
Paciencia, Patia, Patiance, Patient, Patince, Patishia

Patra (Greek, Latin) a form of Petra.

Patrice (French) a form of Patricia.
Patrease, Patrece, Patreece, Patreese, Patreice, Patriece, Patryce, Pattrice

Patricia (Latin) noblewoman. See also Payton, Peyton, Tricia, Trisha, Trissa.
Pat, Patia, Patresa, Patrica, Patrice, Patricea, Patriceia, Patrichea, Patriciana, Patricianna, Patricja, Patricka, Patrickia, Patrisha, Patrishia, Patrisia, Patrissa, Patrizia, Patrizzia, Patrycia, Patrycja, Patsy, Patty

Patsy (Latin) a familiar form of Patricia.
Pat, Patsey, Patsi

Patty (English) a familiar form of Patricia.
Patte, Pattee, Patti, Pattie

Paula (Latin) small. See also Pavla, Polly.
Paliki, Paola, Paulane, Paulann,

Paule, Paulette, Paulina,
Pauline, Paulla, Pavia

Paulette (Latin) a familiar
form of Paula.
Paulet, Paulett, Pauletta,
Paulita, Paullett, Paulletta,
Paullette

Paulina (Slavic) a form of
Paula.
Paulena, Paulene, Paulenia,
Pauliana, Paulianne, Paullena,
Paulyna, Pawlina, Polena,
Polina, Polinia

Pauline (French) a form of
Paula.
Pauleen, Paulene, Paulien,
Paulin, Paulyne, Paulynn,
Pouline

Pausha (Hindi) lunar month
of Capricorn.

Pavla (Czech, Russian) a form
of Paula.
Pavlina, Pavlinka

Paxton (Latin) peaceful town.
Paxtin, Paxtynn

Payge (English) a form of
Paige.

Payton (Irish) a form of
Patricia.
Paydon, Paytan, Payten, Paytin,
Paytn, Paytton

Paz (Spanish) peace.

Pazi (Ponca) yellow bird.

Pazia (Hebrew) golden.
Paz, Paza, Pazice, Pazit

Peace (English) peaceful.

Pearl (Latin) jewel.
Pearle, Pearleen, Pearlena,
Pearlene, Pearlette, Pearlina,
Pearline, Pearlisha, Pearlyn,
Perl, Perla, Perle, Perlette, Perlie,
Perline, Perlline

Peggy (Greek) a familiar form
of Margaret.
Peg, Pegeen, Pegg, Peggey, Peggi,
Peggie, Pegi

Peke (Hawaiian) a form of
Bertha.

Pela (Polish) a short form of
Penelope.
Pele

Pelagia (Greek) sea.
Pelage, Pelageia, Pelagie, Pelga,
Pelgia, Pellagia

Pelipa (Zuni) a form of
Philippa.

Pemba (Bambara) the power
that controls all life.

Penda (Swahili) loved.

Penelope (Greek) weaver.
Mythology: the clever and
loyal wife of Odysseus, a
Greek hero.
Pela, Pen, Penelopa, Penna,
Pennelope, Penny, Pinelopi

Peni (Carrier) mind.

Peninah (Hebrew) pearl.
*Penina, Peninit, Peninnah,
Penny*

Penny (Greek) a familiar form
of Penelope, Peninah.
*Penee, Peni, Penney, Penni,
Pennie*

Peony (Greek) flower.
Peonie

Pepita (Spanish) a familiar
form of Josephine.
Pepa, Pepi, Peppy, Peta

Pepper (Latin) condiment
from the pepper plant.

Perah (Hebrew) flower.

Perdita (Latin) lost. Literature:
a character in Shakespeare's
play *The Winter's Tale*.
Perdida, Perdy

Perfecta (Spanish) flawless.

Peri (Greek) mountain
dweller. (Persian) fairy or elf.
Perita

Perla (Latin) a form of Pearl.
Pearla

Perlie (Latin) a familiar form
of Pearl.
*Pearley, Pearlie, Pearly, Perley,
Perli, Perly, Purley, Purly*

Pernella (Greek, French) rock.
(Latin) a short form of
Petronella.
*Parnella, Pernel, Pernell,
Pernelle*

Perri (Greek, Latin) small
rock; traveler. (French) pear
tree. (Welsh) child of Harry.
(English) a form of Perry.
*Perre, Perrey, Perriann, Perrie,
Perrin, Perrine, Perry*

Persephone (Greek)
Mythology: the goddess of
the underworld.
*Persephanie, Persephany,
Persephonie*

Persis (Latin) from Persia.
Perssis, Persy

Peta (Blackfoot) golden eagle.

Petra (Greek, Latin) small
rock. A short form of
Petronella.
*Patra, Pet, Peta, Petena,
Peterina, Petraann, Petrice,
Petrina, Petrine, Petrova,
Petrovna, Pier, Pierce, Pietra*

Petronella (Greek) small rock.
(Latin) of the Roman clan
Petronius.
*Pernella, Peternella, Petra,
Petrona, Petronela, Petronella,
Petronelle, Petronia, Petronija,
Petronilla, Petronille*

Petula (Latin) seeker.
Petulah

Petunia (Native American)
flower.

Peyton (Irish) a form of
Patricia.
Peyden, Peydon, Peyten, Peytyn

Phaedra (Greek) bright.
*Faydra, Phae, Phaidra, Phe,
Phedre*

Phallon (Irish) a form of
Fallon.
*Phalaine, Phalen, Phallan,
Phallie, Phalon, Phalyn*

Phebe (Greek) a form of
Phoebe.
Pheba, Pheby

Pheodora (Greek, Russian) a
form of Feodora.
*Phedora, Phedorah, Pheodorah,
Pheydora, Pheydorah*

Philana (Greek) lover of
mankind.
*Phila, Philanna, Philene,
Philiane, Philina, Philine*

Philantha (Greek) lover of
flowers.

Philicia (Latin) a form of
Phylicia.
*Philecia, Philesha, Philica,
Philicha, Philycia*

Philippa (Greek) lover of
horses. See also Filippa.
*Phil, Philipa, Philippe,
Phillipina, Phillippine, Phillie,
Philly, Pippa, Pippy*

Philomena (Greek) love song;
loved one. Bible: a first-cen-
tury saint. See also Filomena,
Mena.
Philoméne, Philomina

Phoebe (Greek) shining.
Phaebe, Phebe, Pheobe, Phoebey

Phylicia (Latin) fortunate;
happy. (Greek) a form of
Felicia.
*Philicia, Phylecia, Phylesha,
Phylesia, Phylica, Phylisha,
Phylisia, Phylissa, Phyllecia,
Phyllicia, Phyllisha, Phyllisia,
Phyllissa, Phyllyza*

Phyllida (Greek) a form of
Phyllis.
*Fillida, Philida, Phillida,
Phillyda*

Phyllis (Greek) green bough.
*Filise, Fillys, Fyllis, Philis,
Phillis, Philliss, Philys, Philyss,
Phylis, Phyllida, Phyllis,
Phylliss, Phyllys*

Pia (Italian) devout.

Piedad (Spanish) devoted;
pious.

Pier (French) a form of Petra.
Pierette, Pierrette, Pierra, Pierre

Pierce (English) a form of Petra.

Pilar (Spanish) pillar, column.
Peelar, Pilár, Pillar

Ping (Chinese) duckweed.
(Vietnamese) peaceful.

Pinga (Eskimo) Mythology: the
goddess of game and the hunt.

Piper (English) pipe player.

Pippa (English) a short form
of Phillipa.

Pippi (French) rosy cheeked.
Pippen, Pippie, Pippin, Pippy

Pita (African) fourth daughter.

Placidia (Latin) serene.
Placida

Pleasance (French) pleasant.
Pleasence

Polla (Arabic) poppy.
Pola

Polly (Latin) a familiar form of
Paula.
*Paili, Pali, Pauli, Paulie, Pauly,
Poll, Pollee, Polley, Polli, Pollie*

Pollyam (Hindi) goddess of
the plague. Religion: the
Hindu name invoked to
ward off bad spirits.

Pollyanna (English) a combination of Polly + Anna.
Literature: an overly
optimistic heroine created by
Eleanor Porter.

Poloma (Choctaw) bow.

Pomona (Latin) apple.
Mythology: the goddess of
fruit and fruit trees.

Poni (African) second daughter.

Poppy (Latin) poppy flower.
Popi, Poppey, Poppi, Poppie

Pora, Poria (Hebrew) fruitful.

Porcha (Latin) a form of
Portia.
*Porchae, Porchai, Porche,
Porchia, Porcia*

Porscha, Porsche (German)
forms of Portia.
*Porcsha, Porcshe, Porschah,
Porsché, Porschea, Porschia,
Pourche*

Porsha (Latin) a form of
Portia.
*Porshai, Porshay, Porshe,
Porshea, Porshia*

Portia (Latin) offering.
Literature: the heroine of
Shakespeare's play *The
Merchant of Venice.*
*Porcha, Porsca, Porsche,
Porsha, Portiea*

Precious (French) precious;
dear.
*Pracious, Preciouse, Precisha,
Prescious, Preshious, Presious*

Presley (English) priest's
meadow.
*Preslea, Preslee, Preslei, Presli,
Preslie, Presly, Preslye, Pressley,
Presslie, Pressly*

Prima (Latin) first, beginning;
first child.
*Prema, Primalia, Primetta,
Primina, Priminia*

Primavera (Italian, Spanish)
spring.

Primrose (English) primrose flower.
Primula

Princess (English) daughter of royalty.
Princcess, Princes, Princesa, Princessa, Princetta, Princie, Princilla

Priscilla (Latin) ancient.
Cilla, Piri, Precila, Precilla, Prescilla, Presilla, Pressilia, Pricila, Pricilla, Pris, Prisca, Priscela, Priscella, Priscila, Priscilia, Priscill, Priscille, Priscillia, Prisella, Prisila, Prisilla, Prissila, Prissilla, Prissy, Pryscylla, Prysilla

Prissy (Latin) a familiar form of Priscilla.
Prisi, Priss, Prissi, Prissie

Priya (Hindi) beloved; sweet natured.
Pria

Procopia (Latin) declared leader.

Promise (Latin) promise, pledge.
Promis, Promiss, Promys, Promyse

Pru (Latin) a short form of Prudence.
Prue

Prudence (Latin) cautious; discreet.
Pru, Prudencia, Prudens, Prudy

Prudy (Latin) a familiar form of Prudence.
Prudee, Prudi, Prudie

Prunella (Latin) brown; little plum. See also Nellie.
Prunela

Psyche (Greek) soul. Mythology: a beautiful mortal loved by Eros, the Greek god of love.

Pua (Hawaiian) flower.

Pualani (Hawaiian) heavenly flower.
Puni

Purity (English) purity.
Pura, Pureza, Purisima

Pyralis (Greek) fire.
Pyrene

Q

Qadira (Arabic) powerful.
Kadira

Qamra (Arabic) moon.
Kamra

Qitarah (Arabic) fragrant.

Quaashie (Ewe) born on Sunday.

Quadeisha (American) a combination of Qadira + Aisha.
Qudaisha, Quadaishia, Quadajah, Quadasha, Quadasia, Quadayshia, Quadaza, Quadejah, Quadesha, Quadeshia, Quadiasha, Quaesha

Quaneisha (American) a combination of the prefix Qu + Niesha.
Quaneasa, Quanece, Quanecia, Quaneice, Quanesha, Quanisha, Quansha, Quarnisha, Queisha, Qwanisha, Qynisha

Quanesha (American) a form of Quaneisha.
Quamesha, Quaneesha, Quaneshia, Quanesia, Quanessa, Quanessia, Quannesha, Quanneshia, Quannezia, Quayneshia, Quinesha

Quanika (American) a combination of the prefix Qu + Nika.
Quanikka, Quanikki, Quaniqua, Quanique, Quantenique, Quawanica, Queenika, Queenique

Quanisha (American) a form of Quaneisha.
Quaniesha, Quanishia, Quaynisha, Queenisha, Quenisha, Quenishia

Quartilla (Latin) fourth.
Quantilla

Qubilah (Arabic) agreeable.

Queen (English) queen. See also Quinn.
Queena, Queenie, Quenna

Queenie (English) a form of Queen.
Queenation, Queeneste, Queeny

Queisha (American) a short form of Quaneisha.
Qeysha, Queshia, Queysha

Quenby (Scandinavian) feminine.

Quenisha (American) a combination of Queen + Aisha.
Queneesha, Quenesha, Quennisha, Quensha, Quinesha, Quinisha

Quenna (English) a form of Queen.
Quenell, Quenessa

Querida (Spanish) dear; beloved.

Questa (French) searcher.

Queta (Spanish) a short form of names ending in "queta" or "quetta."
Quenetta, Quetta

Quiana (American) a combination of the prefix Qu + Anna.
Quian, Quianah, Quianda, Quiane, Quiani, Quianita, Quianna, Quianne, Quionna

Quinby (Scandinavian) queen's estate.

Quincy (Irish) fifth.
Quincee, Quincey, Quinci, Quincia, Quincie

Quinella (Latin) a form of Quintana.

Quinesha, Quinisha (American) forms of Quenisha.
Quineshia, Quinessa, Quinessia, Quinisa, Quinishia, Quinnesha, Quinneshia, Quinnisha, Quneasha, Quonesha, Quonisha, Quonnisha

Quinetta (Latin) a form of Quintana.
Queenetta, Queenette, Quinette, Quinita, Quinnette

Quinn (German, English) queen. See also Queen.
Quin, Quinna, Quinne, Quynn

Quinshawna (American) a combination of Quinn + Shauna.
Quinshea

Quintana (Latin) fifth. (English) queen's lawn. See also Quinella, Quinetta.
Quinntina, Quinta, Quintanna, Quintara, Quintarah, Quintia, Quintila, Quintilla, Quintina, Quintona, Quintonice

Quintessa (Latin) essence. See also Tess.
Quintaysha, Quintesa, Quintesha, Quintessia,

Quintice, Quinticia, Quintisha, Quintosha

Quintrell (American) a combination of Quinn + Trella.
Quintela, Quintella, Quintrelle

Quiterie (Latin, French) tranquil.
Quita

Qwanisha (American) a form of Quaneisha.
Qwanechia, Qwanesha, Qwanessia, Qwantasha

R

Rabecca (Hebrew) a form of Rebecca.
Rabecka, Rabeca, Rabekah

Rabi (Arabic) breeze.
Rabia, Rabiah

Rachael (Hebrew) a form of Rachel.
Rachaele, Rachaell, Rachail, Rachalle

Racheal (Hebrew) a form of Rachel.

Rachel (Hebrew) female sheep. Bible: the second wife of Jacob. See also Lahela, Rae, Rochelle.
Racha, Rachael, Rachal, Racheal, Rachela, Rachelann, Rachele, Rachelle, Racquel, Raechel, Rahel, Rahela, Rahil, Raiche, Raquel, Rashel,

Rachel *(cont.)*
*Rashelle, Ray, Raycene,
Raychel, Raychelle, Rey, Ruchel*

Rachelle (French) a form of
Rachel. See also Shelley.
*Rachalle, Rachell, Rachella,
Raechell, Raechelle, Raeshelle,
Rashel, Rashele, Rashell,
Rashelle, Raychell, Rayshell,
Ruchelle*

Racquel (French) a form of
Rachel.
*Rackel, Racquell, Racquella,
Racquelle*

Radella (German) counselor.

Radeyah (Arabic) content,
satisfied.
*Radeeyah, Radhiya, Radiah,
Radiyah*

Radinka (Slavic) full of life;
happy, glad.

Radmilla (Slavic) worker for
the people.

Rae (English) doe. (Hebrew) a
short form of Rachel.
*Raeh, Raeneice, Raeneisha,
Raesha, Ray, Raye, Rayetta,
Rayette, Rayma, Rey*

Raeann (American) a combi-
nation of Rae + Ann. See
also Rayanne.
*Raea, Raean, Raeanna,
Raeannah, Raeona, Reanna,
Raeanne*

Raechel (Hebrew) a form of
Rachel.
*Raechael, Raechal, Raechele,
Raechell, Raechyl*

Raeden (Japanese) Mythology:
Raiden was the god of thun-
der and lightning.
Raeda, Raedeen

Raegan (Irish) a form of
Reagan.
*Raegen, Raegene, Raegine,
Raegyn*

Raelene (American) a combi-
nation of Rae + Lee.
*Rael, Raela, Raelani, Raele,
Raeleah, Raelee, Raeleen,
Raeleia, Raeleigh, Raeleigha,
Raelein, Raelene, Raelennia,
Raelesha, Raelin, Raelina,
Raelle, Raelyn, Raelynn*

Raelyn, Raelynn (American)
forms of Raelene.
Raelynda, Raelyne, Raelynne

Raena (German) a form of
Raina.
*Raenah, Raenia, Raenie,
Raenna, Raeonna, Raeyauna,
Raeyn, Raeyonna*

Raeven (English) a form of
Raven.
*Raevin, Raevion, Raevon,
Raevonna, Raevyn, Raevynne,
Raewyn, Raewynne, Raivan,
Raiven, Raivin, Raivyn*

Rafa (Arabic) happy; prosperous.

Rafaela (Hebrew) a form of
Raphaela.
Rafaelia, Rafaella

Ragan (Irish) a form of
Reagan.
*Ragean, Rageane, Rageen,
Ragen, Ragene, Rageni,
Ragenna, Raggan, Raygan,
Raygen, Raygene, Rayghan,
Raygin*

Ragine (English) a form of
Regina.
*Raegina, Ragin, Ragina,
Raginee*

Ragnild (Scandinavian) battle
counsel.
*Ragna, Ragnell, Ragnhild,
Rainell, Renilda, Renilde*

Raheem (Punjabi) compassionate God.
Raheema, Rahima

Ráidah (Arabic) leader.

Raina (German) mighty.
(English) a short form of
Regina. See also Rayna.
*Raeinna, Raena, Raheena,
Rain, Rainah, Rainai, Raine,
Rainea, Rainna, Reanna*

Rainbow (English) rainbow.
*Rainbeau, Rainbeaux, Rainbo,
Raynbow*

Raine (Latin) a short form of
Regina. A form of Raina,
Rane.
*Rainee, Rainey, Raini, Rainie,
Rainy, Reyne*

Raisa (Russian) a form of
Rose.
*Raisah, Raissa, Raiza, Raysa,
Rayza, Razia*

Raizel (Yiddish) a form of
Rose.
Rayzil, Razil, Reizel, Resel

Raja (Arabic) hopeful.
*Raia, Rajaah, Rajae, Rajah,
Rajai*

Raku (Japanese) pleasure.

Raleigh (Irish) a form of
Riley.
Ralea, Raleiah, Raley

Rama (Hebrew) lofty, exalted.
(Hindi) godlike. Religion: an
incarnation of the Hindu
god Vishnu.
Ramah

Raman (Spanish) a form of
Ramona.

Ramandeep (Sikh) covered by
the light of the Lord's love.

Ramla (Swahili) fortuneteller.
Ramlah

Ramona (Spanish) mighty;
wise protector. See also
Mona.
*Raman, Ramonda, Raymona,
Romona, Romonda*

Ramsey (English) ram's island.
*Ramsha, Ramsi, Ramsie,
Ramza*

Ran (Japanese) water lily.
(Scandinavian) destroyer.
Mythology: the Norse sea
goddess who destroys.

Rana (Sanskrit) royal. (Arabic)
gaze, look.
Rahna, Rahni, Rani

Ranait (Irish) graceful; prosperous.
Rane, Renny

Randall (English) protected.
*Randa, Randah, Randal,
Randalee, Randel, Randell,
Randelle, Randi, Randilee,
Randilynn, Randlyn, Randy,
Randyl*

Randi, Randy (English) famil-
iar forms of Miranda,
Randall.
*Rande, Randee, Randeen,
Randene, Randey, Randie,
Randii*

Rane (Scandinavian) queen.
Raine

Rani (Sanskrit) queen.
(Hebrew) joyful. A short
form of Kerani.
*Rahni, Ranee, Raney, Rania,
Ranie, Ranice, Ranique, Ranni,
Rannie*

Ranita (Hebrew) song; joyful.
*Ranata, Ranice, Ranit, Ranite,
Ranitta, Ronita*

Raniyah (Arabic) gazing.
Ranya, Ranyah

Rapa (Hawaiian) moonbeam.

Raphaela (Hebrew) healed by
God.
Rafaella, Raphaella, Raphaelle

Raphaelle (French) a form of
Raphaela.
Rafaelle, Raphael, Raphaele

Raquel (French) a form of
Rachel.
*Rakel, Rakhil, Rakhila,
Raqueal, Raquela, Raquella,
Raquelle, Rickelle, Rickquel,
Ricquel, Ricquelle, Rikell,
Rikelle, Rockell*

Rasha (Arabic) young gazelle.
*Rahshea, Rahshia, Rashae,
Rashai, Rashea, Rashi, Rashia*

Rashawna (American) a com-
bination of the prefix Ra +
Shawna.
*Rashana, Rashanae, Rashanah,
Rashanda, Rashane, Rashani,
Rashanna, Rashanta, Rashaun,
Rashauna, Rashaunda,
Rashaundra, Rashaune,
Rashawn, Rashawnda,
Rashawnna, Rashon, Rashona,
Rashonda, Rashunda*

Rashel, Rashelle (American)
forms of Rachel.
Rashele, Rashell, Rashella

Rashida (Swahili, Turkish)
righteous.
*Rahshea, Rahsheda, Rahsheita,
Rashdah, Rasheda, Rashedah,*

Rasheeda, Rasheedah, Rasheeta, Rasheida, Rashidah, Rashidi

Rashieka (Arabic) descended from royalty.
Rasheeka, Rasheika, Rasheka, Rashika, Rasika

Rasia (Greek) rose.

Ratana (Tai) crystal.
Ratania, Ratanya, Ratna, Rattan, Rattana

Ratri (Hindi) night. Religion: the goddess of the night.

Raula (French) wolf counselor.
Raoula, Raulla, Raulle

Raven (English) blackbird.
Raeven, Raveen, Raveena, Raveenn, Ravena, Ravene, Ravenn, Ravenna, Ravennah, Ravenne, Raveon, Ravin, Ravon, Ravyn, Rayven, Revena

Ravin (English) forms of Raven.
Ravi, Ravina, Ravine, Ravinne, Ravion,

Ravyn (English) a form of Raven.
Ravynn

Rawnie (Gypsy) fine lady.
Rawan, Rawna, Rhawnie

Raya (Hebrew) friend.
Raia, Raiah, Raiya, Ray, Rayah

Rayanne (American) a form of Raeann.
Rayane, Ray-Ann, Rayan, Rayana, Rayann, Rayanna, Rayeanna, Rayona, Rayonna, Reyan, Reyana, Reyann, Reyanna, Reyanne

Raychel, Raychelle (Hebrew) forms of Rachel.
Raychael, Raychele, Raychell, Raychil

Raylene (American) forms of Raylyn.
Ralina, Rayel, Rayele, Rayelle, Rayleana, Raylee, Rayleen, Rayleigh, Raylena, Raylin, Raylinn, Raylona, Raylyn, Raylynn, Raylynne

Raymonde (German) wise protector.
Rayma, Raymae, Raymie

Rayna (Scandinavian) mighty. (Yiddish) pure, clean. (English) king's advisor. (French) a familiar form of Lorraine. See also Raina.
Raynah, Rayne, Raynell, Raynelle, Raynette, Rayona, Rayonna, Reyna

Rayven (English) a form of Raven.
Rayvan, Rayvana, Rayvein, Rayvenne, Rayveona, Rayvin, Rayvon, Rayvonia

Rayya (Arabic) thirsty no longer.

Razi (Aramaic) secretive.
*Rayzil, Rayzilee, Raz, Razia,
Raziah, Raziela, Razilee,
Razili*

Raziya (Swahili) agreeable.

Rea (Greek) poppy flower.
Reah

Reagan (Irish) little ruler.
Reagen, Reaghan, Reagine

Reanna (German, English) a
form of Raina. (American) a
form of Raeann.
Reannah

Reanne (American) a form of
Raeann, Reanna.
*Reana, Reane, Reann,
Reannan, Reanne, Reannen,
Reannon, Reeana*

Reba (Hebrew) fourth-born
child. A short form of
Rebecca. See also Reva,
Riva.
Rabah, Reeba, Rheba

Rebeca (Hebrew) an alernate
form of Rebecca.
Rebbeca, Rebecah

Rebecca (Hebrew) tied,
bound. Bible: the wife of
Isaac. See also Becca, Becky.
*Rabecca, Reba, Rebbecca,
Rebeca, Rebeccah, Rebeccea,
Rebeccka, Rebecha, Rebecka,
Rebeckah, Rebeckia, Rebecky,
Rebekah, Rebeque, Rebi,
Reveca, Riva, Rivka*

Rebekah (Hebrew) a form of
Rebecca.
*Rebeka, Rebekha, Rebekka,
Rebekkah, Rebekke, Revecca,
Reveka, Revekka, Rifka*

Rebi (Hebrew) a familiar form
of Rebecca.
*Rebbie, Rebe, Rebie, Reby, Ree,
Reebie*

Reena (Greek) peaceful.
(English) a form of Rina.
(Hebrew) a form of Rinah.
Reen, Reenie, Rena, Reyna

Reet (Estonian) a form of
Margaret.
Reatha, Reta, Retha

Regan (Irish) a form of
Reagan.
Regane, Reghan

Reganne (Irish) a form of
Reagan.
Raegan, Ragan, Reagan, Regin

Reggie (English) a familiar
form of Regina.
*Reggi, Reggy, Regi, Regia,
Regie*

Regina (Latin) queen.
(English) king's advisor.
Geography: the capital of
Saskatchewan. See also Gina.
*Ragine, Raina, Raine, Rega,
Regena, Regennia, Reggie,
Regiena, Regine, Reginia, Regis,
Reina, Rena*

Regine (Latin) a form of
Regina.
Regin

Rei (Japanese) polite, well
behaved.
Reiko

Reilly (Irish) a form of Riley.
*Reilee, Reileigh, Reiley, Reili,
Reilley, Reily*

Reina (Spanish) a short form
of Regina. See also Reyna.
*Reinah, Reine, Reinette, Reinie,
Reinna, Reiny, Reiona, Renia,
Rina*

Rekha (Hindi) thin line.
Reka, Rekia, Rekiah, Rekiya

Remedios (Spanish) remedy.

Remi (French) from Rheims,
France.
Raymi, Remee, Remie, Remy

Remington (English) raven
estate.
Remmington

Ren (Japanese) arranger; water
lily; lotus.

Rena (Hebrew) song; joy. A
familiar form of Irene,
Regina, Renata, Sabrina,
Serena.
Reena, Rina, Rinna, Rinnah

Renae (French) a form of
Renée.
Renay

Renata (French) a form of
Renée.
*Ranata, Rena, Renada,
Renatta, Renita, Rennie,
Renyatta, Rinada, Rinata*

Rene (Greek) a short form of
Irene, Renée.
Reen, Reenie, Reney, Rennie

Renée (French) born again.
*Renae, Renata, Renay, Rene,
Renea, Reneigh, Renell,
Renelle, Renne*

Renita (French) a form of
Renata.
Reneeta, Renetta, Renitza

Rennie (English) a familiar
form of Renata.
Reni, Renie, Renni

Reseda (Spanish) fragrant
mignonette blossom.

Reshawna (American) a com-
bination of the prefix Re +
Shawna.
*Resaunna, Reshana,
Reshaunda, Reshawnda,
Reshawnna, Reshonda,
Reshonn, Reshonta*

Resi (German) a familiar form
of Theresa.
*Resia, Ressa, Resse, Ressie,
Reza, Rezka, Rezi*

Reta (African) shaken.
Reeta, Retta, Rheta, Rhetta

Reubena (Hebrew) behold a child.
Reubina, Reuvena, Rubena, Rubenia, Rubina, Rubine, Rubyna

Reva (Latin) revived. (Hebrew) rain; one-fourth. A form of Reba, Riva.
Ree, Reeva, Revia, Revida

Reveca, Reveka (Slavic) forms of Rebecca, Rebekah.
Reve, Revecca, Revekka, Rivka

Rexanne (American) queen.
Rexan, Rexana, Rexann, Rexanna

Reyhan (Turkish) sweet-smelling flower.

Reyna (Greek) peaceful. (English) a form of Reina.
Reyana, Reyanna, Reyni, Reynna

Reynalda (German) king's advisor.

Réz (Latin, Hungarian) copper-colored hair.

Reza (Czech) a form of Theresa.
Rezi, Rezka

Rhea (Greek) brook, stream. Mythology: the mother of Zeus.
Rheá, Rhéa, Rhealyn, Rheanna, Rhia, Rhianna

Rheanna, Rhianna (Greek) forms of Rhea.
Rheana, Rheann, Rheanne, Rhiana, Rhiauna

Rhian (Welsh) a short form of Rhiannon.
Rhianne, Rhyan, Rhyann, Rhyanne, Rian, Riane, Riann, Rianne, Riayn

Rhiannon (Welsh) witch; nymph; goddess.
Rheannan, Rheannin, Rheannon, Rheanon, Rhian, Rhianen, Rhianna, Rhiannan, Rhiannen, Rhianon, Rhianwen, Rhinnon, Rhyanna, Riana, Riannon, Rianon

Rhoda (Greek) from Rhodes, Greece.
Rhode, Rhodeia, Rhodie, Rhody, Roda, Rodi, Rodie, Rodina

Rhona (Scottish) powerful, mighty. (English) king's advisor.
Rhonae, Rhonnie

Rhonda (Welsh) grand.
Rhondene, Rhondiesha, Ronda, Ronelle, Ronnette

Ria (Spanish) river.
Riah

Riana, Rianna (Irish) short forms of Briana. (Arabic) forms of Rihana.
Reana, Reanna, Rhianna, Rhyanna, Riana, Rianah

Rica (Spanish) a short form of Erica, Frederica, Ricarda. See also Enrica, Sandrica, Terrica, Ulrica.
Ricca, Rieca, Riecka, Rieka, Rikka, Riqua, Rycca

Ricarda (Spanish) rich and powerful ruler.
Rica, Richanda, Richarda, Richi, Ricki

Richael (Irish) saint.

Richelle (German, French) a form of Ricarda.
Richel, Richela, Richele, Richell, Richella, Richia

Rickelle (American) a form of Raquel.
Rickel, Rickela, Rickell

Ricki, Rikki (American) familiar forms of Erica, Frederica, Ricarda.
Rica, Ricci, Riccy, Rici, Rickee, Rickia, Rickie, Rickilee, Rickina, Rickita, Ricky, Ricquie, Riki, Rikia, Rikita, Rikka, Rikke, Rikkia, Rikkie, Rikky, Riko

Ricquel (American) a form of Raquel.
Rickquell, Ricquelle, Rikell, Rikelle

Rida (Arabic) favored by God.

Rihana (Arabic) sweet basil.
Rhiana, Rhianna, Riana, Rianna

Rika (Swedish) ruler.
Ricka

Rilee (Irish) a form of Riley.
Rielee, Rielle

Riley (Irish) valiant.
Raleigh, Reilly, Rieley, Rielly, Riely, Rilee, Rileigh, Rilie

Rilla (German) small brook.

Rima (Arabic) white antelope.
Reem, Reema, Reemah, Rema, Remah, Rhymia, Rim, Ryma

Rimona (Hebrew) pomegranate. See also Mona.

Rin (Japanese) park. Geography: a Japanese village.
Rini, Rynn

Rina (English) a short form of names ending in "rina." (Hebrew) a form of Rena, Rinah.
Reena, Rena

Rinah (Hebrew) joyful.
Rina

Riona (Irish) saint.

Risa (Latin) laughter.
Reesa, Resa

Risha (Hindi) born during the lunar month of Taurus.
Rishah, Rishay

Rishona (Hebrew) first.
Rishina, Rishon

Rissa (Greek) a short form of Nerissa.
Risa, Rissah, Ryssa, Ryssah

Rita (Sanskrit) brave; honest. (Greek) a short form of Margarita.
Reatha, Reda, Reeta, Reida, Reitha, Rheta, Riet, Ritah, Ritamae, Ritamarie

Ritsa (Greek) a familiar form of Alexandra.
Ritsah, Ritsi, Ritsie, Ritsy

Riva (French) river bank. (Hebrew) a short form of Rebecca. See also Reba, Reva.
Rivalee, Rivi, Rivvy

River (Latin, French) stream, water.
Rivana, Rivanna, Rivers, Riviane

Rivka (Hebrew) a short form of Rebecca.
Rivca, Rivcah, Rivkah

Riza (Greek) a form of Theresa.
Riesa, Rizus, Rizza

Roanna (American) a form of Rosana.
Ranna, Roana, Roanda, Roanne

Robbi, Robbie (English) familiar forms of Roberta.
Robby, Robbye, Robey, Robi, Robia, Roby

Roberta (English) famous brilliance.
Roba, Robbi, Robbie, Robena, Robertena, Robertina

Robin (English) robin. A form of Roberta.
Robann, Robbin, Robeen, Roben, Robena, Robian, Robina, Robine, Robinette, Robinia, Robinn, Robinta, Robyn

Robinette (English) a familiar form of Robin.
Robernetta, Robinet, Robinett, Robinita

Robyn (English) a form of Robin.
Robbyn, Robbynn, Robyne, Robynn, Robynne

Rochelle (French) large stone. (Hebrew) a form of Rachel. See also Shelley.
Reshelle, Roch, Rocheal, Rochealle, Rochel, Rochele, Rochell, Rochella, Rochette, Rockelle, Roshele, Roshell, Roshelle

Rocio (Spanish) dewdrops.
Rocío

Roderica (German) famous ruler.
Rica, Rika, Rodericka, Roderika, Rodreicka, Rodricka, Rodrika

Rodnae (English) island clearing.
Rodna, Rodnetta, Rodnicka

Rodneisha (American) a combination of Rodnae + Aisha.
Rodesha, Rodisha, Rodishah,

Rodnecia, Rodnesha,
Rodneshia, Rodneycia,
Rodneysha, Rodnisha

Rohana (Hindi) sandalwood.
(American) a combination of
Rose + Hannah.
Rochana, Rohena

Rohini (Hindi) woman.

Rolanda (German) famous
throughout the land.
Ralna, Rolande, Rolando,
Rolaunda, Roleesha, Rolene,
Rolinda, Rollande, Rolonda

Rolene (German) a form of
Rolanda.
Rolaine, Rolena, Rolleen,
Rollene

Roma (Latin) from Rome.
Romai, Rome, Romeise,
Romeka, Romelle, Romesha,
Rometta, Romia, Romilda,
Romilla, Romina, Romini,
Romma, Romonia

Romaine (French) from Rome.
Romana, Romanda, Romanelle,
Romania, Romanique, Romany,
Romayne, Romona, Romy

Romy (French) a familiar form
of Romaine. (English) a
familiar form of Rosemary.
Romi, Romie

Rona (Scandinavian) short
forms of Ronalda.
Rhona, Roana, Ronalda,
Ronna, Ronnae, Ronnay,
Ronne, Ronni, Ronsy

Ronaele (Greek) the name
Eleanor spelled backwards.
Ronalee, Ronni, Ronnie, Ronny

Ronda (Welsh) a form of
Rhonda.
Rondai, Rondesia, Rondi,
Rondie, Ronelle, Ronnette,
Ronni, Ronnie, Ronny

Rondelle (French) short poem.
Rhondelle, Rondel, Ronndelle

Roneisha (American) a com-
bination of Rhonda + Aisha.
Roneasha, Ronecia, Ronee,
Roneeka, Roneesha, Roneice,
Ronese, Ronesha, Roneshia,
Ronesia, Ronessa, Ronessia,
Ronichia, Ronicia, Roniesha,
Ronisha, Ronneisha, Ronnesa,
Ronnesha, Ronneshia, Ronni,
Ronnie, Ronniesha, Ronny

Ronelle (Welsh) a form of
Rhonda, Ronda.
Ranell, Ranelle, Ronel, Ronella,
Ronielle, Ronnella, Ronnelle

Ronisha (American) a form of
Roneisha.
Ronise, Ronnise, Ronnisha,
Ronnishia

Ronli (Hebrew) joyful.
Ronia, Ronice, Ronit, Ronlee,
Ronlie, Ronni, Ronnie, Ronny

Ronnette (Welsh) a familiar
form of Rhonda, Ronda.
Ronetta, Ronette, Ronit,
Ronita, Ronnetta, Ronni,
Ronnie, Ronny

Ronni, Ronnie, Ronny
(American) familiar forms of
Veronica and names begin-
ning with "Ron."
Rone, Ronee, Roni, Ronnee,
Ronney

Rori, Rory (Irish) famous brilliance; famous ruler.
Rorie

Ros, Roz (English) short forms
of Rosalind, Rosalyn.
Rozz, Rozzey, Rozzi, Rozzie,
Rozzy

Rosa (Italian, Spanish) a form
of Rose. History: Rosa Parks
inspired the American Civil
Rights movement by refusing
to give up her bus seat to a
white man in Montgomery,
Alabama. See also Charo,
Roza.

Rosabel (French) beautiful
rose.
Rosabelia, Rosabella, Rosabelle,
Rosebelle

Rosalba (Latin) white rose.
Rosalva, Roselba

Rosalie (English) a form of
Rosalind.
Rosalea, Rosalee, Rosaleen,
Rosaleigh, Rosalene, Rosalia,
Rosealee, Rosealie, Roselee,
Roseli, Roselia, Roselie, Roseley,
Rosely, Rosilee, Rosli, Rozali,
Rozália, Rozalie, Rozele

Rosalind (Spanish) fair rose.
Ros, Rosalie, Rosalinda,
Rosalinde, Rosalyn, Rosalynd,
Rosalynde, Roselind, Roselyn,
Rosie, Roz, Rozalind, Rozland

Rosalinda (Spanish) a form of
Rosalind.
Rosalina

Rosalyn (Spanish) a form of
Rosalind.
Ros, Rosaleen, Rosalin,
Rosaline, Rosalyne, Rosalynn,
Rosalynne, Rosilyn, Roslin,
Roslyn, Roslyne, Roslynn, Roz,
Rozalyn, Rozlyn

Rosamond (German) famous
guardian.
Rosamund, Rosamunda,
Rosemonde, Rozamond

Rosanna, Roseanna (English)
combinations of Rose + Anna.
Ranna, Roanna, Rosana,
Rosannah, Roseana,
Roseannah, Rosehanah,
Rosehannah, Rosie, Rossana,
Rossanna, Rozana, Rozanna

Rosanne, Roseanne (English)
combinations of Rose +
Ann.
Roanne, Rosan, Rosann,
Roseann, Rose Ann, Rose
Anne, Rossann, Rossanne,
Rozann, Rozanne

Rosario (Filipino, Spanish)
rosary.
Rosarah, Rosaria, Rosarie,
Rosary, Rosaura

Rose (Latin) rose. See also
Chalina, Raisa, Raizel, Roza.
Rada, Rasia, Rasine, Rois,
Róise, Rosa, Rosea, Rosella,
Roselle, Roses, Rosetta, Rosie,
Rosina, Rosita, Rosse

Roselani (Hawaiian) heavenly
rose.

Roselyn (Spanish) a form of
Rosalind.
Roseleen, Roselene, Roselin,
Roseline, Roselyne, Roselynn,
Roselynne

Rosemarie (English) a combi-
nation of Rose + Marie.
Rosamaria, Rosamarie,
Rosemari, Rosemaria, Rose
Marie

Rosemary (English) a combination of Rose + Mary.
Romi, Romy

Rosetta (Italian) a form of
Rose.
Roseta, Rosette

Roshan (Sanskrit) shining
light.

Roshawna (American) a com-
bination of Rose + Shawna.
Roshan, Roshana, Roshanda,
Roshani, Roshann, Roshanna,
Roshanta, Roshaun, Roshauna,
Roshaunda, Roshawn,
Roshawnda, Roshawnna,
Roshona, Roshonda, Roshowna,
Roshunda

Rosie (English) a familiar form
of Rosalind, Rosanna, Rose.
Rosey, Rosi, Rosio, Rosse, Rosy,
Rozsi, Rozy

Rosina (English) a familiar
form of Rose.
Rosena, Rosenah, Rosene,
Rosheen, Rozena, Rozina

Rosita (Spanish) a familiar
form of Rose.
Roseeta, Roseta, Rozeta,
Rozita, Rozyte

Roslyn (Scottish) a form of
Rossalyn.
Roslin, Roslynn, Rosslyn,
Rosslynn

Rossalyn (Scottish) cape;
promontory.
Roslyn, Rosselyn, Rosylin,
Roszaliyn

Rowan (English) tree with red
berries. (Welsh) a form of
Rowena.
Rowana

Rowena (Welsh) fair-haired.
(English) famous friend.
Literature: Ivanhoe's love
interest in Sir Walter Scott's
novel *Ivanhoe*.
Ranna, Ronni, Row, Rowan,
Rowe, Roweena, Rowen,
Rowina

Roxana, Roxanna (Persian)
forms of Roxann.
Rocsana, Roxannah

Roxann, Roxanne (Persian)
sunrise. Literature: Roxanne
is the heroine of Edmond
Rostand's play *Cyrano de
Bergerac.*
*Rocxann, Roxan, Roxana,
Roxane, Roxanna, Roxianne,
Roxy*

Roxy (Persian) a familiar form
of Roxann.
Roxi, Roxie

Royale (English) royal.
*Royal, Royalene, Royalle,
Roylee, Roylene, Ryal, Ryale*

Royanna (English) queenly,
royal.
Roya

Roza (Slavic) a form of Rosa.
*Roz, Rozalia, Roze, Rozel,
Rozele, Rozell, Rozella,
Rozelli, Rozia, Rozsa, Rozsi,
Rozyte, Rozza, Rozzie*

Rozene (Native American)
rose blossom.
*Rozena, Rozina, Rozine,
Ruzena*

Ruana (Hindi) stringed musical instrument.
Ruan, Ruon

Rubena (Hebrew) a form of
Reubena.
*Rubenia, Rubina, Rubine,
Rubinia, Rubyn, Rubyna*

Rubi (French) a form of Ruby.
*Ruba, Rubbie, Rubee, Rubia,
Rubie*

Ruby (French) precious stone.
*Rubby, Rubetta, Rubette,
Rubey, Rubi, Rubiann,
Rubyann, Rubye*

Ruchi (Hindi) one who wishes
to please.

Rudee (German) famous wolf.
*Rudeline, Rudell, Rudella,
Rudi, Rudie, Rudina, Rudy*

Rudra (Hindi) seeds of the
rudraksha plant.

Rue (German) famous.
(French) street. (English)
regretful; strong-scented
herbs.
Ru, Ruey

Ruffina (Italian) redhead.
*Rufeena, Rufeine, Rufina,
Ruphyna*

Rui (Japanese) affectionate.

Rukan (Arabic) steady; confi-
dent.

Rula (Latin, English) ruler.

Runa (Norwegian) secret;
flowing.
Runna

Ruperta (Spanish) a form of
Roberta.

Rupinder (Sanskrit) beautiful.

Ruri (Japanese) emerald.
Ruriko

Rusalka (Czech) wood nymph. (Russian) mermaid.

Russhell (French) redhead; fox colored.
Rushell, Rushelle, Russellynn, Russhelle

Rusti (English) redhead.
Russet, Rustie, Rusty

Ruth (Hebrew) friendship. Bible: daughter-in-law of Naomi.
Rutha, Ruthalma, Ruthe, Ruthella, Ruthetta, Ruthie, Ruthven

Ruthann (American) a combination of Ruth + Ann.
Ruthan, Ruthanna, Ruthannah, Ruthanne, Ruthina, Ruthine

Ruthie (Hebrew) a familiar form of Ruth.
Ruthey, Ruthi, Ruthy

Ruza (Czech) rose.
Ruzena, Ruzenka, Ruzha, Ruzsa

Ryan, Ryann (Irish) little ruler.
Raiann, Raianne, Rhyann, Riana, Riane, Ryana, Ryane, Ryanna, Ryanne, Rye, Ryen, Ryenne

Ryba (Czech) fish.

Rylee (Irish) valiant.
Rye, Ryelee, Rylea, Ryleigh, Ryley, Rylie, Rylina, Rylyn

Ryleigh, Rylie (Irish) forms of Rylee.
Ryelie, Ryli, Rylleigh, Ryllie

Ryley (Irish) a form of Rylee.
Ryeley, Rylly, Ryly

Ryo (Japanese) dragon.
Ryoko

S

Saarah (Arabic) princess.

Saba (Arabic) morning. (Greek) a form of Sheba.
Sabaah, Sabah, Sabba, Sabbah

Sabi (Arabic) young girl.

Sabina (Latin) History: the Sabine were a tribe in ancient Italy. See also Bina.
Sabeen, Sabena, Sabienne, Sabin, Sabine, Sabinka, Sabinna, Sabiny, Saby, Sabyne, Savina, Sebina, Sebinah

Sabiya (Arabic) morning; eastern wind.
Saba, Sabaya, Sabiyah

Sable (English) sable; sleek.
Sabel, Sabela, Sabella

Sabra (Hebrew) thorny cactus fruit. (Arabic) resting. History: a name for native-born Israelis, who were said to be hard on the outside and soft and sweet on the inside.
Sabera, Sabira, Sabrah, Sabre, Sabrea, Sabreah, Sabree, Sabreea, Sabri, Sabria, Sabriah, Sabriya, Sebra

Sabreena (English) a form of
Sabrina.
Sabreen, Sabrena, Sabrene

Sabrina (Latin) boundary line.
(English) princess. (Hebrew) a
familiar form of Sabra. See also
Bree, Brina, Rena, Zabrina.
Sabre, Sabreena, Sabrinas,
Sabrinah, Sabrine, Sabrinia,
Sabrinna, Sabryna, Sebree,
Sebrina, Subrina

Sabryna (English) a form of
Sabrina.
Sabrynna

Sacha (Russian) a form of Sasha.
Sache, Sachia

Sachi (Japanese) blessed; lucky.
Saatchi, Sachie, Sachiko

Sada (Japanese) chaste.
(English) a form of Sadie.
Sadá, Sadah, Sadako

Sade (Hebrew) a form of
Chadee, Sarah, Shardae,
Sharday.
Sáde, Sadé, Sadea, Sadee, Shaday

Sadella (American) a combi-
nation of Sade + Ella.
Sadelle, Sydel, Sydell, Sydella,
Sydelle

Sadhana (Hindi) devoted.

Sadie (Hebrew) a familiar
form of Sarah. See also Sada.
Saddie, Sadee, Sadey, Sadi,
Sadiey, Sady, Sadye, Saide,
Saidee, Saidey, Saidi, Saidia,

Saidie, Saidy, Sayde, Saydee,
Seidy

Sadira (Persian) lotus tree.
(Arabic) star.
Sadra

Sadiya (Arabic) lucky, fortu-
nate.
Sadi, Sadia, Sadiah, Sadiyah,
Sadiyyah, Sadya

Sadzi (Carrier) sunny disposi-
tion.

Saffron (English) Botany: a
plant with purple or white
flowers whose orange stigmas
are used as a spice.
Safron

Safiya (Arabic) pure; serene;
best friend.
Safa, Safeya, Saffa, Safia,
Safiyah

Sagara (Hindi) ocean.

Sage (English) wise. Botany:
an herb used as a seasoning.
Sagia, Saige, Salvia

Sahara (Arabic) desert;
wilderness.
Sahar, Saharah, Sahari, Saheer,
Saher, Sahira, Sahra, Sahrah

Sai (Japanese) talented.
Saiko

Saida (Hebrew) a form of
Sarah. (Arabic) happy; fortu-
nate.
Saidah

Saige (English) a form of Sage.

Saira (Hebrew) a form of Sara.
Sairah, Sairi

Sakaë (Japanese) prosperous.

Sakari (Hindi) sweet.
Sakkara

Saki (Japanese) cloak; rice wine.

Sakti (Hindi) energy, power.

Sakuna (Native American) bird.

Sakura (Japanese) cherry blossom; wealthy; prosperous.

Sala (Hindi) sala tree.
Religion: the sacred tree under which Buddha died.

Salali (Cherokee) squirrel.

Salama (Arabic) peaceful. See also Zulima.

Salena (French) a form of Salina.
Saleana, Saleen, Saleena, Salene, Salenna, Sallene

Salima (Arabic) safe and sound; healthy.
Saleema, Salema, Salim, Salimah, Salma

Salina (French) solemn, dignified.
Salena, Salin, Salinah, Salinda, Saline

Salliann (English) a combination of Sally + Ann.
Sallian, Sallianne, Sallyann, Sally-Ann, Sallyanne, Sally-Anne

Sally (English) princess.
History: Sally Ride, an American astronaut, became the first U. S. woman in space.
Sal, Salaid, Sallee, Salletta, Sallette, Salley, Salli, Sallie

Salome (Hebrew) peaceful.
History: Salome Alexandra was a ruler of ancient Judea. Bible: the niece of King Herod.
Saloma, Salomé, Salomey, Salomi

Salvadora (Spanish) savior.

Salvia (Spanish) healthy; saved. (Latin) a form of Sage.
Sallvia, Salviana, Salviane, Salvina, Salvine

Samala (Hebrew) asked of God.
Samale, Sammala

Samanta (Hebrew) a form of Samantha.
Samantah, Smanta

Samantha (Aramaic) listener. (Hebrew) told by God.
Sam, Samana, Samanath, Samanatha, Samanitha, Samanithia, Samanta, Samanth, Samanthe, Samanthi, Samanthia, Samatha, Sami, Sammanth, Sammantha, Semantha, Simantha, Smantha, Symantha

Samara (Latin) elm-tree seed.
Saimara, Samaira, Samar,
Samarah, Samari, Samaria,
Samariah, Samarie, Samarra,
Samarrea, Samary, Samera,
Sameria, Samira, Sammar,
Sammara, Samora

Samatha (Hebrew) a form of
Samantha.
Sammatha

Sameh (Hebrew) listener.
(Arabic) forgiving.
Samaiya, Samaya

Sami (Arabic) praised.
(Hebrew) a short form of
Samantha, Samuela.
Samia, Samiah, Samiha,
Samina, Sammey, Sammi,
Sammie, Sammijo, Sammy,
Sammyjo, Samya, Samye

Samira (Arabic) entertaining.
Samirah, Samire, Samiria,
Samirra, Samyra

Samone (Hebrew) a form of
Simone.
Samoan, Samoane, Samon,
Samona, Samoné, Samonia

Samuela (Hebrew) heard
God, asked of God.
Samala, Samelia, Samella,
Sami, Samielle, Samille,
Sammile, Samuelle

Samuelle (Hebrew) a form of
Samuela.
Samuella

Sana (Arabic) mountaintop;
splendid; brilliant.
Sanaa, Sanáa, Sanaah, Sane,
Sanah

Sancia (Spanish) holy, sacred.
Sanceska, Sancha, Sancharia,
Sanchia, Sancie, Santsia, Sanzia

Sandeep (Punjabi) enlightened.
Sandip

Sandi (Greek) a familiar form
of Sandra.
Sandee, Sandia, Sandie,
Sandiey, Sandine, Sanndie

Sandra (Greek) defender of
mankind. A short form of
Cassandra. History: Sandra
Day O'Connor was the first
woman appointed to the
U.S. Supreme Court. See also
Zandra.
Sahndra, Sandi, Sandira,
Sandrea, Sandria, Sandrica,
Sandy, Sanndra, Saundra

Sandrea (Greek) a form of
Sandra.
Sandreea, Sandreia, Sandrell,
Sandria, Sanndria

Sandrica (Greek) a form of
Sandra. See also Rica.
Sandricka, Sandrika

Sandrine (Greek) a form of
Alexandra.
Sandreana, Sandrene,
Sandrenna, Sandrianna,
Sandrina

Sandy (Greek) a familiar form of Cassandra, Sandra.
Sandya, Sandye

Sanne (Hebrew, Dutch) lily.
Sanea, Saneh, Sanna, Sanneen

Santana (Spanish) saint.
Santa, Santaniata, Santanna, Santanne, Santena, Santenna, Shantana

Santina (Spanish) little saint.
Santinia

Sanura (Swahili) kitten.
Sanora

Sanuye (Moquelumnan) red clouds at sunset.

Sanya (Sanskrit) born on Saturday.
Saneiya, Sania, Sanyia

Sanyu (Luganda) happiness.

Sapata (Native American) dancing bear.

Sapphira (Hebrew) a form of Sapphire.
Safira, Sapheria, Saphira, Saphyra, Sephira

Sapphire (Greek) blue gemstone.
Saffire, Saphire, Saphyre, Sapphira

Sara (Hebrew) a form of Sarah.
Saira, Sarae, Saralee, Sarra, Sera

Sarah (Hebrew) princess. Bible: the wife of Abraham and mother of Isaac. See also Sadie, Saida, Sally, Saree, Sharai, Shari, Zara, Zarita.
Sahra, Sara, Saraha, Sarahann, Sarahi, Sarai, Sarann, Saray, Sarha, Sariah, Sarina, Sarita, Sarolta, Sarotte, Sarrah, Sasa, Sayra, Sorcha

Sarai, Saray (Hebrew) forms of Sarah.
Saraya

Saralyn (American) a combination of Sarah + Lynn.
Saralena, Saraly, Saralynn

Saree (Arabic) noble. (Hebrew) a familiar form of Sarah.
Sareeka, Sareka, Sari, Sarika, Sarka, Sarri, Sarrie, Sary

Sariah (Hebrew) forms of Sarah.
Saria, Sarie

Sarila (Turkish) waterfall.

Sarina (Hebrew) a familiar form of Sarah.
Sareen, Sareena, Saren, Sarena, Sarene, Sarenna, Sarin, Sarine, Sarinna, Sarinne

Sarita (Hebrew) a familiar form of Sarah.
Saretta, Sarette, Sarit, Saritia, Saritta

Sarolta (Hungarian) a form of Sarah.

Sarotte (French) a form of Sarah.

Sarrah (Hebrew) a form of Sarah.
Sarra

Sasa (Japanese) assistant. (Hungarian) a form of Sarah, Sasha.

Sasha (Russian) defender of mankind. See also Zasha.
Sacha, Sahsha, Sasa, Sascha, Saschae, Sashae, Sashah, Sashai, Sashana, Sashay, Sashea, Sashel, Sashenka, Sashey, Sashi, Sashia, Sashira, Sashsha, Sashya, Sasjara, Sauscha, Sausha, Shasha, Shashi, Shashia

Sass (Irish) Saxon.
Sassie, Sassoon, Sassy

Satara (American) a combination of Sarah + Tara.
Sataria, Satarra, Sateriaa, Saterra, Saterria

Satin (French) smooth, shiny.
Satinder

Satinka (Native American) sacred dancer.

Sato (Japanese) sugar.
Satu

Saundra (English) a form of Sandra, Sondra.
Saundee, Saundi, Saundie, Saundy

Saura (Hindi) sun worshiper.

Savana, Savanna (Spanish) forms of Savannah.
Saveena, Savhana, Savhanna, Savina, Savine, Savona, Savonna

Savanah (Spanish) a form of Savannah.
Savhannah

Savannah (Spanish) treeless plain.
Sahvannah, Savana, Savanah, Savanha, Savanna, Savannha, Savauna, Savonnah, Savonne, Sevan, Sevanah, Sevanh, Sevann, Sevanna, Svannah

Sawa (Japanese) swamp. (Moquelumnan) stone.

Sawyer (English) wood worker.
Sawyar, Sawyor

Sayde, Saydee (Hebrew) forms of Sadie.
Saydi, Saydia, Saydie, Saydy

Sayo (Japanese) born at night.

Sayra (Hebrew) a form of Sarah.
Sayrah, Sayre, Sayri

Scarlett (English) bright red. Literature: Scarlett O'Hara is the heroine of Margaret Mitchell's novel *Gone with the Wind.*
Scarlet, Scarlette, Scarlotte, Skarlette

Schyler (Dutch) sheltering.
*Schuyla, Schuyler, Schuylia,
Schylar*

Scotti (Scottish) from
Scotland.
Scota, Scotia, Scottie, Scotty

Seana, Seanna (Irish) forms
of Jane. See also Shauna,
Shawna.
*Seaana, Sean, Seane, Seann,
Seannae, Seannah, Seannalisa,
Seanté, Sianna, Sina*

Sebastiane (Greek) venerable.
(Latin) revered. (French) a
form of Sebastian (see Boys'
Names).
*Sebastene, Sebastia, Sebastian,
Sebastiana, Sebastien,
Sebastienne*

Seble (Ethiopian) autumn.

Sebrina (English) a form of
Sabrina.
*Sebrena, Sebrenna, Sebria,
Sebriana*

Secilia (Latin) a form of
Cecilia.
Saselia, Sasilia, Sesilia, Sileas

Secunda (Latin) second.

Seda (Armenian) forest
voices.

Sedna (Eskimo) well-fed.
Mythology: the goddess of
sea animals.

Seelia (English) a form of
Sheila.

Seema (Greek) sprout.
(Afghan) sky; profile.
Seemah, Sima, Simah

Sefa (Swiss) a familiar form of
Josefina.

Seirra (Irish) a form of Sierra.
Seiara, Seiarra, Seira, Seirria

Seki (Japanese) wonderful.
Seka

Sela (English) a short form of
Selena.
Seeley, Selah

Selam (Ethiopian) peaceful.

Selda (German) a short form
of Griselda. (Yiddish) a form
of Zelda.
Seldah, Selde, Sellda, Selldah

Selena (Greek) moon.
Mythology: Selene was the
goddess of the moon. See
also Celena.
*Saleena, Sela, Selana, Seleana,
Seleena, Selen, Selenah, Selene,
Séléné, Selenia, Selenna, Selina,
Sena, Syleena, Sylena*

Selene (Greek) a form of
Selena.
Seleni, Selenie, Seleny

Selia (Latin) a short form of
Cecilia.
Seel, Seil, Sela, Silia

Selima (Hebrew) peaceful.
Selema, Selemah, Selimah

Selina (Greek) a form of Celina, Selena.
Selie, Selin, Selinda, Seline, Selinia, Selinka, Sellina, Selyna, Selyne, Selynne, Sylina

Selma (German) devine protector. (Irish) fair, just. (Scandinavian) divinely protected. (Arabic) secure. See also Zelma.
Sellma, Sellmah, Selmah

Sema (Turkish) heaven; divine omen.
Semaj

Sen (Japanese) Mythology: a magical forest elf that lives for thousands of years.

Senalda (Spanish) sign.
Sena, Senda, Senna

Seneca (Iroquoian) a tribal name.
Senaka, Seneka, Senequa, Senequae, Senequai, Seneque

Septima (Latin) seventh.

Sequoia (Cherokee) giant redwood tree.
Seqoiyia, Seqouyia, Seqoya, Sequoi, Sequoiah, Sequora, Sequoya, Sequoyah, Sikoya

Serafina (Hebrew) burning; ardent. Bible: seraphim are an order of angels.
Sarafina, Serafine, Seraphe, Seraphin, Seraphina, Seraphine, Seraphita, Serapia, Serofina

Serena (Latin) peaceful. See also Rena.
Sarina, Saryna, Seraina, Serana, Sereen, Sereina, Seren, Serenah, Serene, Serenea, Serenia, Serenna, Serina, Serreana, Serrena, Serrenna

Serenity (Latin) peaceful.
Serenidy, Serenitee, Serenitey, Sereniti, Serenitiy, Serinity, Serrennity

Serilda (Greek) armed warrior woman.

Serina (Latin) a form of Serena.
Sereena, Serin, Serine, Serreena, Serrin, Serrina, Seryna

Sevilla (Spanish) from Seville.
Seville

Shaba (Spanish) rose.
Shabana, Shabina

Shada (Native American) pelican.
Shadae, Shadea, Shadeana, Shadee, Shadi, Shadia, Shadiah, Shadie, Shadiya, Shaida

Shaday (American) a form of Sade.
Shadai, Shadaia, Shadaya, Shadayna, Shadei, Shadeziah, Shaiday

Shadrika (American) a combination of the prefix Sha + Rika.
Shadreeka, Shadreka, Shadrica, Shadricka, Shadrieka

Shae (Irish) a form of Shea.
Shaenel, Shaeya, Shai, Shaia

Shaelee (Irish) a form of
Shea.
*Shaeleigh, Shaeley, Shaelie,
Shaely*

Shaelyn (Irish) a form of
Shea.
*Shael, Shaelaine, Shaelan,
Shaelanie, Shaelanna, Shaeleen,
Shaelene, Shaelin, Shaeline,
Shaelyne, Shaelynn, Shae-Lynn,
Shaelynne*

Shafira (Swahili)
distinguished.
Shaffira

Shahar (Arabic) moonlit.
Shahara

Shahina (Arabic) falcon.
*Shaheen, Shaheena, Shahi,
Shahin*

Shahla (Afghani) beautiful
eyes.
Shaila, Shailah, Shalah

Shaianne (Cheyenne) a form
of Cheyenne.
*Shaeen, Shaeine, Shaian,
Shaiana, Shaiandra, Shaiane,
Shaiann, Shaianna*

Shaila (Latin) a form of
Sheila.
*Shaela, Shaelea, Shaeyla,
Shailah, Shailee, Shailey, Shaili,
Shailie, Shailla, Shaily, Shailyn,
Shailynn*

Shaina (Yiddish) beautiful.
*Shaena, Shainah, Shaine,
Shainna, Shajna, Shanie, Shayna,
Shayndel, Sheina, Sheindel*

Shajuana (American) a com-
bination of the prefix Sha +
Juanita. See also Shawanna.
*Shajuan, Shajuanda,
Shajuanita, Shajuanna,
Shajuanza*

Shaka (Hindi) a form of
Shakti. A short form of
names beginning with
"Shak." See also Chaka.
Shakah, Shakha

Shakarah (American) a combi-
nation of the prefix Sha +
Kara.
*Shacara, Shacari, Shaccara, Shaka,
Shakari, Shakkara, Shikara*

Shakayla (Arabic) a form of
Shakila.
*Shakaela, Shakail, Shakaila,
Shakala*

Shakeena (American) a com-
bination of the prefix Sha +
Keena.
*Shaka, Shakeina, Shakeyna,
Shakina, Shakyna*

Shakeita (American) a combi-
nation of the prefix Sha +
Keita. See also Shaqueita.
*Shaka, Shakeeta, Shakeitha,
Shakeithia, Shaketa, Shaketha,
Shakethia, Shaketia, Shakita,
Shakitra, Sheketa, Shekita,
Shikita, Shikitha*

Shakera (Arabic) a form of Shakira.
Chakeria, Shakeira, Shakeirra, Shakerah, Shakeria, Shakeriah, Shakeriay, Shakerra, Shakerri, Shakerria, Shakerya, Shakeryia, Shakeyra

Shakia (American) a combination of the prefix Sha + Kia.
Shakeeia, Shakeeyah, Shakeia, Shakeya, Shakiya, Shekeia, Shekia, Shekiah, Shikia

Shakila (Arabic) pretty.
Chakila, Shaka, Shakayla, Shakeela, Shakeena, Shakela, Shakelah, Shakilah, Shakyla, Shekila, Shekilla, Shikeela

Shakira (Arabic) thankful.
Shaakira, Shacora, Shaka, Shakeera, Shakeerah, Shakeeria, Shakera, Shakiera, Shakierra, Shakir, Shakirah, Shakirat, Shakirea, Shakirra, Shakora, Shakuria, Shakyra, Shaquira, Shekiera, Shekira, Shikira

Shakti (Hindi) energy, power. Religion: a form of the Hindu goddess Devi.
Sakti, Shaka, Sita

Shakyra (Arabic) a form of Shakira.
Shakyria

Shalana (American) a combination of the prefix Sha + Lana.
Shalaana, Shalain, Shalaina, Shalaine, Shaland, Shalanda, Shalane, Shalann, Shalaun, Shalauna, Shalayna, Shalayne, Shalaynna, Shallan, Shelan, Shelanda

Shaleah (American) a combination of the prefix Sha + Leah.
Shalea, Shalee, Shaleea, Shalia, Shaliah

Shaleisha (American) a combination of the prefix Sha + Aisha.
Shalesha, Shalesia, Shalicia, Shalisha

Shalena (American) a combination of the prefix Sha + Lena.
Shaleana, Shaleen, Shaleena, Shalen, Shálena, Shalene, Shalené, Shalenna, Shalina, Shalinda, Shaline, Shalini, Shalinna, Shelayna, Shelayne, Shelena

Shalisa (American) a combination of the prefix Sha + Lisa.
Shalesa, Shalese, Shalessa, Shalice, Shalicia, Shaliece, Shalise, Shalisha, Shalishea, Shalisia, Shalissa, Shalisse, Shalyce, Shalys, Shalyse

Shalita (American) a combination of the prefix Sha + Lita.
Shaleta, Shaletta, Shalida, Shalitta

Shalona (American) a combination of the prefix Sha + Lona.
Shalon, Shalone, Shálonna, Shalonne

Shalonda (American) a combination of the prefix Sha + Ondine.
Shalonde, Shalondine, Shalondra, Shalondria

Shalyn (American) a combination of the prefix Sha + Lynn.
Shalin, Shalina, Shalinda, Shaline, Shalyna, Shalynda, Shalyne, Shalynn, Shalynne

Shamara (Arabic) ready for battle.
Shamar, Shamarah, Shamare, Shamarea, Shamaree, Shamari, Shamaria, Shamariah, Shamarra, Shamarri, Shammara, Shamora, Shamori, Shamorra, Shamorria, Shamorriah

Shameka (American) a combination of the prefix Sha + Meka.
Shameaka, Shameakah, Shameca, Shamecca, Shamecha, Shamecia, Shameika, Shameke, Shamekia

Shamika (American) a combination of the prefix Sha + Mika.
Shameeca, Shameeka, Shamica, Shamicia, Shamicka, Shamieka, Shamikia

Shamira (Hebrew) precious stone.
Shamir, Shamiran, Shamiria, Shamyra

Shamiya (American) a combination of the prefix Sha + Mia.
Shamea, Shamia, Shamiah, Shamiyah, Shamyia, Shamyiah, Shamyne

Shana (Hebrew) God is gracious. (Irish) a form of Jane.
Shaana, Shan, Shanae, Shanda, Shandi, Shane, Shania, Shanna, Shannah, Shauna, Shawna

Shanae (Irish) a form of Shana.
Shanay, Shanea

Shanda (American) a form of Chanda, Shana.
Shandae, Shandah, Shandra, Shannda

Shandi (English) a familiar form of Shana.
Shandee, Shandeigh, Shandey, Shandice, Shandie

Shandra (American) a form of Shanda. See also Chandra.
Shandrea, Shandreka, Shandri, Shandria, Shandriah, Shandrice, Shandrie, Shandry

Shane (Irish) a form of Shana.
Shanea, Shaneah, Shanee, Shanée, Shanie

Shaneisha (American) a combination of the prefix Sha + Aisha.
Shanesha, Shaneshia, Shanessa, Shanisha, Shanissha

Shaneka (American) a form of Shanika.
Shanecka, Shaneekah, Shaneequa, Shaneeque, Shaneika, Shaneikah, Shanekia, Shanequa, Shaneyka, Shonneka

Shanel, Shanell, Shanelle
(American) forms of Chanel.
Schanel, Schanell, Shanella, Shanelly, Shannel, Shannell, Shannelle, Shenel, Shenela, Shenell, Shenelle, Shenelly, Shinelle, Shonelle, Shynelle

Shaneta (American) a combination of the prefix Sha + Neta.
Seanette, Shaneeta, Shanetha, Shanethis, Shanetta, Shanette, Shineta, Shonetta

Shani (Swahili) a form of Shany.

Shania (American) a form of Shana.
Shanasia, Shanaya, Shaniah, Shaniya, Shanya, Shenia

Shanice (American) a form of Janice. See also Chanise.
Chenise, Shanece, Shaneese, Shaneice, Shanese, Shanicea, Shaniece, Shanise, Shanneice, Shannice, Shanyce, Sheneice

Shanida (American) a combination of the prefix Sha + Ida.
Shaneeda, Shannida

Shanika (American) a combination of the prefix Sha + Nika.
Shaneka, Shanica, Shanicca, Shanicka, Shanieka, Shanike, Shanikia, Shanikka, Shanikqua, Shanikwa, Shaniqua, Shenika, Shineeca, Shonnika

Shaniqua (American) a form of Shanika.
Shaniqa, Shaniquah, Shanique, Shaniquia, Shaniquwa, Shaniqwa, Shenequa, Sheniqua, Shinequa, Shiniqua

Shanise (American) a form of Shanice.
Shanisa, Shanisha, Shanisia, Shanissa, Shanisse, Shineese

Shanita (American) a combination of the prefix Sha + Nita.
Shanitha, Shanitra, Shanitta, Shinita

Shanley (Irish) hero's child.
Shanlee, Shanleigh, Shanlie, Shanly

Shanna (Irish) a form of Shana, Shannon.
Shanea, Shannah, Shannea

Shannen (Irish) a form of Shannon.
Shanen, Shanena, Shanene

Shannon (Irish) small and wise.
Shanan, Shanadoah, Shann, Shanna, Shannan, Shanneen, Shannen, Shannie, Shannin, Shannyn, Shanon

Shanta, Shantae, Shante (French) forms of Chantal.
Shantai, Shantay, Shantaya, Shantaye, Shanté, Shantea, Shantee, Shantée, Shanteia

Shantal (American) a form of Shantel.
Shantall, Shontal

Shantana (American) a form of Santana.
Shantan, Shantanae, Shantanell, Shantanickia, Shantanika, Shantanna

Shantara (American) a combination of the prefix Sha + Tara.
Shantaria, Shantarra, Shantera, Shanteria, Shanterra, Shantira, Shontara, Shuntara

Shanteca (American) a combination of the prefix Sha + Teca.
Shantecca, Shanteka, Shantika, Shantikia

Shantel, Shantell (American) song.
Seantelle, Shanntell, Shanta, Shantal, Shantae, Shantale, Shante, Shanteal, Shanteil, Shantele, Shantella, Shantelle, Shantrell, Shantyl, Shantyle,
Shauntel, Shauntell, Shauntelle, Shauntrel, Shauntrell, Shauntrella, Shentel, Shentelle, Shontal, Shontalla, Shontalle, Shontel, Shontelle

Shanteria (American) a form of Shantara.
Shanterica, Shanterria, Shanterrie, Shantieria, Shantirea, Shonteria

Shantesa (American) a combination of the prefix Sha + Tess.
Shantese, Shantice, Shantise, Shantisha, Shontecia, Shontessia

Shantia (American) a combination of the prefix Sha + Tia.
Shanteya, Shanti, Shantida, Shantie, Shaunteya, Shauntia, Shontia

Shantille (American) a form of Chantilly.
Shanteil, Shantil, Shantilli, Shantillie, Shantilly, Shantyl, Shantyle

Shantina (American) a combination of the prefix Sha + Tina.
Shanteena, Shontina

Shantora (American) a combination of the prefix Sha + Tory.
Shantoia, Shantori, Shantoria, Shantory, Shantorya, Shantoya, Shanttoria

Shantrice (American) a combination of the prefix Sha + Trice. See also Chantrice.
Shantrece, Shantrecia, Shantreece, Shantreese, Shantrese, Shantress, Shantrezia, Shantricia, Shantriece, Shantris, Shantrisse, Shontrice

Shany (Swahili) marvelous, wonderful.
Shaney, Shannai, Shannea, Shanni, Shannia, Shannie, Shanny, Shanya

Shappa (Native American) red thunder.

Shaquanda (American) a combination of the prefix Sha + Wanda.
Shaquan, Shaquana, Shaquand, Shaquandey, Shaquandra, Shaquandria, Shaquanera, Shaquani, Shaquania, Shaquanna, Shaquanta, Shaquantae, Shaquantay, Shaquante, Shaquantia, Shaquona, Shaquonda, Shaquondra, Shaquondria

Shaqueita, Shaquita (American) forms of Shakeita.
Shaqueta, Shaquetta, Shaquette, Shaquitta, Shequida, Shequita, Shequittia

Shaquila, Shaquilla (American) forms of Shakila.
Shaquail, Shaquia, Shaquil, Shaquilah, Shaquile, Shaquill,

Shaquillah, Shaquille, Shaquillia, Shequela, Shequele, Shequila, Shquiyla

Shaquira (American) a form of Shakira.
Shaquirah, Shaquire, Shaquirra, Shaqura, Shaqurah, Shaquri

Shara (Hebrew) a short form of Sharon.
Shaara, Sharah, Sharal, Sharala, Sharalee, Sharlyn, Sharlynn, Sharra, Sharrah

Sharai (Hebrew) princess. See also Sharon.
Sharae, Sharaé, Sharah, Sharaiah, Sharay, Sharaya, Sharayah

Sharan (Hindi) protector.
Sharaine, Sharanda, Sharanjeet

Shardae, Sharday (Punjabi) charity. (Yoruba) honored by royalty. (Arabic) runaway. A form of Chardae.
Sade, Shadae, Sharda, Shar-Dae, Shardai, Shar-Day, Sharde, Shardea, Shardee, Shardée, Shardei, Shardeia, Shardey

Sharee (English) a form of Shari.
Shareen, Shareena, Sharine

Shari (French) beloved, dearest. (Hungarian) a form of Sarah. See also Sharita, Sheree, Sherry.
Shara, Share, Sharee, Sharia,

*Shariah, Sharian, Shariann,
Sharianne, Sharie, Sharra,
Sharree, Sharri, Sharrie, Sharry,
Shary*

Sharice (French) a form of
Cherice.
*Shareese, Sharesse, Sharese,
Sharica, Sharicka, Shariece,
Sharis, Sharise, Sharish, Shariss,
Sharissa, Sharisse, Sharyse*

Sharik (African) child of God.

Sharissa (American) a form of
Sharice.
*Sharesa, Sharessia, Sharisa,
Sharisha, Shereeza, Shericia,
Sherisa, Sherissa*

Sharita (French) a familiar form
of Shari. (American) a form of
Charity. See also Sherita.
Shareeta, Sharrita

Sharla (French) a short form
of Sharlene, Sharlotte.

Sharlene (French) little and
strong.
*Scharlane, Scharlene, Shar,
Sharla, Sharlaina, Sharlaine,
Sharlane, Sharlanna, Sharlee,
Sharleen, Sharleine, Sharlena,
Sharleyne, Sharline, Sharlyn,
Sharlyne, Sharlynn, Sharlynne,
Sherlean, Sherleen, Sherlene,
Sherline*

Sharlotte (American) a form
of Charlotte.
*Sharlet, Sharlett, Sharlott,
Sharlotta*

Sharma (American) a short
form of Sharmaine.
Sharmae, Sharme

Sharmaine (American) a form
of Charmaine.
*Sharma, Sharmain, Sharman,
Sharmane, Sharmanta,
Sharmayne, Sharmeen,
Sharmene, Sharmese, Sharmin,
Sharmine, Sharmon, Sharmyn*

Sharna (Hebrew) a form of
Sharon.
*Sharnae, Sharnay, Sharne,
Sharnea, Sharnease, Sharnee,
Sharneese, Sharnell, Sharnelle,
Sharnese, Sharnett, Sharnetta,
Sharnise*

Sharon (Hebrew) desert plain.
A form of Sharai.
*Shaaron, Shara, Sharai, Sharan,
Shareen, Sharen, Shari, Sharin,
Sharna, Sharonda, Sharone,
Sharran, Sharren, Sharrin,
Sharron, Sharrona, Sharyn,
Sharyon, Sheren, Sheron,
Sherryn*

Sharonda (Hebrew) a form of
Sharon.
*Sharronda, Sheronda,
Sherrhonda*

Sharrona (Hebrew) a form of
Sharon.
*Sharona, Sharone, Sharonia,
Sharonna, Sharony, Sharronne,
Sheron, Sherona, Sheronna,
Sherron, Sherronna, Sherronne,
Shirona*

Shatara (Hindi) umbrella.
(Arabic) good; industrious.
(American) a combination of
Sharon + Tara.
*Shatarea, Shatari, Shataria,
Shatarra, Shataura, Shateira,
Shatera, Shaterah, Shateria,
Shaterra, Shaterri, Shaterria,
Shatherian, Shatierra, Shatiria*

Shatoria (American) a combi-
nation of the prefix Sha +
Tory.
*Shatora, Shatorea, Shatori,
Shatorri, Shatorria, Shatory,
Shatorya, Shatoya*

Shauna (Hebrew) God is gra-
cious. (Irish) a form of
Shana. See also Seana, Shona.
*Shaun, Shaunah, Shaunda,
Shaune, Shaunee, Shauneen,
Shaunelle, Shaunette, Shauni,
Shaunice, Shaunicy, Shaunie,
Shaunika, Shaunisha, Shaunna,
Shaunnea, Shaunta, Shaunua,
Shaunya*

Shaunda (Irish) a form of
Shauna. See also Shanda,
Shawnda, Shonda.
*Shaundal, Shaundala,
Shaundel, Shaundela,
Shaundell, Shaundelle,
Shaundra, Shaundrea,
Shaundree, Shaundria,
Shaundrice*

Shaunta (Irish) a form of
Shauna. See also Shawnta,
Shonta.
Schunta, Shauntae, Shauntay,
*Shaunte, Shauntea, Shauntee,
Shauntée, Shaunteena,
Shauntei, Shauntia, Shauntier,
Shauntrel, Shauntrell,
Shauntrella*

Shavon (American) a form of
Shavonne.
*Schavon, Schevon, Shavan,
Shavana, Shavaun, Shavona,
Shavonda, Shavone, Shavonia,
Shivon*

Shavonne (American) a com-
bination of the prefix Sha +
Yvonne. See also Siobhan.
*Shavanna, Shavon, Shavondra,
Shavonn, Shavonna, Shavonni,
Shavonnia, Shavonnie,
Shavontae, Shavonte, Shavonté,
Shavoun, Shivaun, Shivawn,
Shivonne, Shyvon, Shyvonne*

Shawanna (American) a com-
bination of the prefix Sha +
Wanda. See also Shajuana,
Shawna.
*Shawan, Shawana, Shawanda,
Shawante, Shiwani*

Shawna (Hebrew) God is gra-
cious. (Irish) a form of Jane.
A form of Shana, Shauna.
See also Seana, Shona.
*Sawna, Shaw, Shawn, Shawnae,
Shawnai, Shawnea, Shawnee,
Shawneen, Shawneena,
Shawnell, Shawnette, Shawnna,
Shawnra, Shawnta, Sheona,
Siân, Siana, Sianna*

Shawnda (Irish) a form of
Shawna. See also Shanda,
Shaunda, Shonda.
*Shawndal, Shawndala,
Shawndan, Shawndel,
Shawndra, Shawndrea,
Shawndree, Shawndreel,
Shawndrell, Shawndria*

Shawnee (Irish) a form of
Shawna.
*Shawne, Shawneea, Shawney,
Shawni, Shawnie*

Shawnika (American) a com-
bination of Shawna + Nika.
*Shawnaka, Shawnequa,
Shawneika, Shawnicka*

Shawnta (Irish) a form of
Shawna. See also Shaunta,
Shonta.
*Shawntae, Shawntay, Shawnte,
Shawnté, Shawntee, Shawntell,
Shawntelle, Shawnteria,
Shawntia, Shawntil, Shawntile,
Shawntill, Shawntille,
Shawntina, Shawntish,
Shawntrese, Shawntriece*

Shay, Shaye (Irish) forms of
Shea.
*Shaya, Shayah, Shayda, Shayha,
Shayia, Shayla, Shey, Sheye*

Shayla (Irish) a form of Shay.
*Shaylagh, Shaylah, Shaylain,
Shaylan, Shaylea, Shayleah,
Shaylla, Shaylyn, Sheyla*

Shaylee (Irish) a form of Shea.
*Shaylei, Shayleigh, Shayley,
Shayli, Shaylie, Shayly, Shealy*

Shaylyn (Irish) a form of
Shea.
*Shaylin, Shaylina, Shaylinn,
Shaylynn, Shaylynne, Shealyn,
Sheylyn*

Shayna (Hebrew) beautiful.
*Shaynae, Shaynah, Shayne,
Shaynee, Shayney, Shayni,
Shaynie, Shaynna, Shaynne,
Shayny, Sheana, Sheanna*

Shea (Irish) fairy palace.
*Shae, Shay, Shaylee, Shaylyn,
Shealy, Shaelee, Shaelyn,
Shealyn, Sheann, Sheannon,
Sheanta, Sheaon, Shearra,
Sheatara, Sheaunna, Sheavon*

Sheba (Hebrew) a short form
of Bathsheba. Geography: an
ancient country of south
Arabia.
Saba, Sabah, Shebah, Sheeba

Sheena (Hebrew) God is gra-
cious. (Irish) a form of Jane.
*Sheenagh, Sheenah, Sheenan,
Sheeneal, Sheenika, Sheenna,
Sheina, Shena, Shiona*

Sheila (Latin) blind. (Irish) a
form of Cecelia. See also
Cheyla, Zelizi.
*Seelia, Seila, Selia, Shaila,
Sheela, Sheelagh, Sheelah,
Sheilagh, Sheilah, Sheileen,
Sheiletta, Sheilia, Sheillynn,
Sheilya, Shela, Shelagh, Shelah,
Shelia, Shiela, Shila, Shilah,
Shilea, Shyla*

Shelbi, Shelbie (English)
forms of Shelby.
Shelbbie, Shellbi, Shellbie

Shelby (English) ledge estate.
*Chelby, Schelby, Shel, Shelbe,
Shelbee, Shelbey, Shelbi, Shelbie,
Shelbye, Shellby*

Sheldon (English) farm on
the ledge.
*Sheldina, Sheldine, Sheldrina,
Sheldyn, Shelton*

Shelee (English) a form of
Shelley.
*Shelee, Sheleen, Shelena, Sheley,
Sheli, Shelia, Shelina, Shelinda,
Shelita*

Shelisa (American) a combi-
nation of Shelley + Lisa.
*Sheleza, Shelica, Shelicia,
Shelise, Shelisse, Sheliza*

Shelley, Shelly (English)
meadow on the ledge.
(French) familiar forms of
Michelle. See also Rochelle.
*Shelee, Shell, Shella, Shellaine,
Shellana, Shellany, Shellee,
Shellene, Shelli, Shellian,
Shelliann, Shellie, Shellina*

Shelsea (American) a form of
Chelsea.
*Shellsea, Shellsey, Shelsey,
Shelsie, Shelsy*

Shena (Irish) a form of
Sheena.
*Shenada, Shenae, Shenah,
Shenay, Shenda, Shene, Shenea,*
*Sheneda, Shenee, Sheneena,
Shenica, Shenika, Shenina,
Sheniqua, Shenita, Shenna,
Shennae, Shennah, Shenoa*

Shera (Aramaic) light.
*Sheera, Sheerah, Sherae, Sherah,
Sheralee, Sheralle, Sheralyn,
Sheralynn, Sheralynne, Sheray,
Sheraya*

Sheree (French) beloved, dearest.
*Scherie, Sheeree, Shere, Shereé,
Sherrelle, Shereen, Shereena*

Sherelle (French) a form of
Cherelle, Sheryl.
*Sherel, Sherell, Sheriel, Sherrel,
Sherrell, Sherrelle, Shirelle*

Sheri, Sherri (French) forms
of Sherry.
Sheria, Sheriah, Sherie, Sherrie

Sherian (American) a combination of Sheri + Ann.
Sherianne, Sherrina

Sherice (French) a form of
Cherice.
*Scherise, Sherece, Shereece,
Sherees, Shereese, Sherese,
Shericia, Sherise, Sherisse,
Sherrish, Sherryse, Sheryce*

Sheridan (Irish) wild.
*Sherida, Sheridane, Sherideen,
Sheriden, Sheridian, Sheridon,
Sherridan, Sherridon*

Sherika (Punjabi) relative.
(Arabic) easterner.
*Shereka, Sherica, Shericka,
Sherrica, Sherricka, Sherrika*

Sherissa (French) a form of
Sherry, Sheryl.
*Shereeza, Sheresa, Shericia,
Sherrish*

Sherita (French) a form of
Sherry, Sheryl. See also
Sharita.
*Shereta, Sheretta, Sherette,
Sherrita*

Sherleen (French, English) a
form of Sheryl, Shirley.
*Sherileen, Sherlene, Sherlin,
Sherlina, Sherline, Sherlyn,
Sherlyne, Sherlynne, Shirlena,
Shirlene, Shirlina, Shirlyn*

Sherry (French) beloved,
dearest. A familiar form of
Sheryl. See also Sheree.
*Sherey, Sheri, Sherissa, Sherrey,
Sherri, Sherria, Sherriah,
Sherrie, Sherye, Sheryy*

Sheryl (French) beloved. A
familiar form of Shirley. See
also Sherry.
*Sharel, Sharil, Sharilyn, Sharyl,
Sharyll, Sheral, Sherell, Sheriel,
Sheril, Sherill, Sherily, Sherilyn,
Sherissa, Sherita, Sherleen,
Sherral, Sherrelle, Sherril,
Sherrill, Sherryl, Sherylly*

Sherylyn (American) a com-
bination of Sheryl + Lynn.
See also Cherilyn.
*Sharolin, Sharolyn, Sharyl-
Lynn, Sheralyn, Sherilyn,
Sherilynn, Sherilynne,
Sherralyn, Sherralynn,*

*Sherrilyn, Sherrilynn,
Sherrilynne, Sherrylyn, Sherryn,
Sherylanne*

Shevonne (American) a com-
bination of the prefix She +
Yvonne.
*Shevaun, Shevon, Shevonda,
Shevone*

Sheyenne (Cheyenne) a form
of Cheyenne. See also
Shyann, Shyanne.
*Shayhan, Sheyan, Sheyane,
Sheyann, Sheyanna,
Sheyannah, Sheyanne, Sheyen,
Sheyene, Shiante, Shyanne*

Shianne (Cheyenne) a form
of Cheyenne.
*She, Shian, Shiana, Shianah,
Shianda, Shiane, Shiann,
Shianna, Shiannah, Shiany,
Shieana, Shieann, Shieanne,
Shiena, Shiene, Shienna*

Shifra (Hebrew) beautiful.
Schifra, Shifrah

Shika (Japanese) gentle deer.
Shi, Shikah, Shikha

Shilo (Hebrew) God's gift.
Bible: a sanctuary for the
Israelites where the Ark of
the Covenant was kept.
Shiloh

Shina (Japanese) virtuous,
good; wealthy. (Chinese) a
form of China.
Shinae, Shinay, Shine, Shinna

Shino (Japanese) bamboo stalk.

Shiquita (American) a form of Chiquita.
Shiquata, Shiquitta

Shira (Hebrew) song.
Shirah, Shiray, Shire, Shiree, Shiri, Shirit, Shyra

Shirlene (English) a form of Shirley.
Shirleen, Shirline, Shirlynn

Shirley (English) bright meadow. See also Sheryl.
Sherlee, Sherleen, Sherley, Sherli, Sherlie, Shir, Shirl, Shirlee, Shirlie, Shirly, Shirlly, Shurlee, Shurley

Shivani (Hindi) life and death.
Shiva, Shivana, Shivanie, Shivanna

Shizu (Japanese) silent.
Shizue, Shizuka, Shizuko, Shizuyo

Shona (Irish) a form of Jane. A form of Shana, Shauna, Shawna.
Shiona, Shonagh, Shonah, Shonalee, Shonda, Shone, Shonee, Shonette, Shoni, Shonie, Shonna, Shonnah, Shonta

Shonda (Irish) a form of Shona. See also Shanda, Shaunda, Shawnda.
Shondalette, Shondalyn, Shondel, Shondelle, Shondi,
Shondia, Shondie, Shondra, Shondreka, Shounda

Shonta (Irish) a form of Shona. See also Shaunta, Shawnta.
Shontá, Shontae, Shontai, Shontalea, Shontasia, Shontavia, Shontaviea, Shontay, Shontaya, Shonte, Shonté, Shontedra, Shontee, Shonteral, Shonti, Shontol, Shontoy, Shontrail, Shountáe

Shoshana (Hebrew) a form of Susan.
Shosha, Shoshan, Shoshanah, Shoshane, Shoshanha, Shoshann, Shoshanna, Shoshannah, Shoshauna, Shoshaunah, Shoshawna, Shoshona, Shoshone, Shoshonee, Shoshoney, Shoshoni, Shoushan, Shushana, Sosha, Soshana

Shu (Chinese) kind, gentle.

Shug (American) a short form of Sugar.

Shula (Arabic) flaming, bright.
Shulah

Shulamith (Hebrew) peaceful. See also Sula.
Shulamit, Sulamith

Shunta (Irish) a form of Shonta.
Shuntae, Shunté, Shuntel, Shuntell, Shuntelle, Shuntia

Shura (Russian) a form of Alexandra.
Schura, Shurah, Shuree,

Shureen, Shurelle, Shuritta,
Shurka, Shurlana

Shyann, Shyanne (Cheyenne)
forms of Cheyenne. See also
Sheyenne.
Shyan, Shyana, Shyandra,
Shyane, Shynee, Shyanna,
Shyannah, Shye, Shyene,
Shyenna, Shyenne

Shyla (English) a form of Sheila.
Shya, Shyah, Shylah, Shylan,
Shylayah, Shylana, Shylane,
Shyle, Shyleah, Shylee, Shyley,
Shyli, Shylia, Shylie, Shylo,
Shyloe, Shyloh, Shylon, Shylyn

Shyra (Hebrew) a form of
Shira.
Shyrae, Shyrah, Shyrai, Shyrie,
Shyro

Siara (Irish) a form of Sierra.
Siarah, Siarra, Siarrah, Sieara

Sianna (Irish) a form of
Seana.
Sian, Siana, Sianae, Sianai,
Sianey, Siannah, Sianne,
Sianni, Sianny, Siany

Sibeta (Moquelumnan) find-
ing a fish under a rock.

Sibley (English) sibling; friendly.
(Greek) a form of Sybil.
Sybley

Sidney (French) a form of
Sydney.
Sidne, Sidnee, Sidnei, Sidneya,
Sidni, Sidnie, Sidny, Sidnye

Sidonia (Hebrew) enticing.
Sydania, Syndonia

Sidonie (French) from Saint-
Denis, France. See also Sydney.
Sedona, Sidaine, Sidanni, Sidelle,
Sidoine, Sidona, Sidonae, Sidonia,
Sidony

Sidra (Latin) star child.
Sidrah, Sidras

Sienna (American) a form of
Ciana.
Seini, Siena

Siera (Irish) an alternte form
of Sierra.
Sierah, Sieria

Sierra (Irish) black. (Spanish)
saw toothed. Geography: any
rugged range of mountains
that, when viewed from a
distance, has a jagged profile.
See also Ciara.
Seara, Searria, Seera, Seirra,
Siara, Siearra, Siera, Sierrah,
Sierre, Sierrea, Sierriah, Syerra

Sigfreda (German) victorious
peace. See also Freda.
Sigfreida, Sigfrida, Sigfrieda,
Sigfryda

Sigmunda (German) victorious protector.
Sigmonda

Signe (Latin) sign, signal.
(Scandinavian) a short form
of Sigourney.
Sig, Signa, Signy, Singna,
Singne

Sigourney (English) victorious conquerer.
Signe, Sigournee, Sigourny

Sigrid (Scandinavian) victorious counselor.
Siegrid, Siegrida, Sigritt

Sihu (Native American) flower; bush.

Siko (African) crying baby.

Silvia (Latin) a form of Sylvia.
Silivia, Silva, Silvya

Simcha (Hebrew) joyful.

Simone (Hebrew) she heard. (French) a form of Simon (see Boys' Names).
Samone, Siminie, Simmi, Simmie, Simmona, Simmone, Simoane, Simona, Simonetta, Simonette, Simonia, Simonina, Simonne, Somone, Symone

Simran (Sikh) absorbed in God.
Simren, Simrin, Simrun

Sina (Irish) a form of Seana.
Seena, Sinai, Sinaia, Sinan, Sinay

Sinclaire (French) prayer.
Sinclair

Sindy (American) a form of Cindy.
Sinda, Sindal, Sindee, Sindi, Sindia, Sindie, Sinnedy, Synda, Syndal, Syndee, Syndey, Syndi, Syndia, Syndie, Syndy

Sinead (Irish) a form of Jane.
Seonaid, Sine, Sinéad

Siobhan (Irish) a form of Joan. See also Shavonne.
Shibahn, Shibani, Shibhan, Shioban, Shobana, Shobha, Shobhana, Siobahn, Siobhana, Siobhann, Siobhon, Siovaun, Siovhan

Sirena (Greek) enchanter. Mythology: Sirens were sea nymphs whose singing enchanted sailors and made them crash their ships into nearby rocks.
Sireena, Sirene, Sirine, Syrena, Syrenia, Syrenna, Syrina

Sisika (Native American) songbird.

Sissy (American) a familiar form of Cecelia.
Sisi, Sisie, Sissey, Sissie

Sita (Hindi) a form of Shakti.
Sitah, Sitarah, Sitha, Sithara

Siti (Swahili) respected woman.

Skye (Arabic) water giver. (Dutch) a short form of Skyler. Geography: an island in the Hebrides, Scotland.
Ski, Skie, Skii, Skky, Sky, Skya, Skyy

Skylar (Dutch) a form of Skyler.
Skyela, Skyelar, Skyla, Skylair, Skyylar

Skyler (Dutch) sheltering.
Skila, Skilah, Skye, Skyeler,
Skyelur, Skyla, Skylar, Skylee,
Skylena, Skyli, Skylia, Skylie,
Skylin, Skyllar, Skylor, Skylyn,
Skylynn, Skylyr, Skyra

Sloane (Irish) warrior.
Sloan, Sloanne

Socorro (Spanish) helper.

Sofia (Greek) a form of Sophia.
See also Zofia, Zsofia.
Sofeea, Sofeeia, Soffi, Sofi, Soficita,
Sofie, Sofija, Sofiya, Sofka, Sofya

Solada (Tai) listener.

Solana (Spanish) sunshine.
Solande, Solanna, Soleil,
Solena, Soley, Solina, Solinda

Solange (French) dignified.

Soledad (Spanish) solitary.
Sole, Soleda

Solenne (French) solemn, dig-
nified.
Solaine, Solene, Soléne, Solenna,
Solina, Soline, Solonez, Souline,
Soulle

Soma (Hindi) lunar.

Sommer (English) summer;
summoner. (Arabic) black.
See also Summer.
Somara, Somer, Sommar,
Sommara, Sommers

Sondra (Greek) defender of
mankind.
Saundra, Sondre, Sonndra, Sonndre

Sonia (Russian, Slavic) a form
of Sonya.
Sonica, Sonida, Sonita, Sonna,
Sonni, Sonnia, Sonnie, Sonny

Sonja (Scandinavian) a form
of Sonya.
Sonjae, Sonjia

Sonya (Greek) wise. (Russian,
Slavic) a form of Sophia.
Sonia, Sonja, Sonnya, Sonyae,
Sunya

Sook (Korean) pure.

Sopheary (Cambodian) beautiful girl.

Sophia (Greek) wise. See also
Sonya, Zofia.
Sofia, Sophie

Sophie (Greek) a familiar form
of Sophia. See also Zocha.
Sophey, Sophi, Sophy

Sophronia (Greek) wise; sensible.
Soffrona, Sofronia

Sora (Native American)
chirping songbird.

Soraya (Persian) princess.
Suraya

Sorrel (French) reddish
brown. Botany: a plant
whose leaves are used as salad
greens.

Soso (Native American) tree
squirrel dining on pine nuts;
chubby-cheeked baby.

Souzan (Persian) burning fire.
Sousan, Souzanne

Spencer (English) dispenser of
provisions.
Spenser

Speranza (Italian) a form of
Esperanza.
Speranca

Spring (English) springtime.
Spryng

Stacey, Stacy (Greek) resur-
rection. (Irish) a short form
of Anastasia, Eustacia,
Natasha.
*Stace, Stacee, Staceyan,
Staceyann, Staicy, Stasey,
Stasya, Stayce, Staycee, Staci,
Steacy*

Staci, Stacie (Greek) forms of
Stacey.
Stacci, Stacia, Stayci

Stacia (English) a short form
of Anastasia.
Stasia, Staysha

Starla (English) a form of
Starr.
Starrla

Starleen (English) a form of
Starr.
*Starleena, Starlena, Starlene,
Starlin, Starlyn, Starlynn, Starrlen*

Starley (English) a familiar
form of Starr.
Starle, Starlee, Staly

Starling (English) bird.

Starr (English) star.
*Star, Staria, Starisha, Starla,
Starleen, Starlet, Starlette,
Starley, Starlight, Starre, Starri,
Starria, Starrika, Starrsha,
Starsha, Starshanna, Startish*

Stasya (Greek) a familiar form
of Anastasia. (Russian) a form
of Stacey.
*Stasa, Stasha, Stashia, Stasia,
Stasja, Staska*

Stefani, Steffani (Greek)
forms of Stephanie.
*Stafani, Stefanni, Steffane,
Steffanee, Stefini, Stefoni*

Stefanie (Greek) a form of
Stephanie.
*Stafanie, Staffany, Stefane,
Stefanee, Stefaney, Stefania,
Stefanié, Stefanija, Stefannie,
Stefcia, Stefenie, Steffanie, Steffi,
Stefinie, Stefka*

Stefany, Steffany (Greek)
forms of Stephanie.
Stefanny, Stefanya, Steffaney

Steffi (Greek) a familiar form
of Stefanie, Stephanie.
*Stefa, Stefcia, Steffee, Steffie,
Steffy, Stefi, Stefka, Stefy,
Stepha, Stephi, Stephie, Stephy*

Stella (Latin) star. (French) a
familiar form of Estelle.
Steile, Stellina

Stepania (Russian) a form of
Stephanie.
Stepa, Stepahny, Stepanida,

Stepanie, Stepanyda, Stepfanie,
Stephana

Stephani (Greek) a form of
Stephanie.
Stephania, Stephanni

Stephanie (Greek) crowned.
See also Estefani, Estephanie,
Panya, Stevie, Zephania.
Stamatios, Stefani, Stefanie,
Stefany, Steffie, Stepania,
Stephaija, Stephaine, Stephanas,
Stephane, Stephanee, Stephani,
Stephanida, Stéphanie,
Stephanine, Stephann,
Stephannie, Stephany, Stephene,
Stephenie, Stephianie, Stephney,
Stesha, Steshka, Stevanee

Stephany (Greek) a form of
Stephanie.
Stephaney, Stephanye

Stephene (Greek) a form of
Stephanie.
Stephina, Stephine, Stephyne

Stephenie (Greek) a form of
Stephanie.
Stephena, Stephenee, Stepheney,
Stepheni, Stephenny, Stepheny,
Stephine, Stephinie

Stephney (Greek) a form of
Stephanie.
Stephne, Stephni, Stephnie,
Stephny

Sterling (English) valuable;
silver penny.

Stevie (Greek) a familiar form
of Stephanie.
Steva, Stevana, Stevanee, Stevee,
Stevena, Stevey, Stevi, Stevy,
Stevye

Stina (German) a short form
of Christina.
Steena, Stena, Stine, Stinna

Stockard (English) stockyard.

Stormie (English) a form of
Stormy.
Stormee, Stormi, Stormii

Stormy (English) impetuous
by nature.
Storm, Storme, Stormey,
Stormie, Stormm

Suchin (Tai) beautiful
thought.

Sue (Hebrew) a short form of
Susan, Susanna.

Sueann, Sueanna (American)
combinations of Sue + Ann,
Sue + Anna.
Suann, Suanna, Suannah,
Suanne, Sueanne

Suela (Spanish) consolation.
Suelita

Sugar (American) sweet as
sugar.
Shug

Sugi (Japanese) cedar tree.

Suke (Hawaiian) a form of
Susan.

Sukey (Hawaiian) a familiar form of Susan.
Suka, Sukee, Suki, Sukie, Suky

Sukhdeep (Sikh) light of peace and bliss.
Sukhdip

Suki (Japanese) loved one. (Moquelumnan) eagle-eyed.
Sukie

Sula (Icelandic) large sea bird. (Greek, Hebrew) a short form of Shulamith, Ursula. Suletu (Moquelumnan) soaring bird.

Sulia (Latin) a form of Julia.
Suliana

Sulwen (Welsh) bright as the sun.

Sumalee (Tai) beautiful flower.

Sumati (Hindi) unity.

Sumaya (American) a combination of Sue + Maya.
Sumayah, Sumayya, Sumayyah

Sumi (Japanese) elegant, refined.
Sumiko

Summer (English) summertime. See also Sommer.
Sumer, Summar, Summerann, Summerbreeze, Summerhaze, Summerine, Summerlee, Summerlin, Summerlyn, Summerlynn, Summers, Sumrah, Summyr, Sumyr

Sun (Korean) obedient.
Suncance, Sundee, Sundeep, Sundi, Sundip, Sundrenea, Sunta, Sunya

Sunee (Tai) good.
Suni

Sun-Hi (Korean) good; joyful.

Suni (Zuni) native; member of our tribe.
Sunita, Sunitha, Suniti, Sunne, Sunni, Sunnie, Sunnilei

Sunki (Hopi) swift.
Sunkia

Sunny (English) bright, cheerful.
Sunni, Sunnie

Sunshine (English) sunshine.
Sunshyn, Sunshyne

Surata (Pakistani) blessed joy.

Suri (Todas) pointy nose.
Suree, Surena, Surenia

Surya (Sanskrit) Mythology: a sun god.
Suria, Suriya, Surra

Susammi (French) a combination of Susan + Aimee.
Suzami, Suzamie, Suzamy

Susan (Hebrew) lily. See also Shoshana, Sukey, Zsa Zsa, Zusa.
Sawsan, Siusan, Sosan, Sosana, Sue, Suesan, Sueva, Suisan, Suke, Susana, Susann, Susanna, Suse, Susen, Susette,

Susie, Suson, Suzan, Suzanna, Suzannah, Suzanne, Suzette

Susana (Hebrew) a form of Susan.
Susanah, Susane

Susanna, Susannah (Hebrew) forms of Susan. See also Xuxa, Zanna, Zsuzsanna.
Sonel, Sosana, Sue, Suesanna, Susana, Susanah, Susanka, Susette, Susie, Suzanna

Suse (Hawaiian) a form of Susan.

Susette (French) a familiar form of Susan, Susanna.
Susetta

Susie, Suzie (American) familiar forms of Susan, Susanna.
Suse, Susey, Susi, Sussi, Sussy, Susy, Suze, Suzi, Suzy, Suzzie

Suzanna, Suzannah (Hebrew) forms of Susan.
Suzana, Suzenna, Suzzanna

Suzanne (English) a form of Susan.
Susanne, Suszanne, Suzane, Suzann, Suzzane, Suzzann, Suzzanne

Suzette (French) a form of Susan.
Suzetta, Suzzette

Suzu (Japanese) little bell.
Suzue, Suzuko

Suzuki (Japanese) bell tree.

Svetlana (Russian) bright light.
Sveta, Svetochka

Syá (Chinese) summer.

Sybella (English) a form of Sybil.
Sebila, Sibbella, Sibeal, Sibel, Sibell, Sibella, Sibelle, Sibilla, Sibylla, Sybel, Sybelle, Sybila, Sybilla

Sybil (Greek) prophet. Mythology: sibyls were oracles who relayed the messages of the gods. See also Cybele, Sibley.
Sib, Sibbel, Sibbie, Sibbill, Sibby, Sibeal, Sibel, Sibyl, Sibylle, Sibylline, Sybella, Sybille, Syble

Sydnee (French) a form of Sydney.
Sydne, Sydnea, Sydnei

Sydney (French) from Saint-Denis, France. See also Sidonie.
Cidney, Cydney, Sidney, Sy, Syd, Sydel, Sydelle, Sydna, Sydnee, Sydni, Sydnie, Sydny, Sydnye, Syndona, Syndonah

Sydni, Sydnie (French) forms of Sydney.

Sying (Chinese) star.

Sylvana (Latin) forest.
Silvaine, Silvana, Silvanna, Silviane, Sylva, Sylvaine, Sylvanah, Sylvania, Sylvanna, Sylvie, Sylvina, Sylvinnia, Sylvonah, Sylvonia, Sylvonna

Sylvia (Latin) forest. Literature: Sylvia Plath was a well-known American poet. See also Silvia, Xylia.
Sylvette, Sylvie, Sylwia

Sylvianne (American) a combination of Sylvia + Anne.
Sylvian

Sylvie (Latin) a familiar form of Sylvia.
Silvi, Silvie, Silvy, Sylvi

Symone (Hebrew) a form of Simone.
Symmeon, Symmone, Symona, Symoné, Symonne

Symphony (Greek) symphony, harmonious sound.
Symfoni, Symphanie, Symphany, Symphanée, Symphoni, Symphoni

Syreeta (Hindi) good traditions. (Arabic) companion.
Syretta, Syrrita

T

Tabatha (Greek, Aramaic) a form of Tabitha.
Tabathe, Tabathia, Tabbatha

Tabby (English) a familiar form of Tabitha.
Tabbi

Tabia (Swahili) talented.
Tabea

Tabetha (Greek, Aramaic) a form of Tabitha.

Tabina (Arabic) follower of Muhammad.

Tabitha (Greek, Aramaic) gazelle.
Tabatha, Tabbee, Tabbetha, Tabbey, Tabbi, Tabbie, Tabbitha, Tabby, Tabetha, Tabiatha, Tabita, Tabithia, Tabotha, Tabtha, Tabytha

Tabytha (Greek, Aramaic) a form of Tabitha.
Tabbytha

Tacey (English) a familiar form of Tacita.
Tace, Tacee, Taci, Tacy, Tacye

Taci (Zuni) washtub. (English) a form of Tacey.
Tacia, Taciana, Tacie

Tacita (Latin) silent.
Tacey

Tadita (Omaha) runner.
Tadeta, Tadra

Taelor (English) a form of Taylor.
Taelar, Taeler, Taellor, Taelore, Taelyr

Taesha (Latin) a form of Tisha. (American) a combination of the prefix Ta + Aisha.
Tadasha, Taeshayla, Taeshia, Taheisha, Tahisha, Taiesha,

Taisha, Taishae, Teasha, Teashia, Teisha, Tesha

Taffy (Welsh) beloved.
Taffia, Taffine, Taffye, Tafia, Tafisa, Tafoya

Tahira (Arabic) virginal, pure.
Taheera, Taheerah, Tahera, Tahere, Taheria, Taherri, Tahiara, Tahirah, Tahireh

Tahlia (Greek, Hebrew) a form of Talia.
Tahleah, Tahleia

Tailor (English) a form of Taylor.
Tailar, Tailer, Taillor, Tailyr

Taima (Native American) clash of thunder.
Taimi, Taimia, Taimy

Taipa (Moquelumnan) flying quail.
Taite (English) cheerful.
Tate, Tayte, Tayten

Taja (Hindi) crown.
Taiajára, Taija, Tajae, Tajah, Tahai, Tehya, Teja, Tejah, Tejal

Taka (Japanese) honored.

Takala (Hopi) corn tassel.

Takara (Japanese) treasure.
Takarah, Takaria, Takarra, Takra

Takayla (American) a combination of the prefix Ta + Kayla.
Takayler, Takeyli

Takeisha (American) a combination of the prefix Ta + Keisha.
Takecia, Takesha, Takeshia, Takesia, Takisha, Takishea, Takishia, Tekeesha, Tekeisha, Tekeshi, Tekeysia, Tekisha, Tikesha, Tikisha, Tokesia, Tykeisha

Takenya (Hebrew) animal horn. (Moquelumnan) falcon. (American) a combination of the prefix Ta + Kenya.
Takenia, Takenja

Takeria (American) a form of Takira.
Takera, Takeri, Takerian, Takerra, Takerria, Takierria, Takoria

Taki (Japanese) waterfall.
Tiki

Takia (Arabic) worshiper.
Takeia, Takeiyah, Takeya, Takeyah, Takhiya, Takiah, Takija, Takiya, Takiyah, Takkia, Takya, Takyah, Takyia, Taqiyya, Taquaia, Taquaya, Taquiia, Tekeiya, Tekeiyah, Tekeyia, Tekiya, Tekiyah, Tikia, Tykeia, Tykia

Takila (American) a form of Tequila.
Takayla, Takeila, Takela, Takelia, Takella, Takeyla, Takiela, Takilah, Takilla, Takilya, Takyla, Takylia, Tatakyla, Tehilla, Tekeila, Tekela, Tekelia, Tekilaa, Tekilia, Tekilla, Tekilyah, Tekla

Takira (American) a combination of the prefix Ta + Kira.
Takara, Takarra, Takeara, Takeera, Takeira, Takeirah, Takera, Takiara, Takiera, Takierah, Takierra, Takirah, Takiria, Takirra, Takora, Takyra, Takyrra, Taquera, Taquira, Tekeria, Tikara, Tikira, Tykera

Tala (Native American) stalking wolf.

Talasi (Hopi) corn tassel.
Talasea, Talasia

Taleah (American) a form of Talia.
Talaya, Talayah, Talayia, Talea, Taleana, Taleea, Taleéi, Talei, Taleia, Taleiya, Tylea, Tyleah, Tylee

Taleisha (American) a combination of Talia + Aisha.
Taileisha, Taleise, Talesha, Talicia, Taliesha, Talisa, Talisha, Talysha, Telisha, Tilisha, Tyleasha, Tyleisha, Tylicia, Tylisha, Tylishia

Talena (American) a combination of the prefix Ta + Lena.
Talayna, Talihna, Taline, Tallenia, Talná, Tilena, Tilene, Tylena

Talesha (American) a form of Taleisha.
Taleesha, Talesa, Talese, Taleshia, Talesia, Tallese, Tallesia, Tylesha, Tyleshia, Tylesia

Talia (Greek) blooming. (Hebrew) dew from heaven. (Latin, French) birthday. A short form of Natalie. See also Thalia.
Tahlia, Taleah, Taliah, Taliatha, Taliea, Taliyah, Talley, Tallia, Tallya, Talya, Tylia

Talina (American) a combination of Talia + Lina.
Talin, Talinda, Taline, Tallyn, Talyn, Talynn, Tylina, Tyline

Talisa (English) a form of Tallis.
Talisha, Talishia, Talisia, Talissa, Talysa, Talysha, Talysia, Talyssa

Talitha (Arabic) young girl.
Taleetha, Taletha, Talethia, Taliatha, Talita, Talithia, Taliya, Telita, Tiletha

Taliyah (Greek) a form of Talia.
Taleya, Taleyah, Talieya, Talliyah, Talya, Talyah, Talyia

Talley (French) a familiar form of Talia.
Tali, Talle, Tallie, Tally, Taly, Talye

Tallis (French, English) forest.
Talice, Talisa, Talise, Tallys

Tallulah (Choctaw) leaping water.
Tallou, Talula

Tam (Vietnamese) heart.

Tama (Japanese) jewel.
Tamaa, Tamah, Tamaiah,
Tamala, Tema

Tamaka (Japanese) bracelet.
Tamaki, Tamako, Timaka

Tamar (Hebrew) a short form
of Tamara. (Russian) History:
a twelfth-century Georgian
queen. (Hebrew) a short
form of Tamara.
Tamer, Tamor, Tamour

Tamara (Hebrew) palm tree.
See also Tammy.
Tamar, Tamará, Tamarae,
Tamarah, Tamaria, Tamarin,
Tamarla, Tamarra, Tamarria,
Tamarrian, Tamarsha, Tamary,
Tamera, Tamira, Tamma,
Tammara, Tamora, Tamoya,
Tamra, Tamura, Tamyra, Temara,
Temarian, Thama, Thamar,
Thamara, Thamarra, Timara,
Tomara, Tymara

Tamassa (Hebrew) a form of
Thomasina.
Tamasin, Tamasine, Tamsen,
Tamsin, Tamzen, Tamzin

Tameka (Aramaic) twin.
Tameca, Tamecia, Tamecka,
Tameeka, Tamekia, Tamiecka,
Tamieka, Temeka, Timeeka,
Timeka, Tomeka, Tomekia,
Trameika, Tymeka, Tymmeeka,
Tymmeka

Tamera (Hebrew) a form of
Tamara.
Tamer, Tamerai, Tameran,
Tameria, Tamerra, Tammera,
Thamer, Timera

Tamesha (American) a com-
bination of the prefix Ta +
Mesha.
Tameesha, Tameisha, Tameshia,
Tameshkia, Tameshya, Tamisha,
Tamishia, Tamnesha, Temisha,
Timesha, Timisha, Tomesha,
Tomiese, Tomise, Tomisha,
Tramesha, Tramisha, Tymesha

Tamika (Japanese) a form of
Tamiko.
Tamica, Tamieka, Tamikah,
Tamikia, Tamikka, Tammika,
Tamyka, Timika, Timikia,
Tomika, Tymika, Tymmicka

Tamiko (Japanese) child of the
people.
Tami, Tamika, Tamike, Tamiqua,
Tamiyo, Tammiko

Tamila (American) a combi-
nation of the prefix Ta +
Mila.
Tamala, Tamela, Tamelia,
Tamilla, Tamille, Tamillia,
Tamilya

Tamira (Hebrew) a form of
Tamara.
Tamir, Tamirae, Tamirah,
Tamiria, Tamirra, Tamyra,
Tamyria, Tamyrra

Tammi, Tammie (English)
forms of Tammy.
Tameia, Tami, Tamia, Tamiah,
Tamie, Tamijo, Tamiya

Tammy (English) twin. (Hebrew) a familiar form of Tamara.
Tamilyn, Tamlyn, Tammee, Tammey, Tammi, Tammie, Tamy, Tamya

Tamra (Hebrew) a short form of Tamara.
Tammra, Tamrah

Tamsin (English) a short form of Thomasina.

Tana (Slavic) a short form of Tanya.
Taina, Tanae, Tanaeah, Tanah, Tanairi, Tanairy, Tanalia, Tanara, Tanavia, Tanaya, Tanaz, Tanna, Tannah

Tandy (English) team.
Tanda, Tandalaya, Tandi, Tandie, Tandis, Tandra, Tandrea, Tandria

Taneisha, Tanesha
(American) combinations of the prefix Ta + Nesha.
Tahniesha, Taineshia, Tanasha, Tanashia, Tanaysia, Taneasha, Taneesha, Taneshea, Taneshia, Taneshya, Tanesia, Tanesian, Tanessa, Tanessia, Taniesha, Tannesha, Tanneshia, Tanniecia, Tanniesha, Tantashea

Taneya (Russian, Slavic) a form of Tanya.
Tanea, Taneah, Tanee, Taneé, Taneia

Tangia (American) a combination of the prefix Ta + Angela.
Tangela, Tangi, Tangie, Tanja, Tanji, Tanjia, Tanjie

Tani (Japanese) valley. (Slavic) stand of glory. A familiar form of Tania.
Tahnee, Tahni, Tahnie, Tanee, Taney, Tanie, Tany

Tania (Russian, Slavic) fairy queen.
Taneea, Tani, Taniah, Tanija, Tanika, Tanis, Taniya, Tannia, Tannis, Tanniya, Tannya, Tarnia

Taniel (American) a combination of Tania + Danielle.
Taniele, Tanielle, Teniel, Teniele, Tenielle

Tanika (American) a form of Tania.
Tanikka, Tanikqua, Taniqua, Tanique, Tannica, Tianeka, Tianika

Tanis, Tannis (Slavic) forms of Tania, Tanya.
Tanas, Tanese, Taniese, Tanise, Tanisia, Tanka, Tannese, Tanniece, Tanniese, Tannis, Tannise, Tannus, Tannyce, Tenice, Tenise, Tenyse, Tiannis, Tonise, Tranice, Tranise, Tynice, Tyniece, Tyniese, Tynise

Tanisha (American) a combination of the prefix Ta + Nisha.
Tahniscia, Tahnisha, Tanasha, Tanashea, Tanicha, Taniesha, Tanish, Tanishah, Tanishia, Tanitia, Tannicia, Tannisha, Tenisha, Tenishka, Tinisha, Tonisha, Tonnisha, Tynisha

Tanissa (American) a combination of the prefix Tania + Nissa.
Tanesa, Tanisa, Tannesa, Tannisa, Tennessa, Tranissa

Tanita (American) a combination of the prefix Ta + Nita.
Taneta, Tanetta, Tanitra, Tanitta, Teneta, Tenetta, Tenita, Tenitta, Tyneta, Tynetta, Tynette, Tynita, Tynitra, Tynitta

Tanith (Phoenician) Mythology: Tanit is the goddess of love.
Tanitha

Tanner (English) leather worker, tanner.
Tannor

Tansy (Greek) immortal. (Latin) tenacious, persistent.
Tancy, Tansee, Tansey, Tanshay, Tanzey

Tanya (Russian, Slavic) fairy queen.
Tahnee, Tahnya, Tana, Tanaya, Taneya, Tania, Tanis, Taniya, Tanka, Tannis, Tannya, Tanoya, Tany, Tanyia, Taunya, Tawnya, Thanya

Tao (Chinese, Vietnamese) peach.

Tara (Aramaic) throw; carry. (Irish) rocky hill. (Arabic) a measurement.
Taira, Tairra, Taraea, Tarah, Taráh, Tarai, Taralee, Tarali, Tarasa, Tarasha, Taraya, Tarha, Tari, Tarra, Taryn, Tayra, Tehra

Taraneh (Persian) melody.

Taree (Japanese) arching branch.
Tarea, Tareya, Tari, Taria

Tari (Irish) a familiar form of Tara.
Taria, Tarika, Tarila, Tarilyn, Tarin, Tarina, Tarita

Tarissa (American) a combination of Tara + Rissa.
Taris, Tarisa, Tarise, Tarisha

Tarra (Irish) a form of Tara.
Tarrah

Taryn (Irish) a form of Tara.
Taran, Tareen, Tareena, Taren, Tarene, Tarin, Tarina, Tarren, Tarrena, Tarrin, Tarrina, Tarron, Tarryn, Taryna

Tasarla (Gypsy) dawn.

Tasha (Greek) born on Christmas day. (Russian) a short form of Natasha. See also Tashi, Tosha.
Tacha, Tachiana, Tahsha, Tasenka, Tashae, Tashana, Tashay, Tashe, Tashee, Tasheka, Tashka, Tasia, Taska, Taysha, Thasha, Tiaisha, Tysha

Tashana (American) a combination of the prefix Ta + Shana.
Tashan, Tashanda, Tashani, Tashanika, Tashanna, Tashiana, Tashianna, Tashina, Tishana, Tishani, Tishanna, Tishanne, Toshanna, Toshanti, Tyshana

Tashara (American) a combination of the prefix Ta + Shara.
Tashar, Tasharah, Tasharia, Tasharna, Tasharra, Tashera, Tasherey, Tasheri, Tasherra, Tashira, Tashirah

Tashawna (American) a combination of the prefix Ta + Shawna.
Tashauna, Tashauni, Tashaunie, Tashaunna, Tashawanna, Tashawn, Tashawnda, Tashawnna, Tashawnnia, Tashonda, Tashondra, Tiashauna, Tishawn, Tishunda, Tishunta, Toshauna, Toshawna, Tyshauna, Tyshawna

Tasheena (American) a combination of the prefix Ta + Sheena.
Tasheana, Tasheeana, Tasheeni, Tashena, Tashenna, Tashennia, Tasheona, Tashina, Tisheena, Tosheena, Tysheana, Tysheena, Tyshyna

Tashelle (American) a combination of the prefix Ta + Shelley.
Tachell, Tashell, Techell, Techelle, Teshell, Teshelle, Tochell, Tochelle, Toshelle, Tychell, Tychelle, Tyshell, Tyshelle

Tashi (Hausa) a bird in flight. (Slavic) a form of Tasha.
Tashia, Tashie, Tashika, Tashima, Tashiya

Tasia (Slavic) a familiar form of Tasha.
Tachia, Tashea, Tasiya, Tassi, Tassia, Tassiana, Tassie, Tasya

Tassos (Greek) a form of Theresa.

Tata (Russian) a familiar form of Tatiana.
Tate, Tatia

Tate (English) a short form of Tatum. A form of Taite, Tata.

Tatiana (Slavic) fairy queen. See also Tanya, Tiana.
Tata, Tatania, Tatanya, Tateana, Tati, Tatia, Tatianna, Tatie, Tatihana, Tatiyana, Tatjana, Tatyana, Tiatiana

Tatianna (Slavic) a form of Tatiana.
Taitiann, Taitianna, Tateanna, Tateonna, Tationna

Tatiyana (Slavic) a form of Tatiana.
Tateyana, Tatiayana, Tatiyanna, Tatiyona, Tatiyonna

Tatum (English) cheerful.
Tate, Tatumn

Tatyana (Slavic) a form of Tatiana.
Tatyanah, Tatyani, Tatyanna, Tatyannah, Tatyona, Tatyonna

Taura (Latin) bull. Astrology: Taurus is a sign of the zodiac.
Taurae, Tauria, Taurina

Tauri (English) a form of Tory.
Taure, Taurie, Taury

Tavia (Latin) a short form of
Octavia. See also Tawia.
*Taiva, Tauvia, Tava, Tavah,
Tavita*

Tavie (Scottish) twin.
Tavey, Tavi

Tawanna (American) a combi-
nation of the prefix Ta +
Wanda.
*Taiwana, Taiwanna, Taquana,
Taquanna, Tawan, Tawana,
Tawanda, Tawanne, Tequana,
Tequanna, Tequawna, Tewanna,
Tewauna, Tiquana, Tiwanna,
Tiwena, Towanda, Towanna,
Tywania, Tywanna*

Tawia (African) born after
twins. (Polish) a form of
Tavia.

Tawni (English) a form of
Tawny.
*Tauni, Taunia, Tawnia, Tawnie,
Tawnnie, Tiawni*

Tawny (Gypsy) little one.
(English) brownish yellow,
tan.
*Tahnee, Tany, Tauna, Tauné,
Taunisha, Tawnee, Tawnesha,
Tawney, Tawni, Tawnyell,
Tiawna*

Tawnya (American) a combination of Tawny + Tonya.
Tawna

Taya, Taye (English) short
forms of Taylor.
*Tay, Tayah, Tayana, Tayiah,
Tayna, Tayra, Taysha, Taysia,
Tayva, Tayvonne, Teya, Teyanna,
Teyona, Teyuna, Tiaya, Tiya,
Tiyah, Tiyana, Tye*

Tayla (English) a short form of
Taylor.
*Taylah, Tayleah, Taylee, Tayleigh,
Taylie, Teila*

Taylar (English) a form of
Taylor.
*Talar, Tayla, Taylah, Taylare,
Tayllar*

Tayler (English) a form of Taylor.
Tayller

Taylor (English) tailor.
*Taelor, Tailor, Taiylor, Talor,
Talora, Taya, Taye, Tayla, Taylar,
Tayler, Tayllor, Tayllore, Tayloir,
Taylorann, Taylore, Taylorr,
Taylour, Taylur, Teylor*

Tazu (Japanese) stork; longevity.
Taz, Tazi, Tazia

Teagan (Welsh) beautiful,
attractive.
*Taegen, Teage, Teagen, Teaghan,
Teaghanne, Teaghen, Teagin,
Teague, Teegan, Teeghan, Tegan,
Tegwen, Teigan, Tejan, Tiegan,
Tigan, Tijan, Tijana*

Teaira (Latin) a form of Tiara.
*Teairra, Teairre, Teairria, Teara,
Tearah, Teareya, Teari, Tearia,
Teariea, Tearra, Tearria*

Teal (English) river duck; blue green.
Teala, Teale, Tealia, Tealisha

Teanna (American) a combination of the prefix Te + Anna. A form of Tiana.
Tean, Teana, Teanah, Teann, Teannah, Teanne, Teaunna, Teena, Teuana

Teca (Hungarian) a form of Theresa.
Techa, Teka, Tica, Tika

Tecla (Greek) God's fame.
Tekla, Theckla

Teddi (Greek) a familiar form of Theodora.
Tedde, Teddey, Teddie, Teddy, Tedi, Tediah, Tedy

Tedra (Greek) a short form of Theodora.
Teddra, Teddreya, Tedera, Teedra, Teidra

Tegan (Welsh) a form of Teagan.
Tega, Tegen, Teggan, Teghan, Tegin, Tegyn, Teigen

Telisha (American) a form of Taleisha.
Teleesha, Teleisia, Telesa, Telesha, Teleshia, Telesia, Telicia, Telisa, Telishia, Telisia, Telissa, Telisse, Tellisa, Tellisha, Telsa, Telysa

Temira (Hebrew) tall.
Temora, Timora

Tempest (French) stormy.
Tempesta, Tempeste, Tempestt, Tempist, Tempistt, Tempress, Tempteste

Tenesha, Tenisha (American) combinations of the prefix Te + Niesha. Tenecia, Teneesha, Teneisha, Teneshia, Tenesia, Tenessa, Teneusa, Teniesha, Tenishia

Tennille (American) a combination of the prefix Te + Nellie.
Taniel, Tanille, Teneal, Teneil, Teneille, Teniel, Tenille, Tenneal, Tenneill, Tenneille, Tennia, Tennie, Tennielle, Tennile, Tineal, Tiniel, Tonielle, Tonille

Teodora (Czech) a form of Theodora.
Teadora

Teona, Teonna (Greek) forms of Tiana, Tianna.
Teon, Teoni, Teonia, Teonie, Teonney, Teonnia, Teonnie

Tequila (Spanish) a kind of liquor. See also Takila.
Taquela, Taquella, Taquila, Taquilla, Tequilia, Tequilla, Tiquila, Tiquilia

Tera, Terra (Latin) earth. (Japanese) swift arrow. (American) forms of Tara.
Terah, Terai, Teria, Terrae, Terrah, Terria, Tierra

Teralyn (American) a combi-
nation of Terri + Lynn.
*Taralyn, Teralyn, Teralynn,
Terralin, Terralyn*

Teresa (Greek) a form of
Theresa. See also Tressa.
*Taresa, Taressa, Tarissa, Terasa,
Tercza, Tereasa, Tereatha, Terese,
Teresea, Teresha, Teresia,
Teresina, Teresita, Tereska,
Tereson, Teressa, Teretha, Tereza,
Terezia, Terezie, Terezilya,
Terezinha, Terezka, Terezsa,
Terisa, Terisha, Teriza, Terrasa,
Terresa, Terresha, Terresia,
Terressa, Terrosina, Tersa, Tersea,
Teruska, Terza, Tété, Tyresa,
Tyresia*

Terese (Greek) a form of
Teresa.
*Tarese, Taress, Taris, Tarise,
Tereece, Tereese, Teress, Terez,
Teris, Terrise*

Teri (Greek) reaper. A familiar
form of Theresa.
Terie

Terrelle (Greek) a form of
Theresa.
*Tarrell, Teral, Terall, Terel, Terell,
Teriel, Terral, Terrall, Terrell,
Terrella, Terriel, Terriell, Terrielle,
Terrill, Terryelle, Terryl, Terryll,
Terrylle, Teryl, Tyrell, Tyrelle*

Terrene (Latin) smooth.
*Tareena, Tarena, Teran, Teranee,
Tereena, Terena, Terencia, Terene,
Terenia, Terentia, Terina, Terran,*
*Terren, Terrena, Terrin, Terrina,
Terron, Terrosina, Terryn, Terun,
Teryn, Teryna, Terynn, Tyreen,
Tyrene*

Terri (Greek) reaper. A familiar
form of Theresa.
Terree, Terria, Terrie

Terriann (American) a combi-
nation of Terri + Ann.
*Teran, Terian, Teriann, Terianne,
Teriyan, Terria, Terrian,
Terrianne, Terryann*

Terrianna (American) a com-
bination of Terri + Anna.
*Teriana, Terianna, Terriana,
Terriauna, Terrina, Terriona,
Terrionna, Terriyana, Terriyanna,
Terryana, Terryauna, Tyrina*

Terrica (American) a combi-
nation of Terri + Erica. See
also Rica.
*Tereka, Terica, Tericka, Terika,
Terreka, Terricka, Terrika, Tyrica,
Tyricka, Tyrika, Tyrikka,
Tyronica*

Terry (Greek) a short form of
Theresa.
*Tere, Teree, Terelle, Terene, Teri,
Terie, Terrey, Terri, Terrie, Terrye,
Tery*

Terry-Lynn (American) a
combination of Terry +
Lynn.
*Terelyn, Terelynn, Terri-Lynn,
Terrilynn, Terrylynn*

Tertia (Latin) third.
Tercia, Tercina, Tercine, Terecena,
Tersia, Terza

Tess (Greek) a short form of
Quintessa, Theresa.
Tes, Tese

Tessa (Greek) reaper.
Tesa, Tesah, Tesha, Tesia, Tessah,
Tessia, Tezia

Tessie (Greek) a familiar form
of Theresa.
Tesi, Tessey, Tessi, Tessy, Tezi

Tetsu (Japanese) strong as iron.

Tetty (English) a familiar form
of Elizabeth.

Tevy (Cambodian) angel.
Teva

Teylor (English) a form of
Taylor.
Teighlor, Teylar

Thaddea (Greek) courageous.
(Latin) praiser.
Thada, Thadda

Thalassa (Greek) sea, ocean.

Thalia (Greek) a form of Talia.
Mythology: the Muse of
comedy.
Thaleia, Thalie, Thalya

Thana (Arabic) happy occa-
sion.
Thaina, Thania, Thanie

Thanh (Vietnamese) bright
blue. (Punjabi) good place.
Thantra, Thanya

Thao (Vietnamese) respectful
of parents.

Thea (Greek) goddess. A short
form of Althea.
Theo

Thelma (Greek) willful.
Thelmalina

Thema (African) queen.

Theodora (Greek) gift of
God. See also Dora, Dorothy,
Feodora.
Taedra, Teddi, Tedra, Teodora,
Teodory, Teodosia, Theda,
Thedorsha, Thedrica, Theo,
Theodore, Theodoria,
Theodorian, Theodosia, Theodra

Theone (Greek) gift of God.
Theondra, Theoni, Theonie

Theophania (Greek) God's
appearance. See also Tiffany.
Theo, Theophanie

Theophila (Greek) loved by
God.
Theo

Theresa (Greek) reaper. See
also Resi, Reza, Riza, Tassos,
Teca, Terrelle, Tracey, Tracy,
Zilya.
Teresa, Teri, Terri, Terry, Tersea,
Tess, Tessa, Tessie, Theresia,
Theresina, Theresita, Theressa,
Thereza, Therisa, Therissie,
Thersa, Thersea, Tresha, Tressa,
Trice

Therese (Greek) a form of
Theresa.
*Terese, Thérèse, Theresia,
Theressa, Therra, Therressa,
Thersa*

Theta (Greek) Linguistics: a
letter in the Greek alphabet.

Thetis (Greek) disposed.
Mythology: the mother of
Achilles.

Thi (Vietnamese) poem.
Thia, Thy, Thya

Thirza (Hebrew) pleasant.
*Therza, Thirsa, Thirzah,
Thursa, Thurza, Thyrza,
Tirshka, Tirza*

Thomasina (Hebrew) twin.
See also Tamassa.
*Tamsin, Thomasa, Thomasia,
Thomasin, Thomasine,
Thomazine, Thomencia,
Thomethia, Thomisha,
Thomsina, Toma, Tomasa,
Tomasina, Tomasine, Tomina,
Tommie, Tommina*

Thora (Scandinavian) thunder.
*Thordia, Thordis, Thorri, Thyra,
Tyra*

Thuy (Vietnamese) gentle.

Tia (Greek) princess. (Spanish)
aunt.
*Téa, Teah, Teeya, Teia, Ti,
Tiakeisha, Tialeigh, Tiamarie,
Tianda, Tiandria, Tiante, Tiia,
Tiye, Tyja*

Tiana, Tianna (Greek)
princess. (Latin) short forms
of Tatiana.
*Teana, Teanna, Tiahna, Tianah,
Tiane, Tianea, Tianee, Tiani,
Tiann, Tiannah, Tianne, Tianni,
Tiaon, Tiauna, Tiena, Tiona,
Tionna, Tiyana*

Tiara (Latin) crowned.
*Teair, Teaira, Teara, Téare, Tearia,
Tearria, Teearia, Teira, Teirra,
Tiaira, Tiare, Tiarea, Tiareah,
Tiari, Tiaria, Tiarra, Tiera,
Tierra, Tyara*

Tiarra (Latin) a form of Tiara.
Tiairra, Tiarrah, Tyarra

Tiauna (Greek) a form of
Tiana.
Tiaunah, Tiaunia, Tiaunna

Tiberia (Latin) Geography: the
Tiber River in Italy.
Tib, Tibbie, Tibby

Tichina (American) a combi-
nation of the prefix Ti +
China.
Tichian, Tichin, Tichinia

Tida (Tai) daughter.
Tiera, Tierra (Latin) forms of
Tiara.
*Tieara, Tiéra, Tierah, Tierre,
Tierrea, Tierria*

Tierney (Irish) noble.
*Tieranae, Tierani, Tieranie,
Tieranni, Tierany, Tiernan,
Tiernee, Tierny*

Tiff (Latin) a short form of
Tiffani, Tiffanie, Tiffany.

Tiffani, Tiffanie (Latin) forms
of Tiffany.
*Tephanie, Tifanee, Tifani,
Tifanie, Tiff, Tiffanee, Tiffayne,
Tiffeni, Tiffenie, Tiffennie,
Tiffiani, Tiffianie, Tiffine, Tiffini,
Tiffinie, Tiffni, Tiffy, Tiffynie,
Tifni*

Tiffany (Latin) trinity. (Greek)
a short form of Theophania.
See also Tyfany.
*Taffanay, Taffany, Tifaney, Tifany,
Tiff, Tiffaney, Tiffani, Tiffanie,
Tiffanny, Tiffeney, Tiffiany,
Tiffiney, Tiffiny, Tiffnay, Tiffney,
Tiffny, Tiffy, Tiphanie, Triffany*

Tiffy (Latin) a familiar form
of Tiffani, Tiffany.
Tiffey, Tiffi, Tiffie

Tijuana (Spanish) Geography:
a border town in Mexico.
*Tajuana, Tajuanna, Thejuana,
Tiajuana, Tiajuanna, Tiawanna*

Tilda (German) a short form
of Matilda.
Tilde, Tildie, Tildy, Tylda, Tyldy

Tillie (German) a familiar
form of Matilda.
*Tilia, Tilley, Tilli, Tillia, Tilly,
Tillye*

Timi (English) a familiar form
of Timothea.
Timia, Timie, Timmi, Timmie

Timothea (English) honoring
God.
Thea, Timi

Tina (Spanish, American) a
short form of Augustine,
Martina, Christina, Valentina.
*Teanna, Teena, Teina, Tena,
Tenae, Tinai, Tine, Tinea, Tinia,
Tiniah, Tinna, Tinnia, Tyna,
Tynka*

Tinble (English) sound bells
make.
Tynble

Tinesha (American) a combi-
nation of the prefix Ti +
Niesha.
*Timnesha, Tinecia, Tineisha,
Tinesa, Tineshia, Tinessa,
Tinisha, Tinsia*

Tinisha (American) a form of
Tenisha.
*Tiniesha, Tinieshia, Tinishia,
Tinishya*

Tiona, Tionna (American)
forms of Tiana.
*Teona, Teonna, Tionda, Tiondra,
Tiondre, Tioné, Tionette, Tioni,
Tionia, Tionie, Tionja, Tionnah,
Tionne, Tionya, Tyonna*

Tiphanie (Latin) a form of
Tiffany.
Tiphanee, Tiphani, Tiphany

Tiponya (Native American)
great horned owl.
Tipper

Tipper (Irish) water pourer.
(Native American) a short
form of Tiponya.

Tira (Hindi) arrow.
Tirah, Tirea, Tirena

Tirtha (Hindi) ford.

Tirza (Hebrew) pleasant.
*Thersa, Thirza, Tierza, Tirsa,
Tirzah, Tirzha, Tyrzah*

Tisa (Swahili) ninth-born.
Tisah, Tysa, Tyssa

Tish (Latin) a short form of
Tisha.

Tisha (Latin) joy. A short form
of Leticia.
*Taesha, Tesha, Teisha, Tiesha,
Tieshia, Tish, Tishal, Tishia,
Tysha, Tyshia*

Tita (Greek) giant. (Spanish) a
short form of names ending
in "tita." A form of Titus (see
Boys' Names).

Titania (Greek) giant.
Mythology: the Titans were a
race of giants.
*Tania, Teata, Titanna, Titanya,
Titiana, Tiziana, Tytan, Tytania,
Tytiana*

Titiana (Greek) a form of
Titania.
*Titianay, Titiania, Titianna,
Titiayana, Titionia, Titiyana,
Titiyanna, Tityana*

Tivona (Hebrew) nature lover.

Tiwa (Zuni) onion.

Tiyana (Greek) a form of
Tiana.
*Tiyan, Tiyani, Tiyania,
Tiyanna, Tiyonna*

Tobi (Hebrew) God is good.
*Tobe, Tobee, Tobey, Tobie, Tobit,
Toby, Tobye, Tova, Tovah, Tove,
Tovi, Tybi, Tybie*

Tocarra (American) a combination of the prefix To + Cara.
Tocara, Toccara

Toinette (French) a short
form of Antoinette.
*Toinetta, Tola, Tonetta, Tonette,
Toni, Toniette, Twanette*

Toki (Japanese) hopeful.
Toko, Tokoya, Tokyo

Tola (Polish) a form of Toinette.
Tolsia

Tomi (Japanese) rich.
Tomie, Tomiju

Tommie (Hebrew) a short
form of Thomasina.
*Tomme, Tommi, Tommia,
Tommy*

Tomo (Japanese) intelligent.
Tomoko

Tonesha (American) a combi-
nation of the prefix To +
Niesha.
*Toneisha, Toneisheia, Tonesha,
Tonesia, Toniece, Tonisha,
Tonneshia*

Toni (Greek) flourishing. (Latin) praiseworthy.
Tonee, Toney, Tonia, Tonie, Toniee, Tonni, Tonnie, Tony, Tonye

Tonia (Latin, Slavic) a form of Toni, Tonya.
Tonea, Toniah, Toniea, Tonja, Tonje, Tonna, Tonni, Tonnia, Tonnie, Tonnja

Tonisha (American) a form of Toneisha.
Toniesha, Tonisa, Tonise, Tonisia, Tonnisha

Tonya (Slavic) fairy queen.
Tonia, Tonnya, Tonyea, Tonyetta, Tonyia

Topaz (Latin) golden yellow gem.

Topsy (English) on top. Literature: a slave in Harriet Beecher Stowe's novel *Uncle Tom's Cabin.*
Toppsy, Topsey, Topsie

Tora (Japanese) tiger.

Tori (Japanese) bird. (English) a form of Tory.
Toria, Toriana, Torie, Torri, Torrie, Torrita

Toria (English) a form of Tori, Tory.
Toriah, Torria

Toriana (English) a form of Tori.
Torian, Toriane, Toriann, Torianna, Torianne, Toriauna,
Torin, Torina, Torine, Torinne, Torion, Torionna, Torionne, Toriyanna, Torrina

Torie, Torrie (English) forms of Tori.
Tore, Toree, Torei, Torre, Torree

Torilyn (English) a combination of Tori + Lynn.
Torilynn, Torrilyn, Torrilynn

Torri (English) a form of Tori.

Tory (English) victorious. (Latin) a short form of Victoria.
Tauri, Torey, Tori, Torrey, Torreya, Torry, Torrye, Torya, Torye, Toya

Tosha (Punjabi) armaments. (Polish) a familiar form of Antonia. (Russian) a form of Tasha.
Toshea, Toshia, Toshiea, Toshke, Tosia, Toska

Toshi (Japanese) mirror image.
Toshie, Toshiko, Toshikyo

Toski (Hopi) squashed bug.

Totsi (Hopi) moccasins.

Tottie (English) a familiar form of Charlotte.
Tota, Totti, Totty

Tovah (Hebrew) good.
Tova, Tovia

Toya (Spanish) a form of Tory.
Toia, Toyanika, Toyanna, Toyea, Toylea, Toyleah, Toylenn, Toylin, Toylyn

Tracey (Greek) a familiar form
of Theresa. (Latin) warrior.
*Trace, Tracee, Tracell, Traci, Tracie,
Tracy, Traice, Trasey, Treesy*

Traci, Tracie (Latin) forms of
Tracey.
*Tracia, Tracilee, Tracilyn,
Tracilynn, Tracina, Traeci*

Tracy (Greek) a familiar form
of Theresa. (Latin) warrior.
Treacy

Tralena (Latin) a combination
of Tracy + Lena.
*Traleen, Tralene, Tralin, Tralinda,
Tralyn, Tralynn, Tralynne*

Tranesha (American) a com-
bination of the prefix Tra +
Niesha.
*Traneice, Traneis, Traneise,
Traneisha, Tranese, Traneshia,
Tranice, Traniece, Traniesha,
Tranisha, Tranishia*

Trashawn (American) a com-
bination of the prefix Tra +
Shawn.
*Trashan, Trashana, Trashauna,
Trashon, Trayshauna*

Trava (Czech) spring grasses.

Treasure (Latin) treasure,
wealth; valuable.
Treasa, Treasur, Treasuré, Treasury

Trella (Spanish) a familiar
form of Estelle.

Tresha (Greek) a form of
Theresa.
Trescha, Trescia, Treshana, Treshia

Tressa (Greek) a short form of
Theresa. See also Teresa.
*Treaser, Tresa, Tresca, Trese,
Treska, Tressia, Tressie, Trez,
Treza, Trisa*

Trevina (Irish) prudent.
(Welsh) homestead.
*Treva, Trevanna, Trevena,
Trevenia, Treveon, Trevia,
Treviana, Trevien, Trevin, Trevona*

Trevona (Irish) a form of
Trevina.
*Trevion, Trevon, Trevonia,
Trevonna, Trevonne, Trevonye*

Triana (Latin) third. (Greek) a
form of Trina.
Tria, Triann, Trianna, Trianne

Trice (Greek) a short form of
Theresa.
Treece

Tricia (Latin) a form of Trisha.
*Trica, Tricha, Trichelle, Tricina,
Trickia*

Trilby (English) soft hat.
Tribi, Trilbie, Trillby

Trina (Greek) pure.
*Treena, Treina, Trenna, Triana,
Trinia, Trinchen, Trind, Trinda,
Trine, Trinette, Trini, Trinica,
Trinice, Triniece, Trinika,
Trinique, Trinisa, Tryna*

Trini (Greek) a form of Trina.
Trinia, Trinie

Trinity (Latin) triad. Religion:
the Father, the Son, and the
Holy Spirit.
*Trinita, Trinite, Trinitee, Triniti,
Trinnette, Trinty*

Trish (Latin) a short form of
Beatrice, Trisha.
Trishell, Trishelle

Trisha (Latin) noblewoman.
(Hindi) thirsty. See also
Tricia.
*Treasha, Trish, Trishann,
Trishanna, Trishanne, Trishara,
Trishia, Trishna, Trissha, Trycia*

Trissa (Latin) a familiar form
of Patricia.
*Trisa, Trisanne, Trisia, Trisina,
Trissi, Trissie, Trissy, Tryssa*

Trista (Latin) a short form of
Tristen.
*Trisatal, Tristess, Tristia, Trysta,
Trystia*

Tristan (Latin) bold.
*Trista, Tristane, Tristanni,
Tristany, Tristen, Tristian,
Tristiana, Tristin, Triston,
Trystan, Trystyn*

Tristen (Latin) a form of
Tristan.
Tristene, Trysten

Tristin (Latin) a form of
Tristan.
*Tristina, Tristine, Tristinye,
Tristn, Trystin*

Triston, Trystyn (Latin) forms
of Tristan.
Tristony, Trystyn

Trixie (American) a familiar
form of Beatrice.
*Tris, Trissie, Trissina, Trix, Trixi,
Trixy*

Troya (Irish) foot soldier.
Troi, Troia, Troiana, Troiya, Troy

Trudel (Dutch) a form of
Trudy.

Trudy (German) a familiar
form of Gertrude.
*Truda, Trude, Trudel, Trudessa,
Trudey, Trudi, Trudie*

Trycia (Latin) a form of Trisha.

Tryna (Greek) a form of Trina.
Tryane, Tryanna, Trynee

Tryne (Dutch) pure.
Trine

Tsigana (Hungarian) a form
of Zigana.
Tsigane, Tzigana, Tzigane

Tu (Chinese) jade.

Tuesday (English) born on the
third day of the week.
*Tuesdae, Tuesdea, Tuesdee,
Tuesdey, Tusdai*

Tula (Hindi) born in the lunar
month of Capricorn.
Tulah, Tulla, Tullah, Tuula

Tullia (Irish) peaceful, quiet.
Tulia, Tulliah

Tulsi (Hindi) basil, a sacred Hindi herb.
Tulsia

Turquoise (French) blue-green semi-precious stone.
Turkois, Turkoise, Turkoys, Turkoyse

Tusa (Zuni) prairie dog.

Tuyen (Vietnamese) angel.

Tuyet (Vietnamese) snow.

Twyla (English) woven of double thread.
Twila, Twilla

Tyanna (American) a combination of the prefix Ty + Anna.
Tya, Tyana, Tyann, Tyannah, Tyanne, Tyannia

Tyeisha (American) a form of Tyesha.
Tyeesha, Tyeishia, Tyieshia, Tyisha, Tyishea, Tyishia

Tyesha (American) a combination of Ty + Aisha.
Tyasha, Tyashia, Tyasia, Tyasiah, Tyeisha, Tyeshia, Tyeyshia, Tyisha

Tyfany (American) a short form of Tiffany.
Tyfani, Tyfanny, Tyffani, Tyffanni, Tyffany, Tyffini, Typhanie, Typhany

Tykeisha (American) a form of Takeisha.
Tkeesha, Tykeisa, Tykeishia, Tykesha, Tykeshia, Tykeysha, Tykeza, Tykisha

Tykera (American) a form of Takira.
Tykeira, Tykeirah, Tykereiah, Tykeria, Tykeriah, Tykerria, Tykiera, Tykierra, Tykira, Tykiria, Tykirra

Tyler (English) tailor.
Tyller, Tylor

Tyna (Czech) a short form of Kristina.
Tynae, Tynea, Tynia

Tyne (English) river.
Tine, Tyna, Tynelle, Tynessa, Tynetta

Tynesha (American) a combination of Ty + Niesha.
Tynaise, Tynece, Tyneicia, Tynesa, Tynesha, Tyneshia, Tynessia, Tyniesha, Tynisha, Tyseisha

Tynisha (American) a form of Tynesha.
Tyneisha, Tyneisia, Tynisa, Tynise, Tynishi

Tyra (Scandinavian) battler. Mythology: Tyr was the god of war. A form of Thora. (Hindi) a form of Tira.
Tyraa, Tyrah, Tyran, Tyree, Tyria

Tyshanna (American) a combination of Ty + Shawna.
Tyshana, Tyshanae, Tyshane, Tyshaun, Tyshaunda, Tyshawn, Tyshawna, Tyshawnah, Tyshawnda, Tyshawnna, Tysheann, Tysheanna, Tyshonia, Tyshonna, Tyshonya

Tytiana (Greek) a form of Titania.
Tytana, Tytanna, Tyteana, Tyteanna, Tytianna, Tytianni, Tytionna, Tytiyana, Tytiyanna, Tytyana, Tytyauna

U

U (Korean) gentle.

Udele (English) prosperous.
Uda, Udella, Udelle, Yudelle

Ula (Irish) sea jewel. (Scandinavian) wealthy. (Spanish) a short form of Eulalia.
Uli, Ulla

Ulani (Polynesian) cheerful.
Ulana, Ulane

Ulima (Arabic) astute; wise.
Ullima

Ulla (German, Swedish) willful. (Latin) a short form of Ursula. Ulli

Ulrica (German) wolf ruler; ruler of all. See also Rica.
Ulka, Ullrica, Ullricka, Ullrika, Ulrika, Ulrike

Ultima (Latin) last, endmost, farthest.

Ululani (Hawaiian) heavenly inspiration.

Ulva (German) wolf.

Uma (Hindi) mother. Religion: another name for the Hindu goddess Devi.

Umay (Turkish) hopeful.
Umai

Umeko (Japanese) plum-blossom child; patient.
Ume, Umeyo

Una (Latin) one; united. (Hopi) good memory. (Irish) a form of Agnes. See also Oona.
Unna, Uny

Undine (Latin) little wave. Mythology: the undines were water spirits. See also Ondine.
Undeen, Undene

Unice (English) a form of Eunice.

Unika (American) a form of Unique.
Unica, Unicka, Unik, Unikqua, Unikue

Unique (Latin) only one.
Unika, Uniqia, Uniqua, Uniquia

Unity (English) unity.
Uinita, Unita, Unitee

Unn (Norwegian) she who is loved.

Unna (German) woman.

Urania (Greek) heavenly.
Mythology: the Muse of
astronomy.
*Urainia, Uranie, Uraniya,
Uranya*

Urbana (Latin) city dweller.
Urbanah, Urbanna

Urika (Omaha) useful to
everyone.
Ureka

Urit (Hebrew) bright.
Urice

Ursa (Greek) a short form of
Ursula. (Latin) a form of
Orsa.
Ursey, Ursi, Ursie, Ursy

Ursula (Greek) little bear. See
also Sula, Ulla, Vorsila.
*Irsaline, Ursa, Ursala, Ursel,
Ursela, Ursella, Ursely, Ursilla,
Ursillane, Ursola, Ursule,
Ursulina, Ursuline, Urszula,
Urszuli, Urzula*

Usha (Hindi) sunrise.

Ushi (Chinese) ox. Astrology: a
sign of the Chinese zodiac.

Uta (German) rich. (Japanese)
poem.
Utako

Utina (Native American)
woman of my country.
Utahna, Utona, Utonna

V

Vail (English) valley.
Vale, Vayle

Val (Latin) a short form of
Valentina, Valerie.

Vala (German) singled out.
Valla

Valarie (Latin) a form of
Valerie.
*Valarae, Valaree, Valarey, Valari,
Valaria, Vallarie*

Valda (German) famous ruler.
Valida, Velda

Valencia (Spanish) strong.
Geography: a region in east-
ern Spain.
*Valecia, Valence, Valenica,
Valentia, Valenzia*

Valene (Latin) a short form of
Valentina.
*Valaine, Valean, Valeda, Valeen,
Valen, Valena, Valeney, Valien,
Valina, Valine, Vallan, Vallen*

Valentina (Latin) strong.
History: Valentina Tereshkova,
a Soviet cosmonaut, was the
first woman in space. See also
Tina, Valene, Valli.
*Val, Valantina, Vale, Valenteen,
Valentena, Valentijn, Valentin,
Valentine, Valiaka, Valtina,
Valyn, Valynn*

Valera (Russian) a form of Valerie. See also Lera.

Valeria (Latin) a form of Valerie.
Valaria, Valeriana, Valeriane, Veleria

Valerie (Latin) strong.
Vairy, Val, Valarie, Vale, Valera, Valeree, Valeri, Valeria, Valérie, Valery, Valka, Valleree, Valleri, Vallerie, Valli, Vallirie, Valora, Valorie, Valry, Valya, Velerie, Waleria

Valery (Latin) a form of Valerie.
Valerye, Vallary, Vallery

Valeska (Slavic) glorious ruler.
Valesca, Valese, Valeshia, Valeshka, Valezka, Valisha

Valli (Latin) a familiar form of Valentina, Valerie. Botany: a plant native to India.
Vallie, Vally

Valma (Finnish) loyal defender.

Valonia (Latin) shadow valley.
Vallon, Valona

Valora (Latin) a form of Valerie.
Valoria, Valorya, Velora

Valorie (Latin) a form of Valerie.
Vallori, Vallory, Valori, Valory

Vanda (German) a form of Wanda.
Vandana, Vandella, Vandetta, Vandi, Vannda

Vanesa (Greek) a form of Vanessa.
Vanesha, Vaneshah, Vanesia, Vanisa

Vanessa (Greek) butterfly. Literature: a name invented by Jonathan Swift as a nickname for Esther Vanhomrigh. See also Nessie.
Van, Vanassa, Vanesa, Vaneshia, Vanesse, Vanessia, Vanessica, Vanetta, Vaneza, Vaniece, Vaniessa, Vanija, Vanika, Vanissa, Vanita, Vanna, Vannesa, Vannessa, Vanni, Vannie, Vanny, Varnessa, Venessa

Vanetta (English) a form of Vanessa.
Vaneta, Vanita, Vanneta, Vannetta, Vannita, Venetta

Vania, Vanya (Russian) familiar forms of Anna.
Vanija, Vanina, Vaniya, Vanja, Vanka, Vannia

Vanity (English) vain.
Vaniti, Vanitty

Vanna (Cambodian) golden. (Greek) a short form of Vanessa.
Vana, Vanae, Vanelly, Vannah, Vannalee, Vannaleigh, Vannie, Vanny

Vannesa, Vannessa (Greek) forms of Vanessa.
Vannesha, Vanneza

Vanora (Welsh) white wave.
Vannora

Vantrice (American) a combi-
nation of the prefix Van +
Trice.
*Vantrece, Vantricia, Vantrisa,
Vantrissa*

Varda (Hebrew) rose.
*Vadit, Vardia, Vardice, Vardina,
Vardis, Vardit*

Varvara (Slavic) a form of
Barbara.
*Vara, Varenka, Varina, Varinka,
Varya, Varyusha, Vava, Vavka*

Vashti (Persian) lovely. Bible:
the wife of Ahasuerus, king
of Persia.
Vashtee, Vashtie, Vashty

Veanna (American) a combi-
nation of the prefix Ve +
Anna.
Veeana, Veena, Veenaya, Veeona

Veda (Sanskrit) sacred lore;
knowledge. Religion: the
Vedas are the sacred writings
of Hinduism.
*Vedad, Vedis, Veeda, Veida,
Veleda, Vida*

Vedette (Italian) sentry; scout.
(French) movie star.
Vedetta

Vega (Arabic) falling star.

Velda (German) a form of
Valda.

Velika (Slavic) great,
wondrous.

Velma (German) a familiar
form of Vilhelmina.
Valma, Vellma, Vilma, Vilna

Velvet (English) velvety.

Venecia (Italian) from Venice,
Italy.
*Vanecia, Vanetia, Veneise, Venesa,
Venesha, Venesher, Venesse,
Venessia, Venetia, Venette,
Venezia, Venice, Venicia, Veniece,
Veniesa, Venise, Venisha,
Venishia, Venita, Venitia, Venize,
Vennesa, Vennice, Vennisa,
Vennise, Vonitia, Vonizia*

Venessa (Latin) a form of
Vanessa.
*Veneese, Venesa, Venese,
Veneshia, Venesia, Venisa,
Venissa, Vennessa*

Venus (Latin) love. Mythology:
the goddess of love and
beauty.
Venis, Venusa, Venusina, Vinny

Vera (Latin) true. (Slavic) faith.
A short form of Elvera,
Veronica. See also Verena,
Wera.
*Vara, Veera, Veira, Veradis,
Verasha, Vere, Verka, Verla,
Viera, Vira*

Verbena (Latin) sacred plants.
Verbeena, Verbina

Verda (Latin) young, fresh.
Verdi, Verdie, Viridiana, Viridis

Verdad (Spanish) truthful.

Verena (Latin) truthful. A
familiar form of Vera, Verna.
*Verene, Verenis, Vereniz, Verina,
Verine, Verinka, Veroshka,
Verunka, Verusya, Virna*

Verenice (Latin) a form of
Veronica.
Verenis, Verenise, Vereniz

Verity (Latin) truthful.
Verita, Veritie

Verlene (Latin) a combination
of Veronica + Lena.
*Verleen, Verlena, Verlin, Verlina,
Verlinda, Verline, Verlyn*

Verna (Latin) springtime.
(French) a familiar form of
Laverne. See also Verena,
Wera.
*Verasha, Verla, Verne, Vernetia,
Vernetta, Vernette, Vernia,
Vernice, Vernita, Verusya, Viera,
Virida, Virna, Virnell*

Vernice (Latin) a form of
Bernice, Verna.
*Vernese, Vernesha, Verneshia,
Vernessa, Vernica, Vernicca,
Verniece, Vernika, Vernique,
Vernis, Vernise, Vernisha,
Vernisheia, Vernissia*

Veronica (Latin) true image.
See also Ronni, Weronika.
*Varonica, Vera, Veranique,
Verenice, Verhonica, Verinica,*
*Verohnica, Veron, Verona, Verone,
Veronic, Véronic, Veronice,
Veronika, Veronique, Véronique,
Veronne, Veronnica, Veruszhka,
Vironica, Vron, Vronica*

Veronika (Latin) a form of
Veronica.
*Varonika, Veronick, Véronick,
Veronik, Veronike, Veronka,
Veronkia, Veruka*

Veronique, Véronique
(French) forms of Veronica.
Vespera (Latin) evening star.

Vesta (Latin) keeper of the
house. Mythology: the goddess of the home.
Vessy, Vest, Vesteria

Veta (Slavic) a familiar form of
Elizabeth.
Veeta, Vita

Vi (Latin, French) a short form
of Viola, Violet.
Vye

Vianca (Spanish) a form of
Bianca.
Vianeca, Vianica

Vianey (American) a familiar
form of Vianna.
Vianney, Viany

Vianna (American) a combination of Vi + Anna.
Viana, Vianey, Viann, Vianne

Vica (Hungarian) a form of
Eve.

Vicki, Vickie (Latin) familiar
forms of Victoria.
Vic, Vicci, Vicke, Vickee,
Vickiana, Vickilyn, Vickki,
Vicky, Vika, Viki, Vikie, Vikki,
Vikky

Vicky (Latin) a familiar form
of Victoria.
Viccy, Vickey, Viky, Vikkey,
Vikky

Victoria (Latin) victorious. See
also Tory, Wicktoria, Wisia.
Vicki, Vicky, Victoire, Victoriana,
Victorianna, Victorie, Victorina,
Victorine, Victoriya, Victorria,
Victorriah, Victory, Victorya,
Viktoria, Vitoria, Vyctoria

Vida (Sanskrit) a form of Veda.
(Hebrew) a short form of
Davida.
Vidamarie

Vidonia (Portuguese) branch
of a vine.
Vedonia, Vidonya

Vienna (Latin) Geography: the
capital of Austria.
Veena, Vena, Venna, Vienette,
Vienne, Vina

Viktoria (Latin) a form of
Victoria.
Viktorie, Viktorija, Viktorina,
Viktorine, Viktorka

Vilhelmina (German) a form
of Wilhelmina.
Velma, Vilhelmine, Vilma

Villette (French) small town.
Vietta

Vilma (German) a short form
of Vilhemina.

Vina (Hindi) Mythology: a
musical instrument played by
the Hindu goddess of wis-
dom. (Spanish) vineyard.
(Hebrew) a short form of
Davina. (English) a short
form of Alvina. See also
Lavina.
Veena, Vena, Viña, Vinesha,
Vinessa, Vinia, Viniece, Vinique,
Vinisha, Viñita, Vinna, Vinni,
Vinnie, Vinny, Vinora, Vyna

Vincentia (Latin) victor, con-
queror.
Vicenta, Vincenta, Vincentena,
Vincentina, Vincentine,
Vincenza, Vincy, Vinnie

Viñita (Spanish) a form of
Vina.
Viñeet, Viñeeta, Viñetta, Viñette,
Viñitha, Viñta, Viñti, Viñtia,
Vyñetta, Vyñette

Viola (Latin) violet; stringed
instrument in the violin fam-
ily. Literature: the heroine of
Shakespeare's play *Twelfth*
Night.
Vi, Violaine, Violanta, Violante,
Viole, Violeine

Violet (French) Botany: a plant
with purplish blue flowers.
Vi, Violeta, Violette, Vyolet,
Vyoletta, Vyolette

Violeta (French) a form of
Violet.
Violetta

Virgilia (Latin) rod bearer, staff
bearer.
Virgillia

Virginia (Latin) pure, virginal.
Literature: Virginia Woolf was
a well-known British writer.
See also Gina, Ginger, Ginny,
Jinny.
*Verginia, Verginya, Virge, Virgen,
Virgenia, Virgenya, Virgie,
Virgine, Virginie, Virginië,
Virginio, Virginnia, Virgy,
Virjeana*

Virginie (French) a form of
Virginia.

Viridiana (Latin) a form of
Viridis.

Viridis (Latin) green.
Virdis, Virida, Viridia, Viridiana

Virtue (Latin) virtuous.

Vita (Latin) life.
*Veeta, Veta, Vitaliana, Vitalina,
Vitel, Vitella, Vitia, Vitka, Vitke*

Vitoria (Spanish) a form of
Victoria.
Vittoria

Viv (Latin) a short form of
Vivian.

Viva (Latin) a short form of
Aviva, Vivian.
Vica, Vivan, Vivva

Viveca (Scandinavian) a form
of Vivian.
*Viv, Vivecca, Vivecka, Viveka,
Vivica, Vivieca, Vyveca*

Vivian (Latin) full of life.
*Vevay, Vevey, Viv, Viva, Viveca,
Vivee, Vivi, Vivia, Viviana,
Viviane, Viviann, Vivianne,
Vivie, Vivien, Vivienne, Vivina,
Vivion, Vivyan, Vivyann,
Vivyanne, Vyvyan, Vyvyann,
Vyvyanne*

Viviana (Latin) a form of
Vivian.
*Viv, Vivianna, Vivyana,
Vyvyana*

Vondra (Czech) loving
woman.
Vonda, Vondrea

Voneisha (American) a combination of Yvonne + Aisha.
Voneishia, Vonesha, Voneshia

Vonna (French) a form of
Yvonne.
Vona

Vonny (French) a familiar
form of Yvonne.
Vonney, Vonni, Vonnie

Vontricia (American) a com-
bination of Yvonne + Tricia.
*Vontrece, Vontrese, Vontrice,
Vontriece*

Vorsila (Greek) a form of
Ursula.
*Vorsilla, Vorsula, Vorsulla,
Vorsyla*

W

Wadd (Arabic) beloved.

Waheeda (Arabic) one and only.

Wainani (Hawaiian) beautiful water.

Wakana (Japanese) plant.

Wakanda (Dakota) magical power.
Wakenda

Wakeisha (American) a combination of the prefix Wa + Keisha.
Wakeishia, Wakesha, Wakeshia, Wakesia

Walad (Arabic) newborn.
Waladah, Walidah

Walda (German) powerful; famous.
Waldina, Waldine, Walida, Wallda, Welda

Waleria (Polish) a form of Valerie.
Wala

Walker (English) cloth; walker.
Wallker

Wallis (English) from Wales.
Wallie, Walliss, Wally, Wallys

Wanda (German) wanderer. See also Wendy.
Vanda, Wahnda, Wandah, Wandely, Wandie, Wandis, Wandja, Wandzia, Wannda, Wonda, Wonnda

Wandie (German) a familiar form of Wanda.
Wandi, Wandy

Waneta (Native American) charger. See also Juanita.
Waneeta, Wanita, Wanite, Wanneta, Waunita, Wonita, Wonnita, Wynita

Wanetta (English) pale face.
Wanette, Wannetta, Wannette

Wanika (Hawaiian) a form of Juanita.
Wanicka

Warda (German) guardian.
Wardah, Wardeh, Wardena, Wardenia, Wardia, Wardine

Washi (Japanese) eagle.

Wattan (Japanese) homeland.

Wauna (Moquelumnan) snow geese honking.
Waunakee

Wava (Slavic) a form of Barbara.

Waverly (English) quaking aspen-tree meadow.
Waverley, Waverli, Wavierlee

Waynesha (American) a combination of Waynette + Niesha.
Wayneesha, Wayneisha, Waynie, Waynisha

Waynette (English) wagon maker.
Waynel, Waynelle, Waynetta, Waynlyn

Weeko (Dakota) pretty girl.

Wehilani (Hawaiian) heavenly adornment.

Wenda (Welsh) a form of Wendy.
Wendaine, Wendayne

Wendelle (English) wanderer.
Wendaline, Wendall, Wendalyn, Wendeline, Wendella, Wendelline, Wendelly

Wendi (Welsh) a form of Wendy.
Wendie

Wendy (Welsh) white; light skinned. A familiar form of Gwendolyn, Wanda.
Wenda, Wende, Wendee, Wendey, Wendi, Wendye, Wuendy

Wera (Polish) a form of Vera. See also Verna.
Wiera, Wiercia, Wierka

Weronika (Polish) a form of Veronica.
Weronikra

Wesisa (Musoga) foolish.

Weslee (English) western meadow.
Weslea, Wesleigh, Weslene, Wesley, Wesli, Weslia, Weslie, Weslyn

Whitley (English) white field.
Whitely, Whitlee, Whitleigh, Whitlie, Whittley

Whitney (English) white island.
Whiteney, Whitne, Whitné, Whitnee, Whitneigh, Whitnie, Whitny, Whitnye, Whytne, Whytney, Witney

Whitnie (English) a form of Whitney.
Whitani, Whitnei, Whitni, Whytni, Whytnie

Whittney (English) a form of Whitney.
Whittaney, Whittanie, Whittany, Whitteny, Whittnay, Whittnee, Whittney, Whittni, Whittnie

Whoopi (English) happy; excited.
Whoopie, Whoopy

Wicktoria (Polish) a form of Victoria.
Wicktorja, Wiktoria, Wiktorja

Wilda (German) untamed. (English) willow.
Willda, Wylda

Wileen (English) a short form of Wilhelmina.
Wilene, Willeen, Willene

Wilhelmina (German) a form of Wilhelm (see Boys' Names). See also Billie, Guillerma, Helma, Minka, Minna, Minnie.
Vilhelmina, Wileen, Wilhelmine, Willa, Willamina, Willamine,

Willemina, Willette, Williamina,
Willie, Willmina, Willmine,
Wilma, Wimina

Wilikinia (Hawaiian) a form of
Virginia.

Willa (German) a short form
of Wilhelmina.
Willabella, Willette, Williabelle

Willette (English) a familiar
form of Wilhelmina, Willa.
Wiletta, Wilette, Willetta,
Williette

Willie (English) a familiar
form of Wilhelmina.
Willi, Willina, Willisha,
Willishia, Willy

Willow (English) willow tree.
Willough

Wilma (German) a short form
of Wilhelmina.
Williemae, Wilmanie, Wilmayra,
Wilmetta, Wilmette, Wilmina,
Wilmyne, Wylma

Wilona (English) desired.
Willona, Willone, Wilone

Win (German) a short form of
Winifred. See also Edwina.
Wyn

Winda (Swahili) hunter.

Windy (English) windy.
Windee, Windey, Windi,
Windie, Wyndee, Wyndy

Winema (Moquelumnan)
woman chief.

Winifred (German) peaceful
friend. (Welsh) a form of
Guinevere. See also Freddi,
Una, Winnie.
Win, Winafred, Winefred,
Winefride, Winfreda, Winfrieda,
Winiefrida, Winifrid, Winifryd,
Winnafred, Winnefred,
Winniefred, Winnifred,
Winnifrid, Wynafred, Wynifred,
Wynnifred

Winna (African) friend.
Winnah

Winnie (English) a familiar
form of Edwina, Gwyneth,
Winnifred, Winona, Wynne.
History: Winnie Mandela
kept the anti-apartheid
movement alive in South
Africa while her then-hus-
band, Nelson Mandela, was
imprisoned. Literature: the
lovable bear in A. A. Milne's
children's story *Winnie-the-
Pooh.*
Wina, Winne, Winney, Winni,
Winny, Wynnie

Winola (German) charming
friend.
Wynola

Winona (Lakota) oldest
daughter.
Wanona, Wenona, Wenonah,
Winnie, Winonah, Wynonna

Winter (English) winter.
Wintr, Wynter

Wira (Polish) a form of Elvira.
Wiria, Wirke

Wisia (Polish) a form of
Victoria.
Wicia, Wikta

Wren (English) wren, songbird.

Wyanet (Native American)
legendary beauty.
Wyaneta, Wyanita, Wynette

Wynne (Welsh) white, light
skinned. A short form of
Blodwyn, Guinivere,
Gwyneth.
Winnie, Wyn, Wynn

Wynonna (Lakota) a form of
Winona.
Wynnona, Wynona

Wynter (English) a form of
Winter.
Wynteria

Wyoming (Native American)
Geography: a western U. S.
state.
Wy, Wye, Wyoh, Wyomia

Xandra (Greek) a form of
Zandra. (Spanish) a short
form of Alexandra.
Xander, Xandrea, Xandria

Xanthe (Greek) yellow, blond.
See also Zanthe.
*Xanne, Xantha, Xanthia,
Xanthippe*

Xanthippe (Greek) a form of
Xanthe. History: Socrates's
wife.
Xantippie

Xaviera (Basque) owner of the
new house. (Arabic) bright.
See also Javiera, Zaviera.
*Xavia, Xaviére, Xavyera,
Xiveria*

Xela (Quiché) my mountain
home.

Xena (Greek) a form of
Xenia.

Xenia (Greek) hospitable. See
also Zena, Zina.
*Xeenia, Xena, Xenea, Xenya,
Xinia*

Xiang (Chinese) fragrant.

Xiomara (Teutonic) glorious
forest.
Xiomaris, Xiomayra

Xiu Mei (Chinese) beautiful
plum.

Xochitl (Aztec) place of many
flowers.
*Xochil, Xochilt, Xochilth,
Xochiti*

Xuan (Vietnamese) spring.

Xuxa (Portuguese) a familiar
form of Susanna.

Xylia (Greek) a form of Sylvia.
Xylina, Xylona

Y

Yachne (Hebrew) hospitable.

Yadira (Hebrew) friend.
Yadirah, Yadirha, Yadyra

Yael (Hebrew) strength of
God. See also Jael.
Yaeli, Yaella, Yeala

Yaffa (Hebrew) beautiful. See
also Jaffa.
Yafeal, Yaffit, Yafit

Yahaira (Hebrew) a form of
Yakira.
Yahara, Yahayra, Yahira

Yajaira (Hebrew) a form of
Yakira.
Yahaira, Yajara, Yajayra, Yajhaira

Yakira (Hebrew) precious;
dear.
Yahaira, Yajaira

Yalanda (Greek) a form of
Yolanda.
Yalando, Yalonda, Ylana, Ylanda

Yalena (Greek, Russian) a
form of Helen. See also
Lena, Yelena.

Yaletha (American) a form of
Oletha.
Yelitsa

Yamary (American) a combi-
nation of the prefix Ya +
Mary.
*Yamairy, Yamarie, Yamaris,
Yamayra*

Yamelia (American) a form of
Amelia.
Yameily, Yamelya, Yamelys

Yamila (Arabic) a form of
Jamila.
*Yamela, Yamely, Yamil, Yamile,
Yamilet, Yamiley, Yamilla, Yamille*

Yaminah (Arabic) right,
proper.
*Yamina, Yamini, Yemina,
Yeminah, Yemini*

Yamka (Hopi) blossom.

Yamuna (Hindi) sacred river.

Yana (Slavic) a form of Jana.
*Yanae, Yanah, Yanay, Yanaye,
Yanesi, Yanet, Yaneth, Yaney,
Yani, Yanik, Yanina, Yanis,
Yanisha, Yanitza, Yanixia,
Yanna, Yannah, Yanni, Yannica,
Yannick, Yannina*

Yanaba (Navajo) brave.

Yaneli (American) a combina-
tion of the prefix Ya +
Nellie.
*Yanela, Yanelis, Yaneliz, Yanelle,
Yanelli, Yanely, Yanelys*

Yanet (American) a form of
Janet.
*Yanete, Yaneth, Yanethe, Yanette,
Yannet, Yanneth, Yannette*

Yáng (Chinese) sun.

Yareli (American) a form of
Oralee.
Yarely, Yaresly

Yarina (Slavic) a form of
Irene.
Yaryna

Yaritza (American) a combination of Yana + Ritsa.
Yaritsa, Yaritza

Yarkona (Hebrew) green.

Yarmilla (Slavic) market
trader.

Yashira (Afghan) humble;
takes it easy. (Arabic) wealthy.

Yasmeen (Persian) a form of
Yasmin.
*Yasemeen, Yasemin, Yasmeena,
Yasmen, Yasmene, Yasmeni,
Yasmenne, Yassmeen, Yassmen*

Yasmin, Yasmine (Persian)
jasmine flower.
*Yashmine, Yasiman, Yasimine,
Yasma, Yasmain, Yasmaine,
Yasmina, Yasminda, Yasmon,
Yasmyn, Yazmin, Yesmean,
Yesmeen, Yesmin, Yesmina,
Yesmine, Yesmyn*

Yasu (Japanese) resting, calm.
Yasuko, Yasuyo

Yazmin (Persian) a form of
Yasmin.
*Yazmeen, Yazmen, Yazmene,
Yazmina, Yazmine, Yazmyn,*
*Yazmyne, Yazzmien, Yazzmine,
Yazzmine, Yazzmyn*

Yecenia (Arabic) a form of
Yesenia.

Yehudit (Hebrew) a form of
Judith.
Yudit, Yudita, Yuta

Yei (Japanese) flourishing.

Yeira (Hebrew) light.

Yekaterina (Russian) a form
of Katherine.

Yelena (Russian) a form of
Helen, Jelena. See also Lena,
Yalena.
*Yeleana, Yelen, Yelenna, Yelenne,
Yelina, Ylena, Ylenia, Ylenna*

Yelisabeta (Russian) a form of
Elizabeth.
Yelizaveta

Yemena (Arabic) from Yemen.
Yemina

Yen (Chinese) yearning;
desirous.
Yeni, Yenih, Yenny

Yenene (Native American)
shaman.

Yenifer (Welsh) a form of
Jennifer.
Yenefer, Yennifer

Yeo (Korean) mild.
Yee

Yepa (Native American) snow
girl.

Yesenia (Arabic) flower.
Yasenya, Yecenia, Yesinia, Yesnia, Yessenia

Yesica (Hebrew) a form of Jessica.
Yesika, Yesiko

Yessenia (Arabic) a form of Yesenia.
Yessena, Yessenya, Yissenia

Yessica (Hebrew) a form of Jessica.
Yessika, Yesyka

Yetta (English) a short form of Henrietta.
Yette, Yitta, Yitty

Yeva (Ukrainian) a form of Eve.

Yiesha (Arabic, Swahili) a form of Aisha.
Yiasha

Yín (Chinese) silver.

Ynez (Spanish) a form of Agnes. See also Inez.
Ynes, Ynesita

Yoanna (Hebrew) a form of Joanna.
Yoana, Yohana, Yohanka, Yohanna, Yohannah

Yocelin, Yocelyn (Latin) forms of Jocelyn.
Yoceline, Yocelyne, Yuceli

Yoi (Japanese) born in the evening.

Yoki (Hopi) bluebird.
Yokie

Yoko (Japanese) good girl.
Yo

Yolie (Greek) a familiar form of Yolanda.
Yola, Yoley, Yoli, Yoly

Yolanda (Greek) violet flower. See also Iolanthe, Jolanda, Olinda.
Yalanda, Yolie, Yolaine, Yolana, Yoland, Yolande, Yolane, Yolanna, Yolantha, Yolanthe, Yolette, Yolonda, Yorlanda, Youlanda, Yulanda, Yulonda

Yoluta (Native American) summer flower.

Yomara (American) a combination of Yolanda + Tamara.
Yomaira, Yomarie, Yomira

Yon (Burmese) rabbit. (Korean) lotus blossom.
Yona, Yonna

Yoné (Japanese) wealth; rice.

Yonina (Hebrew) a form of Jonina.
Yona, Yonah

Yonita (Hebrew) a form of Jonita.
Yonat, Yonati, Yonit

Yoomee (Coos) star.
Yoome

Yordana (Basque) descendant. See also Jordana.

Yori (Japanese) reliable.
Yoriko, Yoriyo

Yoselin (Latin) a form of
Jocelyn.
*Yoseline, Yoselyn, Yosselin,
Yosseline, Yosselyn*

Yosepha (Hebrew) a form of
Josephine.
Yosefa, Yosifa, Yuseffa

Yoshi (Japanese) good; respectful.
Yoshie, Yoshiko, Yoshiyo

Yovela (Hebrew) joyful heart;
rejoicer.

Ysabel (Spanish) a form of
Isabel.
*Ysabell, Ysabella, Ysabelle, Ysbel,
Ysbella, Ysobel*

Ysanne (American) a combination of Ysabel + Ann.
Ysande, Ysann, Ysanna

Yseult (German) ice rule.
(Irish) fair; light skinned.
(Welsh) a form of Isolde.
Yseulte, Ysolt

Yuana (Spanish) a form of
Juana.
Yuan, Yuanna

Yudelle (English) a form of
Udele.
Yudela, Yudell, Yudella

Yudita (Russian) a form of
Judith.
Yudit, Yudith, Yuditt

Yuki (Japanese) snow.
Yukie, Yukiko, Yukiyo

Yulene (Basque) a form of
Julia.
Yuleen

Yulia (Russian) a form of Julia.
*Yula, Yulenka, Yulinka, Yulka,
Yulya*

Yuliana (Spanish) a form of
Juliana.
Yulenia, Yuliani

Yuri (Japanese) lily.
Yuree, Yuriko, Yuriyo

Yvanna (Slavic) a form of
Ivana.
Yvan, Yvana, Yvannia

Yvette (French) a familiar
form of Yvonne. See also
Evette, Ivette.
*Yavette, Yevett, Yevette, Yevetta,
Yvet, Yveta, Yvett, Yvetta*

Yvonne (French) young
archer. (Scandinavian) yew
wood; bow wood. See also
Evonne, Ivonne, Vonna,
Vonny, Yvette.
*Yavanda, Yavanna, Yavanne,
Yavonda, Yavonna, Yavonne,
Yveline, Yvon, Yvone, Yvonna,
Yvonnah, Yvonnia, Yvonnie,
Yvonny*

Z

Zabrina (American) a form of
Sabrina.
*Zabreena, Zabrinia, Zabrinna,
Zabryna*

Zacharie (Hebrew) God
remembered.
*Zacari, Zacceaus, Zacchaea,
Zachary, Zachoia, Zackaria,
Zackeisha, Zackeria, Zakaria,
Zakaya, Zakeshia, Zakiah,
Zakiria, Zakiya, Zakiyah,
Zechari*

Zachary (Hebrew) a form of
Zacharie.
Zackery, Zakary

Zada (Arabic) fortunate, prosperous.
Zaida, Zayda, Zayeda

Zafina (Arabic) victorious.

Zafirah (Arabic) successful;
victorious.

Zahar (Hebrew) daybreak;
dawn.
*Zahara, Zaharra, Zahera,
Zahira, Zahirah, Zeeherah*

Zahavah (Hebrew) golden.
*Zachava, Zachavah, Zechava,
Zechavah, Zehava, Zehavi,
Zehavit, Zeheva, Zehuva*

Zahra (Swahili) flower.
(Arabic) white.
*Zahara, Zahraa, Zahrah,
Zahreh, Zahria*

Zaira (Hebrew) a form of
Zara.
Zaire, Zairea, Zirrea

Zakia (Swahili) smart. (Arabic)
chaste.
Zakea, Zakeia, Zakiah, Zakiya

Zakira (Hebrew) a form of
Zacharie.
*Zaakira, Zakiera, Zakierra,
Zakir, Zakirah, Zakiria,
Zakiriya, Zykarah, Zykera,
Zykeria, Zykerria, Zykira,
Zykuria*

Zakiya (Arabic) a form of
Zakia.
*Zakeya, Zakeyia, Zakiyaa,
Zakiyah, Zakiyya, Zakiyyah,
Zakkiyya, Zakkiyyah,
Zakkyyah*

Zalika (Swahili) born to royalty.
Zuleika

Zaltana (Native American)
high mountain.

Zandra (Greek) a form of
Sandra.
*Zahndra, Zandrea, Zandria,
Zandy, Zanndra, Zondra*

Zaneta (Spanish) a form of
Jane.
Zanita, Zanitra

Zanna (Spanish) a form of Jane. (English) a short form of Susanna.
Zaina, Zainah, Zainna, Zana, Zanae, Zanah, Zanella, Zanette, Zannah, Zannette, Zannia, Zannie

Zanthe (Greek) a form of Xanthe.
Zanth, Zantha

Zara (Hebrew) a form of Sarah, Zora.
Zaira, Zarah, Zarea, Zaree, Zareea, Zareen, Zareena, Zareh, Zareya, Zari, Zaria, Zariya, Zarria

Zarifa (Arabic) successful.

Zarita (Spanish) a form of Sarah.

Zasha (Russian) a form of Sasha.
Zascha, Zashenka, Zashka, Zasho

Zaviera (Spanish) a form of Xaviera.
Zavera, Zavirah

Zawati (Swahili) gift.

Zayit (Hebrew) olive.

Zaynah (Arabic) beautiful.
Zayn, Zayna

Zea (Latin) grain.

Zelda (Yiddish) gray haired. (German) a short form of Griselda. See also Selda.
Zelde, Zella, Zellda

Zelene (English) sunshine.
Zeleen, Zelena, Zeline

Zelia (Spanish) sunshine.
Zele, Zelene, Zelie, Zélie, Zelina

Zelizi (Basque) a form of Sheila.

Zelma (German) a form of Selma.

Zemirah (Hebrew) song of joy.

Zena (Greek) a form of Xenia. (Ethiopian) news. (Persian) woman. See also Zina.
Zanae, Zanah, Zeena, Zeenat, Zeenet, Zeenia, Zeenya, Zein, Zeina, Zenah, Zenana, Zenea, Zenia, Zenna, Zennah, Zennia, Zenya

Zenaida (Greek) white-winged dove.
Zenaide, Zenaïde, Zenayda, Zenochka

Zenda (Persian) sacred; feminine.

Zenobia (Greek) sign, symbol. History: a queen who ruled the city of Palmyra in ancient Syria.
Zeba, Zeeba, Zenobie, Zenovia

Zephania, Zephanie (Greek) forms of Stephanie.
Zepania, Zephanas, Zephany

Zephyr (Greek) west wind.
*Zefiryn, Zephra, Zephria,
Zephyer, Zephyrine*

Zera (Hebrew) seeds.
Zerah, Zeriah

Zerdali (Turkish) wild apricot.

Zerlina (Latin, Spanish) beautiful dawn. Music: a character in Mozart's opera *Don Giovanni.*
Zerla, Zerlinda

Zerrin (Turkish) golden.
Zerren

Zeta (English) rose.
Linguistics: a letter in the Greek alphabet.
Zayit, Zetana, Zetta

Zetta (Portuguese) rose.

Zhana, Zhane (Slavic) forms of Jane.
*Zhanae, Zhanay, Zhanaya,
Zhané, Zhanea, Zhanee,
Zhaney, Zhani, Zhaniah,
Zhanna*

Zhen (Chinese) chaste.

Zia (Latin) grain. (Arabic) light.
Zea

Zigana (Hungarian) gypsy girl. See also Tsigana.
Zigane

Zihna (Hopi) one who spins tops.

Zilla (Hebrew) shadow.
Zila, Zillah, Zylla

Zilpah (Hebrew) dignified.
Bible: Jacob's wife.
Zilpha, Zylpha

Zilya (Russian) a form of Theresa.

Zimra (Hebrew) song of praise.
*Zamora, Zemira, Zemora,
Zimria*

Zina (African) secret spirit. (English) hospitable. (Greek) a form of Zena.
Zinah, Zine

Zinnia (Latin) Botany: a plant with beautiful, rayed, colorful flowers.
Zinia, Zinny, Zinnya, Zinya

Zipporah (Hebrew) bird.
Bible: Moses' wife.
*Zipora, Ziporah, Zipporia,
Ziproh*

Zita (Spanish) rose. (Arabic) mistress. A short form of names ending in "sita" or "zita."
Zeeta, Zyta, Zytka

Ziva (Hebrew) bright; radiant.
Zeeva, Ziv, Zivanka, Zivi, Zivit

Zizi (Hungarian) a familiar form of Elizabeth.
Zsi Zsi

Zocha (Polish) a form of Sophie.

Zoe (Greek) life.
Zoé, Zoë, Zoee, Zoelie, Zoeline, Zoelle, Zoey, Zoi, Zoie, Zowe, Zowey, Zowie, Zoya

Zoey (Greek) a form of Zoe.
Zooey

Zofia (Slavic) a form of Sophia. See also Sofia.
Zofka, Zsofia

Zohar (Hebrew) shining, brilliant.
Zoheret

Zohra (Hebrew) blossom.

Zohreh (Persian) happy.
Zahreh, Zohrah

Zola (Italian) piece of earth.
Zoela, Zoila

Zona (Latin) belt, sash.
Zonia

Zondra (Greek) a form of Zandra.
Zohndra

Zora (Slavic) aurora; dawn. See also Zara.
Zorah, Zorana, Zoreen, Zoreena, Zorna, Zorra, Zorrah, Zorya

Zorina (Slavic) golden.
Zorana, Zori, Zorie, Zorine, Zorna, Zory

Zoya (Slavic) a form of Zoe.
Zoia, Zoyara, Zoyechka, Zoyenka, Zoyya

Zsa Zsa (Hungarian) a familiar form of Susan.
Zhazha

Zsofia (Hungarian) a form of Sofia.
Zofia, Zsofi, Zsofika

Zsuzsanna (Hungarian) a form of Susanna.
Zsuska, Zsuzsa, Zsuzsi, Zsuzsika, Zsuzska

Zudora (Sanskrit) laborer.

Zuleika (Arabic) brilliant.
Zeleeka, Zul, Zulay, Zulekha, Zuleyka

Zulima (Arabic) a form of Salama.
Zuleima, Zulema, Zulemah, Zulimah

Zurafa (Arabic) lovely.
Ziraf, Zuruf

Zuri (Basque) white; light skinned. (Swahili) beautiful.
Zuria, Zurie, Zurisha, Zury

Zusa (Czech, Polish) a form of Susan.
Zuzana, Zuzanka, Zuzia, Zuzka, Zuzu

Zuwena (Swahili) good.
Zwena

Zytka (Polish) rose.

Boys

Aakash (Hindi) a form of
Akash.

Aaron (Hebrew) enlightened.
(Arabic) messenger. Bible: the
brother of Moses and the
first high priest. See also
Ron.
*Aahron, Aaran, Aaren, Aareon,
Aarin, Aaronn, Aarron, Aaryn,
Aeron, Aharon, Ahran, Ahren,
Aranne, Arek, Aren, Ari, Arin,
Aron, Aronek, Aronne, Aronos,
Arran, Arron*

Aban (Persian) Mythology: a
figure associated with water
and the arts.

Abasi (Swahili) stern.

Abbey (Hebrew) a familiar
form of Abe.
Abey, Abbie, Abby

Abbott (Hebrew) father;
abbot.
*Ab, Abba, Abbah, Abbán, Abbé,
Abbot, Abott*

Abbud (Arabic) devoted.

Abdirahman (Arabic) a form
of Abdulrahman.
Abdirehman

Abdul (Arabic) servant.
*Abdal, Abdeel, Abdel, Abdoul,
Abdual, Abdull, Abul*

Abdulaziz (Arabic) servant of
the Mighty.
*Abdelazim, Abdelaziz,
Abdulazaz, Abdulazeez*

Abdullah (Arabic) servant of
Allah.
*Abdalah, Abdalla, Abdallah,
Abduala, Abdualla, Abduallah,
Abdulah, Abdulahi, Abdulha,
Abdulla, Abdullahi*

Abdulrahman (Arabic) servant
of the Merciful.
*Abdelrahim, Abdelrahman,
Abdirahman, Abdolrahem,
Abdularahman, Abdurrahman,
Abdurram*

Abe (Hebrew) a short form of
Abel, Abraham.

Abel (Hebrew) breath.
(Assyrian) meadow.
(German) a short form of
Abelard. Bible: Adam and
Eve's second son.
*Abe, Abele, Abell, Able, Adal,
Avel*

Abelard (German) noble; res-
olute.
*Ab, Abalard, Abel, Abelardo,
Abelhard, Abilard, Adalard,
Adelard*

Abi (Turkish) older brother.

Abiah (Hebrew) God is my
father.
*Abia, Abiel, Abija, Abijah,
Abisha, Abishai, Aviya, Aviyah*

Abie (Hebrew) a familiar form of Abraham.

Abiel (Hebrew) a form of Abiah.

Abir (Hebrew) strong.

Abisha (Hebrew) gift of God.
Abijah, Abishai

Abner (Hebrew) father of light. Bible: the commander of Saul's army.
Ab, Avner, Ebner

Abraham (Hebrew) father of many nations. Bible: the first Hebrew patriarch. See also Avram, Bram, Ibrahim.
Abarran, Abe, Aberham, Abey, Abhiram, Abie, Abrahaim, Abrahame, Abrahamo, Abrahan, Abrahán, Abraheem, Abrahem, Abrahim, Abrahm, Abram, Abramo, Abrán, Abrao, Arram, Avram

Abrahan (Spanish) a form of Abraham.
Abrahon

Abram (Hebrew) a short form of Abraham. See also Bram.
Abramo, Abrams, Avram

Absalom (Hebrew) father of peace. Bible: the rebellious third son of King David. See also Avshalom, Axel.
Absalaam, Absalon, Abselon, Absolum

Acar (Turkish) bright.

Ace (Latin) unity.
Acer, Acey, Acie

Achilles (Greek) Mythology: a hero of the Trojan War. Literature: the hero of Homer's epic poem *Iliad.*
Achill, Achille, Achillea, Achillios, Akil, Akili, Akilles

Ackerley (English) meadow of oak trees.
Accerley, Ackerlea, Ackerleigh, Ackersley, Acklea, Ackleigh, Ackley, Acklie

Acton (English) oak-tree settlement.

Adahy (Cherokee) in the woods.

Adair (Scottish) oak-tree ford.
Adaire, Adare

Adam (Phoenician) man; mankind. (Hebrew) earth; man of the red earth. Bible: the first man created by God. See also Adamson, Addison, Damek, Keddy, Macadam.
Ad, Adama, Adamec, Adamo, Adão, Adas, Addam, Addams, Addis, Addy, Adem, Adham, Adhamh, Adné, Adok, Adomas

Adamec (Czech) a form of Adam.
Adamek, Adamik, Adamka, Adamko, Adamok

Adamson (Hebrew) son of Adam.
Adams, Adamsson, Addamson

Adan (Irish) a form of Aidan.
Aden, Adian, Adin

Adar (Syrian) ruler; prince.
(Hebrew) noble; exalted.
Addar

Adarius (American) a combi-
nation of Adam + Darius.
*Adareus, Adarias, Adarrius,
Adarro, Adarruis, Adaruis,
Adauris*

Addison (English) son of
Adam.
*Addis, Addisen, Addisun,
Addyson, Adison, Adisson,
Adyson*

Addy (Hebrew) a familiar
form of Adam, Adlai.
(German) a familiar form of
Adelard.
Addey, Addi, Addie, Ade, Adi

Ade (Yoruba) royal.

Adelard (German) noble;
courageous.
*Adal, Adalar, Adalard, Addy,
Adel, Adél, Adelar*

Aden (Arabic) Geography: a
region in southern Yemen.
(Irish) a form of Aidan,
Aiden.

Adham (Arabic) black.

Adil (Arabic) just; wise.
Adeel, Adeele

Adin (Hebrew) pleasant.

Adir (Hebrew) majestic; noble.
Adeer

Adiv (Hebrew) pleasant; gentle.
Adeev

Adlai (Hebrew) my ornament.
Ad, Addy, Adley

Adler (German) eagle.
Ad, Addler, Adlar

Adli (Turkish) just; wise.

Admon (Hebrew) peony.

Adnan (Arabic) pleasant.
Adnaan

Adney (English) noble's island.
Adny

Adolf (German) noble wolf.
History: Adolf Hitler's
German army was defeated
in World War II. See also
Dolf.
Ad, Adolfo, Adolfus, Adolph

Adolfo (Spanish) a form of
Adolf.
Adolpho

Adolph (German) a form of
Adolf.
*Adolphe, Adolpho, Adolphus,
Adulphus*

Adom (Akan) help from God.

Adon (Hebrew) Lord. (Greek)
a short form of Adonis.

Adonis (Greek) highly attractive. Mythology: the attrac-

tive youth loved by
Aphrodite.
Adon, Adonnis, Adonys

Adri (Indo-Pakistani) rock.
Adrey

Adrian (Greek) rich. (Latin)
dark. (Swedish) a short form
of Hadrian.
*Adarian, Ade, Adorjan, Adrain,
Adreian, Adreyan, Adri,
Adriaan, Adriane, Adriann,
Adrianne, Adriano, Adriean,
Adrien, Adrik, Adrion, Adrionn,
Adrionne, Adron, Adryan,
Adryn, Adryon*

Adriano (Italian) a form of
Adrian.
Adrianno

Adriel (Hebrew) member of
God's flock.
Adrial

Adrien (French) a form of
Adrian.
Adriene, Adrienne

Adrik (Russian) a form of
Adrian.
Adric

Aeneas (Greek) praised.
(Scottish) a form of Angus.
Literature: the Trojan hero of
Vergil's epic poem *Aeneid*.
See also Eneas.

Afram (African) Geography: a
river in Ghana, Africa.

Afton (English) from Afton,
England.
Affton

Agamemnon (Greek) resolute.
Mythology: the king of
Mycenae who led the
Greeks in the Trojan War.

Agni (Hindi) Religion: the
Hindu fire god.

Agu (Ibo) leopard.

Agustin (Latin) a form of
Augustine.
*Agostino, Agoston, Aguistin,
Agustine, Agustis, Agusto,
Agustus*

Ahab (Hebrew) father's
brother. Literature: the cap-
tain of the Pequod in
Herman Melville's novel
Moby-Dick.

Ahanu (Native American)
laughter.

Ahdik (Native American) cari-
bou; reindeer.

Ahearn (Scottish) lord of the
horses. (English) heron.
*Ahearne, Aherin, Ahern,
Aherne, Hearn*

Ahir (Turkish) last.

Ahmad (Arabic) most highly
praised. See also Muhammad.
*Achmad, Achmed, Ahamad,
Ahamada, Ahamed, Ahmaad,
Ahmaud, Amad, Amahd, Amed*

Ahmed (Swahili) praiseworthy.

Ahsan (Arabic) charitable.

Aidan (Irish) fiery.
Adan, Aden, Aiden, Aydan, Ayden, Aydin

Aiden, Ayden (Irish) a form of Aidan.
Aden, Aidon, Aidyn, Aydean

Aiken (English) made of oak.
Aicken, Aikin, Ayken, Aykin

Aimery (French) a form of Emery.
Aime, Aimerey, Aimeric, Amerey, Aymeric, Aymery

Aimon (French) house. (Irish) a form of Eamon.

Aindrea (Irish) a form of Andrew.
Aindreas

Ainsley (Scottish) my own meadow.
Ainsleigh, Ainslie, Ansley, Aynslee, Aynsley, Aynslie

Aizik (Russian) a form of Isaac.

Ajala (Yoruba) potter.

Ajay (Punjabi) victorious; undefeatable. (American) a combination of the initials A. + J.
Aj, Aja, Ajae, Ajai, Ajaye, Ajaz, Ajé, Ajee, Ajit

Ajit (Sanskrit) unconquerable.
Ajeet, Ajith

Akar (Turkish) flowing stream.
Akara

Akash (Hindi) sky.
Aakash, Akasha, Akshay

Akbar (Arabic) great.

Akecheta (Sioux) warrior.

Akeem, Akim (Hebrew) short forms of Joachim.
Achim, Ackeem, Ackim, Ahkieme, Akeam, Akee, Akiem, Akima, Arkeem

Akemi (Japanese) dawn.

Akil (Arabic) intelligent. (Greek) a form of Achilles.
Ahkeel, Akeel, Akeil, Akeyla, Akhil, Akiel, Akila, Akilah, Akile, Akili

Akins (Yoruba) brave.

Akira (Japanese) intelligent.
Akihito, Akio, Akiyo

Akiva (Hebrew) a form of Jacob.
Akiba, Kiva

Akmal (Arabic) perfect.

Aksel (Norwegian) father of peace.
Aksell

Akshay (American) a form of Akash.
Akshaj, Akshaya

Akshat (Sanskrit) uninjurable.

Akule (Native American) he looks up.

Al (Irish) a short form of Alan, Albert, Alexander.

Aladdin (Arabic) height of faith. Literature: the hero of a story in the *Arabian Nights*.
Ala, Alaa, Alaaddin, Aladean, Aladin, Aladino

Alain (French) a form of Alan.
Alaen, Alainn, Alayn, Allain

Alaire (French) joyful.

Alam (Arabic) universe.

Alan (Irish) handsome; peaceful.
Ailan, Ailin, Al, Alaan, Alain, Alair, Aland, Alande, Alando, Alani, Alann, Alano, Alanson, Alante, Alao, Allan, Allen, Alon, Alun

Alaric (German) ruler of all. See also Ulrich.
Alarick, Alarico, Alarik, Aleric, Allaric, Allarick, Alric, Alrick, Alrik

Alastair (Scottish) a form of Alexander.
Alaisdair, Alaistair, Alaister, Alasdair, Alasteir, Alaster, Alastor, Aleister, Alester, Alistair, Allaistar, Allastair, Allaster, Allastir, Allysdair, Alystair

Alban (Latin) from Alba, Italy.
Albain, Albany, Albean, Albein, Alby, Auban, Auben

Albern (German) noble; courageous.

Albert (German, French) noble and bright. See also Elbert, Ulbrecht.
Adelbert, Ailbert, Al, Albertik, Alberto, Alberts, Albie, Albrecht, Alby, Alvertos, Aubert

Alberto (Italian) a form of Albert.
Berto

Albie, Alby (German, French) familiar forms of Albert.
Albee, Albi

Albin (Latin) a form of Alvin.
Alben, Albeno, Albinek, Albino, Albins, Albinson, Alby, Auben

Albion (Latin) white cliffs. Geography: a reference to the white cliffs in Dover, England.

Alcandor (Greek) manly; strong.

Alcott (English) old cottage.
Alcot, Alkot, Alkott, Allcot, Allcott, Allkot, Allkott

Aldair (German, English) a form of Alder.
Aldahir, Aldayr

Alden (English) old; wise protector.
Aldan, Aldean, Aldin, Aldous, Elden

Alder (German, English) alder tree.
Aldair

Aldo (Italian) old; elder.
(German) a short form of
Aldous.

Aldous (German) a form of
Alden.
Aldis, Aldo, Aldon, Aldus, Elden

Aldred (English) old; wise
counselor.
Alldred, Eldred

Aldrich (English) wise.
*Aldric, Aldrick, Aldridge,
Aldrige, Aldritch, Alldric,
Alldrich, Alldrick, Alldridge,
Eldridge*

Aldwin (English) old friend.
Aldwyn, Eldwin

Alec, Alek (Greek) short
forms of Alexander.
Aleck, Alekko, Elek

Alejándro (Spanish) a form of
Alexander.
Alejándra, Aléjo, Alexjándro

Aleksandar, Aleksander
(Greek) forms of Alexander.
*Aleksandor, Aleksandr,
Aleksandras, Aleksandur*

Aleksei (Russian) a short form
of Alexander.
*Aleks, Aleksey, Aleksi, Aleksis,
Aleksy, Alexei, Alexey*

Alekzander, Alexzander
(Greek) forms of Alexander.
*Alekxander, Alekxzander,
Alexkzandr, Alexzandr,
Alexzandyr*

Alem (Arabic) wise.

Aleric (German) a form of
Alaric.
Alerick, Alleric, Allerick

Aleron (Latin) winged.

Alessandro (Italian) a form of
Alexander.
Alessand, Allessandro

Alex (Greek) a short form of
Alexander.
Alax, Alix, Allax, Allex, Elek

Alexander (Greek) defender
of mankind. History:
Alexander the Great was the
conqueror of the civilized
world. See also Alastair,
Alistair, Iskander, Jando, Leks,
Lex, Lexus, Macallister,
Oleksandr, Olés, Sander,
Sándor, Sandro, Sandy, Sasha,
Xan, Xander, Zander, Zindel.
*Al, Alec, Alecsandar, Alejándro,
Alek, Alekos, Aleksandar,
Aleksander, Aleksei, Alekzander,
Alessandro, Alex, Alexandar,
Alexandor, Alexandr, Alexandre,
Alexandro, Alexandros, Alexi,
Alexis, Alexxander, Alexzander,
Alic, Alick, Alisander, Alixander*

Alexandre (French) a form of
Alexander.

Alexandro (Greek) a form of
Alexander.
*Alexandras, Alexandros,
Alexandru*

Alexi (Russian) a form of
Aleksei. (Greek) a short form
of Alexander.
*Alexe, Alexee, Alexey, Alexie,
Alexio, Alexy*

Alexis (Greek) a short form of
Alexander.
*Alexei, Alexes, Alexey, Alexios,
Alexius, Alexiz, Alexsis,
Alexsus, Alexus*

Alfie (English) a familiar form
of Alfred.
Alfy

Alfonso (Italian, Spanish) a
form of Alphonse.
*Affonso, Alfons, Alfonse,
Alfonsus, Alfonza, Alfonzo,
Alfonzus*

Alford (English) old river ford.

Alfred (English) elf counselor;
wise counselor. See also
Fred.
*Ailfrid, Ailfryd, Alf, Alfeo, Alfie,
Alfredo, Alured*

Alfredo (Italian, Spanish) a
form of Alfred.
Alfrido

Alger (German) noble spearman. (English) a short form
of Algernon. See also Elger.
Algar, Allgar

Algernon (English) bearded,
wearing a moustache.
*Algenon, Alger, Algie, Algin,
Algon*

Algie (English) a familiar form
of Algernon.
Algee, Algia, Algy

Algis (German) spear.

Ali (Arabic) greatest. (Swahili)
exalted.
Aly

Alic (Greek) a short form of
Alexander.
Alick, Aliek, Alik, Aliko

Alim (Arabic) scholar. (Arabic)
a form of Alem.

Alisander (Greek) a form of
Alexander.
*Alissander, Alissandre, Alsandair,
Alsandare, Alsander*

Alistair (English) a form of
Alexander.
*Alisdair, Alistaire, Alistar, Alister,
Allistair, Allistar, Allister, Allistir,
Alstair*

Alixander (Greek) a form of
Alexander.
*Alixandre, Alixandru,
Alixzander*

Allan (Irish) a form of Alan.
Allayne

Allard (English) noble, brave.
Alard, Ellard

Allen (Irish) a form of Alan.
*Alen, Alley, Alleyn, Alleyne,
Allie, Allin, Allon, Allyn*

Almon (Hebrew) widower.

Alois (German) a short form
of Aloysius.
Aloys

Aloisio (Spanish) a form of
Louis.

Alok (Sanskrit) victorious cry.

Alon (Hebrew) oak.

Alonso, Alonzo (Spanish)
forms of Alphonse.
*Alano, Alanzo, Alon, Alonza,
Elonzo, Lon, Lonnie, Lonso,
Lonzo*

Aloysius (German) a form of
Louis.
Alaois, Alois, Aloisius, Aloisio

Alphonse (German) noble
and eager.
*Alf, Alfie, Alfonso, Alonzo,
Alphons, Alphonsa, Alphonso,
Alphonsus, Alphonza,
Alphonzus, Fonzie*

Alphonso (Italian) a form of
Alphonse.
Alphanso, Alphonzo, Fonso

Alpin (Irish) attractive.
Alpine

Alroy (Spanish) king.

Alston (English) noble's settlement.
Allston, Alstun

Altair (Greek) star. (Arabic)
flying.

Altman (German) old man.
Altmann, Atman

Alton (English) old town.
Alten

Alva (Hebrew) sublime.
Alvah

Alvan (German) a form of
Alvin.
Alvand

Alvar (English) army of elves.
Alvara

Alvaro (Spanish) just; wise.

Alvern (Latin) spring.
Elvern

Alvin (Latin) white; light
skinned. (German) friend to
all; noble friend; friend of
elves. See also Albin, Elvin.
*Aloin, Aluin, Aluino, Alvan,
Alven, Alvie, Alvino, Alvy,
Alvyn, Alwin, Elwin*

Alvis (Scandinavian) all-know-
ing.

Alwin (German) a form of
Alvin.
*Ailwyn, Alwyn, Alwynn,
Aylwin*

Amadeo (Italian) a form of
Amadeus.

Amadeus (Latin) loves God.
Music: Wolfgang Amadeus
Mozart was a famous eigh-
teenth-century Austrian
composer.
*Amad, Amadeaus, Amadée,
Amadeo, Amadei, Amadio,
Amadis, Amado, Amador,*

Amadou, Amando, Amedeo,
Amodaos

Amal (Hebrew) worker.
(Arabic) hopeful.

Amandeep (Punjabi) light of
peace.
Amandip, Amanjit, Amanjot,
Amanpreet

Amando (French) a form of
Amadeus.
Amand, Amandio, Amaniel,
Amato

Amani (Arabic) believer.
(Yoruba) strength; builder.
Amanee

Amar (Punjabi) immortal.
(Arabic) builder.
Amare, Amaree, Amari, Amario,
Amaris, Amarjit, Amaro,
Amarpreet, Amarri, Ammar,
Ammer

Amato (French) loved.
Amatto

Ambar (Sanskrit) sky.
Amber

Ambrose (Greek) immortal.
Ambie, Ambroise, Ambros,
Ambrosi, Ambrosio, Ambrosius,
Ambrus, Amby

Ameer (Hebrew) a form of
Amir.
Ameir, Amer, Amere

Amerigo (Teutonic) industrious. History: Amerigo
Vespucci was the Italian
explorer for whom America
is named.
Americo, Americus

Ames (French) friend.

Amicus (English, Latin)
beloved friend.
Amico

Amiel (Hebrew) God of my
people.
Ammiel

Amin (Hebrew, Arabic) trustworthy; honest. (Hindi) faithful.
Amine

Amir (Hebrew) proclaimed.
(Punjabi) wealthy; king's
minister. (Arabic) prince.
Aamer, Aamir, Ameer, Amire,
Amiri

Amish (Sanskrit) honest.

Amit (Punjabi) unfriendly.
(Arabic) highly praised.
Amitan, Amreet

Ammon (Egyptian) hidden.
Mythology: the ancient god
associated with reproduction.
Amman

Amol (Hindi) priceless, valuable.
Amul

Amon (Hebrew) trustworthy;
faithful.

Amory (German) a form of
Emory.
Amery, Amor

Amos (Hebrew) burdened,
troubled. Bible: an Old
Testament prophet.
Amose

Amram (Hebrew) mighty
nation.
Amarien, Amran, Amren

Amrit (Sanskrit) nectar.
(Punjabi, Arabic) a form of
Amit.

An (Chinese, Vietnamese)
peaceful.
Ana

Anand (Hindi) blissful.
Ananda, Anant, Ananth

Anastasius (Greek) resurrec-
tion.
Anas, Anastacio, Anastacios,
Anastagio, Anastas, Anastase,
Anastasi, Anastasio, Anastasios,
Anastice, Anastisis, Anaztáz,
Athanasius

Anatole (Greek) east.
Anatol, Anatoley, Anatoli,
Anatolijus, Anatolio, Anatoliy,
Anatoly, Anitoly

Anchali (Taos) painter.

Anders (Swedish) a form of
Andrew.
Ander

Anderson (Swedish) son of
Andrew.
Andersen

Andonios (Greek) a form of
Anthony.
Andoni, Andonis, Andonny

Andor (Hungarian) a form of
Andrew.

András (Hungarian) a form of
Andrew.
Andraes, Andri, Andris, Andrius,
Andriy, Aundras, Aundreas

Andre, André (French) forms
of Andrew.
Andra, Andrae, Andrecito,
Andree, Andrei, Aundre, Aundré

Andrea (Greek) a form of
Andrew.
Andrean, Andreani, Andrian

Andreas (Greek) a form of
Andrew.
Andres, Andries

Andrei (Bulgarian, Romanian,
Russian) a form of Andrew.
Andreian, Andrej, Andrey,
Andreyan, Andrie, Aundrei

Andres (Spanish) a form of
Andrew.
Andras, Andrés, Andrez

Andrew (Greek) strong;
manly; courageous. Bible:
one of the Twelve Apostles.
See also Bandi, Drew, Endre,
Evangelos, Kendrew, Ondro.
Aindrea, Anders, Andery,

Andonis, Andor, András, Andre, André, Andrea, Andreas, Andrei, Andres, Andrews, Andru, Andrue, Andrus, Andy, Anker, Anndra, Antal, Audrew

Andros (Polish) sea. Mythology: the god of the sea.
Andris, Andrius, Andrus

Andy (Greek) a short form of Andrew.
Andino, Andis, Andje

Aneurin (Welsh) honorable; gold. See also Nye.
Aneirin

Anfernee (Greek) a form of Anthony.
Anferney, Anfernie, Anferny, Anfranee, Anfrene, Anfrenee, Anpherne

Angel (Greek) angel. (Latin) messenger. See also Gotzon.
Ange, Angell, Angelo, Angie, Angy

Angelo (Italian) a form of Angel.
Angeleo, Angelito, Angello, Angelos, Anglo

Angus (Scottish) exceptional; outstanding. Mythology: Angus Og was the Celtic god of youth, love, and beauty. See also Ennis, Gus.
Aeneas, Aonghas

Anh (Vietnamese) peace; safety.

Anibal (Phoenician) a form of Hannibal.

Anil (Hindi) wind god.
Aneel, Anel, Aniel, Aniello

Anka (Turkish) phoenix.

Anker (Danish) a form of Andrew.
Ankur

Annan (Scottish) brook. (Swahili) fourth-born son.

Annas (Greek) gift from God.
Anis, Anish, Anna, Annais

Anno (German) a familiar form of Johann.

Anoki (Native American) actor.

Ansel (French) follower of a nobleman.
Ancell, Ansa, Ansell

Anselm (German) divine protector. See also Elmo.
Anse, Anselme, Anselmi, Anselmo

Ansis (Latvian) a form of Janis.

Ansley (Scottish) a form of Ainsley.
Anslea, Anslee, Ansleigh, Anslie, Ansly, Ansy

Anson (German) divine. (English) Anne's son.
Ansun

Antal (Hungarian) a form of Anthony.
Antek, Anti, Antos

Antares (Greek) giant, red star. Astronomy: the brightest star in the constellation Scorpio.
Antar, Antario, Antarious, Antarius, Antarr, Antarus

Antavas (Lithuanian) a form of Anthony.
Antae, Antaeus, Antavious, Antavius, Ante, Anteo

Anthany (Latin, Greek) a form of Anthony.
Antanee, Antanie, Antenee, Anthan, Antheny, Anthine, Anthney

Anthonie (Latin, Greek) a form of Anthony.
Anthone, Anthonee, Anthoni, Anthonia

Anthony (Latin) praiseworthy. (Greek) flourishing. See also Tony.
Anathony, Andonios, Andor, András, Anothony, Antal, Antavas, Anfernee, Anthany, Anthawn, Anthey, Anthian, Anthino, Anthone, Anthoney, Anthonie, Anthonio, Anthonu, Anthonysha, Anthoy, Anthyoine, Anthyonny, Antione, Antjuan, Antoine, Anton, Antonio, Antony, Antwan, Antwon

Antione (French) a form of Anthony.
Antion, Antionio, Antionne, Antiono

Antjuan (Spanish) a form of Anthony.
Antajuan, Anthjuan, Antuan, Antuane

Antoan (Vietnamese) safe, secure.

Antoine (French) a form of Anthony.
Anntoin, Anthoine, Antoiné, Antoinne, Atoine

Anton (Slavic) a form of Anthony.
Anthon, Antone, Antonn, Antonne, Antons, Antos

Antonio (Italian) a form of Anthony. See also Tino, Tonio.
Anthonio, Antinio, Antoinio, Antoino, Antonello, Antoneo, Antonin, Antonín, Antonino, Antonnio, Antonios, Antonius, Antonyia, Antonyio, Antonyo

Antony (Latin) a form of Anthony.
Antin, Antini, Antius, Antoney, Antoni, Antonie, Antonin, Antonios, Antonius, Antonyia, Antonyio, Antonyo, Anty

Antti (Finnish) manly.
Anthey, Anthi, Anti

Antwan (Arabic) a form of Anthony.
Antaw, Antawan, Antawn, Anthawn, Antowan, Antowaun, Antowine, Antowne, Antowyn, Antuwan, Antwain, Antwaina, Antwaine, Antwainn, Antwaion, Antwane, Antwann, Antwanne, Antwarn, Antwaun, Antwen, Antwian, Antwine, Antwuan, Antwun, Antwyné

Antwon (Arabic) a form of Anthony.
Antown, Antuwon, Antwion, Antwione, Antwoan, Antwoin, Antwoine, Antwone, Antwonn, Antwonne, Antwoun, Antwyon, Antwyone, Antyon, Antyonne, Antywon

Anwar (Arabic) luminous.
Anour, Anouar, Anwi

Apiatan (Kiowa) wooden lance.

Apollo (Greek) manly. Mythology: the god of prophecy, healing, music, poetry, and light. See also Polo.
Apolinar, Apolinario, Apollos, Apolo, Apolonio, Appollo

Aquila (Latin, Spanish) eagle.
Acquilla, Aquil, Aquilas, Aquileo, Aquiles, Aquilino, Aquilla, Aquille, Aquillino

Araldo (Spanish) a form of Harold.
Aralodo, Aralt, Aroldo, Arry

Aram (Syrian) high, exalted.
Ara, Aramia, Arra, Arram

Aramis (French) Literature: one of the title characters in Alexandre Dumas's novel *The Three Musketeers.*
Airamis, Aramith, Aramys

Aran (Tai) forest. (Danish) a form of Aren. (Hebrew, Scottish) a form of Arran.

Archer (English) bowman.
Archie

Archibald (German) bold. See also Arkady.
Arch, Archaimbaud, Archambault, Archibaldo, Archibold, Archie

Archie (German, English) a familiar form of Archer, Archibald.
Archy

Ardal (Irish) a form of Arnold.
Ardale

Ardell (Latin) eager; industrious.
Ardel

Arden (Latin) ardent; fiery.
Ard, Ardan, Ardene, Ardian, Ardie, Ardin, Ardn, Arduino

Ardon (Hebrew) bronzed.

Aren (Danish) eagle; ruler. (Hebrew, Arabic) a form of Aaron.

Aretino (Greek, Italian) victorious.

Argus (Danish) watchful, vigilant.
Agos

Ari (Hebrew) a short form of Ariel. (Greek) a short form of Aristotle.
Aria, Arias, Arie, Arieh, Arih, Arij, Ario, Arri, Ary, Arye

Arian (Greek) a form of Arion.
Ariana, Ariane, Ariann, Arianne, Arrian, Aryan

Aric (German) a form of Richard. (Scandinavian) a form of Eric.
Aaric, Arec, Areck, Arich, Arick, Ariek, Arik, Arrek, Arric, Arrick, Arrik, Aryk

Ariel (Hebrew) lion of God. Bible: another name for Jerusalem. Literature: the name of a sprite in the Shakespearean play *The Tempest*.
Airel, Arel, Areli, Ari, Ariell, Ariya, Ariyel, Arrial, Arriel

Aries (Latin) ram. Astrology: the first sign of the zodiac.
Ares, Arie, Ariez

Arif (Arabic) knowledgeable.
Areef

Arion (Greek) enchanted. (Hebrew) melodious.
Arian, Arien, Ario, Arione, Aryon

Aristides (Greek) son of the best.
Aris, Aristedes, Aristeed, Aristide, Aristides, Aristidis

Aristotle (Greek) best; wise. History: a third-century B.C. philosopher who tutored Alexander the Great.
Ari, Aris, Aristito, Aristo, Aristokles, Aristotelis

Arjun (Hindi) white; milk colored.
Arjen, Arjin, Arju, Arjuna, Arjune

Arkady (Russian) a form of Archibald.
Arcadio, Arkadi, Arkadij, Arkadiy

Arkin (Norwegian) son of the eternal king.
Aricin, Arkeen, Arkyn

Arledge (English) lake with the hares.
Arlidge, Arlledge

Arlen (Irish) pledge.
Arlan, Arland, Arlend, Arlin, Arlinn, Arlyn, Arlynn

Arley (English) a short form of Harley.
Arleigh, Arlie, Arly

Arlo (Spanish) barberry. (English) fortified hill. A form of Harlow. (German) a form of Charles.

Arman (Persian) desire, goal.
Armaan, Armahn, Armaine

Armand (Latin, German) a form of Herman. See also Mandek.
Armad, Arman, Armanda, Armando, Armands, Armanno, Armaude, Armenta, Armond

Armando (Spanish) a form of Armand.
Armondo

Armani (Hungarian) sly. (Hebrew) a form of Armon.
Arman, Armann, Armoni, Armonie, Armonio, Armonni, Armony

Armon (Hebrew) high fortress, stronghold.
Armani, Armen, Armin, Armino, Armonn, Armons

Armstrong (English) strong arm. History: astronaut Neil Armstrong was the commander of Apollo 11 and the first person to walk on the moon.

Arnaud (French) a form of Arnold.
Arnauld, Arnault, Arnoll

Arne (German) a form of Arnold.
Arna, Arnay, Arnel, Arnele, Arnell, Arnelle

Arnette (English) little eagle.
Arnat, Arnet, Arnett, Arnetta, Arnot, Arnott

Arnie (German) a familiar form of Arnold.
Arney, Arni, Arnny, Arny

Arno (German) a short form of Arnold. (Czech) a short form of Ernest.
Arnou, Arnoux

Arnold (German) eagle ruler.
Ardal, Arnald, Arnaldo, Arnaud, Arne, Arnie, Arno, Arnol, Arnoldas, Arnoldo, Arnoll, Arndt, Arnulfo

Arnon (Hebrew) rushing river.
Arnan

Arnulfo (German) a form of Arnold.

Aron, Arron (Hebrew) forms of Aaron. (Danish) forms of Aren.
Arrion

Aroon (Tai) dawn.

Arran (Scottish) island dweller. Geography: an island off the west coast of Scotland. (Hebrew) a form of Aaron.
Arren, Arrin, Arryn, Aryn

Arrigo (Italian) a form of Harry.
Alrigo, Arrighetto

Arrio (Spanish) warlike.
Ario, Arrow, Arryo, Aryo

Arsenio (Greek) masculine; virile. History: Saint Arsenius was a teacher in the Roman Empire.
Arsen, Arsène, Arsenius, Arseny, Arsinio

Arsha (Persian) venerable.

Art (English) a short form of Arthur.

Artemus (Greek) gift of Artemis. Mythology: Artemis was the goddess of the hunt and the moon.
Artemas, Artemio, Artemis, Artimas, Artimis, Artimus

Arthur (Irish) noble; lofty hill. (Scottish) bear. (English) rock. (Icelandic) follower of Thor. See also Turi.
Art, Artair, Artek, Arth, Arther, Arthor, Artie, Artor, Arturo, Artus, Aurthar, Aurther, Aurthur

Artie (English) a familiar form of Arthur.
Arte, Artian, Artis, Arty, Atty

Arturo (Italian) a form of Arthur.
Arthuro, Artur

Arun (Cambodian, Hindi) sun.
Aruns

Arundel (English) eagle valley.

Arve (Norwegian) heir, inheritor.

Arvel (Welsh) wept over.
Arval, Arvell, Arvelle

Arvid (Hebrew) wanderer. (Norwegian) eagle tree. See also Ravid.
Arv, Arvad, Arve, Arvie, Arvind, Arvinder, Arvydas

Arvin (German) friend of the people; friend of the army.
Arv, Arvie, Arvind, Arvinder, Arvon, Arvy

Aryeh (Hebrew) lion.

Asa (Hebrew) physician, healer. (Yoruba) falcon.
Asaa, Ase

Asád (Arabic) lion.
Asaad, Asad, Asid, Assad, Azad

Asadel (Arabic) prosperous.
Asadour, Asadul, Asael

Ascot (English) eastern cottage; style of necktie. Geography: a village near London and the site of the Royal Ascot horseraces.

Asgard (Scandinavian) court of the gods.

Ash (Hebrew) ash tree.
Ashby

Ashanti (Swahili) from a tribe in West Africa.
Ashan, Ashani, Ashante, Ashantee, Ashaunte

Ashby (Scandinavian) ash-tree farm. (Hebrew) a form of Ash.
Ashbey

Asher (Hebrew) happy;
blessed.
Ashar, Ashor, Ashur

Ashford (English) ash-tree
ford.
Ash, Ashtin

Ashley (English) ash-tree
meadow.
*Ash, Asheley, Ashelie, Ashely,
Ashlan, Ashlee, Ashleigh,
Ashlen, Ashlie, Ashlin, Ashling,
Ashlinn, Ashlone, Ashly, Ashlyn,
Ashlynn, Aslan*

Ashon (Swahili) seventh-born
son.

Ashton (English) ash-tree set-
tlement.
*Ashtan, Ashten, Ashtian,
Ashtin, Ashtion, Ashtonn,
Ashtun, Ashtyn*

Ashur (Swahili) Mythology:
the principal Assyrian deity.

Ashwani (Hindi) first.
Religion: the first of the
twenty-seven galaxies revolv-
ing around the moon.
Ashwan

Ashwin (Hindi) star.

Asiel (Hebrew) created by
God.

Asker (Turkish) soldier.

Aspen (English) aspen tree.

Aston (English) eastern town.
Asten, Astin

Aswad (Arabic) dark skinned,
black.

Ata (Fante) twin.

Atek (Polish) a form of Tanek.

Athan (Greek) immortal.

Atherton (English) town by a
spring.

Atid (Tai) sun.

Atif (Arabic) caring.
Ateef, Atef

Atlas (Greek) lifted; carried.
Mythology: Atlas was forced
by Zeus to carry the heavens
on his shoulders as a punishment for his share of the war
of the Titans.

Atley (English) meadow.
Atlea, Atlee, Atleigh, Atli, Attley

Attila (Gothic) little father.
History: the Hun leader who
invaded the Roman Empire.
*Atalik, Atila, Atilio, Atilla,
Atiya, Attal, Attilio*

Atwater (English) at the
water's edge.

Atwell (English) at the well.

Atwood (English) at the forest.

Atworth (English) at the
farmstead.

Auberon (German) a form of
Oberon.
Auberron, Aubrey

Aubrey (German) noble; bear-like. (French) a familiar form of Auberon. See also Avery.
Aubary, Aube, Aubery, Aubie, Aubré, Aubree, Aubreii, Aubrie, Aubry, Aubury

Auburn (Latin) reddish brown.

Auden (English) old friend.

Audie (German) noble; strong. (English) a familiar form of Edward.
Audi, Audiel, Audley, Audy

Audon (French) old; rich.
Audelon

Audrey (English) noble strength.
Audra, Audre, Audrea, Audrius, Audry

Audric (English) wise ruler.
Audrick, Audrik

Audun (Scandinavian) deserted, desolate.

Augie (Latin) a familiar form of August.
Auggie, Augy

August (Latin) a short form of Augustine, Augustus.
Agosto, Augie, Auguste, Augusto

Augustine (Latin) majestic. Religion: Saint Augustine was the first archbishop of Canterbury. See also Austin, Gus, Tino.
August, Agustin, Augustin,
Augustinas, Augustino, Austen, Austin, Auston, Austyn

Augustus (Latin) majestic; venerable. History: an honorary title given to the first Roman emperor, Octavius Caesar.
August

Aukai (Hawaiian) seafarer.

Aundre (Greek) a form of Andre.
Aundrae, Aundray, Aundrea, Aundrey, Aundry

Aurek (Polish) golden haired.

Aurelio (Latin) a short form of Aurelius.
Aurel, Aurele, Aureli, Aurellio

Aurelius (Latin) golden. History: Marcus Aurelius was a second-century A.D. philosopher and emperor of Rome.
Arelian, Areliano, Aurèle, Aureliano, Aurelien, Aurélien, Aurelio, Aurey, Auriel, Aury

Aurick (German) protecting ruler.
Auric

Austen, Auston, Austyn (Latin) short forms of Augustine.
Austan, Austun, Austyne

Austin (Latin) a short form of Augustine.
Astin, Austine, Oistin, Ostin

Avel (Greek) breath.

Avent (French) born during Advent.
Aventin, Aventino

Averill (French) born in April.
Ave, Averel, Averell, Averiel, Averil, Averyl, Averyll, Avrel, Avrell, Avrill, Avryll

Avery (English) a form of Aubrey.
Avary, Aveary, Avere, Averee, Averey, Averi, Averie, Avrey, Avry

Avi (Hebrew) God is my father.
Avian, Avidan, Avidor, Aviel, Avion

Aviv (Hebrew) youth; springtime.

Avner (Hebrew) a form of Abner.
Avneet, Avniel

Avram (Hebrew) a form of Abraham, Abram.
Arram, Avraam, Avraham, Avrahom, Avrohom, Avrom, Avrum

Avshalom (Hebrew) father of peace. See also Absalom.
Avsalom

Awan (Native American) somebody.

Axel (Latin) axe. (German) small oak tree; source of life. (Scandinavian) a form of Absalom.
Aksel, Ax, Axe, Axell, Axil, Axill, Axl, Axle, Axyle

Aydin (Turkish) intelligent.

Ayers (English) heir to a fortune.

Ayinde (Yoruba) we gave praise and he came.

Aylmer (English) a form of Elmer.
Aillmer, Ailmer, Allmer, Ayllmer

Aymil (Greek) a form of Emil.

Aymon (French) a form of Raymond.

Ayo (Yoruba) happiness.

Azad (Turkish) free.

Azeem (Arabic) a form of Azim.
Aseem, Asim

Azi (Nigerian) youth.

Azim (Arabic) defender.
Azeem

Aziz (Arabic) strong.

Azizi (Swahili) precious.

Azriel (Hebrew) God is my aid.

Azuriah (Hebrew) aided by God.
Azaria, Azariah, Azuria

B

Baden (German) bather.
Baeden, Bayden, Baydon

Bahir (Arabic) brilliant, dazzling.

Bahram (Persian) ancient king.

Bailey (French) bailiff, steward.
Bail, Bailee, Bailie, Bailio, Baillie, Baily, Bailye, Baley, Bayley

Bain (Irish) a short form of Bainbridge.
Baine, Bayne, Baynn

Bainbridge (Irish) fair bridge.
Bain, Baynbridge, Bayne, Baynebridge

Baird (Irish) traveling minstrel, bard; poet.
Bairde, Bard

Bakari (Swahili) noble promise.
Bacari, Baccari, Bakarie

Baker (English) baker. See also Baxter.
Bakir, Bakory, Bakr

Bal (Sanskrit) child born with lots of hair.

Balasi (Basque) flat footed.

Balbo (Latin) stammerer.
Bailby, Balbi, Ballbo

Baldemar (German) bold; famous.
Baldemer, Baldomero, Baumar, Baumer

Balder (Scandinavian) bald. Mythology: the Norse god of light, summer, purity, and innocence.
Baldier, Baldur, Baudier

Baldric (German) brave ruler.
Baldrick, Baudric

Baldwin (German) bold friend.
Bald, Baldovino, Balduin, Baldwinn, Baldwyn, Baldwynn, Balldwin, Baudoin

Balfour (Scottish) pastureland.
Balfor, Balfore

Balin (Hindi) mighty soldier.
Bali, Baylen, Baylin, Baylon, Valin

Ballard (German) brave; strong.
Balard

Balraj (Hindi) strongest.

Baltazar (Greek) a form of Balthasar.
Baltasar

Balthasar (Greek) God save the king. Bible: one of the three wise men who bore gifts for the infant Jesus.
Badassare, Baldassare, Baltazar,

Balthasaar, Balthazar,
Balthazzar, Baltsaros, Belshazar,
Belshazzar, Boldizsár

Bancroft (English) bean field.
Ban, Bancrofft, Bank, Bankroft,
Banky, Binky

Bandi (Hungarian) a form of
Andrew.
Bandit

Bane (Hawaiian) a form of
Bartholomew.

Banner (Scottish, English) flag
bearer.
Bannor, Banny

Banning (Irish) small and fair.
Bannie, Banny

Barak (Hebrew) lightning
bolt. Bible: the valiant warrior who helped Deborah.
Barrak

Baran (Russian) ram.
Baren

Barasa (Kikuyu) meeting
place.

Barclay (Scottish, English)
birch-tree meadow.
Bar, Barcley, Barklay, Barkley,
Barklie, Barrclay, Berkeley

Bard (Irish) a form of Baird.
Bar, Barde, Bardia, Bardiya,
Barr

Bardolf (German) bright wolf.
Bardo, Bardolph, Bardou,
Bardoul, Bardulf, Bardulph

Bardrick (Teutonic) axe ruler.
Bardric, Bardrik

Baris (Turkish) peaceful.

Barker (English) lumberjack;
advertiser at a carnival.

Barlow (English) bare hillside.
Barlowe, Barrlow, Barrlowe

Barnabas (Greek, Hebrew,
Aramaic, Latin) son of the
missionary. Bible: Christian
apostle and companion of
Paul on his first missionary
journey.
Bane, Barna, Barnaba,
Barnabus, Barnaby, Barnebas,
Barnebus, Barney

Barnaby (English) a form of
Barnabas.
Barnabe, Barnabé, Barnabee,
Barnabey, Barnabi, Barnabie,
Bernabé, Burnaby

Barnard (French) a form of
Bernard.
Barn, Barnard, Barnhard,
Barnhardo

Barnes (English) bear; son of
Barnett.

Barnett (English) nobleman;
leader.
Barn, Barnet, Barney, Baronet,
Baronett, Barrie, Barron, Barry

Barney (English) a familiar
form of Barnabas, Barnett.
Barnie, Barny

Barnum (German) barn; storage place. (English) baron's home.
Barnham

Baron (German, English) nobleman, baron.
Baaron, Barion, Baronie, Barrin, Barrion, Barron, Baryn, Bayron, Berron

Barrett (German) strong as a bear.
Bar, Baret, Barrat, Barret, Barretta, Barrette, Barry, Berrett, Berrit

Barric (English) grain farm.
Barrick, Beric, Berric, Berrick, Berrik

Barrington (English) fenced town. Geography: a town in England.

Barry (Welsh) son of Harry. (Irish) spear, marksman. (French) gate, fence.
Baris, Barri, Barrie, Barris, Bary

Bart (Hebrew) a short form of Bartholomew, Barton.
Barrt, Bartel, Bartie, Barty

Bartholomew (Hebrew) son of Talmaí. Bible: one of the Twelve Apostles. See also Jerney, Parlan, Parthalán.
Balta, Bane, Bart, Bartek, Barth, Barthel, Barthelemy, Barthélemy, Barthélmy, Bartho, Bartholo, Bartholomaus, Bartholome, Bartholomeo, Bartholomeus, Bartholomieu, Bartimous, Bartlet, Barto, Bartolome, Bartolomé, Bartolomeo, Bartolomeß, Bartolommeo, Bartome, Bartz, Bat

Bartlet (English) a form of Bartholomew.
Bartlett, Bartley

Barto (Spanish) a form of Bartholomew.
Bardo, Bardol, Bartol, Bartoli, Bartolo, Bartos

Barton (English) barley town; Bart's town.
Barrton, Bart

Bartram (English) a form of Bertram.
Barthram

Baruch (Hebrew) blessed.
Boruch

Basam (Arabic) smiling.
Basem, Basim, Bassam

Basil (Greek, Latin) royal, kingly. Religion: a saint and founder of monasteries. Botany: an herb often used in cooking. See also Vasilis, Wasili.
Bas, Basal, Base, Baseal, Basel, Basle, Basile, Basilio, Basilios, Basilius, Bassel, Bazek, Bazel, Bazil, Bazyli

Basir (Turkish) intelligent, discerning.
Bashar, Basheer, Bashir, Bashiyr, Bechir, Bhasheer

Bassett (English) little person.
Basett, Basit, Basset, Bassit

Bastien (German) a short form of Sebastian.
Baste, Bastiaan, Bastian, Bastion

Bat (English) a short form of Bartholomew.

Baul (Gypsy) snail.

Bavol (Gypsy) wind; air.

Baxter (English) a form of Baker.
Bax, Baxie, Baxty, Baxy

Bay (Vietnamese) seventh son. (French) chestnut brown color; evergreen tree. (English) howler.

Bayard (English) reddish brown hair.
Baiardo, Bay, Bayardo, Bayerd, Bayrd

Bayley (French) a form of Bailey.
Baylee, Bayleigh, Baylie, Bayly

Beacan (Irish) small.
Beacán, Becan

Beacher (English) beech trees.
Beach, Beachy, Beech, Beecher, Beechy

Beagan (Irish) small.
Beagen, Beagin

Beale (French) a form of Beau.
Beal, Beall, Bealle, Beals

Beaman (English) beekeeper.
Beamann, Beamen, Beeman, Beman

Beamer (English) trumpet player.

Beasley (English) field of peas.

Beattie (Latin) blessed; happy; bringer of joy.
Beatie, Beatty, Beaty

Beau (French) handsome.
Beale, Beaux, Bo

Beaufort (French) beautiful fort.

Beaumont (French) beautiful mountain.

Beauregard (French) handsome; beautiful; well regarded.

Beaver (English) beaver.
Beav, Beavo, Beve, Bevo

Bebe (Spanish) baby.

Beck (English, Scandinavian) brook.
Beckett

Bede (English) prayer. Religion: the patron saint of lectors.

Bela (Czech) white.
(Hungarian) bright.
*Béla, Belaal, Belal, Belall,
Belay, Bellal*

Belden (French, English)
pretty valley.
Beldin, Beldon, Bellden, Belldon

Belen (Greek) arrow.

Bell (French) handsome.
(English) bell ringer.

Bellamy (French) beautiful
friend.
Belamy, Bell, Bellamey, Bellamie

Bello (African) helper or pro-
moter of Islam.

Belmiro (Portuguese) good-
looking; attractive.

Bem (Tiv) peace.
Behm

Ben (Hebrew) a short form of
Benjamin.
*Behn, Benio, Benn, Benne,
Benno*

Ben-ami (Hebrew) son of my
people.
Baram, Barami

Benedict (Latin) blessed. See
also Venedictos, Venya.
*Benci, Bendick, Bendict,
Bendino, Bendix, Bendrick,
Benedetto, Benedick, Benedicto,
Benedictus, Benedikt, Bengt,
Benito, Benoit*

Benedikt (German, Slavic) a
form of Benedict.
*Bendek, Bendik, Benedek,
Benedik*

Bengt (Scandinavian) a form
of Benedict.
Beng, Benke, Bent

Beniam (Ethiopian) a form of
Benjamin.
Beneyam, Beniamin, Beniamino

Benito (Italian) a form of
Benedict. History: Benito
Mussolini led Italy during
World War II.
*Benedo, Benino, Benno, Beno,
Betto, Beto*

Benjamen (Hebrew) a form
of Benjamin.
*Benejamen, Benjermen,
Benjjmen*

Benjamin (Hebrew) son of
my right hand. See also
Peniamina, Veniamin.
*Behnjamin, Bejamin,
Bemjiman, Ben, Benejaminas,
Bengamin, Beniam, Benja,
Benjahmin, Benjaim, Benjam,
Benjamaim, Benjaman,
Benjamen, Benjamine,
Benjaminn, Benjamino,
Benjamon, Benjamyn,
Benjamynn, Benjemin,
Benjermain, Benjermin, Benji,
Benjie, Benjiman, Benjy,
Benkamin, Bennjamin, Benny,
Benyamin, Benyamino,
Binyamin, Mincho*

Benjiman (Hebrew) a form of Benjamin.
Benjimen, Benjimin, Benjimon, Benjmain

Benjiro (Japanese) enjoys peace.

Bennett (Latin) little blessed one.
Benet, Benett, Bennet, Benette, Bennete, Bennette

Benny (Hebrew) a familiar form of Benjamin.
Bennie

Beno (Hebrew) son. (Mwera) band member.

Benoit (French) a form of Benedict.
Benott

Benoni (Hebrew) son of my sorrow. Bible: Ben-oni was the son of Jacob and Rachel.
Ben-Oni

Benson (Hebrew) son of Ben. A short form of Ben Zion.
Bensan, Bensen, Benssen, Bensson

Bentley (English) moor; coarse grass meadow.
Bent, Bentlea, Bentlee, Bentlie, Lee

Benton (English) Ben's town; town on the moors.
Bent

Benzi (Hebrew) a familiar form of Ben Zion.

Ben Zion (Hebrew) son of Zion.
Benson, Benzi

Beppe (Italian) a form of Joseph.
Beppy

Ber (English) boundary. (Yiddish) bear.

Beredei (Russian) a form of Hubert.
Berdry, Berdy, Beredej, Beredy

Berg (German) mountain.
Berdj, Berge, Bergh, Berje

Bergen (German, Scandinavian) hill dweller.
Bergin, Birgin

Berger (French) shepherd.

Bergren (Scandinavian) mountain stream.
Berg

Berk (Turkish) solid, rugged.

Berkeley (English) a form of Barclay.
Berk, Berkely, Berkie, Berkley, Berklie, Berkly, Berky

Berl (German) a form of Burl.
Berle, Berlie, Berlin, Berlyn

Berlyn (German) boundary line. See also Burl.
Berlin, Burlin

Bern (German) a short form of Bernard.
Berne

Bernal (German) strong as a
bear.
*Bernald, Bernaldo, Bernel,
Bernhald, Bernhold, Bernold*

Bernard (German) brave as a
bear. See also Bjorn.
*Barnard, Bear, Bearnard, Benek,
Ber, Berend, Bern, Bernabé,
Bernadas, Bernardel, Bernardin,
Bernardo, Bernardus, Bernardyn,
Bernarr, Bernat, Bernek, Bernal,
Bernel, Bernerd, Berngards,
Bernhard, Bernhards, Bernhardt,
Bernie, Bjorn, Burnard*

Bernardo (Spanish) a form of
Bernard.
*Barnardino, Barnardo,
Barnhardo, Benardo, Bernardino,
Bernhardo, Berno, Burnardo,
Nardo*

Bernie (German) a familiar
form of Bernard.
*Berney, Berni, Berny, Birney,
Birnie, Birny, Burney*

Berry (English) berry; grape.
Berrie

Bersh (Gypsy) one year.

Bert (German, English)
bright, shining. A short form
of Berthold, Berton,
Bertram, Bertrand, Egbert,
Filbert.
Bertie, Bertus, Birt, Burt

Berthold (German) bright;
illustrious; brilliant ruler.
Bert, Berthoud, Bertold, Bertolde

Bertie (English) a familiar
form of Bert, Egbert.
Berty, Birt, Birtie, Birty

Bertín (Spanish) distinguished
friend.
Berti

Berto (Spanish) a short form
of Alberto.

Berton (English) bright settlement; fortified town.
Bert

Bertram (German) bright;
illustrious. (English) bright
raven. See also Bartram.
*Beltran, Beltrán, Beltrano, Bert,
Berton, Bertrae, Bertraim,
Bertraum, Bertron*

Bertrand (German) bright
shield.
*Bert, Bertran, Bertrando,
Bertranno*

Berwyn (Welsh) white head.
Berwin, Berwynn, Berwynne

Bevan (Welsh) son of Evan.
*Beavan, Beaven, Beavin, Bev,
Beve, Beven, Bevin, Bevo, Bevon*

Beverly (English) beaver
meadow.
*Beverlea, Beverleigh, Beverley,
Beverlie*

Bevis (French) from Beauvais,
France; bull.
Beauvais, Bevys

Bhagwandas (Hindi) servant
of God.

Bickford (English) axe-man's ford.

Bienvenido (Filipino) welcome.

Bijan (Persian) ancient hero.
Bihjan, Bijann, Bijhan, Bijhon, Bijon

Bilal (Arabic) chosen.
Bila, Bilaal, Bilale, Bile, Bilel, Billaal, Billal

Bill (German) a short form of William.
Bil, Billee, Billijo, Billye, Byll, Will

Billy (German) a familiar form of Bill, William.
Bille, Billey, Billie, Billy, Bily, Willie

Binah (Hebrew) understanding; wise.
Bina

Bing (German) kettle-shaped hollow.

Binh (Vietnamese) peaceful.

Binkentios (Greek) a form of Vincent.

Binky (English) a familiar form of Bancroft, Vincent.
Bink, Binkentios, Binkie

Birch (English) white; shining; birch tree.
Birk, Burch

Birger (Norwegian) rescued.

Birkey (English) island with birch trees.
Birk, Birkie, Birky

Birkitt (English) birch-tree coast.
Birk, Birket, Birkit, Burket, Burkett, Burkitt

Birley (English) meadow with the cow barn.
Birlee, Birlie, Birly

Birney (English) island with a brook.
Birne, Birnie, Birny, Burney, Burnie, Burny

Birtle (English) hill with birds.

Bishop (Greek) overseer. (English) bishop.
Bish, Bishup

Bjorn (Scandinavian) a form of Bernard.
Bjarne

Blackburn (Scottish) black brook.

Blade (English) knife, sword.
Bladen, Bladon, Bladyn, Blae, Blaed, Blayde

Bladimir (Russian) a form of Vladimir.
Bladimer

Blaine (Irish) thin, lean. (English) river source.
Blain, Blane, Blayne

Blair (Irish) plain, field.
(Welsh) place.
Blaire, Blare, Blayr, Blayre

Blaise, Blaize (French) forms
of Blaze.
*Ballas, Balyse, Blais, Blaisot,
Blas, Blase, Blasi, Blasien,
Blasius, Blass, Blaz, Blaze,
Blayz, Blayze, Blayzz*

Blake (English) attractive;
dark.
*Blaik, Blaike, Blakely,
Blakeman, Blakey, Blayke*

Blakely (English) dark
meadow.
*Blakelee, Blakeleigh, Blakeley,
Blakelie, Blakelin, Blakelyn,
Blakeny, Blakley, Blakney*

Blanco (Spanish) light
skinned; white; blond.

Blane (Irish) a form of Blaine.
Blaney, Blanne

Blayne (Irish) a form of
Blaine.
Blayn, Blayney

Blaze (Latin) stammerer.
(English) flame; trail mark
made on a tree.
*Balázs, Biaggio, Biagio, Blaise,
Blaize, Blazen, Blazer*

Bliss (English) blissful; joyful.

Bly (Native American) high.

Blythe (English) carefree;
merry, joyful.
Blithe, Blyth

Bo (English) a form of Beau,
Beauregard. (German) a form
of Bogart.
Boe

Boaz (Hebrew) swift; strong.
Bo, Boas, Booz, Bos, Boz

Bob (English) a short form of
Robert.
Bobb, Bobby, Bobek, Rob

Bobby (English) a familiar
form of Bob, Robert.
*Bobbey, Bobbi, Bobbie, Bobbye,
Boby*

Bobek (Czech) a form of
Bob, Robert.

Boden (Scandinavian) shel-
tered. (French) messenger,
herald.
*Bodie, Bodin, Bodine, Bodyne,
Boe*

Bodie (Scandinavian) a famil-
iar form of Boden.
*Boddie, Bode, Bodee, Bodey,
Bodhi, Bodi, Boedee, Boedi,
Boedy*

Bodil (Norwegian) mighty
ruler.

Bodua (Akan) animal's tail.

Bogart (German) strong as a
bow. (Irish, Welsh) bog,
marshland.
Bo, Bogey, Bogie, Bogy

Bohdan (Ukrainian) a form of Donald.
Bogdan, Bogdashka, Bogdon, Bohden, Bohdon

Bonaro (Italian, Spanish) friend.
Bona, Bonar

Bonaventure (Italian) good luck.

Bond (English) tiller of the soil.
Bondie, Bondon, Bonds, Bondy

Boniface (Latin) do-gooder.
Bonifacio, Bonifacius, Bonifacy

Booker (English) bookmaker; book lover; Bible lover.
Bookie, Books, Booky

Boone (Latin, French) good. History: Daniel Boone was an American pioneer.
Bon, Bone, Bonne, Boonie, Boony

Booth (English) hut. (Scandinavian) temporary dwelling.
Boot, Boote, Boothe

Borak (Arabic) lightning. Mythology: the horse that carried Muhammed to seventh heaven.

Borden (French) cottage. (English) valley of the boar; boar's den.
Bord, Bordie, Bordy

Borg (Scandinavian) castle.

Boris (Slavic) battler, warrior. Religion: the patron saint of Moscow, princes, and Russia.
Boriss, Borja, Borris, Borya, Boryenka, Borys

Borka (Russian) fighter.
Borkinka

Boseda (Tiv) born on Saturday.

Bosley (English) grove of trees.

Botan (Japanese) blossom, bud.

Bourey (Cambodian) country.

Bourne (Latin, French) boundary. (English) brook, stream.

Boutros (Arabic) a form of Peter.

Bowen (Welsh) son of Owen.
Bow, Bowe, Bowie

Bowie (Irish) yellow haired. History: James Bowie was an American-born Mexican colonist who died during the defense of the Alamo.
Bow, Bowen

Boyce (French) woods, forest.
Boice, Boise, Boy, Boycey, Boycie

Boyd (Scottish) yellow haired.
Boid, Boyde

Brad (English) a short form of Bradford, Bradley.
Bradd, Brade

Bradburn (English) broad stream.

Braden (English) broad valley. *Bradan, Bradden, Bradeon, Bradin, Bradine, Bradyn, Braeden, Braiden, Brayden, Bredan, Bredon*

Bradford (English) broad river crossing. *Brad, Braddford, Ford*

Bradlee (English) a form of Bradley. *Bradlea, Bradleigh, Bradlie*

Bradley (English) broad meadow. *Brad, Braddly, Bradlay, Bradlee, Bradly, Bradlyn, Bradney*

Bradly (English) a form of Bradley.

Bradon (English) broad hill. *Braedon, Braidon, Braydon*

Bradshaw (English) broad forest.

Brady (Irish) spirited. (English) broad island. *Bradey, Bradi, Bradie, Bradye, Braidy*

Bradyn (English) a form of Braden. *Bradynne, Breidyn*

Braeden, Braiden (English) forms of Braden. *Braedan, Braedin, Braedyn, Braidyn*

Braedon (English) a form of Bradon. *Breadon*

Bragi (Scandinavian) poet. Mythology: the god of poetry, eloquence, and song. *Brage*

Braham (Hindi) creator. *Braheem, Braheim, Brahiem, Brahima, Brahm*

Brainard (English) bold raven; prince. *Brainerd*

Bram (Scottish) bramble, brushwood. (Hebrew) a short form of Abraham, Abram. *Brame, Bramm, Bramdon*

Bramwell (English) bramble spring. *Brammel, Brammell, Bramwel, Bramwyll*

Branch (Latin) paw; claw; tree branch.

Brand (English) firebrand; sword. A short form of Brandon. *Brandall, Brande, Brandel, Brandell, Brander, Brandley, Brandol, Brandt, Brandy, Brann*

Brandeis (Czech) dweller on a burned clearing. *Brandis*

Branden (English) beacon val-
ley.
Brandden, Brandene, Brandin,
Brandine, Brandyn, Breandan

Brandon (English) beacon
hill.
Bran, Brand, Brandan,
Branddon, Brandone, Brandonn,
Brandyn, Branndan, Branndon,
Brannon, Breandon, Brendon

Brandt (English) a form of
Brant.

Brandy (Dutch) brandy.
(English) a familiar form of
Brand.
Branddy, Brandey, Brandi,
Brandie

Brandyn (English) a form of
Branden, Brandon.
Brandynn

Brannon (Irish) a form of
Brandon.
Branen, Brannan, Brannen,
Branon

Branson (English) son of
Brandon, Brant. A form of
Bronson.
Bransen, Bransin, Brantson

Brant (English) proud.
Brandt, Brannt, Brante,
Brantley, Branton

Brantley (English) a form of
Brant.
Brantlie, Brantly, Brentlee,
Brentley, Brently

Braulio (Italian) a form of
Brawley.
Brauli, Brauliuo

Brawley (English) meadow on
the hillside.
Braulio, Brawlee, Brawly

Braxton (English) Brock's town.
Brax, Braxdon, Braxston,
Braxten, Braxtin, Braxxton

Brayan (Irish, Scottish) a form
of Brian.
Brayn, Brayon

Brayden (English) a form of
Braden.
Braydan, Braydn, Bradyn,
Breydan, Breyden, Brydan,
Bryden

Braydon (English) a form of
Bradon.
Braydoon, Brydon, Breydon

Breck (Irish) freckled.
Brec, Breckan, Brecken, Breckie,
Breckin, Breckke, Breckyn, Brek,
Brexton

Brede (Scandinavian) iceberg,
glacier.

Brencis (Latvian) a form of
Lawrence.
Brence

Brendan (Irish) little raven.
(English) sword.
Breandan, Bren, Brenden,
Brendis, Brendon, Brendyn,
Brenn, Brennan, Brennen,
Brenndan, Brenyan, Bryn

Brenden (Irish) a form of
Brendan.
*Bren, Brendene, Brendin,
Brendine, Brennden*

Brendon (English) a form of
Brandon. (Irish, English) a
form of Brendan.
Brenndon

Brennan, Brennen (English,
Irish) forms of Brendan.
*Bren, Brenan, Brenen, Brenin,
Brenn, Brenna, Brennann,
Brenner, Brennin, Brennon,
Brennor, Brennyn, Brenon*

Brent (English) a short form
of Brenton.
Brendt, Brente, Brentson, Brentt

Brenton (English) steep hill.
*Brent, Brentan, Brenten,
Brentin, Brentten, Brentton,
Brentyn*

Bret, Brett (Scottish) from
Great Britain. See also
Britton.
*Bhrett, Braten, Braton, Brayton,
Bretin, Bretley, Bretlin, Breton,
Brettan, Brette, Bretten, Bretton,
Brit, Britt*

Brewster (English) brewer.
Brew, Brewer, Bruwster

Breyon (Irish, Scottish) a form
of Brian.
Breon, Breyan

Brian (Irish, Scottish) strong;
virtuous; honorable. History:
Brian Boru was an eleventh-
century Irish king and
national hero. See also
Palaina.
*Brayan, Breyon, Briana, Briann,
Brianna, Brianne, Briano,
Briant, Briante, Briaun,
Briayan, Brien, Brience, Brient,
Brin, Briny, Brion, Bryan,
Bryen*

Briar (French) heather.
Brier, Brierly, Bryar, Bryer, Bryor

Brice (Welsh) alert; ambitious.
(English) son of Rice.
Bricen, Briceton, Bryce

Brick (English) bridge.
*Bricker, Bricklen, Brickman,
Brik*

Bridger (English) bridge
builder.
*Bridd, Bridge, Bridgeley,
Bridgely*

Brigham (English) covered
bridge. (French) troops,
brigade.
Brig, Brigg, Briggs, Brighton

Brighton (English) bright
town.
*Breighton, Bright, Brightin,
Bryton*

Brion (Irish, Scottish) a form
of Brian.
Brieon, Brione, Brionn, Brionne

Brit, Britt (Scottish) forms of
Bret, Brett. See also Britton.
Brit, Brityce

Britton (Scottish) from Great
Britain. See also Bret, Brett,
Brit, Britt.
*Britain, Briten, Britian, Britin,
Briton, Brittain, Brittan,
Britten, Brittian, Brittin, Britton*

Brock (English) badger.
*Broc, Brocke, Brockett, Brockie,
Brockley, Brockton, Brocky,
Brok, Broque*

Brod (English) a short form of
Broderick.
Brode, Broden

Broderick (Welsh) son of the
famous ruler. (English) broad
ridge. See also Roderick.
*Brod, Broddie, Brodderick,
Brodderrick, Broddy, Broderic,
Broderrick, Brodrick,*

Brodie (Irish) a form of
Brody.
Brodi, Broedi

Brodrick (Welsh, English) a
form of Broderick.
Broddrick, Brodric, Brodryck

Brody (Irish) ditch; canal
builder.
*Brodee, Broden, Brodey, Brodie,
Broedy*

Brogan (Irish) a heavy work
shoe.
Brogen, Broghan, Broghen

Bromley (English) brushwood
meadow.

Bron (Afrikaans) source.

Bronislaw (Polish) weapon of
glory.

Bronson (English) son of
Brown.
*Bransen, Bransin, Branson,
Bron, Bronnie, Bronnson,
Bronny, Bronsan, Bronsen,
Bronsin, Bronsonn, Bronsson,
Bronsun, Bronsyn, Brunson*

Brook (English) brook, stream.
*Brooke, Brooker, Brookin,
Brooklyn*

Brooks (English) son of
Brook.
Brookes, Broox

Brown (English) brown; bear.

Bruce (French) brushwood
thicket; woods.
Brucey, Brucy, Brue, Bruis

Bruno (German, Italian)
brown haired; brown
skinned.
Brunon, Bruns

Bryan (Irish) a form of Brian.
Brayan, Bryann, Bryant, Bryen

Bryant (Irish) a form of
Bryan.
Bryent

Bryce (Welsh) a form of
Brice.
*Brycen, Bryceton, Bryson,
Bryston*

Bryon (German) cottage.
(English) bear.
Bryeon, Bryn, Bryne, Brynn,
Brynne, Bryone

Bryson (Welsh) son of Brice.
Brysan, Brysen, Brysun, Brysyn

Bryton (English) a form of
Brighton.
Brayten, Brayton, Breyton,
Bryeton, Brytan, Bryten, Brytin,
Brytten, Brytton

Bubba (German) a boy.
Babba, Babe, Bebba

Buck (German, English) male
deer.
Buckie, Buckley, Buckner,
Bucko, Bucky

Buckley (English) deer
meadow.
Bucklea, Bucklee

Buckminster (English)
preacher.

Bud (English) herald, messenger.
Budd, Buddy

Buddy (American) a familiar
form of Bud.
Budde, Buddey, Buddie

Buell (German) hill dweller.
(English) bull.

Buford (English) ford near the
castle.
Burford

Burgess (English) town
dweller; shopkeeper.
Burg, Burges, Burgh, Burgiss,
Burr

Burian (Ukrainian) lives near
weeds.

Burke (German, French)
fortress, castle.
Berk, Berke, Birk, Bourke,
Burk, Burkley

Burl (English) cup bearer;
wine servant; knot in a tree.
(German) a short form of
Berlyn
Berl, Burley, Burlie, Byrle

Burleigh (English) meadow
with knotted tree trunks.
Burlee, Burley, Burlie, Byrleigh,
Byrlee

Burne (English) brook.
Beirne, Burn, Burnell, Burnett,
Burney, Byrn, Byrne

Burney (English) island with a
brook. A familiar form of
Rayburn.

Burr (Swedish) youth.
(English) prickly plant.

Burris (English) town dweller.

Burt (English) a form of Bert.
A short form of Burton.
Burrt, Burtt, Burty

Burton (English) fortified
town.
Berton, Burt

C

Busby (Scottish) village in the thicket; tall military hat made of fur.
Busbee, Buzby, Buzz

Buster (American) hitter, puncher.

Butch (American) a short form of Butcher.

Butcher (English) butcher.
Butch

Buzz (Scottish) a short form of Busby.
Buzzy

Byford (English) by the ford.

Byram (English) cattle yard.

Byrd (English) birdlike.
Bird, Birdie, Byrdie

Byrne (English) a form of Burne.
Byrn, Byrnes

Byron (French) cottage. (English) barn.
Beyren, Beyron, Biren, Biron, Buiron, Byram, Byran, Byrann, Byren, Byrom, Byrone

Cable (French, English) rope maker.
Cabell

Cadao (Vietnamese) folksong.

Cadby (English) warrior's settlement.

Caddock (Welsh) eager for war.

Cade (Welsh) a short form of Cadell.
Cady

Cadell (Welsh) battler.
Cade, Cadel, Cedell

Caden (American) a form of Kadin.
Cadan, Caddon, Cadian, Cadien, Cadin, Cadon, Cadyn, Caeden, Caedon, Caid, Caiden, Cayden

Cadmus (Greek) from the east. Mythology: a Phoenician prince who founded Thebes and introduced writing to the Greeks.

Caelan (Scottish) a form of Nicholas.
Cael, Caelon, Caelyn, Cailan, Cailean, Caillan, Cailun, Cailyn, Calan, Calen, Caleon, Caley, Calin, Callan, Callon, Callyn, Calon, Calyn, Caylan, Cayley

Caesar (Latin) long-haired.
History: a title for Roman
emperors. See also Kaiser,
Kesar, Sarito.
*Caesarae, Caesear, Caeser, Caezar,
Caseare, Ceasar, Cesar, Ceseare,
Cezar, Cézar, Czar, Seasar*

Cahil (Turkish) young, naive.

Cai (Welsh) a form of Gaius.
Caio, Caius, Caw

Cain (Hebrew) spear; gatherer.
Bible: Adam and Eve's oldest
son. See also Kabil, Kane,
Kayne.
*Cainaen, Cainan, Caine, Cainen,
Caineth, Cayn, Cayne*

Cairn (Welsh) landmark made
of a mound of stones.
Cairne, Carn, Carne

Cairo (Arabic) Geography: the
capital of Egypt.
Kairo

Cal (Latin) a short form of
Calvert, Calvin.

Calder (Welsh, English)
brook, stream.

Caldwell (English) cold well.

Cale (Hebrew) a short form
of Caleb.

Caleb (Hebrew) dog; faithful.
(Arabic) bold, brave. Bible: one
of the twelve spies sent by
Moses. See also Kaleb, Kayleb.
*Caeleb, Calab, Calabe, Cale,
Caley, Calib, Calieb, Callob,*

*Calob, Calyb, Cayleb, Caylebb,
Caylib, Caylob*

Calen, Calin (Scottish) forms
of Caelan.
*Caelen, Caelin, Caellin, Cailen,
Cailin, Caillin, Calean, Callen,
Caylin*

Caley (Irish) a familiar form
of Caleb.
Calee, Caleigh

Calhoun (Irish) narrow
woods. (Scottish) warrior.
Colhoun, Colhoune, Colquhoun

Callahan (Irish) descendant of
Ceallachen.
Calahan, Callaghan

Callum (Irish) dove.
Callam, Calum, Calym

Calvert (English) calf herder.
Cal, Calbert, Calvirt

Calvin (Latin) bald. See also
Kalvin, Vinny.
*Cal, Calv, Calvien, Calvon,
Calvyn*

Cam (Gypsy) beloved.
(Scottish) a short form of
Cameron. (Latin, French,
Scottish) a short form of
Campbell.
*Camm, Cammie, Cammy,
Camy*

Camaron (Scottish) a form of
Cameron.
*Camar, Camari, Camaran,
Camaren*

Camden (Scottish) winding
valley.
Kamden

Cameron (Scottish) crooked
nose. See also Kameron.
*Cam, Camaron, Cameran,
Cameren, Camerin, Cameroun,
Camerron, Camerson,
Camerun, Cameryn, Camiren,
Camiron, Cammeron, Camron*

Camille (French) young cere-
monial attendant.
Camile

Camilo (Latin) child born to
freedom; noble.
Camiel, Camillo, Camillus

Campbell (Latin, French)
beautiful field. (Scottish)
crooked mouth.
Cam, Camp, Campy

Camron (Scottish) a short
form of Cameron.
*Camren, Cammrin, Cammron,
Camran, Camreon, Camrin,
Camryn, Camrynn*

Canaan (French) a form of
Cannon. History: an ancient
region between the Jordan
River and the
Mediterranean.
Canan, Canen, Caynan

Candide (Latin) pure; sincere.
Candid, Candido, Candonino

Cannon (French) church offi-
cial; large gun. See also
Kannon.
*Canaan, Cannan, Cannen,
Cannin, Canning, Canon*

Canute (Latin) white haired.
(Scandinavian) knot. History:
a Danish king who became
king of England after 1016.
See also Knute.
Cnut, Cnute

Cappi (Gypsy) good fortune.

Car (Irish) a short form of
Carney.

Carey (Greek) pure. (Welsh)
castle; rocky island. See also
Karey.
*Care, Caree, Cari, Carre,
Carree, Carrie, Cary*

Carl (German, English) a short
form of Carlton. A form of
Charles. See also Carroll,
Kale, Kalle, Karl, Karlen,
Karol.
*Carle, Carles, Carless, Carlis,
Carll, Carlo, Carlos, Carlson,
Carlston, Carlus, Carolos*

Carlin (Irish) little champion.
*Carlan, Carlen, Carley, Carlie,
Carling, Carlino, Carly*

Carlisle (English) Carl's island.
Carlyle, Carlysle

Carlito (Spanish) a familiar
form of Carlos.
Carlitos

Carlo (Italian) a form of Carl,
Charles.
Carolo

Carlos (Spanish) a form of
Carl, Charles.
Carlito

Carlton (English) Carl's town.
*Carl, Carleton, Carllton,
Carlston, Carltonn, Carltton,
Charlton*

Carmel (Hebrew) vineyard,
garden. See also Carmine.
Carmello, Carmelo, Karmel

Carmichael (Scottish) follower
of Michael.

Carmine (Latin) song; crim-
son. (Italian) a form of
Carmel.
*Carmain, Carmaine, Carman,
Carmen, Carmon*

Carnelius (Greek, Latin) a
form of Cornelius.
*Carnealius, Carneilius,
Carnellius, Carnilious*

Carnell (English) defender of
the castle. (French) a form of
Cornell.

Carney (Irish) victorious.
(Scottish) fighter. See also
Kearney.
Car, Carny, Karney

Carr (Scandinavian) marsh.
See also Kerr.
Karr

Carrick (Irish) rock.
Carooq, Carricko

Carrington (Welsh) rocky
town.

Carroll (Irish) champion.
(German) a form of Carl.
*Carel, Carell, Cariel, Cariell,
Carol, Carole, Carolo, Carols,
Carollan, Carolus, Carrol, Cary,
Caryl*

Carson (English) son of Carr.
*Carsen, Carsino, Carrson,
Karson*

Carsten (Greek) a form of
Karsten.
Carston

Carter (English) cart driver.
Cart

Cartwright (English) cart
builder.

Carvell (French, English) village on the marsh.
Carvel, Carvelle, Carvellius

Carver (English) wood-carver;
sculptor.

Cary (Welsh) a form of Carey.
(German, Irish) a form of
Carroll.
Carray, Carry

Case (Irish) a short form of
Casey. (English) a short form
of Casimir.

Casey (Irish) brave.
*Case, Casie, Casy, Cayse,
Caysey, Kacey, Kasey*

Cash (Latin) vain. (Slavic) a
short form of Casimir.
Cashe

Casimir (Slavic) peacemaker.
*Cachi, Cas, Case, Cash,
Cashemere, Cashi, Cashmeire,
Cashmere, Casimere, Casimire,
Casimiro, Castimer, Kasimir,
Kazio*

Casper (Persian) treasurer.
(German) imperial. See also
Gaspar, Jasper, Kasper.
Caspar, Cass

Cass (Irish, Persian) a short
form of Casper, Cassidy.

Cassidy (Irish) clever; curly
haired. See also Kazio.
*Casidy, Cass, Cassady, Cassie,
Kassidy*

Cassie (Irish) a familiar form
of Cassidy.
*Casi, Casie, Casio, Cassey,
Cassy, Casy*

Cassius (Latin, French) box;
protective cover.
Cassia, Cassio, Cazzie

Castle (Latin) castle.
Cassle, Castel

Castor (Greek) beaver.
Astrology: one of the twins
in the constellation Gemini.
Mythology: one of the
patron saints of mariners.
Caster, Caston

Cater (English) caterer.

Cato (Latin) knowledgeable,
wise.
Caton, Catón

Cavan (Irish) handsome. See
also Kevin.
Caven, Cavin, Cavan, Cawoun

Cayden (American) a form of
Caden.
Cayde, Caydin

Caylan (Scottish) a form of
Caelan.
Caylans, Caylen, Caylon

Cazzie (American) a familiar
form of Cassius.
Caz, Cazz, Cazzy

Ceasar (Latin) a form of Caesar.
Ceaser

Cecil (Latin) blind.
*Cece, Cecile, Cecilio, Cecilius,
Cecill, Celio, Siseal*

Cedric (English) battle chief-
tain. See also Kedrick, Rick.
*Cad, Caddaric, Ced, Cederic,
Cedrec, Cédric, Cedrick,
Cedryche, Sedric*

Cedrick (English) a form of
Cedric.
*Ceddrick, Cederick, Cederrick,
Cedirick, Cedrik*

Ceejay (American) a combination of the initials C. + J.
Cejay, C.J.

Cemal (Arabic) attractive.

Cephas (Latin) small rock.
Bible: the term used by Jesus
to describe Peter.
Cepheus, Cephus

Cerdic (Welsh) beloved.
*Caradoc, Caradog, Ceredig,
Ceretic*

Cerek (Polish) lordly. (Greek)
a form of Cyril.

Cesar (Spanish) a form of
Caesar.
*Casar, César, Cesare, Cesareo,
Cesario, Cesaro, Cessar*

Cestmir (Czech) fortress.

Cezar (Slavic) a form of
Caesar.
*Cézar, Cezary, Cezek,
Chezrae, Sezar*

Chace (French) a form of
Chase.
Chayce

Chad (English) warrior. A
short form of Chadwick.
Geography: a country in
north-central Africa.
*Ceadd, Chaad, Chadd,
Chaddie, Chaddy, Chade,*

*Chadleigh, Chadler, Chadley,
Chadlin, Chadlyn, Chadmen,
Chado, Chadron, Chady*

Chadrick (German) mighty
warrior.
*Chaddrick, Chaderic,
Chaderick, Chadrack, Chadric*

Chadwick (English) warrior's
town.
*Chad, Chaddwick, Chadvic,
Chadwyck*

Chago (Spanish) a form of
Jacob.
Chango, Chanti

Chaim (Hebrew) life. See also
Hyman.
Chai, Chaimek, Haim, Khaim

Chaise (French) a form of
Chase.
Chais, Chaisen, Chaison

Chal (Gypsy) boy; son.
Chalie, Chalin

Chalmers (Scottish) son of the
lord.
*Chalmer, Chalmr, Chamar,
Chamarr*

Cham (Vietnamese) hard
worker.
Chams

Chan (Sanskrit) shining.
(English) a form of
Chauncey. (Spanish) a form
of Juan.
Chann, Chano, Chayo

Chanan (Hebrew) cloud.

Chance (English) a short form of Chancellor, Chauncey.
Chanc, Chancee, Chancey, Chancie, Chancy, Chanse, Chansy, Chants, Chantz, Chanze, Chanz, Chaynce

Chancellor (English) record keeper.
Chance, Chancelar, Chancelen, Chanceleor, Chanceler, Chanceller, Chancelor, Chanselor, Chanslor

Chander (Hindi) moon.
Chand, Chandan, Chandany, Chandara, Chandon

Chandler (English) candle maker.
Chandelar, Chandlan, Chandlar, Chandlier, Chandlor, Chandlyr

Chane (Swahili) dependable.

Chaney (French) oak.
Chayne, Cheaney, Cheney, Cheyn, Cheyne, Cheyney

Chankrisna (Cambodian) sweet smelling tree.

Channing (English) wise. (French) canon; church official.
Chane, Chann

Chanse (English) a form of Chance.
Chans, Chansey

Chante (French) singer.
Chant, Chantha, Chanthar, Chantra, Chantry, Shantae

Chapman (English) merchant.
Chap, Chappie, Chappy

Charles (German) farmer. (English) strong and manly. See also Carl, Searlas, Tearlach, Xarles.
Arlo, Chareles, Charels, Charlese, Carlo, Carlos, Charl, Charle, Charlen, Charlie, Charlot, Charlz, Charlzell, Chaz, Chick, Chip, Chuck

Charlie (German, English) a familiar form of Charles.
Charle, Charlee, Charley, Charli, Charly

Charlton (English) a form of Carlton.
Charlesten, Charleston, Charleton, Charlotin

Charro (Spanish) cowboy.

Chase (French) hunter.
Chace, Chaise, Chasen, Chason, Chass, Chasse, Chastan, Chasten, Chastin, Chastinn, Chaston, Chasyn, Chayse

Chaska (Sioux) first-born son.

Chauncey (English) chancellor; church official.
Chan, Chance, Chancey, Chaunce, Chauncei, Chauncy, Chaunecy, Chaunesy, Chaunszi

Chavez (Hispanic) a surname
used as a first name.
*Chavaz, Chaves, Chaveze,
Chavies, Chavis, Chavius,
Chevez, Cheveze, Cheviez,
Chevious, Chevis, Chivass,
Chivez*

Chayse (French) a form of
Chase.
*Chaysea, Chaysen, Chayson,
Chaysten*

Chayton (Lakota) falcon.

Chaz (English) a familiar form
of Charles.
*Chas, Chasz, Chaze,
Chazwick, Chazy, Chazz,
Chez*

Ché (Spanish) a familiar form
of José. History: Ernesto
"Che" Guevara was a revolu-
tionary who fought at Fidel
Castro's side in Cuba.
Chay

Checha (Spanish) a familiar
form of Jacob.

Cheche (Spanish) a familiar
form of Joseph.

Chen (Chinese) great, tremen-
dous.

Chencho (Spanish) a familiar
form of Lawrence.

Chepe (Spanish) a familiar
form of Joseph.
Cepito

Cherokee (Cherokee) people
of a different speech.
Cherrakee

Chesmu (Native American)
gritty.

Chester (English) a short
form of Rochester.
Ches, Cheslav, Cheston, Chet

Chet (English) a short form of
Chester.
Chett, Chette

Cheung (Chinese) good luck.

Chevalier (French) horseman,
knight.
Chev, Chevy

Chevy (French) a familiar form
of Chevalier. Geography:
Chevy Chase is a town in
Maryland. Culture: a short
form of Chevrolet, an
American automobile
company.
*Chev, Chevey, Chevi, Chevie,
Chevvy, Chewy*

Cheyenne (Cheyenne) a tribal
name.
*Chayann, Chayanne,
Cheyeenne, Cheyene, Chyenne,
Shayan*

Chi (Chinese) younger generation. (Nigerian) personal
guardian angel.

Chick (English) a familiar
form of Charles.
Chic, Chickie, Chicky

Chico (Spanish) boy.

Chik (Gypsy) earth.

Chike (Ibo) God's power.

Chiko (Japanese) arrow; pledge.

Chilo (Spanish) a familiar form of Francisco.

Chilton (English) farm by the spring.
Chil, Chill, Chillton, Chilt

Chim (Vietnamese) bird.

Chinua (Ibo) God's blessing.
Chino, Chinou

Chioke (Ibo) gift of God.

Chip (English) a familiar form of Charles.
Chipman, Chipper

Chiram (Hebrew) exalted; noble.

Chris (Greek) a short form of Christian, Christopher. See also Kris.
Chriss, Christ, Chrys, Cris, Crist

Christain (Greek) a form of Christian.
Christai, Christan, Christane, Christaun, Christein

Christian (Greek) follower of Christ; anointed. See also Jaan, Kerstan, Khristian, Kit, Krister, Kristian, Krystian.
Chretien, Chris, Christa, Christain, Christé, Christen, Christensen, Christiaan,

Christiana, Christiane, Christiann, Christianna, Christianno, Christiano, Christianos, Christien, Christin, Christino, Christion, Christon, Christos, Christyan, Christyon, Chritian, Chrystian, Cristian, Crystek

Christien (Greek) a form of Christian.
Christienne, Christinne, Chrystien

Christofer (Greek) a form of Christopher.
Christafer, Christafur, Christefor, Christerfer, Christifer, Christoffer, Christofher, Christofper, Chrystofer

Christoff (Russian) a form of Christopher.
Chrisof, Christif, Christof, Cristofe

Christophe (French) a form of Christopher.
Christoph

Christopher (Greek) Christ-bearer. Religion: the patron saint of travelers. See also Cristopher, Kester, Kit, Kristopher, Risto, Stoffel, Tobal, Topher.
Chris, Chrisopherson, Christapher, Christepher, Christerpher, Christhoper, Christipher, Christobal, Christofer, Christoff, Christoforo, Christoher, Christopehr, Christoper, Christophe,

Christopher *(cont.)*
Christopherr, Christophor,
Christophoros, Christophr,
Christophre, Christophyer,
Christophyr, Christorpher,
Christos, Christovao, Christpher,
Christphere, Christphor,
Christpor, Christrpher,
Chrystopher, Cristobal

Christophoros (Greek) a
form of Christopher.
Christoforo, Christoforos,
Christophor, Christophorus,
Christphor, Cristoforo,
Cristopher

Christos (Greek) a form of
Christopher. See also
Khristos.

Chucho (Hebrew) a familiar
form of Jesus.

Chuck (American) a familiar
form of Charles.
Chuckey, Chuckie, Chucky

Chui (Swahili) leopard.

Chul (Korean) firm.

Chuma (Ibo) having many
beads, wealthy. (Swahili) iron.

Chuminga (Spanish) a familiar
form of Dominic.
Chumin

Chumo (Spanish) a familiar
form of Thomas.

Chun (Chinese) spring.

Chung (Chinese) intelligent.
Chungo, Chuong

Churchill (English) church on
the hill. History: Sir Winston
Churchill served as British
prime minister and won a
Nobel Prize for literature.

Cian (Irish) ancient.
Céin, Cianán, Kian

Cicero (Latin) chickpea.
History: a famous Roman
orator, philosopher, and
statesman.
Cicerón

Cid (Spanish) lord. History:
title for Rodrigo Díaz de
Vivar, an eleventh-century
Spanish soldier and national
hero.
Cyd

Ciqala (Dakota) little.

Cirrillo (Italian) a form of Cyril.
Cirilio, Cirillo, Cirilo, Ciro

Cisco (Spanish) a short form
of Francisco.

Clancy (Irish) redheaded
fighter.
Clancey, Claney

Clare (Latin) a short form of
Clarence.
Clair, Clarey, Clary

Clarence (Latin) clear; victori-
ous.
Clarance, Clare, Clarrance,
Clarrence, Clearence

Clark (French) cleric; scholar.
Clarke, Clerc, Clerk

Claude (Latin, French) lame.
*Claud, Claudan, Claudel,
Claudell, Claudey, Claudi,
Claudian, Claudianus, Claudie,
Claudien, Claudin, Claudio,
Claudis, Claudius, Claudy*

Claudio (Italian) a form of
Claude.

Claus (German) a short form
of Nicholas. See also Klaus.
Claas, Claes, Clause

Clay (English) clay pit. A short
form of Clayborne, Clayton.
Klay

Clayborne (English) brook
near the clay pit.
*Claibern, Claiborn, Claiborne,
Claibrone, Clay, Claybon,
Clayborn, Claybourn,
Claybourne, Clayburn,
Clebourn*

Clayton (English) town built
on clay.
*Clay, Clayten, Cleighton,
Cleyton, Clyton, Klayton*

Cleary (Irish) learned.

Cleavon (English) cliff.
*Clavin, Clavion, Clavon,
Clavone, Clayvon, Claywon,
Clévon, Clevonn, Clyvon*

Clem (Latin) a short form of
Clement.
Cleme, Clemmy, Clim

Clement (Latin) merciful.
Bible: a coworker of Paul.
See also Klement, Menz.
*Clem, Clemens, Clément,
Clemente, Clementius,
Clemmons*

Clemente (Italian, Spanish) a
form of Clement.
Clemento, Clemenza

Cleon (Greek) famous.
Kleon

Cletus (Greek) illustrious.
History: a Roman pope and
martyr.
*Cleatus, Cledis, Cleotis, Clete,
Cletis*

Cleveland (English) land of
cliffs.
*Cleaveland, Cleavland,
Cleavon, Cleve, Clevelend,
Clevelynn, Clevey, Clevie,
Clevon*

Cliff (English) a short form of
Clifford, Clifton.
*Clif, Clift, Clive, Clyff, Clyph,
Kliff*

Clifford (English) cliff at the
river crossing.
Cliff, Cliford, Clyfford, Klifford

Clifton (English) cliff town.
*Cliff, Cliffton, Clift, Cliften,
Clyfton*

Clint (English) a short form of
Clinton.
Klint

Clinton (English) hill town.
*Clenten, Clint, Clinten,
Clintion, Clintton, Clynton,
Klinton*

Clive (English) a form of Cliff.
*Cleve, Clivans, Clivens, Clyve,
Klyve*

Clovis (German) famous soldier. See also Louis.

Cluny (Irish) meadow.

Clyde (Welsh) warm.
(Scottish) Geography: a river
in Scotland.
Cly, Clywd, Klyde

Coby (Hebrew) a familiar
form of Jacob.
*Cob, Cobby, Cobe, Cobey, Cobi,
Cobia, Cobie*

Cochise (Apache) hardwood.
History: a famous Chiricahua
Apache leader.

Coco (French) a familiar form
of Jacques.
Coko, Koko

Codey (English) a form of
Cody.
Coday

Codi, Codie (English) forms
of Cody.
Coadi, Codea

Cody (English) cushion.
History: William "Buffalo
Bill" Cody was an American
frontier scout who toured
America and Europe with

his Wild West show. See also
Kody.
*Coady, Coddy, Code, Codee,
Codell, Codey, Codi, Codiak,
Codie, Coedy*

Coffie (Ewe) born on Friday.

Cola (Italian) a familiar form
of Nicholas, Nicola.
Colas

Colar (French) a form of
Nicholas.

Colbert (English) famous seafarer.
Cole, Colt, Colvert, Culbert

Colby (English) dark; dark
haired.
*Colbey, Colbi, Colbie, Colbin,
Colebee, Coleby, Collby, Kolby*

Cole (Latin) cabbage farmer.
(English) a short form of
Coleman.
Colet, Coley, Colie, Kole

Coleman (Latin) cabbage
farmer. (English) coal miner.
*Cole, Colemann, Colm,
Colman, Koleman*

Colin (Irish) young cub.
(Greek) a short form of
Nicholas.
*Cailean, Colan, Cole, Colen,
Coleon, Colinn, Collin, Colyn,
Kolin*

Colley (English) black haired;
swarthy.
Colee, Collie, Collis

Collier (English) miner.
Colier, Collayer, Collie, Collyer, Colyer

Collin (Scottish) a form of
Colin, Collins.
Collan, Collen, Collian, Collon, Collyn

Collins (Greek) son of Colin.
(Irish) holly.
Collin, Collis

Colson (Greek, English) son
of Nicholas.
Colsen, Coulson

Colt (English) young horse;
frisky. A short form of
Colter, Colton.
Colte

Colten (English) a form of
Colton.

Colter (English) herd of colts.
Colt

Colton (English) coal town.
Colt, Coltan, Colten, Coltin, Coltinn, Coltn, Coltrane, Colttan, Coltton, Coltun, Coltyn, Coltyne, Kolton

Columba (Latin) dove.
Coim, Colum, Columbia, Columbus

Colwyn (Welsh) Geography: a
river in Wales.
Colwin, Colwinn

Coman (Arabic) noble. (Irish)
bent.
Comán

Conall (Irish) high, mighty.
Conal, Connal, Connel, Connell, Connelly, Connolly

Conan (Irish) praised; exalted.
(Scottish) wise.
Conant, Conary, Connen, Connie, Connon, Connor, Conon

Conary (Irish) a form of
Conan.
Conaire

Conlan (Irish) hero.
Conlen, Conley, Conlin, Conlyn

Conner (Irish) a form of
Connor.
Connar, Connary, Conneer, Connery, Konner

Connie (English, Irish) a
familiar form of Conan,
Conrad, Constantine,
Conway.
Con, Conn, Conney, Conny

Connor (Scottish) wise. (Irish)
a form of Conan.
Conner, Connoer, Connory, Connyr, Conor, Konner, Konnor

Conor (Irish) a form of
Connor.
Conar, Coner, Conour, Konner

Conrad (German) brave
counselor.
Connie, Conrade, Conrado, Corrado, Konrad

Conroy (Irish) wise.
Conry, Roy

Constant (Latin) a short form
of Constantine.

Constantine (Latin) firm, con-
stant. History: Constantine
the Great was the Roman
emperor who adopted the
Christian faith. See also
Dinos, Konstantin, Stancio.
*Connie, Constadine,
Constandine, Constandios,
Constanstine, Constant,
Constantin, Constantino,
Constantinos, Constantios, Costa*

Conway (Irish) hound of the
plain.
Connie, Conwy

Cook (English) cook.
Cooke

Cooper (English) barrel
maker. See also Keiffer.
Coop, Couper

Corbett (Latin) raven.
*Corbbitt, Corbet, Corbette,
Corbit, Corbitt*

Corbin (Latin) raven.
*Corban, Corben, Corbey,
Corbie, Corbon, Corby, Corbyn,
Korbin*

Corcoran (Irish) ruddy.

Cordaro (Spanish) a form of
Cordero.
*Coradaro, Cordairo, Cordara,
Cordarel, Cordarell, Cordarelle,
Cordareo, Cordarin, Cordario,
Cordarion, Cordarious,
Cordarius, Cordarrel, Cordarrell,
Cordarris, Cordarrius, Cordarro,
Cordarrol, Cordarus, Cordarryl,
Cordaryal, Corddarro, Corrdarl*

Cordell (French) rope maker.
*Cord, Cordae, Cordale, Corday,
Cordeal, Cordeil, Cordel,
Cordele, Cordelle, Cordie,
Cordy, Kordell*

Cordero (Spanish) little lamb.
*Cordaro, Cordeal, Cordeara,
Cordearo, Cordeiro, Cordelro,
Corder, Cordera, Corderall,
Corderias, Corderious, Corderral,
Corderro, Corderryn, Corderun,
Corderus, Cordiaro, Cordierre,
Cordy, Corrderio*

Corey (Irish) hollow. See also
Korey, Kory.
*Core, Coreaa, Coree, Cori,
Corian, Corie, Corio, Correy,
Corria, Corrie, Corry, Corrye,
Cory*

Cormac (Irish) raven's son.
History: a third-century king
of Ireland who was a great
lawmaker.
Cormack, Cormick

Cornelius (Greek) cornel tree.
(Latin) horn colored. See also
Kornel, Kornelius, Nelek.
*Carnelius, Conny, Cornealous,
Corneili, Corneilius, Corneilus,
Corneliaus, Cornelious,
Cornelias, Cornelis, Corneliu,*

Cornell, Cornellious, Cornellis, Cornellius, Cornelous, Corneluis, Cornelus, Corney, Cornie, Cornielius, Corniellus, Corny, Cournelius, Cournelyous, Nelius, Nellie

Cornell (French) a form of Cornelius.
Carnell, Cornall, Corneil, Cornel, Cornelio, Corney, Cornie, Corny, Nellie

Cornwallis (English) from Cornwall.

Corrado (Italian) a form of Conrad.
Carrado

Corrigan (Irish) spearman.
Carrigan, Carrigen, Corrigon, Corrigun, Korrigan

Corrin (Irish) spear carrier.
Corin, Corion

Corry (Latin) a form of Corey.

Cort (German) bold. (Scandinavian) short. (English) a short form of Courtney.
Corte, Cortie, Corty, Kort

Cortez (Spanish) conqueror. History: Hernando Cortés was a Spanish conquistador who conquered Aztec Mexico.
Cartez, Cortes, Cortis, Cortize, Courtes, Courtez, Curtez, Kortez

Corwin (English) heart's companion; heart's delight.
Corwinn, Corwyn, Corwynn, Corwynne

Cory (Latin) a form of Corey. (French) a familiar form of Cornell. (Greek) a short form of Corydon.
Corye

Corydon (Greek) helmet, crest.
Coridon, Corradino, Cory, Coryden, Coryell

Cosgrove (Irish) victor, champion.

Cosmo (Greek) orderly; harmonious; universe.
Cos, Cosimo, Cosme, Cosmé, Cozmo, Kosmo

Costa (Greek) a short form of Constantine.
Costandinos, Costantinos, Costas, Costes

Coty (French) slope, hillside.
Cote, Cotee, Cotey, Coti, Cotie, Cotty, Cotye

Courtland (English) court's land.
Court, Courtlan, Courtlana, Courtlandt, Courtlin, Courtlind, Courtlon, Courtlyn, Kourtland

Courtney (English) court.
Cort, Cortnay, Cortne, Cortney, Court, Courten, Courtenay, Courteney, Courtnay, Courtnee, Curt, Kortney

Cowan (Irish) hillside hollow.
*Coe, Coven, Covin, Cowen,
Cowey, Cowie*

Coy (English) woods.
Coye, Coyie, Coyt

Coyle (Irish) leader in battle.

Coyne (French) modest.
Coyan

Craddock (Welsh) love.
Caradoc, Caradog

Craig (Irish, Scottish) crag;
steep rock.
*Crag, Craige, Craigen, Craigery,
Craigh, Craigon, Creag, Creg,
Cregan, Cregg, Creig, Creigh,
Criag, Kraig*

Crandall (English) crane's val-
ley.
*Cran, Crandal, Crandel,
Crandell, Crendal*

Crawford (English) ford
where crows fly.
Craw, Crow, Ford

Creed (Latin) belief.
Creedon

Creighton (English) town
near the rocks.
*Cray, Crayton, Creighm,
Creight, Creighto, Crichton*

Crepin (French) a form of
Crispin.

Crispin (Latin) curly haired.
Crepin, Cris, Crispian,

*Crispien, Crispino, Crispo,
Krispin*

Cristian (Greek) a form of
Christian.
*Crétien, Cristean, Cristhian,
Cristiano, Cristien, Cristino,
Cristle, Criston, Cristos, Cristy,
Cristyan, Crystek, Crystian*

Cristobal (Greek) a form of
Christopher.
Cristóbal, Cristoval, Cristovao

Cristoforo (Italian) a form of
Christopher.
Cristofor

Cristopher (Greek) a form of
Christopher.
*Cristaph, Cristhofer, Cristifer,
Cristofer, Cristoph, Cristophe,
Crystapher, Crystifer*

Crofton (Irish) town with
cottages.

Cromwell (English) crooked
spring, winding spring.

Crosby (Scandinavian) shrine
of the cross.
Crosbey, Crosbie, Cross

Crosley (English) meadow of
the cross.
Cross

Crowther (English) fiddler.

Cruz (Portuguese, Spanish)
cross.
Cruze, Kruz

Crystek (Polish) a form of Christian.

Cullen (Irish) handsome.
Cull, Cullan, Cullie, Cullin

Culley (Irish) woods.
Cullie, Cully

Culver (English) dove.
Colver, Cull, Cullie, Cully

Cunningham (Irish) village of the milk pail.

Curran (Irish) hero.
Curan, Curon, Curr, Curren, Currey, Curri, Currie, Currin, Curry

Currito (Spanish) a form of Curtis.
Curcio

Curt (Latin) a short form of Courtney, Curtis. See also Kurt.

Curtis (Latin) enclosure. (French) courteous. See also Kurtis.
Curio, Currito, Curt, Curtice, Curtiss, Curtus

Cuthbert (English) brilliant.

Cutler (English) knife maker.
Cut, Cuttie, Cutty

Cy (Persian) a short form of Cyrus.

Cyle (Irish) a form of Kyle.

Cyprian (Latin) from the island of Cyprus.
Ciprian, Cipriano, Ciprien, Cyprien

Cyrano (Greek) from Cyrene, an ancient city in North Africa. Literature: *Cyrano de Bergerac* is a play by Edmond Rostand about a great guardsman and poet whose large nose prevented him from pursuing the woman he loved.

Cyril (Greek) lordly. See also Kiril.
Cerek, Cerel, Cyrell, Ceril, Ciril, Cirillo, Cirrillo, Cyra, Cyrel, Cyrell, Cyrelle, Cyrill, Cyrille, Cyrillus, Syrell, Syril

Cyrus (Persian) sun. Historical: Cyrus the Great was a king in ancient Persia. See also Kir.
Ciro, Cy, Cyress, Cyris, Cyriss, Cyruss, Syris, Syrus

D

Dabi (Basque) a form of David.

Dabir (Arabic) tutor.

Dacey (Latin) from Dacia, an area now in Romania. (Irish) southerner.
Dace, Dache, Dacian, Dacias, Dacio, Dacy, Daicey, Daicy

Dada (Yoruba) curly haired.
Dadi

Daegel (English) from Daegel, England.

Daelen (English) a form of Dale.
Daelan, Daelin, Daelon, Daelyn, Daelyne

Daemon (Greek) a form of Damian. (Greek, Latin) a form of Damon.
Daemean, Daemeon, Daemien, Daemin, Daemion, Daemyen

Daequan (American) a form of Daquan.
Daequane, Daequon, Daequone, Daeqwan

Daeshawn (American) a combination of the prefix Da + Shawn.
Daesean, Daeshaun, Daeshon, Daeshun, Daisean, Daishaun, Daishawn, Daishon, Daishoun

Daevon (American) a form of Davon.
Daevion, Daevohn, Daevonne, Daevonte, Daevontey

Dafydd (Welsh) a form of David.
Dafyd

Dag (Scandinavian) day; bright.
Daeg, Daegan, Dagen, Dagny, Deegan

Dagan (Hebrew) corn; grain.
Daegan, Daegon, Dagen, Dageon, Dagon

Dagwood (English) shining forest.

Dai (Japanese) big.

Daimian (Greek) a form of Damian.
Daiman, Daimean, Daimen, Daimeon, Daimeyon, Daimien, Daimin, Daimion, Daimyan

Daimon (Greek, Latin) a form of Damon.
Daimone

Daiquan (American) a form of Dajuan.
Daekwaun, Daekwon, Daiqone, Daiqua, Daiquane, Daiquawn, Daiquon, Daiqwan, Daiqwon

Daivon (American) a form of Davon.
Daivain, Daivion, Daivonn, Daivonte, Daiwan

Dajon (American) a form of Dajuan.
Dajean, Dajiawn, Dajin, Dajion, Dajn, Dajohn, Dajonae

Dajuan (American) a combination of the prefix Da + Juan. See also Dejuan.
Daejon, Daejuan, Daiquan, Dajon, Da Jon, Da-Juan, Dajwan, Dajwoun, Dakuan, Dakwan, Dawan, Dawaun, Dawawn, Dawon, Dawoyan,

Dijuan, Diuan, Dujuan, D'Juan, D'juan, Dwaun

Dakarai (Shona) happy.
Dakairi, Dakar, Dakaraia, Dakari, Dakarri

Dakoda (Dakota) a form of Dakota.
Dacoda, Dacodah, Dakodah, Dakodas

Dakota (Dakota) friend; partner; tribal name.
Dac, Dack, Dackota, Dacota, DaCota, Dak, Dakcota, Dakkota, Dakoata, Dakoda, Dakotah, Dakotha, Dakotta, Dekota

Dakotah (Dakota) a form of Dakota.
Dakottah

Daksh (Hindi) efficient.

Dalal (Sanskrit) broker.

Dalbert (English) bright, shining. See also Delbert.

Dale (English) dale, valley.
Dael, Daelen, Dal, Dalen, Daley, Dalibor, Dallan, Dallin, Dallyn, Daly, Dayl, Dayle

Dalen (English) a form of Dale.
Dailin, Dalaan, Dalan, Dalane, Daleon, Dalian, Dalibor, Dalione, Dallan, Dalon, Daylan, Daylen, Daylin, Daylon

Daley (Irish) assembly. (English) a familiar form of Dale.
Daily, Daly, Dawley

Dallan (English) a form of Dale.
Dallen, Dallon

Dallas (Scottish) valley of the water; resting place. Geography: a town in Scotland; a city in Texas.
Dal, Dalieass, Dall, Dalles, Dallis, Dalys, Dellis

Dallin, Dallyn (English) pride's people.
Dalin, Dalyn

Dalston (English) Daegel's place.
Dalis, Dallon

Dalton (English) town in the valley.
Dal, Dalaton, Dallton, Dalt, Daltan, Dalten, Daltin, Daltyn, Daulton, Delton

Dalvin (English) a form of Delvin.
Dalven, Dalvon, Dalvyn

Dalziel (Scottish) small field.

Damar (American) a short form of Damarcus, Damario.
Damare, Damari, Damarre, Damauri

Damarcus (American) a combination of the prefix Da + Marcus.
Damacus, Damar, Damarco, Damarcue, Damarick, Damark, Damarkco, Damarkis, Damarko, Damarkus, Damarques, Damarquez, Damarquis, Damarrco

Damario (Greek) gentle.
(American) a combination of
the prefix Da + Mario.
*Damar, Damarea, Damareus,
Damaria, Damarie, Damarino,
Damarion, Damarious,
Damaris, Damarius, Damarrea,
Damarrion, Damarrious,
Damarrius, Damaryo, Dameris,
Damerius*

Damek (Slavic) a form of
Adam.
Damick, Damicke

Dameon (Greek) a form of
Damian.
Damein, Dameion, Dameone

Dametrius (Greek) a form of
Demetrius.
*Dametri, Dametries,
Dametrious, Damitri, Damitric,
Damitrie, Damitrious,
Damitrius*

Damian (Greek) tamer;
soother.
*Daemon, Daimian, Damaiaon,
Damaian, Damaien, Damain,
Damaine, Damaion, Damani,
Damanni, Damaun, Damayon,
Dame, Damean, Dameon,
Damián, Damiane, Damiann,
Damiano, Damianos, Damien,
Damion, Damiyan, Damján,
Damyan, Daymian, Dema,
Demyan*

Damien (Greek) a form of
Damian. Religion: Father
Damien ministered to the
leper colony on the
Hawaiian island Molokai.
*Daemien, Daimien, Damie,
Damienne, Damyen*

Damion (Greek) a form of
Damian.
*Damieon, Damiion, Damin,
Damine, Damionne, Damiyon,
Dammion, Damyon*

Damon (Greek) constant,
loyal. (Latin) spirit, demon.
*Daemen, Daemon, Daemond,
Daimon, Daman, Damen,
Damond, Damone, Damoni,
Damonn, Damonni, Damonta,
Damontae, Damonte,
Damontez, Damontis, Damyn,
Daymon, Daymond*

Dan (Vietnamese) yes. (Hebrew)
a short form of Daniel.
Dahn, Danh, Danne

Dana (Scandinavian) from
Denmark.
Dain, Daina, Dayna

Dandin (Hindi) holy man.

Dandré (French) a combina-
tion of the prefix De +
André.
*D'André, Dandrae, D'andrea,
Dandras, Dandray, Dandre,
Dondrea*

Dane (English) from
Denmark. See also Halden.
*Dain, Daine, Danie, Dayne,
Dhane*

Danek (Polish) a form of Daniel.

Danforth (English) a form of Daniel.

Danial (Hebrew) a form of Daniel.
Danal, Daneal, Danieal, Daniyal, Dannial

Danick, Dannick (Slavic) familiar forms of Daniel.
Danek, Danieko, Danik, Danika, Danyck

Daniel (Hebrew) God is my judge. Bible: a Hebrew prophet. See also Danno, Kanaiela.
Dacso, Dainel, Dan, Daneel, Daneil, Danek, Danel, Danforth, Danial, Danick, Dániel, Daniël, Daniele, Danielius, Daniell, Daniels, Danielson, Danilo, Daniyel, Dan'l, Dannel, Dannick, Danniel, Dannil, Danno, Danny, Dano, Danukas, Dany, Danyel, Danyell, Daoud, Dasco, Dayne, Deniel, Doneal, Doniel, Donois, Dusan, Nelo

Daniele (Hebrew) a form of Daniel.
Danile, Danniele

Danilo (Slavic) a form of Daniel.
Danielo, Danil, Danila, Danilka, Danylo

Danior (Gypsy) born with teeth.

Danladi (Hausa) born on Sunday.

Danno (Hebrew) a familiar form of Daniel. (Japanese) gathering in the meadow. (Hebrew) a familiar form of Daniel.
Dannon, Dano

Dannon (American) a form of Danno.
Daenan, Daenen, Dainon, Danaan, Danen, Danon

Danny, Dany (Hebrew) familiar forms of Daniel.
Daney, Dani, Dannee, Danney, Danni, Dannie, Dannye

Dano (Czech) a form of Daniel.
Danko, Danno

Dante, Danté (Latin) lasting, enduring.
Danatay, Danaté, Dant, Dantae, Dantay, Dantee, Dauntay, Dauntaye, Daunté, Dauntrae, Deante, Dontae, Donté

Dantrell (American) a combination of Dante + Darell.
Dantrel, Dantrey, Dantril, Dantyrell, Dontrell

Danyel (Hebrew) a form of
Daniel.
*Danya, Danyal, Danyale,
Danyele, Danyell, Danyiel,
Danyl, Danyle, Danylets,
Danylo, Donyell*

Daoud (Arabic) a form of
David.
Daudi, Daudy, Dauod, Dawud

Daquan (American) a combi-
nation of the prefix Da +
Quan.
*Daequan, Daqon, Daquain,
Daquaine, Da'quan,
Daquandre, Daquandrey,
Daquane, Daquann,
Daquantae, Daquante,
Daquarius, Daquaun,
Daquawn, Daquin, Daquon,
Daquone, Daquwon, Daqwain,
Daqwan, Daqwane, Daqwann,
Daqwon, Daqwone, Dayquan,
Dequain, Dequan, Dequann,
Dequaun*

Dar (Hebrew) pearl.

Dara (Cambodian) stars.

Daran (Irish) a form of Darren.
*Darann, Darawn, Darian,
Darran, Dayran, Deran*

Darby (Irish) free. (English)
deer park.
*Dar, Darb, Darbee, Darbey,
Darbie, Derby*

Darcy (Irish) dark. (French)
from Arcy, France.
Dar, Daray, D'Aray, Darce,

*Darcee, Darcel, Darcey, Darcio,
D'Arcy, Darsey, Darsy*

Dareh (Persian) wealthy.

Darell (English) a form of
Darrell.
*Darall, Daralle, Dareal, Darel,
Darelle, Darral, Darrall*

Daren (Hausa) born at night.
(Irish, English) a form of
Darren.
Dare, Dayren, Dheren

Darian, Darrian (Irish) forms
of Darren.
Daryan

Darick (German) a form of
Derek.
*Darek, Daric, Darico, Darieck,
Dariek, Darik, Daryk*

Darien, Darrien (Irish) forms
of Darren.

Darin (Irish) a form of
Darren.
*Daryn, Darynn, Dayrin,
Dearin, Dharin*

Dario (Spanish) affluent.

Darion Darrion (Irish) forms
of Darren.
Daryeon, Daryon

Darius (Greek) wealthy.
*Dairus, Dare, Darieus,
Darioush, Dariuse, Dariush,
Dariuss, Dariusz, Darrius*

Darnell (English) hidden place.
Dar, Darn, Darnall, Darneal, Darneil, Darnel, Darnelle, Darnyell, Darnyll

Daron (Irish) a form of Darren.
Daeron, Dairon, Darone, Daronn, Darroun, Dayron, Dearon, Dharon, Diron

Darrell (French) darling, beloved; grove of oak trees.
Dare, Darel, Darell, Darral, Darrel, Darrill, Darrol, Darryl, Derrell

Darren (Irish) great. (English) small; rocky hill.
Daran, Dare, Daren, Darian, Darien, Darin, Darion, Daron, Darran, Darrian, Darrien, Darrience, Darrin, Darrion, Darron, Darryn, Darun, Daryn, Dearron, Deren, Dereon, Derren, Derron

Darrick (German) a form of Derek.
Darrec, Darrek, Darric, Darrik, Darryk

Darrin (Irish) a form of Darren.

Darrion (Irish) a form of Darren.
Dairean, Dairion, Darian, Darien, Darion, Darrian, Darrien, Darrione, Darriyun, Derrian, Derrion

Darrius (Greek) a form of Darius.
Darreus, Darrias, Darrious, Darris, Darriuss, Darrus, Darryus, Derrious, Derris, Derrius

Darron (Irish) a form of Darren.
Darriun, Darroun

Darryl (French) darling, beloved; grove of oak trees. A form of Darrell.
Dahrll, Darryle, Darryll, Daryl, Daryle, Daryll, Derryl

Darshan (Hindi) god; godlike. Religion: another name for the Hindu god Shiva.
Darshaun, Darshon

Darton (English) deer town.
Dartel, Dartrel

Darwin (English) dear friend. History: Charles Darwin was the British naturalist who established the theory of evolution.
Darvin, Darvon, Darwyn, Derwin, Derwynn, Durwin

Daryl (French) a form of Darryl.
Darel, Daril, Darl, Darly, Daryell, Daryle, Daryll, Darylle, Daroyl

Dasan (Pomo) leader of the bird clan.
Dassan

Dashawn (American) a combination of the prefix Da + Shawn.
Dasean, Dashan, Dashane, Dashante, Dashaun, Dashaunte, Dashean, Dashon, Dashonnie, Dashonte, Dashuan, Dashun, Dashwan, Dayshawn

Dauid (Swahili) a form of David.

Daulton (English) a form of Dalton.

Davante (American) a form of Davonte.
Davanta, Davantay, Davinte

Davaris (American) a combination of Dave + Darius.
Davario, Davarious, Davarius, Davarrius, Davarus

Dave (Hebrew) a short form of David, Davis.

Davey (Hebrew) a familiar form of David.
Davee, Davi, Davie, Davy

David (Hebrew) beloved. Bible: the second king of Israel. See also Dov, Havika, Kawika, Taaveti, Taffy, Tevel.
Dabi, Daevid, Dafydd, Dai, Daivid, Daoud, Dauid, Dav, Dave, Daved, Daveed, Daven, Davey, Davidde, Davide, Davidek, Davido, Davon, Davoud, Davyd, Dawid, Dawit, Dawud, Dayvid, Dodya, Dov

Davin (Scandinavian) brilliant Finn.
Daevin, Davion, Davon, Davyn, Dawan, Dawin, Dawine, Dayvon, Deavan, Deaven

Davion (American) a form of Davin.
Davione, Davionne, Daviyon, Davyon, Deaveon

Davis (Welsh) son of David.
Dave, Davidson, Davies, Davison

Davon (American) a form of Davin.
Daevon, Daivon, Davon, Davone, Davonn, Davonne, Deavon, Deavone, Devon

Davonte (American) a combination of Davon + the suffix Te.
Davante, Davonnte, Davonta, Davontae, Davontah, Davontai, Davontay, Davontaye, Davontea, Davontee, Davonti

Dawan (American) a form of Davin.
Dawann, Dawante, Dawaun, Dawayne, Dawon, Dawone, Dawoon, Dawyne, Dawyun

Dawit (Ethiopian) a form of David.

Dawson (English) son of David.
Dawsyn

Dax (French, English) water.
Daylon (American) a form of
Dillon.
*Daylan, Daylen, Daylin,
Daylun, Daylyn*

Daymian (Greek) a form of
Damian.
*Daymayne, Daymen, Daymeon,
Daymiane, Daymien, Daymin,
Dayminn, Daymion, Daymn*

Dayne (Scandinavian) a form
of Dane.
Dayn

Dayquan (American) a form
of Daquan.
*Dayquain, Dayquawane,
Dayquin, Dayqwan*

Dayshawn (American) a form
of Dashawn.
*Daysean, Daysen, Dayshaun,
Dayshon, Dayson*

Dayton (English) day town;
bright, sunny town.
*Daeton, Daiton, Daythan,
Daython, Daytona, Daytonn,
Deyton*

Dayvon (American) a form of
Davin.
*Dayven, Dayveon, Dayvin,
Dayvion, Dayvonn*

De (Chinese) virtuous.

Deacon (Greek) one who
serves.
Deke

Dean (French) leader.
(English) valley. See also
Dino.
*Deane, Deen, Dene, Deyn,
Deyne*

Deandre (French) a combina-
tion of the prefix De +
André.
*D'andre, D'andré, D'André,
D'andrea, Deandra, Deandrae,
Déandre, Deandré, De André,
Deandrea, De Andrea,
Deandres, Deandrey,
Deaundera, Deaundra,
Deaundray, Deaundre, De
Aundre, Deaundrey, Deaundry,
Deondre, Diandre, Dondre*

Deangelo (Italian) a combina-
tion of the prefix De +
Angelo.
*Dang, Dangelo, D'Angelo,
Danglo, Deaengelo, Deangelio,
Deangello, Déangelo, De Angelo,
Deangilio, Deangleo, Deanglo,
Deangulo, Diangelo, Di'angelo*

Deante (Latin) a form of
Dante.
*Deanta, Deantai, Deantay,
Deanté, De Anté, Deanteé,
Deaunta, Diantae, Diante,
Diantey*

Deanthony (Italian) a combi-
nation of the prefix De +
Anthony.
D'anthony, Danton, Dianthony

Dearborn (English) deer brook.
Dearbourn, Dearburne, Deaurburn, Deerborn

Decarlos (Spanish) a combination of the prefix De + Carlos.
Dacarlos, Decarlo, Di'carlos

Decha (Tai) strong.

Decimus (Latin) tenth.

Declan (Irish) man of prayer. Religion: Saint Declan was a fifth-century Irish bishop.
Deklan

Dedrick (German) ruler of the people. See also Derek, Theodoric.
Deadrick, Deddrick, Dederick, Dedrek, Dedreko, Dedric, Dedrix, Dedrrick, Deedrick, Diedrich, Diedrick, Dietrich, Detrick

Deems (English) judge's child.

Deion (Greek) a form of Dion.
Deione, Deionta, Deionte

Dejuan (American) a combination of the prefix De + Juan. See also Dajuan.
Dejan, Dejon, Dejuane, Dejun, Dewan, Dewaun, Dewon, Dijaun, Djuan, D'Juan, Dujuan, Dujuane, D'Won

Dekel (Hebrew, Arabic) palm tree, date tree.

Dekota (Dakota) a form of Dakota.
Decoda, Dekoda, Dekodda, Dekotes

Del (English) a short form of Delbert, Delvin, Delwin.

Delaney (Irish) descendant of the challenger.
Delaine, Delainey, Delainy, Delan, Delane, Delanny, Delany

Delano (French) nut tree. (Irish) dark.
Delanio, Delayno, Dellano

Delbert (English) bright as day. See also Dalbert.
Bert, Del, Dilbert

Delfino (Latin) dolphin.
Delfine

Déli (Chinese) virtuous.

Dell (English) small valley. A short form of Udell.

Delling (Scandinavian) scintillating.

Delmar (Latin) sea.
Dalmar, Dalmer, Delmare, Delmario, Delmarr, Delmer, Delmor, Delmore

Delon (American) a form of Dillon.
Deloin, Delone, Deloni, Delonne

Delroy (French) belonging to the king. See also Elroy, Leroy.
Delray, Delree, Delroi

Delshawn (American) a combination of Del + Shawn.
Delsean, Delshon, Delsin, Delson

Delsin (Native American) he is so.
Delsy

Delton (English) a form of Dalton.
Delten, Deltyn

Delvin (English) proud friend; friend from the valley.
Dalvin, Del, Delavan, Delvian, Delvon, Delvyn, Delwin

Delwin (English) a form of Delvin.
Dalwin, Dalwyn, Del, Dellwin, Dellwyn, Delwyn, Delwynn

Deman (Dutch) man.

Demarco (Italian) a combination of the prefix De + Marco.
Damarco, Demarcco, Demarceo, Demarcio, Demarkco, Demarkeo, Demarko, Demarquo, D'Marco

Demarcus (American) a combination of the prefix De + Marcus.
Damarcius, Damarcus, Demarces, Demarcis, Demarcius, Demarcos, Demarcuse, Demarkes, Demarkis, Demarkos, Demarkus, Demarqus, D'Marcus

Demario (Italian) a combination of the prefix De + Mario.
Demarea, Demaree, Demareo, Demari, Demaria, Demariea, Demarion, Demarreio, Demariez, Demarious, Demaris, Demariuz, Demarrio, Demerio, Demerrio

Demarius (American) a combination of the prefix De + Marius.

Demarquis (American) a combination of the prefix De + Marquis.
Demarques, Demarquez, Demarqui

Dembe (Luganda) peaceful.
Damba

Demetri, Demitri (Greek) short forms of Demetrius.
Dametri, Damitré, Demeter, Demetre, Demetrea, Demetriel, Demitre, Demitrie, Domotor

Demetris (Greek) a short form of Demetrius.
Demeatric, Demeatrice, Demeatris, Demetres, Demetress, Demetric, Demetrice, Demetrick, Demetrics, Demetricus, Demetrik, Demitrez, Demitries, Demitris

Demetrius (Greek) lover of the earth. Mythology: a follower of Demeter, the goddess of the harvest. See also Dimitri, Mimis, Mitsos.
Dametrius, Demeitrius, Demeterious, Demetreus, Demetri, Demetrias, Demetrio, Demetrios, Demetrious, Demetris, Demetriu, Demetrium, Demetrois, Demetruis, Demetrus, Demitirus, Demitri, Demitrias, Demitriu, Demitrius, Demitrus, Demtrius, Demtrus, Dimitri, Dimitrios, Dimitrius, Dmetrius, Dymek

Demichael (American) a combination of the prefix De + Michael.
Dumichael

Demond (Irish) a short form of Desmond.
Demonde, Demonds, Demone, Dumonde

Demont (French) mountain.
Démont, Demonta, Demontae, Demontay, Demontaz, Demonte, Demontez, Demontre

Demorris (American) a combination of the prefix De + Morris.
Demoris, DeMorris, Demorus

Demos (Greek) people.
Demas, Demosthenes

Demothi (Native American) talks while walking.

Dempsey (Irish) proud.
Demp, Demps, Dempsie, Dempsy

Dempster (English) one who judges.
Demster

Denby (Scandinavian) Geography: a Danish village.
Danby, Den, Denbey, Denney, Dennie, Denny

Denham (English) village in the valley.

Denholm (Scottish) Geography: a town in Scotland.

Denis (Greek) a form of Dennis.
Denise, Deniz

Denley (English) meadow; valley.
Denlie, Denly

Denman (English) man from the valley.

Dennis (Greek) Mythology: a follower of Dionysus, the god of wine. See also Dion, Nicho.
Den, Dénes, Denies, Denis, Deniz, Dennes, Dennet, Dennez, Denny, Dennys, Denya, Denys, Deon, Dinis

Dennison (English) son of Dennis. See also Dyson, Tennyson.
Den, Denison, Denisson, Dennyson

Denny (Greek) a familiar form of Dennis.
Den, Denney, Dennie, Deny

Denton (English) happy home.
Dent, Denten, Dentin

Denver (English) green valley. Geography: the capital of Colorado.

Denzel (Cornish) a form of Denzil.
Danzel, Danzell, Dennzel, Denzal, Denzale, Denzall, Denzell, Denzelle, Denzle, Denzsel

Denzell (Cornish) Geography: a location in Cornwall, England.
Dennzil, Dennzyl, Denzel, Denzial, Denziel, Denzil, Denzill, Denzyel, Denzyl, Donzell

Deon (Greek) a form of Dennis. See also Dion.
Deion, Deone, Deonn, Deonno

Deondre (French) a form of Deandre.
Deiondray, Deiondre, Deondra, Deondrae, Deondray, Deondré, Deondrea, Deondree, Deondrei, Deondrey, Diondra, Diondrae, Diondre, Diondrey

Deontae (American) a combination of the prefix De + Dontae.
Deonta, Deontai, Deontay,
Deontaye, Deonte, Deonté, Deontea, Deonteya, Deonteye, Deontia, Deontre, Dionte

Deonte, Deonté (American) forms of Deontae.
D'Ante, Deante, Deontée, Deontie

Deontre (American) forms of Deontae.
Deontrae, Deontrais, Deontray, Deontrea, Deontrey, Deontrez, Deontreze, Deontrus

Dequan (American) a combination of the prefix De + Quan.
Dequain, Dequane, Dequann, Dequante, Dequantez, Dequantis, Dequaun, Dequavius, Dequawn, Dequian, Dequin, Dequine, Dequinn, Dequion, Dequoin, Dequon, Deqwan, Deqwon, Deqwone

Dereck, Derick (German) forms of Derek.
Derekk, Dericka, Derico, Deriek, Derique, Deryck, Deryk, Deryke, Detrek

Derek (German) a short form of Theodoric. See also Dedrick, Dirk.
Darek, Darick, Darrick, Derak, Dereck, Derecke, Derele, Deric, Derick, Derik, Derk, Derke, Derrek, Derrick, Deryek

Deric, Derik (German) forms of Derek.
Deriek, Derikk

Dermot (Irish) free from envy. (English) free. (Hebrew) a short form of Jeremiah. See also Kermit.
Der, Dermod, Dermott, Diarmid, Diarmuid

Deron (Hebrew) bird; freedom. (American) a combination of the prefix De + Ron.
Daaron, Daron, Da-Ron, Darone, Darron, Dayron, Dereon, Deronn, Deronne, Derrin, Derrion, Derron, Derronn, Derronne, Derryn, Diron, Düron, Durron, Dyron

Deror (Hebrew) lover of freedom.
Derori, Derorie

Derrek (German) a form of Derek.
Derrec, Derreck

Derrell (French) a form of Darrell.
Derel, Derele, Derell, Derelle, Derrel, Dérrell, Derriel, Derril, Derrill, Deryl, Deryll

Derren (Irish, English) a form of Darren.
Deren, Derran, Derraun, Derreon, Derrian, Derrien, Derrin, Derrion, Derron, Derryn, Deryan, Deryn, Deryon

Derrick (German) ruler of the people. A form of Derek.
Derric, Derrik, Derryck, Derryk

Derry (Irish) redhead. Geography: a city in Northern Ireland.
Darrie, Darry, Derri, Derrie, Derrye, Dery

Derryl (French) a form of Darryl.
Deryl, Deryll

Derward (English) deer keeper.

Derwin (English) a form of Darwin.
Derwyn

Desean (American) a combination of the prefix De + Sean.
Dasean, D'Sean, Dusean

Deshane (American) a combination of the prefix De + Shane.
Deshan, Deshayne

Deshaun (American) a combination of the prefix De + Shaun.
Deshan, Deshane, Deshann, Deshaon, Deshaune, D'shaun, D'Shaun, Dushaun

Deshawn (American) a combination of the prefix De + Shawn.
Dashaun, Dashawn, Deshauwn, Deshawan, Deshawon, Deshon, D'shawn, D'Shawn, Dushan, Dushawn

Deshea (American) a combination of the prefix De + Shea.
Deshay

Déshì (Chinese) virtuous.

Deshon (American) a form of Deshawn.
Deshondre, Deshone, Deshonn, Deshonte, Deshun, Deshunn

Desiderio (Spanish) desired.

Desmond (Irish) from south Munster.
Demond, Des, Desi, Desimon, Desman, Desmand, Desmane, Desmen, Desmine, Desmon, Desmound, Desmund, Desmyn, Dezmon, Dezmond

Destin (French) destiny, fate.
Destan, Desten, Destine, Deston, Destry, Destyn

Destry (American) a form of Destin.
Destrey, Destrie

Detrick (German) a form of Dedrick.
Detrek, Detric, Detrich, Detrik, Detrix

Devan (Irish) a form of Devin.
Devaan, Devain, Devane, Devann, Devean, Devun, Diwan

Devante (American) a combination of Devan + the suffix Te.
Devanta, Devantae, Devantay, Devanté, Devantée, Devantez, Devanty, Devaughntae, Devaughnte, Devaunte, Deventae, Deventay, Devente, Divante

Devaughn (American) a form of Devin.
Devaugh, Devaun

Devayne (American) a form of Dewayne.
Devain, Devaine, Devan, Devane, Devayn, Devein, Deveion

Deven (Hindi) for God. (Irish) a form of Devin.
Deaven, Deiven, Devein, Devenn, Devven, Diven

Deverell (English) riverbank.

Devin (Irish) poet.
Deavin, Deivin, Dev, Devan, Devaughn, Deven, Devlyn, Devon, Devvin, Devy, Devyn, Dyvon

Devine (Latin) divine. (Irish) ox.
Davon, Devinn, Devon, Devyn, Devyne, Dewine

Devlin (Irish) brave, fierce.
Dev, Devlan, Devland, Devlen, Devlon, Devlyn

Devon (Irish) a form of Devin.
Deavon, Deivon, Deivone, Deivonne, Deveon, Deveone, Devion, Devoen, Devohn, Devonae, Devone, Devoni, Devonio, Devonn, Devonne, Devontaine, Devvon, Devvonne, Dewon, Dewone, Divon, Diwon

Devonta (American) a combination of Devon + the suffix Ta.
Deveonta, Devonnta, Devonntae, Devontae, Devontai, Devontay, Devontaye

Devonte (American) a combination of Devon + the suffix Te.
Deveonte, Devionte, Devonté, Devontea, Devontee, Devonti, Devontia, Devontre

Devyn (Irish) a form of Devin.
Devyin, Devynn, Devynne

Dewayne (Irish) a form of Dwayne. (American) a combination of the prefix De + Wayne.
Deuwayne, Devayne, Dewain, Dewaine, Dewan, Dewane, Dewaun, Dewaune, Dewayen, Dewean, Dewon, Dewune

Dewei (Chinese) highly virtuous.

Dewey (Welsh) prized.
Dew, Dewi, Dewie

DeWitt (Flemish) blond.
Dewitt, Dwight, Wit

Dexter (Latin) dexterous, adroit. (English) fabric dyer.
Daxter, Decca, Deck, Decka, Dekka, Dex, Dextar, Dextor, Dextrel, Dextron

Dezmon, Dezmond (Irish) forms of Desmond.
Dezman, Dezmand, Dezmen, Dezmin

Diamond (English) brilliant gem; bright guardian.
Diaman, Diamanta, Diamante, Diamend, Diamenn, Diamont, Diamonta, Diamonte, Diamund, Dimond, Dimonta, Dimontae, Dimonte

Dick (German) a short form of Frederick, Richard.
Dic, Dicken, Dickens, Dickie, Dickon, Dicky, Dik

Dickran (Armenian) History: an ancient Armenian king.
Dicran, Dikran

Dickson (English) son of Dick.
Dickenson, Dickerson, Dikerson, Diksan

Didi (Hebrew) a familiar form of Jedidiah, Yedidyah.

Didier (French) desired, longed for.

Diedrich (German) a form of Dedrick, Dietrich.
Didrich, Didrick, Didrik, Diederick

Diego (Spanish) a form of Jacob, James.
Iago, Diaz, Jago

Dietbald (German) a form of Theobald.
Dietbalt, Dietbolt

Dieter (German) army of the people.
Deiter

Dietrich (German) a form of Dedrick.
Deitrich, Deitrick, Deke, Diedrich, Dietrick, Dierck, Dieter, Dieterich, Dieterick, Dietz

Digby (Irish) ditch town; dike town.

Dillan (Irish) a form of Dillon.
Dilan, Dillian, Dilun, Dilyan

Dillon (Irish) loyal, faithful. See also Dylan.
Daylon, Delon, Dil, Dill, Dillan, Dillen, Dillie, Dillin, Dillion, Dilly, Dillyn, Dilon, Dilyn, Dilynn

Dilwyn (Welsh) shady place.
Dillwyn

Dima (Russian) a familiar form of Vladimir.
Dimka

Dimitri (Russian) a form of Demetrius.
Dimetra, Dimetri, Dimetric, Dimetrie, Dimitr, Dimitric, Dimitrie, Dimitrik, Dimitris, Dimitry, Dimmy, Dmitri, Dymitr, Dymitry

Dimitrios (Greek) a form of Demetrius.
Dhimitrios, Dimitrius, Dimos, Dmitrios

Dimitrius (Greek) a form of Demetrius.
Dimetrius, Dimitricus, Dimitrius, Dimetrus, Dmitrius

Dingbang (Chinese) protector of the country.

Dinh (Vietnamese) calm, peaceful.
Din

Dino (German) little sword. (Italian) a form of Dean.
Deano

Dinos (Greek) a familiar form of Constantine, Konstantin.

Dinsmore (Irish) fortified hill.
Dinnie, Dinny, Dinse

Diogenes (Greek) honest. History: an ancient philosopher who searched with a lantern in daylight for an honest man.
Diogenese

Dion (Greek) a short form of Dennis, Dionysus.
Deion, Deon, Dio, Dione, Dionigi, Dionis, Dionn, Dionne, Diontae, Dionte, Diontray

Dionte (American) a form of Deontae.
Diante, Dionta, Diontae, Diontay, Diontaye, Dionté, Diontea

Dionysus (Greek) celebration. Mythology: the god of wine.
Dion, Dionesios, Dionicio, Dionisio, Dionisios, Dionusios, Dionysios, Dionysius, Dunixi

Diquan (American) a combination of the prefix Di + Quan.
Diqawan, Diqawn, Diquane

Dirk (German) a short form of Derek, Theodoric.
Derk, Dirck, Dirke, Durc, Durk, Dyrk

Dixon (English) son of Dick.
Dickson, Dix

Dmitri (Russian) a form of Dimitri.
Dmetriy, Dmitiri, Dmitri, Dmitrik, Dmitriy

Doane (English) low, rolling hills.
Doan

Dob (English) a familiar form of Robert.
Dobie

Dobry (Polish) good.

Doherty (Irish) harmful.
Docherty, Dougherty, Douherty

Dolan (Irish) dark haired.
Dolin, Dolyn

Dolf, Dolph (German) short forms of Adolf, Adolph, Rudolf, Rudolph.
Dolfe, Dolfi, Dolphe, Dolphus

Dom (Latin) a short form of Dominic.
Dome, Domó

Domenic (Latin) an alternate form of Dominic.
Domanick, Domenick

Domenico (Italian) a form of Dominic.
Domenic, Domicio, Dominico, Menico

Domingo (Spanish) born on Sunday. See also Mingo.
Demingo, Domingos

Dominic (Latin) belonging to the Lord. See also Chuminga.
Deco, Demenico, Dom, Domanic, Domeka, Domenic, Domenico, Domini, Dominie, Dominik, Dominique, Dominitric, Dominy, Domminic, Domnenique, Domokos, Domonic, Nick

Dominick (Latin) a form of Dominic.
Domiku, Domineck, Dominick, Dominicke, Dominiek, Dominik, Dominnick, Dominyck, Domminick, Dommonick, Domnick, Domokos, Domonick, Donek, Dumin

Dominik (Latin) an alternte form of Dominic.
Domenik, Dominiko, Dominyk, Domonik

Dominique (French) a form of Dominic.
Domeniq, Domeniqu, Domenique, Domenque, Dominiqu, Dominque, Dominiqueia, Domnenique, Domnique, Domoniqu, Domonique, Domunique

Domokos (Hungarian) a form of Dominic.
Dedo, Dome, Domek, Domok, Domonkos

Don (Scottish) a short form of Donald. See also Kona.
Donn

Donahue (Irish) dark warrior.
Donohoe, Donohue

Donal (Irish) a form of Donald.

Donald (Scottish) world leader; proud ruler. See also Bohdan, Tauno.
Don, Donal, Dónal, Donaldo, Donall, Donalt, Donát, Donaugh, Donnie

Donatien (French) gift.
Donathan, Donathon

Donato (Italian) gift.
Dodek, Donatello, Donati, Donatien, Donatus

Donavan (Irish) a form of Donovan.
Donaven, Donavin, Donavon, Donavyn

Dondre (French) a form of Deandre.
Dondra, Dondrae, Dondray, Dondré, Dondrea

Dong (Vietnamese) easterner.
Duong

Donkor (Akan) humble.

Donnell (Irish) brave; dark.
Doneal, Donel, Donele, Donell, Donelle, Donnel, Donnele, Donnelly, Doniel, Donielle, Donnel, Donnelle, Donniel, Donyel, Donyell

Donnelly (Irish) a form of Donnell.
Donelly, Donlee, Donley

Donnie, Donny (Irish) familiar forms of Donald.

Donovan (Irish) dark warrior.
Dohnovan, Donavan, Donevan, Donevon, Donivan, Donnivan, Donnovan, Donnoven, Donoven, Donovin, Donovon, Donvan

Dontae, Donté (American) forms of Dante.
Donta, Dontai, Dontao, Dontate, Dontavious, Dontavius, Dontay, Dontaye, Dontea, Dontee, Dontez

Dontrell (American) a form
of Dantrell.
*Dontral, Dontrall, Dontray,
Dontre, Dontreal, Dontrel,
Dontrelle, Dontriel, Dontriell*

Donzell (Cornish) a form of
Denzell.
*Donzeil, Donzel, Donzelle,
Donzello*

Dooley (Irish) dark hero.
Dooly

Dor (Hebrew) generation.

Doran (Greek, Hebrew) gift.
(Irish) stranger; exile.
*Dore, Dorin, Dorran, Doron,
Dorren, Dory*

Dorian (Greek) from Doris,
Greece. See also Isidore.
*Dore, Dorey, Dorie, Dorien,
Dorin, Dorion, Dorján, Doron,
Dorrian, Dorrien, Dorrin,
Dorrion, Dorron, Dorryen,
Dory*

Dorrell (Scottish) king's doorkeeper. See also Durell.
Dorrel, Dorrelle

Dotan (Hebrew) law.
Dothan

Doug (Scottish) a short form
of Dougal, Douglas.
*Dougie, Dougy, Dugey, Dugie,
Dugy*

Dougal (Scottish) dark
stranger. See also Doyle.
*Doug, Dougall, Dugal, Dugald,
Dugall, Dughall*

Douglas (Scottish) dark river,
dark stream. See also
Koukalaka.
*Doug, Douglass, Dougles,
Dugaid, Dughlas*

Dov (Yiddish) bear. (Hebrew)
a familiar form of David.
Dovid, Dovidas, Dowid

Dovev (Hebrew) whisper.

Dow (Irish) dark haired.

Doyle (Irish) a form of
Dougal.
Doy, Doyal, Doyel

Drago (Italian) a form of
Drake.

Drake (English) dragon;
owner of the inn with the
dragon trademark.
Drago

Draper (English) fabric maker.
Dray, Draypr

Draven (American) a combi-
nation of the letter D +
Raven.
*Dravian, Dravin, Dravion,
Dravon, Dravone, Dravyn,
Drayven, Drevon*

Dreng (Norwegian) hired
hand; brave.

Dreshawn (American) a combination of Drew + Shawn.
Dreshaun, Dreshon, Dreshown

Drevon (American) a form of Draven.
Drevan, Drevaun, Dreven, Drevin, Drevion, Drevone

Drew (Welsh) wise. (English) a short form of Andrew.
Drewe, Dru

Dru (English) a form of Drew.
Druan, Drud, Drue, Drugi, Drui

Drummond (Scottish) druid's mountain.
Drummund, Drumond, Drumund

Drury (French) loving. Geography: Drury Lane is a street in London's theater district.

Dryden (English) dry valley.
Dry

Duane (Irish) a form of Dwayne.
Deune, Duain, Duaine, Duana

Duarte (Portuguese) rich guard. See also Edward.

Duc (Vietnamese) moral.
Duoc, Duy

Dudd (English) a short form of Dudley.
Dud, Dudde, Duddy

Dudley (English) common field.
Dudd, Dudly

Duer (Scottish) heroic.

Duff (Scottish) dark.
Duffey, Duffie, Duffy

Dugan (Irish) dark.
Doogan, Dougan, Douggan, Duggan

Duke (French) leader; duke.
Dukey, Dukie, Duky

Dukker (Gypsy) fortuneteller.

Dulani (Nguni) cutting.

Dumaka (Ibo) helping hand.

Duman (Turkish) misty, smoky.

Duncan (Scottish) brown warrior. Literature: King Duncan was Macbeth's victim in Shakespeare's play *Macbeth*.
Dunc, Dunn

Dunham (Scottish) brown.

Dunixi (Basque) a form of Dionysus.

Dunley (English) hilly meadow.

Dunlop (Scottish) muddy hill.

Dunmore (Scottish) fortress on the hill.

Dunn (Scottish) a short form of Duncan.
Dun, Dune, Dunne

Dunstan (English) brownstone fortress.
Dun, Dunston

Dunton (English) hill town.

Dur (Hebrew) stacked up. (English) a short form of Durwin.

Durand (Latin) a form of Durant.

Durant (Latin) enduring.
Duran, Durance, Durand, Durante, Durontae, Durrant

Durell (Scottish, English) king's doorkeeper. See also Dorrell.
Durel, Durial, Durreil, Durrell, Durrelle

Durko (Czech) a form of George.

Durriken (Gypsy) fortuneteller.

Durril (Gypsy) gooseberry.
Durrel, Durrell

Durward (English) gatekeeper.
Dur, Ward

Durwin (English) a form of Darwin.

Dushawn (American) a combination of the prefix Du + Shawn.
Dusan, Dusean, Dushan, Dushane, Dushaun, Dushon, Dushun

Dustin (German) valiant fighter. (English) brown rock quarry.
Dust, Dustain, Dustan, Dusten, Dustie, Dustine, Dustion, Duston, Dusty, Dustyn, Dustynn

Dusty (English) a familiar form of Dustin.
Dustyn (English) a form of Dustin.

Dutch (Dutch) from the Netherlands; from Germany.

Duval (French) a combination of the prefix Du + Val.
Duvall, Duveuil

Dwaun (American) a form of Dajuan.
Dwan, Dwaunn, Dwawn, Dwon, Dwuann

Dwayne (Irish) dark. See also Dewayne.
Dawayne, Dawyne, Duane, Duwain, Duwan, Duwane, Duwayn, Duwayne, Dwain, Dwaine, Dwan, Dwane, Dwyane, Dywan, Dywane, Dywayne, Dywone

Dwight (English) a form of DeWitt.

Dyami (Native American) soaring eagle.

Dyer (English) fabric dyer.

Dyke (English) dike; ditch.
Dike

Dylan (Welsh) sea. See also Dillon.
Dylane, Dylann, Dylen, Dylian, Dylin, Dyllan, Dyllen, Dyllian, Dyllin, Dyllyn, Dylon, Dylyn

Dylon (Welsh) a form of Dylan.
Dyllion, Dyllon

Dyre (Norwegian) dear heart.

Dyson (English) a short form of Dennison.
Dysen, Dysonn

E

Ea (Irish) a form of Hugh.

Eachan (Irish) horseman.

Eagan (Irish) very mighty.
Egan, Egon

Eamon (Irish) a form of Edmond, Edmund.
Aimon, Eammon, Eamonn

Ean (English) a form of Ian.
Eaen, Eann, Eayon, Eion, Eon, Eyan, Eyon

Earl (Irish) pledge. (English) nobleman.
Airle, Earld, Earle, Earlie, Earlson, Early, Eorl, Erl, Erle, Errol

Earnest (English) a form of Ernest.
Earn, Earnesto, Earnie, Eranest

Easton (English) eastern town.
Eason, Easten, Eastin, Eastton

Eaton (English) estate on the river.
Eatton, Eton, Eyton

Eb (Hebrew) a short form of Ebenezer.
Ebb, Ebbie, Ebby

Eben (Hebrew) rock.
Eban, Ebin, Ebon

Ebenezer (Hebrew) foundation stone. Literature: Ebenezer Scrooge is a miserly character in Charles Dickens's *A Christmas Carol.*
Eb, Ebbaneza, Eben, Ebeneezer, Ebeneser, Ebenezar, Eveneser

Eberhard (German) courageous as a boar. See also Everett.
Eber, Ebere, Eberardo, Eberhardt, Evard, Everard, Everardo, Everhardt, Everhart

Ebner (English) a form of Abner.

Ebo (Fante) born on Tuesday.

Ed (English) a short form of Edgar, Edsel, Edward.
Edd

Edan (Scottish) fire.
Edain

Edbert (English) wealthy; bright.
Ediberto

Eddie (English) a familiar form of Edgar, Edsel, Edward.
Eddee, Eddy, Edi, Edie

Eddy (English) a form of Eddie.
Eddye, Edy

Edel (German) noble.
Adel, Edell, Edelmar, Edelweiss

Eden (Hebrew) delightful. Bible: the garden that was first home to Adam and Eve.
Eaden, Eadin, Edan, Edenson, Edin, Edyn, Eiden

Eder (Hebrew) flock.
Ederick, Edir

Edgar (English) successful spearman. See also Garek, Gerik, Medgar.
Ed, Eddie, Edek, Edgard, Edgardo, Edgars

Edgardo (Spanish) a form of Edgar.

Edison (English) son of Edward.
Eddison, Edisen, Edson

Edmond (English) a form of Edmund.
Eamon, Edmon, Edmonde, Edmondo, Edmondson, Esmond

Edmund (English) prosperous protector.
Eadmund, Eamon, Edmand, Edmaund, Edmond, Edmun, Edmundo, Edmunds

Edmundo (Spanish) a form of Edmund.
Edmando, Mundo

Edo (Czech) a form of Edward.

Edoardo (Italian) a form of Edward.

Edorta (Basque) a form of Edward.

Edouard (French) a form of Edward.
Édoard, Édouard

Edric (English) prosperous ruler.
Eddric, Eddrick, Ederick, Edrek, Edrice, Edrick, Edrico

Edsel (English) rich man's house.
Ed, Eddie, Edsell

Edson (English) a short form of Edison.
Eddson, Edsen

Eduardo (Spanish) a form of Edward.
Estuardo, Estvardo

Edur (Basque) snow.

Edward (English) prosperous guardian. See also Audie, Duarte, Ekewaka, Ned, Ted,

Teddy.
Ed, Eddie, Edik, Edko, Edo, Edoardo, Edorta, Édouard, Eduard, Eduardo, Edus, Edvard, Edvardo, Edwardo, Edwards, Edwy, Edzio, Ekewaka, Etzio, Ewart

Edwin (English) prosperous friend. See also Ned, Ted.
Eadwinn, Edik, Edlin, Eduino, Edwan, Edwen, Edwon, Edwyn

Efrain (Hebrew) fruitful.
Efran, Efrane, Efrayin, Efren, Efrian, Eifraine

Efrat (Hebrew) honored.

Efrem (Hebrew) a short form of Ephraim.
Efe, Efraim, Efrim, Efrum

Efren (Hebrew) a form of Efrain, Ephraim.

Egan (Irish) ardent, fiery.
Egann, Egen, Egon

Egbert (English) bright sword. See also Bert, Bertie.

Egerton (English) Edgar's town.
Edgarton, Edgartown, Edgerton, Egeton

Egil (Norwegian) awe inspiring.
Eigil

Eginhard (German) power of the sword.
Eginhardt, Einhard, Einhardt, Enno

Egon (German) formidable.

Egor (Russian) a form of George. See also Igor, Yegor.

Ehren (German) honorable.

Eikki (Finnish) ever powerful.

Einar (Scandinavian) individualist.
Ejnar, Inar

Eion (Irish) a form of Ean, Ian.
Eann, Eian, Ein, Eine, Einn

Eitan (Hebrew) a form of Ethan.
Eita, Eithan, Eiton

Ejau (Ateso) we have received.

Ekewaka (Hawaiian) a form of Edward.

Ekon (Nigerian) strong.

Elam (Hebrew) highlands.

Elan (Hebrew) tree. (Native American) friendly.
Elann

Elbert (English) a form of Albert.
Elberto

Elchanan (Hebrew) a form of John.
Elchan, Elchonon, Elhanan, Elhannan

Elden (English) a form of Alden, Aldous.
Eldan, Eldin

Elder (English) dweller near the elder trees.

Eldon (English) holy hill.

Eldred (English) a form of Aldred.
Eldrid

Eldridge (English) a form of Aldrich.
El, Eldred, Eldredge, Eldrege, Eldrid, Eldrige, Elric

Eldwin (English) a form of Aldwin.
Eldwinn, Eldwyn, Eldwynn

Eleazar (Hebrew) God has helped. See also Lazarus.
Elazar, Elazaro, Eleasar, Eléazar, Eliazar, Eliezer

Elek (Hungarian) a form of Alec, Alex.
Elec, Elic, Elik

Elger (German) a form of Alger.
Elger, Ellgar, Ellger

Elgin (English) noble; white.
Elgan, Elgen

Eli (Hebrew) uplifted. A short form of Elijah, Elisha. Bible: the high priest who trained the prophet Samuel. See also Elliot.
Elie, Elier, Ellie, Eloi, Eloy, Ely

Elia (Zuni) a short form of Elijah.
Eliah, Elio, Eliya, Elya

Elian (English) a form of Elijah. See also Trevelyan.
Elion

Elias (Greek) a form of Elijah.
Elia, Eliasz, Elice, Eliyas, Ellias, Ellice, Ellis, Elyas, Elyes

Eliazar (Hebrew) a form of Eleazar.
Eliasar, Eliazer, Elizar, Elizardo

Elie (Hebrew) a form of Eli.

Eliezer (Hebrew) a form of Eleazar.
Elieser

Elihu (Hebrew) a short form of Eliyahu.
Elih, Eliu, Ellihu

Elijah (Hebrew) a form of Eliyahu. Bible: a Hebrew prophet. See also Eli, Elisha, Elliot, Ilias, Ilya.
El, Elia, Elian, Elias, Elija, Elijha, Elijiah, Elijio, Elijuah, Elijuo, Elisjsha, Eliya, Eliyah, Ellis

Elika (Hawaiian) a form of Eric.

Eliseo (Hebrew) a form of Elisha.
Elisee, Elisée, Elisei, Elisiah, Elisio

Elisha (Hebrew) God is my salvation. Bible: a Hebrew prophet, successor to Elijah. See also Eli, Elijah.
Elijsha, Eliseo, Elish, Elishah,

Elisher, Elishia, Elishua, Elysha, Lisha

Eliyahu (Hebrew) the Lord is my God.
Eliyahou, Elihu

Elkan (Hebrew) God is jealous.
Elkana, Elkanah, Elkin, Elkins

Elki (Moquelumnan) hanging over the top.

Ellard (German) sacred; brave.
Allard, Ellerd

Ellery (English) from a surname derived from the name Hilary.
Ellary, Ellerey

Elliot, Elliott (English) forms of Eli, Elijah.
Elio, Eliot, Eliott, Eliud, Eliut, Elliotte, Elyot, Elyott

Ellis (English) a form of Elias.
Elis

Ellison (English) son of Ellis.
Elison, Ellson, Ellyson, Elson

Ellsworth (English) nobleman's estate.
Ellswerth, Elsworth

Elman (German) like an elm tree.
Elmen

Elmer (English) noble; famous.
Aylmer, Elemér, Ellmer, Elmir, Elmo

Elmo (Greek) lovable, friendly. (Italian) guardian. (Latin) a familiar form of Anselm. (English) a form of Elmer.

Elmore (English) moor where the elm trees grow.

Elonzo (Spanish) a form of Alonzo.
Elon, Élon, Elonso

Eloy (Latin) chosen.
Eloi

Elrad (Hebrew) God rules.
Rad, Radd

Elroy (French) a form of Delroy, Leroy.
Elroi

Elsdon (English) nobleman's hill.

Elston (English) noble's town.
Ellston

Elsu (Native American) swooping, soaring falcon.

Elsworth (English) noble's estate.

Elton (English) old town.
Alton, Eldon, Ellton, Elthon, Eltonia

Elvern (Latin) a form of Alvern.
Elver, Elverne

Elvin (English) a form of Alvin.
El, Elvyn, Elwin, Elwyn, Elwynn

Elvio (Spanish) light skinned; blond.

Elvis (Scandinavian) wise.
El, Elviz, Elvys

Elvy (English) elfin warrior.

Elwell (English) old well.

Elwood (English) old forest. See also Wood, Woody.

Ely (Hebrew) a form of Eli. Geography: a region of England with extensive drained fens.
Elya, Elyie

Eman (Czech) a form of Emmanuel.
Emaney, Emani

Emanuel (Hebrew) a form of Emmanuel.
Emaniel, Emannual, Emannuel, Emanual, Emanueal, Emanuele, Emanuell, Emanuell, Emanuelle

Emerson (German, English) son of Emery.
Emmerson, Emreson

Emery (German) industrious leader.
Aimery, Emari, Emarri, Emeri, Emerich, Emerio, Emmerich, Emmerie, Emmery, Emmo, Emory, Emrick, Emry, Inre, Imrich

Emil (Latin) flatterer. (German) industrious. See also Milko, Milo.
Aymil, Emiel, Émile, Emilek,
Emiliano, Emilio, Emill, Emils, Emilyan, Emlyn

Émile (French) a form of Emil.
Emiel, Emile, Emille

Emiliano (Italian) a form of Emil.
Emilian, Emilion

Emilien (Latin) friendly; industrious.

Emilio (Italian, Spanish) a form of Emil.
Emielio, Emileo, Emilio, Emilios, Emillio, Emilo

Emlyn (Welsh) waterfall.
Emelen, Emlen, Emlin

Emmanuel (Hebrew) God is with us. See also Immanuel, Maco, Mango, Manuel.
Eman, Emanuel, Emanuell, Emek, Emmahnuel, Emmanel, Emmaneuol, Emmanle, Emmanual, Emmanueal, Emmanuele, Emmanuell, Emmanuelle, Emmanuil, Enmanuel

Emmett (German) industrious; strong. (English) ant. History: Robert Emmett was an Irish patriot.
Em, Emet, Emett, Emitt, Emmet, Emmette, Emmitt, Emmot, Emmott, Emmy

Emmitt (German, English) a form of Emmett.
Emmit

Emory (German) a form of
Emery.
Amory, Emmory, Emorye

Emre (Turkish) brother.
Emra, Emrah, Emreson

Emrick (German) a form of
Emery.
*Emeric, Emerick, Emric,
Emrique, Emryk*

Enapay (Sioux) brave appearance; he appears.

Endre (Hungarian) a form of
Andrew.
Ender

Eneas (Greek) a form of
Aeneas.
Eneias, Enné

Engelbert (German) bright as
an angel. See also Ingelbert.
Bert, Englebert

Enli (Dene) that dog over
there.

Ennis (Greek) mine. (Scottish)
a form of Angus.
Eni, Enni

Enoch (Hebrew) dedicated,
consecrated. Bible: the father
of Methuselah.
Enoc, Enock, Enok

Enos (Hebrew) man.
Enosh

Enric (Romanian) a form of
Henry.
Enrica

Enrick (Spanish) a form of
Henry.
Enricky

Enrico (Italian) a form of
Henry.
Enzio, Enzo, Rico

Enrikos (Greek) a form of
Henry.

Enrique (Spanish) a form of
Henry. See also Quiqui.
*Enrigué, Enriqué, Enriquez,
Enrrique*

Enver (Turkish) bright; handsome.

Enyeto (Native American)
walks like a bear.

Enzi (Swahili) powerful.

Eoin (Welsh) a form of Evan.

Ephraim (Hebrew) fruitful.
Bible: the second son of
Joseph.
*Efraim, Efrayim, Efrem, Efren,
Ephraen, Ephrain, Ephram,
Ephrem, Ephriam*

Erasmus (Greek) lovable.
Érasme, Erasmo, Rasmus

Erastus (Greek) beloved.
Éraste, Erastious, Ras, Rastus

Erbert (German) a short form
of Herbert.
Ebert, Erberto

Ercole (Italian) splendid gift.

Erek (Scandinavian) a form of
Eric.
Erec

Erhard (German) strong; resolute.
Erhardt, Erhart

Eriberto (Italian) a form of
Herbert.
Erberto, Heriberto

Eric (Scandinavian) ruler of all.
(English) brave ruler.
(German) a short form of
Frederick. History: Eric the
Red was a Norwegian
explorer who founded
Greenland's first colony.
*Aric, Ehrich, Elika, Erek, Éric,
Erica, Ericc, Erich, Erick, Erico,
Erik, Erikur, Erric, Eryc, Rick*

Erich (Czech, German) a form
of Eric.

Erick (English) a form of Eric.
Errick, Eryck

Erickson (English) son of Eric.
*Erickzon, Erics, Ericson, Ericsson,
Erikson, Erikzzon, Eriqson*

Erik (Scandinavian) a form of
Eric.
*Erek, Erike, Eriks, Erikur,
Errick, Errik, Eryk*

Erikur (Icelandic) a form of
Eric, Erik.

Erin (Irish) peaceful. History:
an ancient name for Ireland.
*Erine, Erinn, Erino, Eron,
Errin, Eryn, Erynn*

Erland (English) nobleman's
land.
Erlend

Erling (English) nobleman's
son.

Ermanno (Italian) a form of
Herman.
Erman

Ermano (Spanish) a form of
Herman.
Ermin, Ermine, Erminio, Ermon

Ernest (English) earnest, sincere. See also Arno.
*Earnest, Ernestino, Ernesto,
Ernestus, Ernie, Erno, Ernst*

Ernesto (Spanish) a form of
Ernest.
Ernester, Neto

Ernie (English) a familiar form
of Ernest.
Earnie, Erney, Erny

Erno (Hungarian) a form of
Ernest.
Ernö

Ernst (German) a form of
Ernest.
Erns

Erol (Turkish) strong, courageous.
Eroll

Eron (Irish) a form of Erin.
Erran, Erren, Errion, Erron

Errando (Basque) bold.

Errol (Latin) wanderer.
(English) a form of Earl.
Erol, Erold, Erroll, Erryl

Erroman (Basque) from Rome.

Erskine (Scottish) high cliff.
(English) from Ireland.
Ersin, Erskin, Kinny

Ervin, Erwin (English) sea
friend. Forms of Irving,
Irwin.
*Earvin, Erv, Erven, Ervyn,
Erwan, Erwinek, Erwinn,
Erwyn, Erwynn*

Ervine (English) a form of
Irving.
*Erv, Ervin, Ervince, Erving,
Ervins*

Esau (Hebrew) rough; hairy.
Bible: Jacob's twin brother.
Esaw

Esequiel (Hebrew) a form of
Ezekiel.

Eshkol (Hebrew) grape clusters.

Eskil (Norwegian) god vessel.

Esmond (English) rich protector.

Espen (Danish) bear of the gods.

Essien (Ochi) sixth-born son.

Este (Italian) east.
Estes

Estéban (Spanish) a form of
Stephen.
*Estabon, Esteben, Estefan,
Estefano, Estefen, Estephan,
Estephen*

Estebe (Basque) a form of
Stephen.

Estevan (Spanish) a form of
Stephen.
Esteven, Estevon, Estiven

Estevao (Spanish) a form of
Stephen.
Estevez

Ethan (Hebrew) strong; firm.
*Eathan, Eathen, Eathon,
Eeathen, Eitan, Etan, Ethaen,
Ethe, Ethen, Ethian*

Étienne (French) a form of
Stephen.
Etian, Etien, Étienn, Ettien

Ettore (Italian) steadfast.
Etor, Etore

Etu (Native American) sunny.

Euclid (Greek) intelligent.
History: the founder of
Euclidean geometry.

Eugen (German) a form of
Eugene.

Eugene (Greek) born to
nobility. See also Ewan,
Gene, Gino, Iukini, Jenö,
Yevgenyi, Zenda.
*Eoghan, Eugen, Eugéne,
Eugeni, Eugenio, Eugenius,
Evgeny, Ezven*

Eugenio (Spanish) a form of Eugene.

Eulises (Latin) a form of Ulysses.

Eustace (Greek) productive. (Latin) stable, calm. See also Stacey.
Eustache, Eustachius, Eustachy, Eustashe, Eustasius, Eustatius, Eustazio, Eustis, Eustiss

Evan (Irish) young warrior. (English) a form of John. See also Bevan, Owen.
Eavan, Eoin, Ev, Evaine, Evann, Evans, Even, Evens, Evin, Evon, Evyn, Ewan, Ewen

Evangelos (Greek) a form of Andrew.
Evagelos, Evaggelos, Evangelo

Evelyn (English) hazelnut.
Evelin

Everardo (German) strong as a boar.
Everado

Everett (English) a form of Eberhard.
Ev, Evered, Everet, Everette, Everhett, Everit, Everitt, Everrett, Evert, Evrett

Everley (English) boar meadow.
Everlea, Everlee

Everton (English) boar town.

Evgeny (Russian) a form of Eugene. See also Zhek.
Evgeni, Evgenij, Evgenyi

Evin (Irish) a form of Evan.
Evian, Evinn, Evins

Ewald (German) always powerful. (English) powerful lawman.

Ewan (Scottish) a form of Eugene, Evan. See also Keon.
Euan, Euann, Euen, Ewen, Ewhen

Ewert (English) ewe herder, shepherd.
Ewart

Ewing (English) friend of the law.
Ewin, Ewynn

Exavier (Basque) a form of Xavier.
Exaviar, Exavior, Ezavier

Eyota (Native American) great.

Ezekiel (Hebrew) strength of God. Bible: a Hebrew prophet. See also Haskel, Zeke.
Esequiel, Ezakeil, Ezéchiel, Ezeck, Ezeckiel, Ezeeckel, Ezekeial, Ezekeil, Ezekeyial, Ezekial, Ezekielle, Ezell, Ezequiel, Eziakah, Eziechiele

Ezequiel (Hebrew) a form of Ezekiel.
Esequiel, Eziequel

Ezer (Hebrew) a form of Ezra.

Ezra (Hebrew) helper; strong.
Bible: a Jewish priest who
led the Jews back to
Jerusalem.
*Esdras, Esra, Ezer, Ezera,
Ezrah, Ezri, Ezry*

Ezven (Czech) a form of
Eugene.
Esven, Esvin, Ezavin, Ezavine

F

Faber (German) a form of
Fabian.

Fabian (Latin) bean grower.
*Fabain, Fabayan, Fabe, Fabein,
Fabek, Fabeon, Faber, Fabert,
Fabi, Fabiano, Fabien, Fabin,
Fabio, Fabion, Fabius, Fabiyan,
Fabiyus, Fabyan, Fabyen,
Faybian, Faybien*

Fabiano (Italian) a form of
Fabian.
Fabianno, Fabio

Fabio (Latin) a form of
Fabian. (Italian) a short form
of Fabiano.
Fabbio

Fabrizio (Italian) craftsman.
Fabrice, Fabricio, Fabrizius

Fabron (French) little blacksmith; apprentice.
Fabre, Fabroni

Fadey (Ukrainian) a form of
Thaddeus.
*Faday, Faddei, Faddey, Faddy,
Fade, Fadeyka, Fadie, Fady*

Fadi (Arabic) redeemer.
Fadhi

Fadil (Arabic) generous.
Fadeel, Fadel

Fagan (Irish) little fiery one.
Fagin

Fahd (Arabic) lynx.
Fahaad, Fahad

Fai (Chinese) beginning.

Fairfax (English) blond.
Fair, Fax

Faisal (Arabic) decisive.
*Faisel, Faisil, Faisl, Faiyaz,
Faiz, Faizal, Faize, Faizel,
Faizi, Fasel, Fasil, Faysal,
Fayzal, Fayzel*

Fakhir (Arabic) excellent.
Fahkry, Fakher

Fakih (Arabic) thinker; reader
of the Koran.

Falco (Latin) falconer.
Falcon, Falk, Falke, Falken

Falito (Italian) a familiar form
of Rafael, Raphael.

Falkner (English) trainer of
falcons. See also Falco.
*Falconer, Falconner, Faulconer,
Faulconner, Faulkner*

Fane (English) joyful, glad.
Fanes, Faniel

Faraji (Swahili) consolation.

Farid (Arabic) unique.

Faris (Arabic) horseman.
*Faraz, Fares, Farhaz, Farice,
Fariez, Farris*

Farley (English) bull meadow;
sheep meadow. See also Lee.
*Fairlay, Fairlee, Fairleigh,
Fairley, Fairlie, Far, Farlay,
Farlee, Farleigh, Farlie, Farly,
Farrleigh, Farrley*

Farnell (English) fern-covered
hill.
*Farnall, Fernald, Fernall,
Furnald*

Farnham (English) field of
ferns.
Farnam, Farnum, Fernham

Farnley (English) fern
meadow.
*Farnlea, Farnlee, Farnleigh,
Farnly, Fernlea, Fernlee,
Fernleigh, Fernley*

Faroh (Latin) a form of
Pharaoh.

Farold (English) mighty traveler.

Farquhar (Scottish) dear.
*Fark, Farq, Farquar, Farquarson,
Farque, Farquharson, Farquy,
Farqy*

Farr (English) traveler.
*Faer, Farran, Farren, Farrin,
Farrington, Farron*

Farrell (Irish) heroic; courageous.
Farrel, Farrill, Farryll, Ferrell

Farrow (English) piglet.

Farruco (Spanish) a form of
Francis, Francisco.
Frascuelo

Faruq (Arabic) honest.
*Farook, Farooq, Faroque,
Farouk, Faruqh*

Faste (Norwegian) firm.

Fath (Arabic) victor.

Fatin (Arabic) clever.

Faust (Latin) lucky, fortunate.
History: the sixteenth-cen-
tury German necromancer
who inspired many legends.
*Faustino, Faustis, Fausto,
Faustus*

Faustino (Italian) a form of
Faust.

Fausto (Italian) a form of
Faust.

Favian (Latin) understanding.
Favain, Favio, Favyen

Faxon (German) long-haired.

Federico (Italian, Spanish) a
form of Frederick.
Federic, Federigo, Federoquito

Feivel (Yiddish) God aids.

Feliks (Russian) a form of
Felix.

Felipe (Spanish) a form of
Philip.
*Feeleep, Felipino, Felo, Filip,
Filippo, Filips, Fillip, Flip*

Felippo (Italian) a form of
Philip.
*Felip, Filippo, Lipp, Lippo, Pip,
Pippo*

Felix (Latin) fortunate; happy.
See also Pitin.
*Fee, Felic, Félice, Feliciano,
Felicio, Felike, Feliks, Felo,
Félix, Felizio, Phelix*

Felton (English) field town.
Felten, Feltin

Fenton (English) marshland
farm.
*Fen, Fennie, Fenny, Fintan,
Finton*

Feodor (Slavic) a form of
Theodore.
*Dorek, Fedar, Fedinka, Fedor,
Fedya, Fyodor*

Feoras (Greek) smooth rock.

Ferdinand (German) daring,
adventurous. See also
Hernando.
*Feranado, Ferd, Ferda, Ferdie,
Ferdinánd, Ferdy, Ferdynand,
Fernando, Nando*

Ferenc (Hungarian) a form of
Francis.
Feri, Ferke, Ferko

Fergus (Irish) strong; manly.
*Fearghas, Fearghus, Feargus,
Ferghus, Fergie, Ferguson,
Fergusson*

Fermin (French, Spanish) firm,
strong.
Ferman, Firmin, Furman

Fernando (Spanish) a form of
Ferdinand.
*Ferando, Ferdinando, Ferdnando,
Ferdo, Fernand, Fernandez,
Fernendo*

Feroz (Persian) fortunate.

Ferran (Arabic) baker.
Feran, Feron, Ferrin, Ferron

Ferrand (French) iron gray
hair.
*Farand, Farrand, Farrant,
Ferrant*

Ferrell (Irish) a form of
Farrell.
Ferrel, Ferrill, Ferryl

Ferris (Irish) a form of Peter.
*Fares, Faris, Fariz, Farris,
Farrish, Feris, Ferriss*

Fico (Spanish) a familiar form
of Frederick.

Fidel (Latin) faithful. History:
Fidel Castro was the Cuban
revolutionary who overthrew
a dictatorship in 1959 and
established a communist
regime in Cuba.
*Fidele, Fidèle, Fidelio, Fidelis,
Fidell, Fido*

Field (English) a short form of
Fielding.
Fields

Fielding (English) field; field
worker.
Field

Fife (Scottish) from Fife,
Scotland.
Fyfe

Fifi (Fante) born on Friday.

Fil (Polish) a form of Phil.
Filipek

Filbert (English) brilliant. See
also Bert.
*Filberte, Filberto, Filiberto,
Philbert*

Filiberto (Spanish) a form of
Filbert.

Filip (Greek) a form of Philip.
Filip, Filippo

Fillipp (Russian) a form of
Philip.
*Filip, Filipe, Filipek, Filips, Fill,
Fillip, Filya*

Filmore (English) famous.
*Fillmore, Filmer, Fyllmer,
Fylmer, Philmore*

Filya (Russian) a form of Philip.

Fineas (Irish) a form of Phineas.
Finneas

Finian (Irish) light skinned;
white.
*Finnen, Finnian, Fionan,
Fionn, Phinean*

Finlay (Irish) blond-haired
soldier.
*Findlay, Findley, Finlea, Finlee,
Finley, Finn, Finnlea, Finnley*

Finn (German) from Finland.
(Irish) blond haired; light
skinned. A short form of
Finlay. (Norwegian) from
the Lapland.
Fin, Finnie, Finnis, Finny

Finnegan (Irish) light skinned;
white.
Finegan

Fiorello (Italian) little flower.
Fiore

Firas (Arabic) persistent.

Firman (French) firm; strong.
Ferman, Firmin

Firth (English) woodland.

Fischel (Yiddish) a form of
Phillip.

Fiske (English) fisherman.
Fisk

Fitch (English) weasel, ermine.
Fitche

Fitz (English) son.
Filz

Fitzgerald (English) son of
Gerald.

Fitzhugh (English) son of
Hugh.
Hugh

Fitzpatrick (English) son of Patrick.

Fitzroy (Irish) son of Roy.

Flaminio (Spanish) Religion: Marcantonio Flaminio coauthored one of the most important texts of the Italian Reformation.

Flann (Irish) redhead.
Flainn, Flannan, Flannery

Flavian (Latin) blond, yellow haired.
Flavel, Flavelle, Flavien, Flavio, Flawiusz

Flavio (Italian) a form of Flavian.
Flabio, Flavious, Flavius

Fleming (English) from Denmark; from Flanders.
Flemming, Flemmyng, Flemyng

Fletcher (English) arrow featherer, arrow maker.
Flecher, Fletch

Flint (English) stream; flint stone.
Flynt

Flip (Spanish) a short form of Felipe. (American) a short form of Philip.

Florencio (Italian) a form of Florent.

Florent (French) flowering.
Florenci, Florencio, Florentin,
Florentino, Florentyn, Florentz, Florinio, Florino

Florian (Latin) flowering, blooming.
Florien, Florrian, Flory, Floryan

Floyd (English) a form of Lloyd.

Flurry (English) flourishing, blooming.

Flynn (Irish) son of the red-haired man.
Flin, Flinn, Flyn

Folke (German) a form of Volker.
Folker

Foluke (Yoruba) given to God.

Foma (Bulgarian, Russian) a form of Thomas.
Fomka

Fonso (German, Italian) a short form of Alphonso.
Fonzo

Fontaine (French) fountain.

Fonzie (German) a familiar form of Alphonse.
Fons, Fonsie, Fonsy, Fonz

Forbes (Irish) prosperous.
Forbe

Ford (English) a short form of names ending in "ford."

Fordel (Gypsy) forgiving.

Forest (French) a form of
Forrest.
Forestt, Foryst

Forester (English) forest
guardian.
*Forrester, Forrie, Forry, Forster,
Foss, Foster*

Forrest (French) forest;
woodsman.
*Forest, Forester, Forrestar,
Forrester, Forrestt, Forrie*

Fortino (Italian) fortunate,
lucky.

Fortune (French) fortunate,
lucky.
*Fortun, Fortunato, Fortuné,
Fortunio*

Foster (Latin) a short form of
Forester.

Fowler (English) trapper of
wildfowl.

Fran (Latin) a short form of
Francis.
Franh

Francesco (Italian) a form of
Francis.

Franchot (French) a form of
Francis.

Francis (Latin) free; from
France. Religion: Saint
Francis of Assisi was the
founder of the Franciscan
order. See also Farruco,
Ferenc.
Fran, France, Frances, Francesco,
*Franchot, Francisco, Franciskus,
Franco, François, Frang, Frank,
Frannie, Franny, Frans, Franscis,
Fransis, Franta, Frantisek,
Frants, Franus, Frantisek,
Franz, Frencis*

Francisco (Portuguese,
Spanish) a form of Francis.
See also Chilo, Cisco,
Farruco, Paco, Pancho.
*Franco, Fransisco, Fransysco,
Frasco, Frisco*

Franco (Latin) a short form of
Francis.
Franko

François (French) a form of
Francis.
Francoise

Frank (English) a short form
of Francis, Franklin. See also
Palani, Pancho.
*Franc, Franck, Franek, Frang,
Franio, Franke, Frankie, Franko*

Frankie (English) a familiar
form of Frank.
*Francky, Franke, Frankey,
Franki, Franky, Franqui*

Franklin (English) free
landowner.
*Fran, Francklen, Francklin,
Francklyn, Francylen, Frank,
Frankin, Franklen, Franklinn,
Franklyn, Franquelin*

Franklyn (English) a form of
Franklin.
Franklynn

Frans (Swedish) a form of
Francis.
Frants

Frantisek (Czech) a form of
Francis.
Franta

Franz (German) a form of
Francis.
*Fransz, Frantz, Franzen,
Franzie, Franzin, Franzl,
Franzy*

Fraser (French) strawberry.
(English) curly haired.
*Fraizer, Frasier, Fraze, Frazer,
Frazier*

Frayne (French) dweller at the
ash tree. (English) stranger.
*Fraine, Frayn, Frean, Freen,
Freyne*

Fred (German) a short form
of Alfred, Frederick,
Manfred.
Fredd, Fredde, Fredo, Fredson

Freddie (German) a familiar
form of Frederick.
Freddi, Freddy, Fredi, Fredy

Freddy, Fredy (German)
familiar forms of Frederick.

Frederic (German) a form of
Frederick.
*Frédéric, Frederich, Frederric,
Fredric, Fredrich*

Frederick (German) peaceful
ruler. See also Dick, Eric,
Fico, Peleke, Rick.
*Federico, Fico, Fred, Fredderick,
Freddie, Freddrick, Freddy,
Fredek, Frederic, Fréderick,
Frédérick, Frederik, Frederique,
Frederrick, Fredo, Fredrick,
Fredwick, Fredwyck, Fredy,
Friedrich, Fritz*

Frederico (Spanish) a form of
Frederick.
Fredrico, Frederigo

Frederik (German) a form of
Frederick.
Frédérik, Frederrik, Fredrik

Frederique (French) a form of
Frederick.

Fredo (Spanish) a form of
Fred.

Fredrick (German) a form of
Frederick.
Fredric, Fredricka, Fredricks

Freeborn (English) child of
freedom.
Free

Freeman (English) free.
*Free, Freedman, Freemin,
Freemon, Friedman, Friedmann*

Fremont (German) free; noble
protector.

Frewin (English) free; noble
friend.
Frewen

Frey (English) lord.
(Scandinavian) Mythology:
the Norse god who dispenses
peace and prosperity.

Frick (English) bold.

Fridolf (English) peaceful
wolf.
Freydolf, Freydulf, Fridulf

Friedrich (German) a form of
Frederick.
*Friedel, Friedrick, Fridrich,
Fridrick, Friedrike, Friedryk,
Fryderyk*

Frisco (Spanish) a short form
of Francisco.

Fritz (German) a familiar form
of Frederick.
Fritson, Fritts, Fritzchen, Fritzl

Frode (Norwegian) wise.

Fulbright (German) very
bright.
Fulbert

Fuller (English) cloth thickener.

Fulton (English) field near
town.

Funsoni (Nguni) requested.

Fyfe (Scottish) a form of Fife.
Fyffe

Fynn (Ghanaian) Geography:
another name for the Offin
River in Ghana.

Fyodor (Russian) a form of
Theodore.

G

Gabby (American) a familiar
form of Gabriel.
*Gabbi, Gabbie, Gabi, Gabie,
Gaby*

Gabe (Hebrew) a short form
of Gabriel.

Gabino (American) a form of
Gabriel.
Gabin, Gabrino

Gábor (Hungarian) God is my
strength.
Gabbo, Gabko, Gabo

Gabrial (Hebrew) a form of
Gabriel.
*Gaberial, Gabrael, Gabraiel,
Gabrail, Gabreal, Gabriael,
Gabrieal, Gabryalle*

Gabriel (Hebrew) devoted to
God. Bible: the angel of the
Annunciation.
*Gab, Gabe, Gabby, Gabino,
Gabis, Gábor, Gabreil, Gabrel,
Gabrell, Gabrial, Gabriël,
Gabriele, Gabriell, Gabrielle,
Gabrielli, Gabrile, Gabris,
Gabryel, Gabys, Gavril,
Gebereal, Ghabriel, Riel*

Gabrielli (Italian) a form of
Gabriel.
Gabriello

Gadi (Arabic) God is my fortune.
Gad, Gaddy, Gadiel

Gaetan (Italian) from Gaeta, a region in southern Italy.
Gaetano, Gaetono

Gage (French) pledge.
Gager, Gaige, Gaje

Gaige (French) a form of Gage.

Gair (Irish) small.
Gaer, Gearr, Geir

Gaius (Latin) rejoicer. See also Cai.

Galbraith (Irish) Scotsman in Ireland.
Galbrait, Galbreath

Gale (Greek) a short form of Galen.
Gael, Gail, Gaile, Gayle

Galen (Greek) healer; calm. (Irish) little and lively.
Gaelan, Gaelen, Gaelin, Gaelyn, Gailen, Galan, Gale, Galeno, Galin, Galyn, Gaylen

Galeno (Spanish) illuminated child. (Greek, Irish) a form of Galen.

Gallagher (Irish) eager helper.

Galloway (Irish) Scotsman in Ireland.
Gallway, Galway

Galt (Norwegian) high ground.

Galton (English) owner of a rented estate.
Gallton

Galvin (Irish) sparrow.
Gal, Gall, Gallven, Gallvin, Galvan, Galven

Gamal (Arabic) camel. See also Jamal.
Gamall, Gamel, Gamil

Gamble (Scandinavian) old.

Gan (Chinese) daring, adventurous. (Vietnamese) near.

Gannon (Irish) light skinned, white.
Gannan, Gannen, Gannie, Ganny

Ganya (Zulu) clever.

Gar (English) a short form of Gareth, Garnett, Garrett, Garvin.
Garr

Garcia (Spanish) mighty with a spear.

Gardner (English) gardener.
Gard, Gardener, Gardie, Gardiner, Gardy

Garek (Polish) a form of Edgar.

Garen (English) a form of Garry.
Garan, Garen, Garin, Garion, Garon, Garyn, Garyon

Gareth (Welsh) gentle.
Gar, Garith, Garreth, Garrith, Garth, Garyth

Garett (Irish) a form of Garrett.
Gared, Garet, Garette, Garhett, Garit, Garitt, Garritt

Garfield (English) field of spears; battlefield.

Garland (French) wreath of flowers; prize. (English) land of spears; battleground.
Garlan, Garlen, Garllan, Garlund, Garlyn

Garman (English) spearman.
Garmann, Garrman

Garner (French) army guard, sentry.
Garnier

Garnett (Latin) pomegranate seed; garnet stone. (English) armed with a spear.
Gar, Garnet, Garnie, Garrnett

Garnock (Welsh) dweller by the alder river.

Garrad (English) a form of Garrett.
Gared, Garrard, Garred, Garrod, Gerred, Gerrid, Gerrod, Garrode, Jared

Garret (Irish) a form of Garrett.
Garrit, Garyt, Gerret, Garrid, Gerrit, Gerrot

Garrett (Irish) brave spearman. See also Jarrett.
Gar, Gareth, Garett, Garrad, Garret, Garrette, Gerrett, Gerritt, Gerrott

Garrick (English) oak spear.
Gaerick, Garek, Garick, Garik, Garreck, Garrek, Garric, Garrik, Garryck, Garryk, Gerreck, Gerrick

Garren, Garrin (English) forms of Garry.
Garran, Garrion, Garron, Garyn, Gerren, Gerron, Gerryn

Garrison (French) troops stationed at a fort; garrison.
Garison, Garisson, Garris

Garroway (English) spear fighter.
Garraway

Garry (English) a form of Gary.
Garen, Garrey, Garri, Garrie, Garren, Garrin

Garson (English) son of Gar.

Garth (Scandinavian) garden, gardener. (Welsh) a short form of Gareth.

Garvey (Irish) rough peace.
Garbhán, Garrvey, Garrvie, Garv, Garvan, Garvie, Garvy

Garvin (English) comrade in battle.
Gar, Garvan, Garven, Garvyn,

Garwen, Garwin, Garwyn,
Garwynn

Garwood (English) evergreen
forest. See also Wood, Woody.
Garrwood

Gary (German) mighty spearman. (English) a familiar
form of Gerald. See also
Kali.
Gare, Garey, Gari, Garry

Gaspar (French) a form of
Casper.
*Gáspár, Gaspard, Gaspare,
Gaspari, Gasparo, Gasper,
Gazsi*

Gaston (French) from
Gascony, France.
Gascon, Gastaun

Gaute (Norwegian) great.

Gautier (French) a form of
Walter.
*Galtero, Gaulterio, Gaultier,
Gaultiero, Gauthier*

Gavin (Welsh) white hawk.
*Gav, Gavan, Gaven, Gavinn,
Gavino, Gavn, Gavohn,
Gavon, Gavyn, Gavynn,
Gawain*

Gavriel (Hebrew) man of
God.
*Gav, Gavi, Gavrel, Gavril,
Gavy*

Gavril (Russian) a form of
Gavriel.
Ganya, Gavrilo, Gavrilushka

Gawain (Welsh) a form of
Gavin.
*Gawaine, Gawayn, Gawayne,
Gawen, Gwayne*

Gaylen (Greek) a form of
Galen.
*Gaylin, Gaylinn, Gaylon,
Gaylyn*

Gaylord (French) merry lord;
jailer.
*Gaillard, Gallard, Gay,
Gayelord, Gayler, Gaylor*

Gaynor (Irish) son of the fair-
skinned man.
*Gainer, Gainor, Gay, Gayner,
Gaynnor*

Geary (English) variable,
changeable.
Gearey, Gery

Gedeon (Bulgarian, French) a
form of Gideon.

Geffrey (English) a form of
Geoffrey. See also Jeffrey.
Gefery, Geff, Geffery, Geffrard

Gellert (Hungarian) a form of
Gerald.

Gena (Russian) a short form
of Yevgenyi.
Genka, Genya, Gine

Genaro (Latin) consecrated to
God.
Genereo, Genero, Gennaro

Gene (Greek) a short form of
Eugene.
Genek

Genek (Polish) a form of Gene.

Geno (Italian) a form of John. A short form of Genovese.
Genio, Jeno

Genovese (Italian) from Genoa, Italy.
Geno, Genovis

Gent (English) gentleman.
Gentle, Gentry

Genty (Irish, English) snow.

Geoff (English) a short form of Geoffrey.

Geoffery (English) a form of Geoffrey.
Geofery

Geoffrey (English) a form of Jeffrey. See also Giotto, Godfrey, Gottfried, Jeff.
Geffrey, Geoff, Geoffery, Geoffre, Geoffrie, Geoffroi, Geoffroy, Geoffry, Geofrey, Geofri, Gofery

Geordan (Scottish) a form of Gordon.
Geordann, Geordian, Geordin, Geordon

Geordie (Scottish) a form of George.
Geordi, Geordy

Georg (Scandinavian) a form of George.

George (Greek) farmer. See also Durko, Egor, Iorgos, Jerzy, Jiri, Joji, Jörg, Jorge, Jorgen, Joris, Jorrín, Jur, Jurgis, Keoki, Mahiái, Semer, Yegor, Yorgos, Yoyi, Yrjo, Yuri, Zhora.
Geordie, Georg, Georgas, Georges, Georget, Georgi, Georgii, Georgio, Georgios, Georgiy, Georgy, Gevork, Gheorghe, Giorgio, Giorgos, Goerge, Goran, Gordios, Gorge, Gorje, Gorya, Grzegorz, Gyorgy

Georges (French) a form of George.
Geórges

Georgio (Italian) a form of George.

Georgios (Greek) a form of George.
Georgious, Georgius

Georgy (Greek) a familiar form of George.
Georgie

Geovanni, Geovanny (Italian) forms of Giovanni.
Geovan, Geovani, Geovanne, Geovannee, Geovannhi, Geovany

Geraint (English) old.

Gerald (German) mighty spearman. See also Fitzgerald, Jarell, Jarrell, Jerald, Jerry, Kharald.
Garald, Garold, Garolds, Gary, Gearalt, Gellert, Gérald, Geralde, Geraldo, Gerale,

Geraud, Gerek, Gerick, Gerik,
Gerold, Gerrald, Gerrell,
Gérrick, Gerrild, Gerrin, Gerrit,
Gerrold, Gerry, Geryld, Giraldo,
Giraud, Girauld

Geraldo (Italian, Spanish) a
form of Gerald.

Gerard (English) brave spear-
man. See also Jerard, Jerry.
Garrard, Garrat, Garratt,
Gearard, Gerad, Gerar, Gérard,
Gerardo, Geraro, Géraud, Gerd,
Gerek, Gerhard, Gerrard,
Gerrit, Gerry, Girard

Gerardo (Spanish) a form of
Gerard.
Gherardo

Géraud (French) a form of
Gerard.
Gerrad, Gerraud

Gerek (Polish) a form of
Gerard.

Geremia (Hebrew) exalted by
God. (Italian) a form of
Jeremiah.

Geremiah (Italian) a form of
Jeremiah.
Geremia, Gerimiah, Geromiah

Gerhard (German) a form of
Gerard.
Garhard, Gerhardi, Gerhardt,
Gerhart, Gerhort

Gerik (Polish) a form of
Edgar.
Geric, Gerick

Germain (French) from
Germany. (English) sprout,
bud. See also Jermaine.
Germaine, German, Germane,
Germano, Germayn, Germayne

Gerome (English) a form of
Jerome.

Geronimo (Greek, Italian) a
form of Jerome. History: a
famous Apache chief.
Geronemo

Gerrit (Dutch) a form of
Gerald.

Gerry (English) a familiar
form of Gerald, Gerard. See
also Jerry.
Geri, Gerre, Gerri, Gerrie,
Gerryson

Gershom (Hebrew) exiled.
(Yiddish) stranger in exile.
Gersham, Gersho, Gershon,
Gerson, Geurson, Gursham,
Gurshan

Gerson (English) son of Gar.
Gersan, Gershawn

Gert (German, Danish)
fighter.

Gervaise (French) honorable.
See also Jervis.
Garvais, Garvaise, Garvey,
Gervais, Gervase, Gervasio,
Gervaso, Gervayse, Gervis,
Gerwazy

Gerwin (Welsh) fair love.

Gethin (Welsh) dusky.
Geth

Ghazi (Arabic) conqueror.

Ghilchrist (Irish) servant of
Christ. See also Gil.
*Gilchrist, Gilcrist, Gilie, Gill,
Gilley, Gilly*

Ghislain (French) pledge.

Gi (Korean) brave.

Gia (Vietnamese) family.

Giacinto (Portuguese, Spanish)
a form of Jacinto.
Giacintho

Giacomo (Italian) a form of
Jacob.
*Gaimo, Giacamo, Giaco,
Giacobbe, Giacobo, Giacopo*

Gian (Italian) a form of
Giovanni, John.
*Gianetto, Giann, Gianne,
Giannes, Gianni, Giannis,
Giannos, Ghian*

Giancarlo (Italian) a combination of John + Charles.
Giancarlos, Gianncarlo

Gianluca (Italian) a combination of John + Lucas.

Gianni (Italian) a form of
Johnny.
Giani, Gionni

Gianpaolo (Italian) a combination of John + Paul.
Gianpaulo

Gib (English) a short form of
Gilbert.
Gibb, Gibbie, Gibby

Gibor (Hebrew) powerful.

Gibson (English) son of Gilbert.
*Gibbon, Gibbons, Gibbs, Gillson,
Gilson*

Gideon (Hebrew) tree cutter.
Bible: the judge who
defeated the Midianites.
*Gedeon, Gideone, Gidon,
Hedeon*

Gidon (Hebrew) a form of
Gideon.

Gifford (English) bold giver.
*Giff, Giffard, Gifferd, Giffie,
Giffy*

Gig (English) horse-drawn
carriage.

Gil (Greek) shield bearer.
(Hebrew) happy. (English) a
short form of Ghilchrist,
Gilbert.
*Gili, Gill, Gilli, Gillie, Gillis,
Gilly*

Gilad (Arabic) camel hump;
from Giladi, Saudi Arabia.
Giladi, Gilead

Gilamu (Basque) a form of
William.
Gillen

Gilbert (English) brilliant
pledge; trustworthy. See also
Gil, Gillett.
Gib, Gilberto, Gilburt,

Giselbert, Giselberto, Giselbertus, Guilbert

Gilberto (Spanish) a form of Gilbert.

Gilby (Scandinavian) hostage's estate. (Irish) blond boy.
Gilbey, Gillbey, Gillbie, Gillby

Gilchrist (Irish) a form of Ghilchrist.

Gilen (Basque, German) illustrious pledge.

Giles (French) goatskin shield.
Gide, Gilles, Gyles

Gillean (Irish) Bible: Saint John's servant.
Gillan, Gillen, Gillian

Gillespie (Irish) son of the bishop's servant.
Gillis

Gillett (French) young Gilbert.
Gelett, Gelette, Gillette

Gilmer (English) famous hostage.
Gilmar

Gilmore (Irish) devoted to the Virgin Mary.
Gillmore, Gillmour, Gilmour

Gilon (Hebrew) circle.

Gilroy (Irish) devoted to the king.
Gilderoy, Gildray, Gildroy, Gillroy, Roy

Gino (Greek) a familiar form of Eugene. (Italian) a short form of names ending in "gene," "gino."
Ghino

Giona (Italian) a form of Jonah.

Giordano (Italian) a form of Jordan.
Giordan, Giordana, Giordin, Guordan

Giorgio (Italian) a form of George.

Giorgos (Greek) a form of George.
Georgos, Giorgios

Giosia (Italian) a form of Joshua.

Giotto (Italian) a form of Geoffrey.

Giovani (Italian) a form of Giovanni.
Giavani, Giovan, Giovane, Giovanie, Giovon

Giovanni (Italian) a form of John. See also Jeovanni, Jiovanni.
Geovanni, Geovanny, Gian, Gianni, Giannino, Giovani, Giovann, Giovannie, Giovanno, Giovanny, Giovonathon, Giovonni, Giovonnia, Giovonnie, Givonni

Giovanny (Italian) a form of
Giovanni.
Giovany

Gipsy (English) wanderer.
Gipson, Gypsy

Girvin (Irish) small; tough.
Girvan, Girven, Girvon

Gitano (Spanish) gypsy.

Giuliano (Italian) a form of
Julius.
Giulano, Giulino, Giulliano

Giulio (Italian) a form of
Julius.
Guilano

Giuseppe (Italian) a form of
Joseph.
*Giuseppi, Giuseppino,
Giusseppe, Guiseppe, Guiseppi,
Guiseppie, Guisseppe*

Giustino (Italian) a form of
Justin.
Giusto

Givon (Hebrew) hill; heights.
Givan, Givawn, Givyn

Gladwin (English) cheerful.
See also Win.
*Glad, Gladdie, Gladdy,
Gladwinn, Gladwyn,
Gladwynne*

Glanville (English) village
with oak trees.

Glen (Irish) a form of Glenn.
Glyn

Glendon (Scottish) fortress in
the glen.
*Glenden, Glendin, Glenn,
Glennden, Glennton, Glenton*

Glendower (Welsh) from
Glyndwr, Wales.

Glenn (Irish) a short form of
Glendon.
*Gleann, Glen, Glennie,
Glennis, Glennon, Glenny,
Glynn*

Glentworth (English) from
Glenton, England.

Glenville (Irish) village in the
glen.

Glyn (Welsh) a form of Glen.
Glin, Glynn

Goddard (German) divinely
firm.
*Godard, Godart, Goddart,
Godhardt, Godhart, Gothart,
Gotthard, Gotthardt, Gotthart*

Godfrey (Irish) God's peace.
(German) a form of Jeffrey.
See also Geoffrey, Gottfried.
*Giotto, Godefroi, Godfree,
Godfry, Godofredo, Godoired,
Godrey, Goffredo, Gofraidh,
Gofredo, Gorry*

Godwin (English) friend of
God. See also Win.
*Godewyn, Godwinn, Godwyn,
Goodwin, Goodwyn,
Goodwynn, Goodwynne*

Goel (Hebrew) redeemer.

Goldwin (English) golden
friend. See also Win.
*Golden, Goldewin, Goldewinn,
Goldewyn, Goldwyn,
Goldwynn*

Goliath (Hebrew) exiled.
Bible: the giant Philistine
whom David slew with a
slingshot.
Golliath

Gomda (Kiowa) wind.

Gomer (Hebrew) completed,
finished. (English) famous
battle.

Gonza (Rutooro) love.

Gonzalo (Spanish) wolf.
*Goncalve, Gonsalo, Gonsalve,
Gonzales, Gonzelee, Gonzolo*

Gordon (English) triangular-
shaped hill.
*Geordan, Gord, Gordain,
Gordan, Gorden, Gordonn,
Gordy*

Gordy (English) a familiar
form of Gordon.
Gordie

Gore (English) triangular-
shaped land; wedge-shaped
land.

Gorman (Irish) small; blue
eyed.

Goro (Japanese) fifth.

Gosheven (Native American)
great leaper.

Gottfried (German) a form of
Geoffrey, Godfrey.
Gotfrid, Gotfrids, Gottfrid

Gotzon (German) a form of
Angel.

Govert (Dutch) heavenly
peace.

Gower (Welsh) pure.

Gowon (Tiv) rainmaker.
Gowan

Gozol (Hebrew) soaring bird.
Gozal

Grady (Irish) noble; illustrious.
*Gradea, Gradee, Gradey,
Gradleigh, Graidey, Graidy*

Graeme (Scottish) a form of
Graham.
Graem

Graham (English) grand
home.
*Graeham, Graehame, Graehme,
Graeme, Grahamme, Grahm,
Grahame, Grahme, Gram,
Grame, Gramm, Grayeme,
Grayham*

Granger (French) farmer.
Grainger, Grange

Grant (English) a short form
of Grantland.
*Grand, Grantham, Granthem,
Grantley*

Grantland (English) great
plains.
Grant

Granville (French) large village.
Gran, Granvel, Granvil, Granvile, Granvill, Grenville, Greville

Gray (English) gray haired.
Graye, Grey, Greye

Grayden (English) gray haired.
Graden, Graydan, Graydyn, Greyden

Graydon (English) gray hill.
Gradon, Grayton, Greydon

Grayson (English) bailiff's son. See also Sonny.
Graysen, Greyson

Greeley (English) gray meadow.
Greelea, Greeleigh, Greely

Greenwood (English) green forest.
Green, Greener

Greg, Gregg (Latin) short forms of Gregory.
Graig, Greig, Gregson

Greggory (Latin) a form of Gregory.
Greggery

Gregor (Scottish) a form of Gregory.
Gregoor, Grégor, Gregore

Gregorio (Italian, Portuguese) a form of Gregory.
Gregorios

Gregory (Latin) vigilant watchman. See also Jörn, Krikor.
Gergely, Gergo, Greagoir, Greagory, Greer, Greg, Gregary, Greger, Gregery, Greggory, Grégoire, Gregor, Gregorey, Gregori, Grégorie, Gregorio, Gregorius, Gregors, Gregos, Gregrey, Gregroy, Gregry, Greogry, Gries, Grisha, Grzegorz

Gresham (English) village in the pasture.

Greyson (English) a form of Grayson.
Greysen, Greysten, Greyston

Griffin (Latin) hooked nose.
Griff, Griffen, Griffie, Griffon, Griffy, Gryphon

Griffith (Welsh) fierce chief; ruddy.
Grifen, Griff, Griffeth, Griffie, Griffy, Griffyn, Griffynn, Gryphon

Grigori (Bulgarian) a form of Gregory.
Grigoi, Grigor, Grigore, Grigorios, Grigorov, Grigory

Grimshaw (English) dark woods.

Grisha (Russian) a form of Gregory.

Griswold (German, French) gray forest.
Gris, Griz, Grizwald

Grosvener (French) big
hunter.

Grover (English) grove.
Grove

Guadalupe (Arabic) river of
black stones.
Guadalope

Gualberto (Spanish) a form of
Walter.
Gualterio

Gualtiero (Italian) a form of
Walter.
Gualterio

Guglielmo (Italian) a form of
William.

Guido (Italian) a form of Guy.

Guilford (English) ford with
yellow flowers.
Guildford

Guilherme (Portuguese) a
form of William.

Guillaume (French) a form of
William.
*Guillaums, Guilleaume,
Guilem, Guyllaume*

Guillermo (Spanish) a form of
William.
Guillerrmo

Gunnar (Scandinavian) a form
of Gunther.
Guner, Gunner

Gunther (Scandinavian) battle
army; warrior.
Guenter, Guenther, Gun,

*Gunnar, Guntar, Gunter,
Guntero, Gunthar, Günther*

Guotin (Chinese) polite;
strong leader.

Gurion (Hebrew) young lion.
Gur, Guri, Guriel

Gurpreet (Sikh) devoted to
the guru; devoted to the
Prophet.
Gurjeet, Gurmeet, Guruprit

Gurvir (Sikh) guru's warrior.
Gurveer

Gus (Scandinavian) a short
form of Angus, Augustine,
Gustave.
*Guss, Gussie, Gussy, Gusti,
Gustry, Gusty*

Gustaf (Swedish) a form of
Gustave.
Gustaaf, Gustaff

Gustave (Scandinavian) staff of
the Goths. History: Gustavus
Adolphus was a king of
Sweden. See also Kosti, Tabo,
Tavo.
*Gus, Gustaf, Gustaff, Gustaof,
Gustav, Gustáv, Gustava,
Gustaves, Gustavo, Gustavs,
Gustavus, Gustik, Gustus,
Gusztav*

Gustavo (Italian, Spanish) a
form of Gustave.
Gustabo

Guthrie (German) war hero.
(Irish) windy place.
Guthrey, Guthry

Gutierre (Spanish) a form of
Walter.

Guy (Hebrew) valley.
(German) warrior. (French)
guide. See also Guido.
Guyon

Guyapi (Native American)
candid.

Gwayne (Welsh) a form of
Gawain.
Gwaine, Gwayn

Gwidon (Polish) life.

Gwilym (Welsh) a form of
William.
Gwillym

Gwyn (Welsh) fair; blessed.
Gwynn, Gwynne

Gyasi (Akan) marvelous baby.

Gyorgy (Russian) a form of
George.
*Gyoergy, György, Gyuri,
Gyurka*

Gyula (Hungarian) youth.
Gyala, Gyuszi

H

Habib (Arabic) beloved.

Hackett (German, French)
little wood cutter.
Hacket, Hackit, Hackitt

Hackman (German, French)
wood cutter.

Hadar (Hebrew) glory.

Haddad (Arabic) blacksmith.

Hadden (English) heather-
covered hill.
Haddan, Haddon, Haden

Haden (English) a form of
Hadden.
Hadin, Hadon, Hadyn, Haeden

Hadi (Arabic) guiding to the
right.
Hadee, Hady

Hadley (English) heather-cov-
ered meadow.
*Had, Hadlea, Hadlee, Hadleigh,
Hadly, Lee, Leigh*

Hadrian (Latin, Swedish) dark.
Adrian, Hadrien

Hadwin (English) friend in a
time of war.
*Hadwinn, Hadwyn, Hadwynn,
Hadwynne*

Hagan (German) strong
defense.
Haggan

Hagen (Irish) young, youthful.

Hagley (English) enclosed
meadow.

Hagos (Ethiopian) happy.

Hahnee (Native American) beggar.

Hai (Vietnamese) sea.

Haidar (Arabic) lion.
Haider

Haiden (English) a form of Hayden.
Haidyn

Haig (English) enclosed with hedges.

Hailey (Irish) a form of Haley.
Haile, Haille, Haily, Halee

Haji (Swahili) born during the pilgrimage to Mecca.

Hakan (Native American) fiery.

Hakeem (Arabic) a form of Hakim.
Hakam, Hakem

Hakim (Arabic) wise. (Ethiopian) doctor.
Hakeem, Hakiem

Hakon (Scandinavian) of Nordic ancestry.
Haaken, Haakin, Haakon, Haeo, Hak, Hakan, Hako

Hal (English) a short form of Halden, Hall, Harold.

Halbert (English) shining hero.
Bert, Halburt

Halden (Scandinavian) half-Danish. See also Dane.
Hal, Haldan, Haldane, Halfdan, Halvdan

Hale (English) a short form of Haley. (Hawaiian) a form of Harry.
Hayle, Heall

Halen (Swedish) hall.
Hale, Hallen, Haylan, Haylen

Haley (Irish) ingenious.
Hailey, Hale, Haleigh, Halley, Hayleigh, Hayley, Hayli

Halford (English) valley ford.

Hali (Greek) sea.

Halian (Zuni) young.

Halil (Turkish) dear friend.
Halill

Halim (Arabic) mild, gentle.
Haleem

Hall (English) manor, hall.
Hal, Halstead, Halsted

Hallam (English) valley.

Hallan (English) dweller at the hall; dweller at the manor.
Halin, Hallene, Hallin

Halley (English) meadow near the hall; holy.
Hallie

Halliwell (English) holy well.
Hallewell, Hellewell, Helliwell

Hallward (English) hall guard.

Halsey (English) Hal's island.

Halstead (English) manor grounds.
Halsted

Halton (English) estate on the hill.

Halvor (Norwegian) rock; protector.
Halvard

Ham (Hebrew) hot. Bible: one of Noah's sons.

Hamal (Arabic) lamb. Astronomy: a bright star in the constellation of Aries.

Hamar (Scandinavian) hammer.

Hamid (Arabic) praised. See also Muhammad.
Haamid, Hamaad, Hamadi, Hamd, Hamdrem, Hamed, Hamedo, Hameed, Hamidi, Hammad, Hammed, Humayd

Hamill (English) scarred.
Hamel, Hamell, Hammill

Hamilton (English) proud estate.
Hamel, Hamelton, Hamil, Hamill, Tony

Hamish (Scottish) a form of Jacob, James.

Hamisi (Swahili) born on Thursday.

Hamlet (German, French) little village; home. Literature: one of Shakespeare's tragic heroes.

Hamlin (German, French) loves his home.
Hamblin, Hamelen, Hamelin, Hamlen, Hamlyn, Lin

Hammet (English, Scandinavian) village.
Hammett, Hamnet, Hamnett

Hammond (English) village.
Hamond

Hampton (English) Geography: a town in England.
Hamp

Hamza (Arabic) powerful.
Hamzah, Hamze, Hamzeh, Hamzia

Hanale (Hawaiian) a form of Henry.
Haneke

Hanan (Hebrew) grace.
Hananel, Hananiah, Johanan

Hanbal (Arabic) pure. History: Ahmad Ibn Hanbal founded an Islamic school of thought.

Handel (German, English) a form of John. Music: George Frideric Handel was a German composer whose works include *Messiah* and *Water Music*.

Hanford (English) high ford.

Hanif (Arabic) true believer.
Haneef, Hanef

Hank (American) a familiar form of Henry.

Hanley (English) high meadow.
Handlea, Handleigh, Handley,

*Hanlea, Hanlee, Hanleigh,
Hanly, Henlea, Henlee,
Henleigh, Henley*

Hannes (Finnish) a form of
John.

Hannibal (Phoenician) grace
of God. History: a famous
Carthaginian general who
fought the Romans.
Anibal

Hanno (German) a short form
of Johan.
*Hanna, Hannah, Hannon,
Hannu, Hanon*

Hans (Scandinavian) a form of
John.
Hanschen, Hansel, Hants, Hanz

Hansel (Scandinavian) a form
of Hans.
*Haensel, Hansell, Hansl,
Hanzel*

Hansen (Scandinavian) son of
Hans.
Hanson

Hansh (Hindi) god; godlike.

Hanson (Scandinavian) a form
of Hansen.
Hansen, Hanssen, Hansson

Hanus (Czech) a form of
John.

Haoa (Hawaiian) a form of
Howard.

Hara (Hindi) seizer. Religion:
another name for the Hindu
god Shiva.

Harald (Scandinavian) a form
of Harold.
Haraldo, Haralds, Haralpos

Harb (Arabic) warrior.

Harbin (German, French) little bright warrior.
Harben, Harbyn

Harcourt (French) fortified
dwelling.
Court, Harcort

Hardeep (Punjabi) a form of
Harpreet.

Harden (English) valley of the
hares.
Hardian, Hardin

Harding (English) brave;
hardy.
Hardin

Hardwin (English) brave
friend.

Hardy (German) bold, daring.
Hardie

Harel (Hebrew) mountain of
God.
Harell, Hariel, Harrell

Harford (English) ford of the
hares.

Hargrove (English) grove of
the hares.
Hargreave, Hargreaves

Hari (Hindi) tawny.
Hariel, Harin

Harith (Arabic) cultivator.

Harjot (Sikh) light of God.
Harjeet, Harjit, Harjodh

Harkin (Irish) dark red.
Harkan, Harken

Harlan (English) hare's land;
army land.
*Harland, Harlen, Harlenn,
Harlin, Harlon, Harlyn,
Harlynn*

Harland (English) a form of
Harlan.
Harlend

Harley (English) hare's
meadow; army meadow.
*Arley, Harlea, Harlee, Harleigh,
Harly*

Harlow (English) hare's hill;
army hill. See also Arlo.

Harman, Harmon (English)
forms of Herman.
*Harm, Harmen, Harmond,
Harms*

Harold (Scandinavian) army
ruler. See also Jindra.
*Araldo, Garald, Garold, Hal,
Harald, Haraldas, Haraldo,
Haralds, Harry, Heraldo, Herold,
Heronim, Herrick, Herryck*

Haroun (Arabic) lofty; exalted.
*Haarun, Harin, Haron, Haroon,
Harron, Harun*

Harper (English) harp player.
Harp, Harpo

Harpreet (Punjabi) loves God,
devoted to God.
Hardeep

Harris (English) a short form
of Harrison.
Haris, Hariss

Harrison (English) son of
Harry.
*Harison, Harreson, Harris,
Harrisen, Harrisson*

Harrod (Hebrew) hero; conqueror.

Harry (English) a familiar
form of Harold. See also
Arrigo, Hale, Parry.
*Harm, Harray, Harrey, Harri,
Harrie*

Hart (English) a short form of
Hartley.

Hartley (English) deer
meadow.
*Hart, Hartlea, Hartlee,
Hartleigh, Hartly*

Hartman (German) hard;
strong.

Hartwell (English) deer well.
Harwell, Harwill

Hartwig (German) strong
advisor.

Hartwood (English) deer forest.
Harwood

Harvey (German) army war-
rior.
*Harv, Hervé, Hervey, Hervie,
Hervy*

Harvir (Sikh) God's warrior.
Harvier

Hasad (Turkish) reaper, harvester.

Hasan (Arabic) a form of
Hassan.
*Hasaan, Hasain, Hasaun,
Hashaan, Hason*

Hasani (Swahili) handsome.
*Hasan, Hasanni, Hassani,
Heseny, Hassen, Hassian,
Husani*

Hashim (Arabic) destroyer of
evil.
*Haashim, Hasham, Hasheem,
Hashem*

Hasin (Hindi) laughing.
*Haseen, Hasen, Hassin, Hazen,
Hesen*

Haskel (Hebrew) a form of
Ezekiel.
Haskell

Haslett (English) hazel-tree
land.
Haze, Hazel, Hazlett, Hazlitt

Hassan (Arabic) handsome.
Hasan, Hassen, Hasson

Hassel (German, English)
witches' corner.
*Hassal, Hassall, Hassell,
Hazael, Hazell*

Hastin (Hindi) elephant.

Hastings (Latin) spear.
(English) house council.
Hastie, Hasty

Hatim (Arabic) judge.
Hateem, Hatem

Hauk (Norwegian) hawk.
Haukeye

Havelock (Norwegian) sea
battler.

Haven (Dutch, English) har-
bor, port; safe place.
*Haeven, Havin, Hevin, Hevon,
Hovan*

Havika (Hawaiian) a form of
David.

Hawk (English) hawk.
Hawke, Hawkin, Hawkins

Hawley (English) hedged
meadow.
Hawleigh, Hawly

Hawthorne (English)
hawthorn tree.

Hayden (English) hedged val-
ley.
*Haiden, Haydan, Haydenn,
Haydn, Haydon*

Hayes (English) hedged valley.
Hayse

Hayward (English) guardian of
the hedged area.
Haward, Heyvard, Heyward

Haywood (English) hedged forest.
Heywood, Woody

Hearn (Scottish, English) a short form of Ahearn.
Hearne, Herin, Hern

Heath (English) heath.
Heathe, Heith

Heathcliff (English) cliff near the heath. Literature: the hero of Emily Brontë's novel *Wuthering Heights.*

Heaton (English) high place.

Heber (Hebrew) ally, partner.

Hector (Greek) steadfast. Mythology: the greatest hero of the Trojan War in Homer's epic poem *Iliad.*

Hedley (English) heather-filled meadow.
Headley, Headly, Hedly

Heinrich (German) a form of Henry.
Heindrick, Heiner, Heinreich, Heinrick, Heinrik, Hinrich

Heinz (German) a familiar form of Henry.

Helaku (Native American) sunny day.

Helge (Russian) holy.

Helki (Moquelumnan) touching.

Helmer (German) warrior's wrath.

Helmut (German) courageous.
Helmuth

Heman (Hebrew) faithful.

Henderson (Scottish, English) son of Henry.
Hendrie, Hendries, Hendron, Henryson

Hendrick (Dutch) a form of Henry.
Hendricks, Hendrickson, Hendrik, Hendriks, Hendrikus, Hendrix, Henning

Heniek (Polish) a form of Henry.
Henier

Henley (English) high meadow.

Henning (German) a form of Hendrick, Henry.

Henoch (Yiddish) initiator.
Enoch, Henock, Henok

Henri (French) a form of Henry.
Henrico, Henrri

Henrick (Dutch) a form of Henry.
Heinrick, Henerik, Henrich, Henrik, Henryk

Henrique (Portuguese) a form of Henry.

Henry (German) ruler of the household. See also Arrigo,

Enric, Enrick, Enrico,
Enrikos, Enrique, Hanale,
Honok, Kiki.
*Hagan, Hank, Harro, Harry,
Heike, Heinrich, Heinz,
Hendrick, Henery, Heniek,
Henning, Henraoi, Henri,
Henrick, Henrim, Henrique,
Henrry, Heromin, Hersz*

Heraldo (Spanish) a form of
Harold.
Herald, Hiraldo

Herb (German) a short form
of Herbert.
Herbie, Herby

Herbert (German) glorious
soldier.
*Bert, Erbert, Eriberto, Harbert,
Hebert, Hébert, Heberto, Herb,
Heriberto, Hurbert*

Hercules (Latin) glorious gift.
Mythology: a Greek hero of
fabulous strength, renowned
for his twelve labors.
Herakles, Herc, Hercule, Herculie

Heriberto (Spanish) a form of
Herbert.
Heribert

Herman (Latin) noble.
(German) soldier. See also
Armand, Ermanno, Ermano,
Mandek.
*Harmon, Hermaan, Hermann,
Hermie, Herminio, Hermino,
Hermon, Hermy, Heromin*

Hermes (Greek) messenger.
Mythology: the divine herald
of Greek mythology.

Hernan (German)
peacemaker.

Hernando (Spanish) a form of
Ferdinand.
Hernandes, Hernandez

Herrick (German) war ruler.
Herrik, Herryck

Herschel (Hebrew) a form of
Hershel.
*Herchel, Hersch, Herschel,
Herschell*

Hersh (Hebrew) a short form
of Hershel.
Hersch, Hirsch

Hershel (Hebrew) deer.
*Herschel, Hersh, Hershal,
Hershall, Hershell, Herzl,
Hirschel, Hirshel*

Hertz (Yiddish) my strife.
Herzel

Hervé (French) a form of
Harvey.

Hesperos (Greek) evening
star.
Hespero

Hesutu (Moquelumnan) pick-
ing up a yellow jacket's nest.

Hew (Welsh) a form of Hugh.
Hewe, Huw

Hewitt (German, French) little smart one.
Hewe, Hewet, Hewett, Hewie, Hewit, Hewlett, Hewlitt, Hugh

Hewson (English) son of Hugh.

Hezekiah (Hebrew) God gives strength.
Hezekyah, Hazikiah, Hezikyah

Hiamovi (Cheyenne) high chief.

Hibah (Arabic) gift.

Hideaki (Japanese) smart, clever.
Hideo

Hieremias (Greek) God will uplift.

Hieronymos (Greek) a form of Jerome. Art: Hieronymus Bosch was a fifteenth-century Dutch painter.
Hierome, Hieronim, Hieronimo, Hieronimos, Hieronymo, Hieronymus

Hieu (Vietnamese) respectful.

Hilario (Spanish) a form of Hilary.

Hilary (Latin) cheerful. See also Ilari.
Hi, Hilair, Hilaire, Hilarie, Hilario, Hilarion, Hilarius, Hil, Hill, Hillary, Hillery, Hilliary, Hillie, Hilly

Hildebrand (German) battle sword.
Hildebrando, Hildo

Hilel (Arabic) new moon.

Hillel (Hebrew) greatly praised. Religion: Rabbi Hillel originated the Talmud.

Hilliard (German) brave warrior.
Hillard, Hiller, Hillier, Hillierd, Hillyard, Hillyer, Hillyerd

Hilmar (Swedish) famous noble.

Hilton (English) town on a hill.
Hylton

Hinto (Dakota) blue.

Hinun (Native American) spirit of the storm.

Hippolyte (Greek) horseman.
Hipolito, Hippolit, Hippolitos, Hippolytus, Ippolito

Hiram (Hebrew) noblest; exalted.
Hi, Hirom, Huram, Hyrum

Hiromasa (Japanese) fair, just.

Hiroshi (Japanese) generous.

Hisoka (Japanese) secretive, reserved.

Hiu (Hawaiian) a form of Hugh.

Ho (Chinese) good.

Hoang (Vietnamese) finished.

Hobart (German) Bart's hill.
Hobard, Hobbie, Hobby, Hobie,
Hoebart

Hobert (German) Bert's hill.
Hobey

Hobson (English) son of
Robert.
Hobbs, Hobs

Hoc (Vietnamese) studious.

Hod (Hebrew) a short form of
Hodgson.

Hodgson (English) son of
Roger.
Hod

Hogan (Irish) youth.
Hogin

Holbrook (English) brook in
the hollow.
Brook, Holbrooke

Holden (English) hollow in
the valley.
Holdan, Holdin, Holdon,
Holdun, Holdyn

Holic (Czech) barber.

Holland (French) Geography:
a former province of the
Netherlands.

Holleb (Polish) dove.
Hollub, Holub

Hollis (English) grove of holly
trees.
Hollie, Holly

Holmes (English) river islands.

Holt (English) forest.
Holten, Holton

Homer (Greek) hostage;
pledge; security. Literature: a
renowned Greek epic poet.
Homar, Homere, Homère,
Homero, Homeros, Homerus

Hondo (Shona) warrior.

Honesto (Filipino) honest.

Honi (Hebrew) gracious.
Choni

Honok (Polish) a form of
Henry.

Honon (Moquelumnan) bear.

Honorato (Spanish) honorable.

Honoré (Latin) honored.
Honor, Honoratus, Honoray,
Honorio, Honorius

Honovi (Native American)
strong.

Honza (Czech) a form of
John.

Hop (Chinese) agreeable.

Horace (Latin) keeper of the
hours. Literature: a famous
Roman lyric poet and
satirist.
Horacio, Horaz

Horacio (Latin) a form of
Horace.

Horatio (Latin) clan name. See also Orris.
Horatius, Oratio

Horst (German) dense grove; thicket.
Hurst

Horton (English) garden estate.
Hort, Horten, Orton

Hosa (Arapaho) young crow.

Hosea (Hebrew) salvation. Bible: a Hebrew prophet.
Hose, Hoseia, Hoshea, Hosheah

Hotah (Lakota) white.

Hototo (Native American) whistler.

Houghton (English) settlement on the headland.

Houston (English) hill town. Geography: a city in Texas.
Housten, Houstin, Hustin, Huston

Howard (English) watchman. See also Haoa.
Howie, Ward

Howe (German) high.
Howey, Howie

Howell (Welsh) remarkable.
Howel

Howi (Moquelumnan) turtledove.

Howie (English) a familiar form of Howard, Howland.
Howey

Howin (Chinese) loyal swallow.

Howland (English) hilly land.
Howie, Howlan, Howlen

Hoyt (Irish) mind; spirit.

Hu (Chinese) tiger.

Hubbard (German) a form of Hubert.

Hubert (German) bright mind; bright spirit. See also Beredei, Uberto.
Bert, Hobart, Hubbard, Hubbert, Huber, Hubertek, Huberto, Hubertson, Hubie, Huey, Hugh, Hugibert, Huibert, Humberto

Huberto (Spanish) a form of Hubert.
Humberto

Hubie (English) a familiar form of Hubert.
Hube, Hubi

Hud (Arabic) Religion: a Muslim prophet.

Hudson (English) son of Hud.

Huey (English) a familiar form of Hugh.
Hughey, Hughie, Hughy, Hui

Hugh (English) a short form of Hubert. See also Ea, Hewitt, Huxley, Maccoy, Ugo.
Fitzhugh, Hew, Hiu, Hue, Huey, Hughes, Hugo, Hugues

Hugo (Latin) a form of Hugh.
Ugo

Hulbert (German) brilliant grace.
Bert, Hulbard, Hulburd, Hulburt, Hull

Humbert (German) brilliant strength. See also Umberto.
Hum, Humberto

Humberto (Portuguese) a form of Humbert.

Humphrey (German) peaceful strength. See also Onofrio, Onufry.
Hum, Humfredo, Humfrey, Humfrid, Humfried, Humfry, Hump, Humph, Humphery, Humphry, Humphrys, Hunfredo

Hung (Vietnamese) brave.

Hunt (English) a short form of names beginning with "Hunt."

Hunter (English) hunter.
Hunt, Huntur

Huntington (English) hunting estate.
Hunt, Huntingdon

Huntley (English) hunter's meadow.
Hunt, Huntlea, Huntlee, Huntleigh, Huntly

Hurley (Irish) sea tide.
Hurlee, Hurleigh

Hurst (English) a form of Horst.
Hearst, Hirst

Husam (Arabic) sword.

Husamettin (Turkish) sharp sword.

Huslu (Native American) hairy bear.

Hussain (Arabic) a form of Hussein.
Hossain, Husain, Husani, Husayn, Hussan, Hussayn

Hussein (Arabic) little; handsome.
Hossein, Houssein, Houssin, Huissien, Huossein, Husein, Husien, Hussain, Hussien

Hussien (Arabic) a form of Hussein.
Husian, Hussin

Hutchinson (English) son of the hutch dweller.
Hutcheson

Hute (Native American) star.

Hutton (English) house on the jutting ledge.
Hut, Hutt, Huttan

Huxley (English) Hugh's meadow.
Hux, Huxlea, Huxlee, Huxleigh, Lee

Huy (Vietnamese) glorious.

Hy (Vietnamese) hopeful.
(English) a short form of
Hyman.

Hyacinthe (French) hyacinth.

Hyatt (English) high gate.
Hyat

Hyde (English) cache; measure
of land equal to 120 acres;
animal hide.

Hyder (English) tanner, pre-
parer of animal hides for tan-
ning.

Hyman (English) a form of
Chaim.
*Haim, Hayim, Hayvim,
Hayyim, Hy, Hyam, Hymie*

Hyun-Ki (Korean) wise.

Hyun-Shik (Korean) clever.

I

Iago (Spanish, Welsh) a form
of Jacob, James. Literature:
the villain in Shakespeare's
Othello.
Jago

Iain (Scottish) a form of Ian.

Iakobos (Greek) a form of
Jacob.
Iakov, Iakovos, Iakovs

Ian (Scottish) a form of John.
See also Ean, Eion.
Iain, Iane, Iann

Ianos (Czech) a form of John.
Iannis

Ib (Phoenician, Danish) oath
of Baal.

Iban (Basque) a form of John.

Ibon (Basque) a form of Ivor.

Ibrahim (Hausa) my father is
exalted.
*Ibrahaim, Ibraham, Ibraheem,
Ibrahem, Ibrahiem, Ibrahiim,
Ibrahmim*

Ichabod (Hebrew) glory is
gone. Literature: Ichabod
Crane is the main character
of Washington Irving's story
"The Legend of Sleepy
Hollow."

Idi (Swahili) born during the
Idd festival.

Idris (Welsh) eager lord.
(Arabic) Religion: a Muslim
prophet.
*Idrease, Idrees, Idres, Idress,
Idreus, Idriece, Idriss, Idrissa,
Idriys*

Iestyn (Welsh) a form of
Justin.

Igashu (Native American)
wanderer; seeker.
Igasho

Iggy (Latin) a familiar form of Ignatius.

Ignacio (Italian) a form of Ignatius.
Ignazio

Ignatius (Latin) fiery, ardent. Religion: Saint Ignatius of Loyola founded the Jesuit order. See also Inigo, Neci.
Iggie, Iggy, Ignac, Ignác, Ignace, Ignacio, Ignacius, Ignatios, Ignatious, Ignatz, Ignaz, Ignazio

Igor (Russian) a form of Inger, Ingvar. See also Egor, Yegor.
Igoryok

Ihsan (Turkish) compassionate.

Ike (Hebrew) a familiar form of Isaac. History: the nickname of the thirty-fourth U.S. president Dwight D. Eisenhower.
Ikee, Ikey

Iker (Basque) visitation.

Ilan (Hebrew) tree. (Basque) youth.

Ilari (Basque) a form of Hilary.
Ilario

Ilias (Greek) a form of Elijah.
Illias, Illyas, Ilyas, Ilyes

Illan (Basque, Latin) youth.

Ilom (Ibo) my enemies are many.

Ilya (Russian) a form of Elijah.
Ilia, Ilie, Ilija, Iliya, Ilja, Illia, Illya

Imad (Arabic) supportive; mainstay.

Iman (Hebrew) a short form of Immanuel.
Imani, Imanni

Immanuel (Hebrew) a form of Emmanuel.
Iman, Imanol, Imanuel, Immanual, Immanuele, Immuneal

Imran (Arabic) host.
Imraan

Imre (Hungarian) a form of Emery.
Imri

Imrich (Czech) a form of Emery.
Imrus

Inay (Hindi) god; godlike.

Ince (Hungarian) innocent.

Inder (Hindi) god; godlike.
Inderbir, Inderdeep, Inderjeet, Inderjit, Inderpal, Inderpreet, Inderveer, Indervir, Indra, Indrajit

Indiana (Hindi) from India.
Indi, Indy

Inek (Welsh) a form of Irvin.

Ing (Scandinavian) a short form of Ingmar.
Inge

Ingelbert (German) a form of Engelbert.
Inglebert

Inger (Scandinavian) son's army.
Igor, Ingemar, Ingmar

Ingmar (Scandinavian) famous son.
Ing, Ingamar, Ingamur, Ingemar

Ingram (English) angel.
Inglis, Ingra, Ingraham, Ingrim

Ingvar (Scandinavian) Ing's soldier.
Igor, Ingevar

Inigo (Basque) a form of Ignatius.
Iñaki, Iniego, Iñigo

Iniko (Ibo) born during bad times.

Innis (Irish) island.
Innes, Inness, Inniss

Innocenzio (Italian) innocent.
Innocenty, Inocenci, Inocencio, Inocente, Inosente

Inteus (Native American) proud; unashamed.

Ioakim (Russian) a form of Joachim.
Ioachime, Ioakimo, Iov

Ioan (Greek, Bulgarian, Romanian) a form of John.
Ioane, Ioann, Ioannes, Ioannikios, Ioannis, Ionel

Iokepa (Hawaiian) a form of Joseph.
Keo

Iolo (Welsh) the Lord is worthy.
Iorwerth

Ionakana (Hawaiian) a form of Jonathan.

Iorgos (Greek) a form of George.

Iosif (Greek, Russian) a form of Joseph.

Iosua (Romanian) a form of Joshua.

Ipyana (Nyakyusa) graceful.

Ira (Hebrew) watchful.

Iram (English) bright.

Irumba (Rutooro) born after twins.

Irv (Irish, Welsh, English) a short form of Irvin, Irving.

Irvin (Irish, Welsh, English) a short form of Irving. See also Ervine.
Inek, Irv, Irven, Irvine, Irvinn, Irvon

Irving (Irish) handsome. (Welsh) white river. (English) sea friend. See also Ervin, Ervine.
Irv, Irvin, Irvington, Irwin, Irwing

Irwin (English) a form of Irving. See also Ervin.
Irwinn, Irwyn

Isa (Arabic) a form of Jesus.
Isaah

Isaac (Hebrew) he will laugh. Bible: the son of Abraham and Sarah. See also Itzak, Izak, Yitzchak.
Aizik, Icek, Ike, Ikey, Ikie, Isaak, Isaakios, Isac, Isacc, Isacco, Isack, Isaic, Ishaq, Isiac, Isiacc, Issac, Issca, Itzak, Izak, Izzy

Isaak (Hebrew) a form of Isaac.
Isack, Isak, Isik, Issak

Isaiah (Hebrew) God is my salvation. Bible: a Hebrew prophet.
Isa, Isai, Isaia, Isaias, Isaid, Isaih, Isaish, Ishaq, Isia, Isiah, Isiash, Issia, Issiah, Izaiah, Izaiha, Izaya, Izayah, Izayaih, Izayiah, Izeyah, Izeyha

Isaias (Hebrew) a form of Isaiah.
Isaiahs, Isais, Izayus

Isam (Arabic) safeguard.

Isas (Japanese) meritorious.

Isekemu (Native American) slow-moving creek.

Isham (English) home of the iron one.

Ishan (Hindi) direction.
Ishaan, Ishaun

Ishaq (Arabic) a form of Isaac.
Ishaac, Ishak

Ishmael (Hebrew) God will hear. Literature: the narrator of Herman Melville's novel *Moby-Dick*.
Isamael, Isamail, Ishma, Ishmail, Ishmale, Ishmeal, Ishmeil, Ishmel, Ishmil, Ismael, Ismail

Isidore (Greek) gift of Isis. See also Dorian, Ysidro.
Isador, Isadore, Isadorios, Isidor, Isidro, Issy, Ixidor, Izadore, Izidor, Izidore, Izydor, Izzy

Isidro (Greek) a form of Isidore.
Isidoro, Isidoros

Iskander (Afghan) a form of Alexander.

Ismael (Arabic) a form of Ishmael.

Ismail (Arabic) a form of Ishmael.
Ismeil, Ismiel

Israel (Hebrew) prince of God; wrestled with God. History: the nation of Israel took its name from the name given Jacob after he wrestled with the angel of the Lord. See also Yisrael.
Iser, Isreal, Israhel, Isrell, Isrrael, Isser, Izrael, Izzy, Yisrael

Isreal (Hebrew) a form of
Israel.
Isrieal

Issa (Swahili) God is our salvation.

Issac (Hebrew) a form of Isaac.
Issacc, Issaic, Issiac

Issiah (Hebrew) a form of
Isaiah.
Issaiah, Issia

Istu (Native American) sugar
pine.

István (Hungarian) a form of
Stephen.
Isti, Istvan, Pista

Ithel (Welsh) generous lord.

Ittamar (Hebrew) island of
palms.
Itamar

Itzak (Hebrew) a form of
Isaac, Yitzchak.
Itzik

Iukini (Hawaiian) a form of
Eugene.
Kini

Iustin (Bulgarian, Russian) a
form of Justin.

Ivan (Russian) a form of John.
*Iván, Ivanchik, Ivanichek, Ivann,
Ivano, Ivas, Iven, Ivin, Ivon,
Ivyn, Vanya*

Ivar (Scandinavian) a form of
Ivor. See also Yves, Yvon.
Iv, Iva

Ives (English) young archer.
Ive, Iven, Ivey, Yves

Ivo (German) yew wood; bow
wood.
*Ibon, Ivar, Ives, Ivon, Ivonnie,
Ivor, Yvo*

Ivor (Scandinavian) a form of
Ivo.
Ibon, Ifor, Ivar, Iver, Ivory, Ivry

Iwan (Polish) a form of John.

Iyapo (Yoruba) many trials;
many obstacles.

Iye (Native American) smoke.

Izak (Czech) a form of Isaac.
*Itzhak, Ixaka, Izaac, Izaak,
Izac, Izaic, Izak, Izec, Izeke,
Izick, Izik, Izsak, Izsák, Izzak*

Izzy (Hebrew) a familiar form
of Isaac, Isidore, Israel.
Issy

J

J (American) an initial used as
a first name.
J.

Ja (Korean) attractive,
magnetic.

Jaali (Swahili) powerful.

Jaan (Estonian) a form of
Christian.

Jaap (Dutch) a form of Jim.

Jabari (Swahili) fearless, brave.
Jabaar, Jabahri, Jabar, Jabarae, Jabare, Jabaree, Jabarei, Jabarie, Jabarri, Jabarrie, Jabary, Jabbar, Jabbaree, Jabbari, Jaber, Jabiari, Jabier, Jabori, Jaborie

Jabez (Hebrew) born in pain.
Jabe, Jabes, Jabesh

Jabin (Hebrew) God has created.
Jabain, Jabien, Jabon

Jabir (Arabic) consoler, comforter.
Jabiri, Jabori

Jabril (Arabic) a form of Jibril.
Jabrail, Jabree, Jabreel, Jabrel, Jabrell, Jabrelle, Jabri, Jabrial, Jabrie, Jabriel, Jabrielle, Jabrille

Jabulani (Shona) happy.

Jacan (Hebrew) trouble.
Jachin

Jacari (American) a form of Jacorey.
Jacarey, Jacaris, Jacarius, Jacarre, Jacarri, Jacarrus, Jacarus, Jacary, Jacaure, Jacauri, Jaccar, Jaccari

Jace (American) a combination of the initials J. + C.
JC, J.C., Jacee, Jacek, Jacey, Jacie, Jaice, Jaicee

Jacen (Greek) a form of Jason.
Jaceon

Jacinto (Portuguese, Spanish) hyacinth. See also Giacinto.
Jacindo, Jacint, Jacinta

Jack (American) a familiar form of Jacob, John. See also Keaka.
Jackie, Jacko, Jackub, Jak, Jax, Jock, Jocko

Jackie, Jacky (American) familiar forms of Jack.
Jackey

Jackson (English) son of Jack.
Jacksen, Jacksin, Jacson, Jakson, Jaxon

Jaco (Portuguese) a form of Jacob.

Jacob (Hebrew) supplanter, substitute. Bible: son of Isaac, brother of Esau. See also Akiva, Chago, Checha, Coby, Diego, Giacomo, Hamish, Iago, Iakobos, James, Kiva, Koby, Kuba, Tiago, Yakov, Yasha, Yoakim.
Jaap, Jachob, Jack, Jackob, Jackub, Jaco, Jacobb, Jacobe, Jacobi, Jacobo, Jacoby, Jacolbi, Jacolby, Jacque, Jacques, Jacub, Jaecob, Jago, Jaicob, Jaime, Jake, Jakob, Jalu, Jasha, Jaycob, Jecis, Jeks, Jeska, Jim, Jocek, Jock, Jocob, Jocobb, Jocoby, Jocolby, Jokubas

Jacobi, Jacoby (Hebrew) forms of Jacob.
Jachobi, Jacobbe, Jacobee, Jacobey, Jacobie, Jacobii, Jacobis

Jacobo (Hebrew) a form of Jacob.

Jacobson (English) son of Jacob.
Jacobs, Jacobsen, Jacobsin, Jacobus

Jacorey (American) a combination of Jacob + Corey.
Jacari, Jacori, Jacoria, Jacorie, Jacoris, Jacorius, Jacorrey, Jacorrien, Jacorry, Jacory, Jacouri, Jacourie, Jakari

Jacque (French) a form of Jacob.
Jacquay, Jacqui, Jocque, Jocqui

Jacques (French) a form of Jacob, James. See also Coco.
Jackque, Jackques, Jackquise, Jacot, Jacquan, Jacquees, Jacquese, Jacquess, Jacquet, Jacquett, Jacquez, Jacquis, Jacquise, Jaquez, Jarques, Jarquis

Jacquez, Jaquez (French) forms of Jacques.
Jaques, Jaquese, Jaqueus, Jaqueze, Jaquis, Jaquise, Jaquze, Jocquez

Jacy (Tupi-Guarani) moon.
Jaicy, Jaycee

Jade (Spanish) jade, precious stone.
Jaeid, Jaid, Jaide

Jaden (Hebrew) a form of Jadon.
Jadee, Jadeen, Jadenn, Jadeon, Jadin, Jaeden

Jadon (Hebrew) God has heard.
Jaden, Jadyn, Jaedon, Jaiden, Jaydon

Jadrien (American) a combination of Jay + Adrien.
Jad, Jada, Jadd, Jader, Jadrian

Jadyn (Hebrew) a form of Jadon.
Jadyne, Jaedyn

Jaegar (German) hunter.
Jaager, Jaeger, Jagur

Jae-Hwa (Korean) rich, prosperous.

Jael (Hebrew) mountain goat.
Yael

Jaelen (American) a form of Jalen.
Jaelan, Jaelaun, Jaelin, Jaelon, Jaelyn

Ja'far (Sanskrit) little stream.
Jafar, Jafari, Jaffar, Jaffer, Jafur

Jagger (English) carter.
Jagar, Jager, Jaggar

Jago (English) a form of James.

Jaguar (Spanish) jaguar.
Jagguar

Jahi (Swahili) dignified.

Jahlil (Hindi) a form of Jalil.
Jahlal, Jahlee, Jahleel, Jahliel

Jahmar (American) a form of Jamar.
Jahmare, Jahmari, Jahmarr, Jahmer

Jahvon (Hebrew) a form of
Javan.
*Jahvan, Jahvine, Jahwaan,
Jahwon*

Jai (Tai) heart.
Jaie, Jaii

Jaiden (Hebrew) a form of
Jadon.
Jaidan, Jaidon, Jaidyn

Jailen (American) a form of
Jalen.
*Jailan, Jailani, Jaileen, Jailen,
Jailon, Jailyn, Jailynn*

Jaime (Spanish) a form of
Jacob, James.
*Jaimee, Jaimey, Jaimie, Jaimito,
Jaimy, Jayme, Jaymie*

Jairo (Spanish) God enlight-
ens.
Jair, Jairay, Jaire, Jairus, Jarius

Jaison (Greek) a form of
Jason.
Jaisan, Jaisen, Jaishon, Jaishun

Jaivon (Hebrew) a form of
Javan.
Jaiven, Jaivion, Jaiwon

Jaja (Ibo) honored.

Jajuan (American) a combina-
tion of the prefix Ja + Juan.
*Ja Juan, Jauan, Jawaun, Jejuan,
Jujuan, Juwan*

Jakari (American) a form
of Jacorey.
Jakaire, Jakar, Jakaray, Jakarie,

*Jakarious, Jakarius, Jakarre,
Jakarri, Jakarus*

Jake (Hebrew) a short form of
Jacob.
Jakie, Jayk, Jayke

Jakeem (Arabic) uplifted.

Jakob (Hebrew) a form of
Jacob.
*Jaekob, Jaikab, Jaikob, Jakab,
Jakeb, Jakeob, Jakeub, Jakib,
Jakiv, Jakobe, Jakobi, Jakobus,
Jakoby, Jakov, Jakovian, Jakub,
Jakubek, Jekebs*

Jakome (Basque) a form of
James.
Xanti

Jal (Gypsy) wanderer.

Jalan (American) a form of
Jalen.
*Jalaan, Jalaen, Jalain, Jaland,
Jalane, Jalani, Jalanie, Jalann,
Jalaun, Jalean, Jallan*

Jaleel (Hindi) a form of Jalil.
Jaleell, Jaleil, Jalel

Jalen (American) a combina-
tion of the prefix Ja + Len.
*Jaelen, Jailen, Jalan, Jaleen,
Jalend, Jalene, Jalin, Jallen,
Jalon, Jalyn*

Jalil (Hindi) revered.
Jahlil, Jalaal, Jalal

Jalin, Jalyn (American) forms
of Jalen.
Jalian, Jaline, Jalynn, Jalynne

Jalon (American) a form of
Jalen.
Jalone, Jaloni, Jalun

Jam (American) a short form
of Jamal, Jamar.
Jama

Jamaal (Arabic) a form of
Jamal.

Jamaine (Arabic) a form of
Germain.

Jamal (Arabic) handsome. See
also Gamal.
*Jahmal, Jahmall, Jahmalle,
Jahmeal, Jahmeel, Jahmeil,
Jahmel, Jahmelle, Jahmil,
Jahmile, Jaimal, Jam, Jamaal,
Jamael, Jamahl, Jamail, Jamaile,
Jamala, Jamale, Jamall, Jamalle,
Jamar, Jamaul, Jamel, Jamil,
Jammal, Jamor, Jamual, Jarmal,
Jaumal, Jemal, Jermal, Jomal,
Jomall*

Jamar (American) a form of
Jamal.
*Jam, Jamaar, Jamaari, Jamahrae,
Jamair, Jamara, Jamaras,
Jamaraus, Jamarl, Jamarr,
Jamarre, Jamarrea, Jamarree,
Jamarri, Jamarvis, Jamaur, Jamir,
Jamire, Jamiree, Jammar, Jarmar,
Jarmarr, Jaumar, Jemaar, Jemar,
Jimar, Jomar*

Jamarcus (American) a com-
bination of the prefix Ja +
Marcus.
*Jamarco, Jamarkus, Jemarcus,
Jimarcus*

Jamari (American) a form of
Jamario.
*Jamare, Jamarea, Jamaree,
Jamareh, Jamaria, Jamarie,
Jamaul*

Jamario (American) a combi-
nation of the prefix Ja +
Mario.
*Jamareo, Jamari, Jamariel,
Jamarious, Jamaris, Jamarius,
Jamariya, Jemario, Jemarus*

Jamarquis (American) a com-
bination of the prefix Ja +
Marquis.
*Jamarkees, Jamarkeus, Jamarkis,
Jamarqese, Jamarqueis,
Jamarques, Jamarquez,
Jamarquios, Jamarqus*

Jamel (Arabic) a form of
Jamal.
*Jameel, Jamele, Jamell, Jamelle,
Jammel, Jamuel, Jamul, Jarmel,
Jaumal, Jaumell, Je-Mell, Jimell*

James (Hebrew) supplanter,
substitute. (English) a form of
Jacob. Bible: James the Great
and James the Less were two
of the Twelve Apostles. See
also Diego, Hamish, Iago,
Kimo, Santiago, Seamus,
Seumas, Yago, Yasha.
*Jacques, Jago, Jaime, Jaimes,
Jakome, Jamesie, Jamesy, Jamez,
Jameze, Jamie, Jamies, Jamse,
Jamyes, Jamze, Jas, Jasha, Jay,
Jaymes, Jem, Jemes, Jim*

Jameson (English) son of
James.
Jamerson, Jamesian, Jamison,
Jaymeson

Jamie (English) a familiar form
of James.
Jaime, Jaimey, Jaimie, Jame,
Jamee, Jamey, Jameyel, Jami,
Jamia, Jamiah, Jamian, Jamme,
Jammie, Jamiee, Jammy, Jamy,
Jamye, Jayme, Jaymee, Jaymie

Jamil (Arabic) a form of Jamal.
Jamiel, Jamiell, Jamielle, Jamile,
Jamill, Jamille, Jamyl, Jarmil

Jamin (Hebrew) favored.
Jamen, Jamian, Jamien, Jamion,
Jamionn, Jamon, Jamun, Jamyn,
Jarmin, Jarmon, Jaymin

Jamison (English) son of
James.
Jamiesen, Jamieson, Jamis,
Jamisen, Jamyson, Jaymison

Jamon (Hebrew) a form of
Jamin.
Jamohn, Jamone, Jamoni

Jamond (American) a combi-
nation of James + Raymond.
Jamod, Jamont, Jamonta,
Jamontae, Jamontay, Jamonte,
Jarmond

Jamor (American) a form of
Jamal.
Jamoree, Jamori, Jamorie,
Jamorius, Jamorrio, Jamorris,
Jamory, Jamour

Jamsheed (Persian) from
Persia.
Jamshaid, Jamshed

Jan (Dutch, Slavic) a form of
John.
Jaan, Jana, Janae, Jann, Janne,
Jano, Janson, Jenda, Yan

Janco (Czech) a form of John.
Jancsi, Janke, Janko

Jando (Spanish) a form of
Alexander.
Jandino

Janeil (American) a combina-
tion of the prefix Ja + Neil.
Janal, Janel, Janell, Janelle,
Janiel, Janielle, Janile, Janille,
Jarnail, Jarneil, Jarnell

Janek (Polish) a form of John.
Janak, Janik, Janika, Janka,
Jankiel, Janko

Janis (Latvian) a form of John.
Ansis, Jancis, Zanis

Janne (Finnish) a form of
John.
Jann, Jannes

János (Hungarian) a form of
John.
Jancsi, Jani, Jankia, Jano

Janson (Scandinavian) son of
Jan.
Janse, Jansen, Jansin, Janssen,
Jansun, Jantzen, Janzen, Jensen,
Jenson

Jantzen (Scandinavian) a form of Janson.
Janten, Jantsen, Jantson

Janus (Latin) gate, passageway; born in January. Mythology: the Roman god of beginnings and endings.
Jannese, Jannus, Januario, Janusz

Japheth (Hebrew) handsome. (Arabic) abundant. Bible: a son of Noah. See also Yaphet.
Japeth, Japhet

Jaquan (American) a combination of the prefix Ja + Quan.
Jaequan, Jaiqaun, Jaiquan, Jaqaun, Jaqawan, Jaquaan, Jaquain, Ja'quan, Jaquane, Jaquann, Jaquanne, Jaquavius, Jaquawn, Jaquin, Jaquon, Jaqwan

Jaquarius (American) a combination of Jaquan + Darius.
Jaquari, Jaquarious, Jaquaris

Jaquavius (American) a form of Jaquan.
Jaquavas, Jaquaveis, Jaquaveius, Jaquaveon, Jaquaveous, Jaquavias, Jaquavious, Jaquavis, Jaquavus

Jaquon (American) a form of Jaquan.
Jaequon, Jaqoun, Jaquinn, Jaqune, Jaquoin, Jaquone, Jaqwon

Jarad (Hebrew) a form of Jared.
Jaraad, Jaraed

Jarah (Hebrew) sweet as honey.
Jerah

Jardan (Hebrew) a form of Jordan.
Jarden, Jardin, Jardon

Jareb (Hebrew) contending.
Jarib

Jared (Hebrew) a form of Jordan.
Jahred, Jaired, Jarad, Jaredd, Jareid, Jarid, Jarod, Jarred, Jarrett, Jarrod, Jarryd, Jerad, Jered, Jerod, Jerrad, Jerred, Jerrod, Jerryd, Jordan

Jarek (Slavic) born in January.
Janiuszck, Januarius, Januisz, Jarec, Jarrek, Jarric, Jarrick

Jarell (Scandinavian) a form of Gerald.
Jairell, Jarael, Jareil, Jarel, Jarelle, Jariel, Jarrell, Jarryl, Jayryl, Jerel, Jerell, Jerrell, Jharell

Jaren (Hebrew) a form of Jaron.
Jarian, Jarien, Jarin, Jarion

Jareth (American) a combination of Jared + Gareth.
Jarreth, Jereth, Jarreth

Jarett (English) a form of Jarrett.
Jaret, Jarette

Jarl (Scandinavian) earl, noble-man.

Jarlath (Latin) in control.
Jarl, Jarlen

Jarman (German) from Germany.
Jerman

Jarod (Hebrew) a form of Jared.
Jarodd, Jaroid

Jaron (Hebrew) he will sing; he will cry out.
Jaaron, Jairon, Jaren, Jarone, Jarren, Jarron, Jaryn, Jayron, Jayronn, Je Ronn, J'ron

Jaroslav (Czech) glory of spring.
Jarda

Jarred (Hebrew) a form of Jared.
Ja'red, Jarrad, Jarrayd, Jarrid, Jarrod, Jarryd, Jerrid

Jarrell (English) a form of Gerald.
Jarel, Jarell, Jarrel, Jerall, Jerel, Jerell

Jarren (Hebrew) a form of Jaron.
Jarrain, Jarran, Jarrian, Jarrin

Jarrett (English) a form of Garrett, Jared.
Jairett, Jareth, Jarett, Jaretté, Jarhett, Jarratt, Jarret, Jarrette, Jarrot, Jarrott, Jerrett

Jarrod (Hebrew) a form of Jared.
Jarod, Jerod, Jerrod

Jarryd (Hebrew) a form of Jared.
Jarrayd, Jaryd

Jarvis (German) skilled with a spear.
Jaravis, Jarv, Jarvaris, Jarvas, Jarvaska, Jarvey, Jarvez, Jarvie, Jarvios, Jarvious, Jarvius, Jarvorice, Jarvoris, Jarvous, Jarvus, Javaris, Jervey, Jervis

Jaryn (Hebrew) a form of Jaron.
Jarryn, Jarynn, Jaryon

Jas (Polish) a form of John. (English) a familiar form of James.
Jasio

Jasha (Russian) a familiar form of Jacob, James.
Jascha

Jashawn (American) a combi-nation of the prefix Ja + Shawn.
Jasean, Jashan, Jashaun, Jashion, Jashon

Jaskaran (Sikh) sings praises to the Lord.
Jaskaren, Jaskarn, Jaskiran

Jasmin (Persian) jasmine flower.
Jasman, Jasmanie, Jasmine, Jasmon, Jasmond

Jason (Greek) healer.
Mythology: the hero who
led the Argonauts in search
of the Golden Fleece.
*Jacen, Jaeson, Jahson, Jaison,
Jasan, Jasaun, Jase, Jasen, Jasin,
Jasson, Jasten, Jasun, Jasyn,
Jathan, Jathon, Jay, Jayson*

Jaspal (Punjabi) living a virtuous lifestyle.

Jasper (French) brown, red, or
yellow ornamental stone.
(English) a form of Casper.
See also Kasper.
Jaspar, Jazper, Jespar, Jesper

Jasson (Greek) a form of
Jason.
Jassen, Jassin

Jatinra (Hindi) great Brahmin
sage.

Javan (Hebrew) Bible: son of
Japheth.
*Jaewan, Jahvaughan, Jahvon,
Jaivon, Javante, Javaon,
JaVaughn, Javen, Javian, Javien,
Javin, Javine, Javoanta, Javon,
Javona, Javone, Javonte, Jayvin,
Jayvion, Jayvon, Jevan, Jevon*

Javante (American) a form of
Javan.
*Javantae, Javantai, Javantée,
Javanti*

Javaris (English) a form of
Jarvis.
*Javaor, Javar, Javaras, Javare,
Javares, Javari, Javarias, Javaries,*

*Javario, Javarius, Javaro, Javaron,
Javarous, Javarre, Javarreis,
Javarri, Javarrious, Javarris,
Javarro, Javarous, Javarte, Javarus,
Javorious, Javoris, Javorius,
Javouris*

Javas (Sanskrit) quick, swift.
Jayvas, Jayvis

Javier (Spanish) owner of a
new house. See also Xavier.
Jabier, Javer, Javere, Javiar

Javon (Hebrew) a form of
Javan.
*Jaavon, Jaevin, Jaevon, Jaewon,
Javeon, Javion, Javionne, Javohn,
Javona, Javone, Javoney, Javoni,
Javonn, Javonne, Javonni,
Javonnie, Javonnte, Javoun,
Jayvon*

Javonte (American) a form of
Javan.
*Javona, Javontae, Javontai,
Javontay, Javontaye, Javonté,
Javontee, Javonteh, Javontey*

Jawaun (American) a form of
Jajuan.
*Jawaan, Jawan, Jawann, Jawn,
Jawon, Jawuan*

Jawhar (Arabic) jewel; essence.

Jaxon (English) a form of
Jackson.
*Jaxen, Jaxsen, Jaxson, Jaxsun,
Jaxun*

Jay (French) blue jay. (English)
a short form of James, Jason.
Jae, Jai, Jave, Jaye, Jeays, Jeyes

Jayce (American) a combination of the initials J. + C.
JC, J.C., Jayc, Jaycee, Jay Cee, Jaycey, Jecie

Jaycob (Hebrew) a form of Jacob.
Jaycub, Jaykob

Jayde (American) a combination of the initials J. + D.
JD, J.D., Jayd, Jaydee, Jayden

Jayden (American) a form of Jayde.
Jaydan, Jaydin, Jaydn, Jaydon

Jaylee (American) a combination of Jay + Lee.
Jayla, Jayle, Jaylen

Jaylen (American) a combination of Jay + Len.
Jaylaan, Jaylan, Jayland, Jayleen, Jaylend, Jaylin, Jayln, Jaylon, Jaylun, Jaylund, Jaylyn

Jaylin (American) a form of Jaylen.
Jaylian, Jayline

Jaylon (American) a form of Jaylen.
Jayleon

Jaylyn (American) a form of Jaylen.
Jaylynd, Jaylynn, Jaylynne

Jayme (English) a form of Jamie.
Jaymie

Jaymes (English) a form of James.
Jaymis, Jayms, Jaymz

Jayquan (American) a combination of Jay + Quan.
Jaykwan, Jaykwon, Jayqon, Jayquawn, Jayqunn

Jayson (Greek) a form of Jason.
Jaycent, Jaysean, Jaysen, Jayshaun, Jayshawn, Jayshon, Jayshun, Jaysin, Jaysn, Jayssen, Jaysson, Jaysun

Jayvon (American) a form of Javon.
Jayvion, Jayvohn, Jayvone, Jayvonn, Jayvontay, Jayvonte, Jaywan, Jaywaun, Jaywin

Jazz (American) jazz.
Jaz, Jazze, Jazzlee, Jazzman, Jazzmen, Jazzmin, Jazzmon, Jazztin, Jazzton, Jazzy

Jean (French) a form of John.
Jéan, Jeane, Jeannah, Jeannie, Jeannot, Jeano, Jeanot, Jeanty, Jene

Jeb (Hebrew) a short form of Jebediah.
Jebb, Jebi, Jeby

Jebediah (Hebrew) a form of Jedidiah.
Jeb, Jebadia, Jebadiah, Jebadieh, Jebidiah

Jed (Hebrew) a short form of Jedidiah. (Arabic) hand.
Jedd, Jeddy, Jedi

Jediah (Hebrew) hand of God.
Jedaia, Jedaiah, Jedeiah, Jedi, Yedaya

Jedidiah (Hebrew) friend of God, beloved of God. See also Didi.
Jebediah, Jed, Jedadiah, Jeddediah, Jedediah, Jedediha, Jedidia, Jedidiah, Jedidiyah, Yedidya

Jedrek (Polish) strong; manly.
Jedric, Jedrik, Jedrus

Jeff (English) a short form of Jefferson, Jeffrey. A familiar form of Geoffrey.
Jef, Jefe, Jeffe, Jeffey, Jeffie, Jeffy, Jhef

Jefferson (English) son of Jeff. History: Thomas Jefferson was the third U.S. president.
Jeferson, Jeff, Jeffers

Jeffery (English) a form of Jeffrey.
Jefery, Jeffari, Jeffary, Jeffeory, Jefferay, Jeffereoy, Jefferey, Jefferie, Jeffory

Jefford (English) Jeff's ford.

Jeffrey (English) divinely peaceful. See also Geffrey, Geoffrey, Godfrey.
Jeff, Jefferies, Jeffery, Jeffre, Jeffree, Jeffrie, Jeffrery, Jeffrie, Jeffries, Jeffry, Jefre, Jefri, Jefry, Jeoffroi, Joffre, Joffrey

Jeffry (English) a form of Jeffrey.

Jehan (French) a form of John.
Jehann

Jehu (Hebrew) God lives. Bible: a military commander and king of Israel.
Yehu

Jelani (Swahili) mighty.
Jel, Jelan, Jelanie, Jelaun

Jem (English) a short form of James, Jeremiah.
Jemmie, Jemmy

Jemal (Arabic) a form of Jamal.
Jemaal, Jemael, Jemale, Jemel

Jemel (Arabic) a form of Jemal.
Jemeal, Jemehl, Jemehyl, Jemell, Jemelle, Jemello, Jemeyle, Jemile, Jemmy

Jemond (French) worldly.
Jemon, Jémond, Jemonde, Jemone

Jenkin (Flemish) little John.
Jenkins, Jenkyn, Jenkyns, Jennings

Jenö (Hungarian) a form of Eugene.
Jenci, Jency, Jenoe, Jensi, Jensy

Jens (Danish) a form of John.
Jense, Jensen, Jenson, Jenssen, Jensy, Jentz

Jeovanni (Italian) a form of
Giovanni.
*Jeovahny, Jeovan, Jeovani,
Jeovany*

Jequan (American) a combi-
nation of the prefix Je +
Quan.
Jeqaun, Jequann, Jequon

Jerad, Jerrad (Hebrew) forms
of Jared.
Jeread, Jeredd

Jerahmy (Hebrew) a form of
Jeremy.
Jerahmeel, Jerahmeil, Jerahmey

Jerald (English) a form of
Gerald.
*Jeraldo, Jerold, Jerral, Jerrald,
Jerrold, Jerry*

Jerall (English) a form of
Jarrell.
*Jerael, Jerai, Jerail, Jeraile, Jeral,
Jerale, Jerall, Jerrail, Jerral, Jerrel,
Jerrell, Jerrelle*

Jeramie, Jeramy (Hebrew)
forms of Jeremy.
*Jerame, Jeramee, Jeramey, Jerami,
Jerammie*

Jerard (French) a form of
Gerard.
*Jarard, Jarrard, Jerardo, Jeraude,
Jerrard*

Jere (Hebrew) a short form of
Jeremiah, Jeremy.
Jeré, Jeree

Jered, Jerred (Hebrew) forms
of Jared.
Jereed, Jerid, Jerryd, Jeryd

Jerel, Jerell, Jerrell (English)
forms of Jarell.
*Jerelle, Jeriel, Jeril, Jerrail, Jerral,
Jerrall, Jerrel, Jerrill, Jerrol,
Jerroll, Jerryl, Jerryll, Jeryl, Jeryle*

Jereme, Jeremey (Hebrew)
forms of Jeremy.
Jarame

Jeremiah (Hebrew) God will
uplift. Bible: a Hebrew
prophet. See also Dermot,
Yeremey, Yirmaya.
*Geremiah, Jaramia, Jem,
Jemeriah, Jemiah, Jeramiah,
Jeramiha, Jere, Jereias, Jeremaya,
Jeremi, Jeremia, Jeremial,
Jeremias, Jeremija, Jeremy,
Jerimiah, Jerimiha, Jerimya,
Jermiah, Jermija, Jerry*

Jeremie, Jérémie (Hebrew)
forms of Jeremy.
Jeremi, Jérémie, Jeremii

Jeremy (English) a form of
Jeremiah.
*Jaremay, Jaremi, Jaremy, Jem,
Jemmy, Jerahmy, Jeramie, Jeramy,
Jere, Jereamy, Jereme, Jeremee,
Jeremey, Jeremie, Jérémie,
Jeremry, Jérémy, Jeremye,
Jereomy, Jeriemy, Jerime, Jerimy,
Jermey, Jeromy, Jerremy*

Jeriah (Hebrew) Jehovah has
seen.

Jericho (Arabic) city of the moon. Bible: a city conquered by Joshua.
Jeric, Jerick, Jerico, Jerik, Jerric, Jerrick, Jerrico, Jerricoh, Jerryco

Jermaine (French) a form of Germain. (English) sprout, bud.
Jarman, Jeremaine, Jeremane, Jerimane, Jermain, Jerman, Jermane, Jermanie, Jermanne, Jermany, Jermayn, Jermayne, Jermiane, Jermine, Jer-Mon, Jermone, Jermoney, Jhirmaine

Jermal (Arabic) a form of Jamal.
Jermael, Jermail, Jermall, Jermaul, Jermel, Jermell, Jermil, Jermol, Jermyll

Jermey (English) a form of Jeremy.
Jerme, Jermee, Jermere, Jermery, Jermie, Jermy, Jhermie

Jermiah (Hebrew) a form of Jeremiah.
Jermiha, Jermiya

Jerney (Slavic) a form of Bartholomew.

Jerod, Jerrod (Hebrew) forms of Jarrod.
Jerode, Jeroid

Jerolin (Basque, Latin) holy.

Jerome (Latin) holy. See also Geronimo, Hieronymos.
Gerome, Jere, Jeroen, Jerom, Jérome, Jérôme, Jeromo, Jeromy, Jeron, Jerónimo, Jerrome, Jerromy

Jeromy (Latin) a form of Jerome.
Jeromee, Jeromey, Jeromie

Jeron (English) a form of Jerome.
Jéron, Jerone, Jeronimo, Jerrin, Jerrion, Jerron, Jerrone, J'ron

Jerrett (Hebrew) a form of Jarrett.
Jeret, Jerett, Jeritt, Jerret, Jerrette, Jerriot, Jerritt, Jerrot, Jerrott

Jerrick (American) a combination of Jerry + Derrick.
Jaric, Jarrick, Jerick, Jerrik

Jerry (German) mighty spearman. (English) a familiar form of Gerald, Gerard. See also Gerry, Kele.
Jehri, Jere, Jeree, Jeris, Jerison, Jerri, Jerrie, Jery

Jervis (English) a form of Gervaise, Jarvis.

Jerzy (Polish) a form of George.
Jersey, Jerzey, Jurek

Jeshua (Hebrew) a form of Joshua.
Jeshuah

Jess (Hebrew) a short form of Jesse.

Jesse (Hebrew) wealthy. Bible: the father of David. See also Yishai.
Jese, Jesee, Jesi, Jess, Jessé, Jessee, Jessie, Jessy

Jessie (Hebrew) a form of Jesse.
Jesie, Jessi, Jessi

Jessy (Hebrew) a form of Jesse.
Jescey, Jessey, Jessye, Jessyie, Jesy

Jestin (Welsh) a form of Justin.
Jessten, Jesten, Jeston, Jesstin, Jesston

Jesus (Hebrew) a form of Joshua. Bible: son of Mary and Joseph, believed by Christians to be the Son of God. See also Chucho, Isa, Yosu.
Jecho, Jessus, Jesu, Jesús, Josu

Jesús (Hispanic) a form of Jesus.

Jethro (Hebrew) abundant. Bible: the father-in-law of Moses. See also Yitro.
Jeth, Jethroe, Jetro, Jett

Jett (English) hard, black mineral. (Hebrew) a short form of Jethro.
Jet, Jetson, Jetter, Jetty

Jevan (Hebrew) a form of Javan.
Jevaun, Jeven, Jevin

Jevon (Hebrew) a form of Javan.
Jevion, Jevohn, Jevone, Jevonn, Jevonne, Jevonnie

Jevonte (American) a form of Jevon.
Jevonta, Jevontae, Jevontaye, Jevonté

Jibade (Yoruba) born close to royalty.

Jibben (Gypsy) life.
Jibin

Jibril (Arabic) archangel of Allah.
Jabril, Jibreel, Jibriel

Jilt (Dutch) money.

Jim (Hebrew, English) a short form of James. See also Jaap.
Jimbo, Jimm, Jimmy

Jimbo (American) a familiar form of Jim.
Jimboo

Jimell (Arabic) a form of Jamel.
Jimel, Jimelle, Jimill, Jimmell, Jimmelle, Jimmiel, Jimmil

Jimiyu (Abaluhya) born in the dry season.

Jimmie (English) a form of Jimmy.
Jimi, Jimie, Jimmee, Jimmi

Jimmy (English) a familiar form of Jim.
Jimmey, Jimmie, Jimmye, Jimmyjo, Jimy

Jimoh (Swahili) born on Friday.

Jin (Chinese) gold.
Jinn

Jindra (Czech) a form of Harold.

Jing-Quo (Chinese) ruler of the country.

Jiovanni (Italian) a form of Giovanni.
Jio, Jiovani, Jiovanie, Jiovann, Jiovannie, Jiovanny, Jiovany, Jiovoni, Jivan

Jirair (Armenian) strong; hard working.

Jiri (Czech) a form of George.
Jirka

Jiro (Japanese) second son.

Jivin (Hindi) life giver.
Jivanta

Jo (Hebrew, Japanese) a form of Joe.

Joab (Hebrew) God is father. See also Yoav.
Joabe, Joaby

Joachim (Hebrew) God will establish. See also Akeem, Ioakim, Yehoyakem.
Joacheim, Joakim, Joaquim, Joaquín, Jokin, Jov

João (Portuguese) a form of John.

Joaquim (Portuguese) a form of Joachim.

Joaquín (Spanish) a form of Joachim, Yehoyakem.
Jehoichin, Joaquin, Jocquin, Jocquinn, Joquin, Juaquin

Job (Hebrew) afflicted. Bible: a righteous man whose faith in God survived the test of many afflictions.
Jobe, Jobert, Jobey, Jobie, Joby

Joben (Japanese) enjoys cleanliness.
Joban, Jobin

Jobo (Spanish) a familiar form of Joseph.

Joby (Hebrew) a familiar form of Job.
Jobie

Jock (American) a familiar form of Jacob.
Jocko, Joco, Jocoby, Jocolby

Jocquez (French) a form of Jacquez.
Jocques, Jocquis, Jocquise

Jodan (Hebrew) a combination of Jo + Dan.
Jodahn, Joden, Jodhan, Jodian, Jodin, Jodon, Jodonnis

Jody (Hebrew) a familiar form of Joseph.
Jodey, Jodi, Jodie, Jodiha, Joedy

Joe (Hebrew) a short form of Joseph.
Jo, Joely, Joey

Joel (Hebrew) God is willing.
Bible: an Old Testament
Hebrew prophet.
*Jóel, Joël, Joell, Joelle, Joely, Jole,
Yoel*

Joeseph (Hebrew) a form of
Joseph.
Joesph

Joey (Hebrew) a familiar form
of Joe, Joseph.

Johan, Johann (German)
forms of John. See also
Anno, Hanno, Yoan, Yohan.
*Joahan, Joan, Joannes, Johahn,
Johan, Johanan, Johane,
Johannan, Johannes, Johanthan,
Johatan, Johathan, Johathon,
Johaun, Johon*

Johannes (German) a form of
Johan, Johann.
*Johanes, Johannas, Johannus,
Johansen, Johanson, Johonson*

John (Hebrew) God is
gracious. Bible: the name
honoring John the Baptist
and John the Evangelist. See
also Elchanan, Evan, Geno,
Gian, Giovanni, Handel,
Hannes, Hans, Hanus,
Honza, Ian, Ianos, Iban, Ioan,
Ivan, Iwan, Keoni, Kwam,
Ohannes, Sean, Ugutz, Yan,
Yanka, Yanni, Yochanan,
Yohance, Zane.
*Jack, Jacsi, Jaenda, Jahn, Jan,
Janak, Janco, Janek, Janis, Janne,
János, Jansen, Jantje, Jantzen,*

*Jas, Jean, Jehan, Jen, Jenkin,
Jenkyn, Jens, Jhan, Jhanick,
Jhon, Jian, Joáo, João, Jock, Joen,
Johan, Johann, Johne, Johnl,
Johnlee, Johnnie, Johnny,
Johnson, Jon, Jonam, Jonas, Jone,
Jones, Jonny, Jonté, Jovan, Juan,
Juhana*

Johnathan (Hebrew) a form
of Jonathan.
*Jhonathan, Johathe, Johnatan,
Johnathann, Johnathaon,
Johnathen, Johnathyne,
Johnatten, Johniathin,
Johnothan, Johnthan*

Johnathon (Hebrew) a form
of Jonathon. See also Yanton.
Johnaton

Johnnie (Hebrew) a familiar
form of John.
*Johnie, Johnier, Johnni, Johnsie,
Jonni, Jonnie*

Johnny (Hebrew) a familiar
form of John. See also
Gianni.
*Jantje, Jhonny, Johney, Johnney,
Johny, Jonny*

Johnson (English) son of
John.
Johnston, Jonson

Joji (Japanese) a form of
George.

Jojo (Fante) born on Monday.

Jokim (Basque) a form of
Joachim.

Jolon (Native American) valley of the dead oaks.
Jolyon

Jomar (American) a form of Jamar.
Jomari, Jomarie, Jomarri

Jomei (Japanese) spreads light.

Jon (Hebrew) a form of John. A short form of Jonathan.
J'on, Joni, Jonn, Jonnie, Jonny, Jony

Jonah (Hebrew) dove. Bible: an Old Testament prophet who was swallowed by a large fish.
Giona, Jona, Yonah, Yunus

Jonas (Hebrew) he accomplishes. (Lithuanian) a form of John.
Jonahs, Jonass, Jonaus, Jonelis, Jonukas, Jonus, Jonutis, Joonas

Jonatan (Hebrew) a form of Jonathan.
Jonatane, Jonate, Jonattan, Jonnattan

Jonathan (Hebrew) gift of God. Bible: the son of King Saul who became a loyal friend of David. See also Ionakana, Yanton, Yonatan.
Janathan, Johnathan, Johnathon, Jon, Jonatan, Jonatha, Jonathen, Jonathin, Jonathon, Jonathun, Jonathyn, Jonethen, Jonnatha, Jonnathan, Jonnathun, Jonothan, Jonthan

Jonathon (Hebrew) a form of Jonathan.
Joanathon, Johnathon, Jonnathon, Jonothon, Jonthon, Jounathon, Yanaton

Jones (Welsh) son of John.
Joenns, Joness, Jonesy

Jonny (Hebrew) a familiar form of John.
Jonhy, Joni, Jonnee, Jony

Jontae (French) a combination of Jon + the suffix Tae.
Johntae, Jontay, Jontea, Jonteau, Jontez

Jontay (American) a form of Jontae.
Johntay, Johnte, Johntez, Jontai, Jonte, Jonté, Jontez

Joop (Dutch) a familiar form of Joseph.
Jopie

Joost (Dutch) just.

Joquin (Spanish) a form of Joaquin.
Joquan, Joquawn, Joqunn, Joquon

Jora (Hebrew) teacher.
Yora, Jorah

Joram (Hebrew) Jehovah is exalted.
Joran, Jorim

Jordan (Hebrew) descending. See also Giordano, Yarden.
Jardan, Jared, Jordaan, Jordae, Jordain, Jordaine, Jordane,

*Jordani, Jordanio, Jordann,
Jordanny, Jordano, Jordany,
Jordáo, Jordayne, Jorden, Jordian,
Jordin, Jordon, Jordun, Jordy,
Jordyn, Jorrdan, Jory, Jourdan*

Jorden (Hebrew) a form of
Jordan.
Jordenn

Jordon (Hebrew) a form of
Jordan.
Jeordon, Johordan

Jordy (Hebrew) a familiar
form of Jordan.
Jordi, Jordie

Jordyn (Hebrew) a form of
Jordan.

Jorell (American) he saves.
Literature: a name inspired
by the fictional character Jor-
El, Superman's father.
*Jorel, Jor-El, Jorelle, Jorl, Jorrel,
Jorrell*

Jörg (German) a form of
George.
Jeorg, Juergen, Jungen, Jürgen

Jorge (Spanish) a form of
George.
Jorrín

Jorgen (Danish) a form of
George.
Joergen, Jorgan, Jörgen

Joris (Dutch) a form of
George.

Jörn (German) a familiar form
of Gregory.

Jorrín (Spanish) a form of
George.
Jorian, Jorje

Jory (Hebrew) a familiar form
of Jordan.
Joar, Joary, Jorey, Jori, Jorie, Jorrie

José (Spanish) a form of
Joseph. See also Ché, Pepe.
*Josean, Josecito, Josee, Joseito,
Joselito, Josey*

Josef (German, Portuguese,
Czech, Scandinavian) a form
of Joseph.
*Joosef, Joseff, Josif, Jozef, József,
Juzef*

Joseluis (Spanish) a combination of Jose + Luis.

Joseph (Hebrew) God will
add, God will increase. Bible:
in the Old Testament, the son
of Jacob who came to rule
Egypt; in the New
Testament, the husband of
Mary. See also Beppe,
Cheche, Chepe, Giuseppe,
Iokepa, Iosif, Osip, Pepa,
Peppe, Pino, Sepp, Yeska,
Yosef, Yousef, Youssel, Yusif,
Yusuf, Zeusef.
*Jazeps, Jo, Jobo, Jody, Joe,
Joeseph, Joey, Jojo, Joop, Joos,
Jooseppi, Jopie, José, Joseba, Josef,
Josep, Josephat, Josephe, Josephie,
Josephus, Josheph, Josip, Jóska,
Joza, Joze, Jozef, Jozeph, Jozhe,
Jozio, Jozka, Jozsi, Jozzepi,
Jupp, Juziu*

Josh (Hebrew) a short form of
Joshua.
Joshe

Josha (Hindi) satisfied.

Joshi (Swahili) galloping.

Joshua (Hebrew) God is my
salvation. Bible: led the
Israelites into the Promised
Land. See also Giosia, Iosua,
Jesus, Yehoshua.
*Jeshua, Johsua, Johusa, Josh,
Joshau, Joshaua, Joshauh,
Joshawa, Joshawah, Joshia,
Joshu, Joshuaa, Joshuah,
Joshuea, Joshuia, Joshula, Joshus,
Joshusa, Joshuwa, Joshwa, Josue,
Jousha, Jozshua, Jozsua, Jozua,
Jushua*

Josiah (Hebrew) fire of the
Lord. See also Yoshiyahu.
*Joshiah, Josia, Josiahs, Josian,
Josias, Josie*

Joss (Chinese) luck; fate.
Josse, Jossy

Josue (Hebrew) a form of
Joshua.
*Joshue, Jossue, Josu, Josua,
Josuha, Jozus*

Jotham (Hebrew) may God
complete. Bible: a king of
Judah.

Jourdan (Hebrew) a form of
Jordan.
*Jourdain, Jourden, Jourdin,
Jourdon, Jourdyn*

Jovan (Latin) Jove-like, majes-
tic. (Slavic) a form of John.
Mythology: Jove, also known
as Jupiter, was the supreme
Roman deity.
*Johvan, Johvon, Jovaan, Jovane,
Jovani, Jovanic, Jovann, Jovanni,
Jovannis, Jovanny, Jovany,
Jovaughn, Jovaun, Joven,
Jovenal, Jovenel, Jovi, Jovian,
Jovin, Jovito, Jovoan, Jovon,
Jovone, Jovonn, Jovonne, Jowan,
Jowaun, Yovan, Yovani*

Jovani, Jovanni (Latin) forms
of Jovan.
*Jovanie, Jovannie, Jovoni,
Jovonie, Jovonni*

Jovanny, Jovany (Latin) forms
of Jovan.
Jovony

Jr (Latin) a short form of
Junior.
Jr.

Juan (Spanish) a form of John.
See also Chan.
*Juanch, Juanchito, Juane, Juanito,
Juann, Juaun*

Juancarlos (Spanish) a combination of Juan + Carlos.

Juaquin (Spanish) a form of
Joaquín.
*Juaqin, Juaqine, Juquan,
Juaquine*

Jubal (Hebrew) ram's horn.
Bible: a musician and a
descendant of Cain.

Judah (Hebrew) praised. Bible: the fourth of Jacob's sons. See also Yehudi.
Juda, Judas, Judd, Jude

Judas (Latin) a form of Judah. Bible: Judas Iscariot was the disciple who betrayed Jesus.
Jude

Judd (Hebrew) a short form of Judah.
Jud, Judson

Jude (Latin) a short form of Judah, Judas. Bible: one of the Twelve Apostles, author of "The Epistle of Jude."

Judson (English) son of Judd.

Juhana (Finnish) a form of John.
Juha, Juho

Juku (Estonian) a form of Richard.
Jukka

Jules (French) a form of Julius.
Joles, Jule

Julian (Greek, Latin) a form of Julius.
Jolyon, Julean, Juliaan, Julianne, Juliano, Julien, Jullian, Julyan

Julien (Latin) a form of Julian.
Juliene, Julienn, Julienne, Jullien, Jullin

Julio (Hispanic) a form of Julius.

Julius (Greek, Latin) youthful, downy bearded. History: Julius Caesar was a great Roman dictator. See also Giuliano.
Jolyon, Julas, Jule, Jules, Julen, Jules, Julian, Julias, Julie, Julio, Juliusz, Jullius, Juluis

Jumaane (Swahili) born on Tuesday.

Jumah (Arabic, Swahili) born on Friday, a holy day in the Islamic religion.
Jimoh, Juma

Jumoke (Yoruba) loved by everyone.

Jun (Chinese) truthful. (Japanese) obedient; pure.
Junnie

Junior (Latin) young.
Jr, Junious, Junius, Junor

Jupp (German) a form of Joseph.

Jur (Czech) a form of George.
Juraz, Jurek, Jurik, Jurko, Juro

Jurgis (Lithuanian) a form of George.
Jurgi, Juri

Juro (Japanese) best wishes; long life.

Jurrien (Dutch) God will uplift.
Jore, Jurian, Jurre

Justen (Latin) a form of Justin.
Jasten

Justice (Latin) a form of Justis.
Justic, Justiz, Justyc, Justyce

Justin (Latin) just, righteous.
See also Giustino, Iestyn,
Iustin, Tutu, Ustin, Yustyn.
*Jastin, Jaston, Jestin, Jobst, Joost,
Jost, Jusa, Just, Justain, Justan,
Justas, Justek, Justen, Justian,
Justinas, Justine, Justinian,
Justinius, Justinn, Justino,
Justins, Justinus, Justo, Juston,
Justton, Justukas, Justun, Justyn*

Justis (French) just.
Justice, Justs, Justus, Justyse

Justyn (Latin) a form of Justin.
Justn, Justyne, Justynn

Juvenal (Latin) young.
Literature: a Roman satirist.
Juvon, Juvone

Juwan (American) a form of
Jajuan.
*Juvon, Juvone, Juvaun, Juwaan,
Juwain, Juwane, Juwann,
Juwaun, Juwon, Juwonn,
Juwuan, Juwuane, Juwvan,
Jwan, Jwon*

K

Kabiito (Rutooro) born while
foreigners are visiting.

Kabil (Turkish) a form of
Cain.
Kabel

Kabir (Hindi) History: an
Indian mystic poet.
Kabar, Kabeer, Kabier

Kabonero (Runyankore) sign.

Kabonesa (Rutooro) difficult
birth.

Kacey (Irish) a form of Casey.
(American) a combination of
the initials K. + C. See also
KC.
*Kace, Kacee, Kaci, Kacy, Kaesy,
Kase, Kasey, Kasie, Kasy,
Kaycee*

Kadar (Arabic) powerful.
Kader

Kadarius (American) a com-
bination of Kade + Darius.
*Kadairious, Kadarious, Kadaris,
Kadarrius, Kadarus, Kaddarrius,
Kaderious, Kaderius*

Kade (Scottish) wetlands.
(American) a combination of
the initials K. + D.
*Kadee, Kady, Kaid, Kaide,
Kaydee*

Kadeem (Arabic) servant.
Kadim, Khadeem

Kaden (Arabic) a form of
Kadin.
*Kadeen, Kadein, Kaidan,
Kaiden*

Kadin (Arabic) friend, companion.
Caden, Kaden, Kadyn, Kaeden, Kayden

Kadir (Arabic) spring greening.
Kadeer

Kado (Japanese) gateway.

Kaeden (Arabic) a form of Kadin.
Kaedin, Kaedon, Kaedyn

Kaelan, Kaelin (Irish) forms of Kellen.
Kael, Kaelen, Kaelon, Kaelyn

Kaeleb (Hebrew) a form of Kaleb.
Kaelib, Kaelob, Kaelyb, Kailab, Kaileb

Kaemon (Japanese) joyful; right-handed.
Kaeman, Kaemen, Kaemin

Kaenan (Irish) a form of Keenan.
Kaenen, Kaenin, Kaenyn

Ka'eo (Hawaiian) victorious.

Kafele (Nguni) worth dying for.

Kaga (Native American) writer.

Kagan (Irish) a form of Keegan.
Kage, Kagen, Kaghen, Kaigan

Kahale (Hawaiian) home.

Kahil (Turkish) young; inexperienced; naive.
Cahil, Kaheel, Kale, Kayle

Kahlil (Arabic) a form of Khalíl.
Kahleal, Kahlee, Kahleel, Kahleil, Kahli, Kahliel, Kahlill, Kalel, Kalil

Kaholo (Hawaiian) runner.

Kahraman (Turkish) hero.

Kai (Welsh) keeper of the keys. (German) a form of Kay. (Hawaiian) sea.
Kae, Kaie, Kaii

Kaikara (Runyoro) Religion: a Banyoro deity.

Kailen (Irish) a form of Kellen.
Kail, Kailan, Kailey, Kailin, Kailon, Kailyn

Kaili (Hawaiian) Religion: a Hawaiian god.
Kailli

Kain (Welsh, Irish) a form of Kane.
Kainan, Kaine, Kainen, Kainin, Kainon

Kainoa (Hawaiian) name.

Kaipo (Hawaiian) sweetheart.

Kairo (Arabic) a form of Cairo.
Kaire, Kairee, Kairi

Kaiser (German) a form of Caesar.
Kaesar, Kaisar, Kaizer

Kaiven (American) a form of Kevin.
Kaivan, Kaiven, Kaivon, Kaiwan

Kaj (Danish) earth.
Kai, Kaje

Kakar (Hindi) grass.

Kala (Hindi) black; phase. (Hawaiian) sun.

Kalama (Hawaiian) torch.
Kalam

Kalan (Irish) a form of Kalen.
Kalane, Kallan

Kalani (Hawaiian) sky; chief.
Kalan

Kale (Arabic) a short form of Kahlil. (Hawaiian) a familiar form of Carl.
Kalee, Kalen, Kaleu, Kaley, Kali, Kalin, Kalle, Kayle

Kaleb (Hebrew) a form of Caleb.
Kaeleb, Kal, Kalab, Kalabe, Kalb, Kale, Kaleob, Kalev, Kalib, Kalieb, Kallb, Kalleb, Kalob, Kaloeb, Kalub, Kalyb, Kilab

Kalen, Kalin (Arabic, Hawaiian) forms of Kale. (Irish) forms of Kellen.
Kalan

Kalevi (Finnish) hero.

Kali (Arabic) a short form of Kalil. (Hawaiian) a form of Gary.

Kalil (Arabic) a form of Khalíl.
Kaleel, Kalell, Kali, Kaliel, Kaliil

Kaliq (Arabic) a form of Khaliq.
Kalic, Kalique

Kalkin (Hindi) tenth. Religion: Kalki is the final incarnation of the Hindu god Vishnu.
Kalki

Kalle (Scandinavian) a form of Carl. (Arabic, Hawaiian) a form of Kale.

Kallen (Irish) a form of Kellen.
Kallan, Kallin, Kallion, Kallon, Kallun, Kalun

Kalon, Kalyn (Irish) forms of Kellen.
Kalone, Kalonn, Kalyen, Kalyne, Kalynn

Kaloosh (Armenian) blessed event.

Kalvin (Latin) a form of Calvin.
Kal, Kalv, Kalvan, Kalven, Kalvon, Kalvyn, Vinny

Kamaka (Hawaiian) face.

Kamakani (Hawaiian) wind.

Kamal (Hindi) lotus. (Arabic) perfect, perfection.
Kamaal, Kamel, Kamil

Kamau (Kikuyu) quiet warrior.

Kamden (Scottish) a form of Camden.
Kamdon

Kameron (Scottish) a form of Cameron.
Kam, Kamaren, Kamaron, Kameran, Kameren, Kamerin, Kamerion, Kamerron, Kamerun, Kameryn, Kamey, Kammeren, Kammeron, Kammy, Kamoryn, Kamran, Kamron

Kami (Hindi) loving.

Kamil (Arabic) a form of Kamal.
Kameel

Kamran, Kamron (Scottish) forms of Kameron.
Kammron, Kamrein, Kamren, Kamrin, Kamrun, Kamryn

Kamuela (Hawaiian) a form of Samuel.

Kamuhanda (Runyankore) born on the way to the hospital.

Kamukama (Runyankore) protected by God.

Kamuzu (Nguni) medicine.

Kamya (Luganda) born after twin brothers.

Kana (Japanese) powerful; capable. (Hawaiian) Mythology: a demigod.

Kanaiela (Hawaiian) a form of Daniel.
Kana, Kaneii

Kane (Welsh) beautiful. (Irish) tribute. (Japanese) golden. (Hawaiian) eastern sky. (English) a form of Keene. See Kahan, Kain, Kaney, Kayne.

Kange (Lakota) raven.
Kang, Kanga

Kaniel (Hebrew) stalk, reed.
Kan, Kani, Kannie, Kanny

Kannan (Hindi) Religion: another name for the Hindu god Krishna.
Kanaan, Kanan, Kanen, Kanin, Kanine, Kannen

Kannon (Polynesian) free. (French) A form of Cannon.
Kanon

Kanoa (Hawaiian) free.

Kantu (Hindi) happy.

Kanu (Swahili) wildcat.

Kaori (Japanese) strong.

Kapila (Hindi) ancient prophet.
Kapil

Kapono (Hawaiian) righteous.
Kapena

Kardal (Arabic) mustard seed.
Karandal, Kardell

Kare (Norwegian) enormous.
Karee

Kareem (Arabic) noble; distinguished.
Karee, Karem, Kareme, Karim, Karriem

Karel (Czech) a form of Carl.
Karell, Karil, Karrell

Karey (Greek) a form of Carey.
Karee, Kari, Karry, Kary

Karif (Arabic) born in autumn.
Kareef

Kariisa (Runyankore) herdsman.

Karim (Arabic) a form of
Kareem.

Karl (German) a form of Carl.
Kaarle, Kaarlo, Kale, Kalle, Kalman, Kálmán, Karcsi, Karel, Kari, Karlen, Karlitis, Karlo, Karlos, Karlton, Karlus, Karol, Kjell

Karlen (Latvian, Russian) a
form of Carl.
Karlan, Karlens, Karlik, Karlin, Karlis, Karlon

Karmel (Hebrew) a form of
Carmel.

Karney (Irish) a form of Carney.

Karol (Czech, Polish) a form
of Carl.
Karal, Karolek, Karolis, Karalos, Károly, Karrel, Karrol

Karr (Scandinavian) a form of
Carr.

Karson (English) a form of
Carson.
Karrson, Karsen

Karsten (Greek) anointed.
Carsten, Karstan, Karston

Karu (Hindi) cousin.
Karun

Karutunda (Runyankore) little.

Karwana (Rutooro) born during wartime.

Kaseem (Arabic) divided.
Kasceem, Kaseam, Kaseym, Kasim, Kasseem, Kassem, Kazeem

Kaseko (Rhodesian) mocked,
ridiculed.

Kasem (Tai) happiness.

Kasen (Basque) protected
with a helmet.
Kasean, Kasene, Kaseon, Kasin, Kason, Kassen

Kasey (Irish) a form of Casey.
Kaese, Kaesy, Kasay, Kassey

Kashawn (American) a combination of the prefix Ka +
Shawn.
Kashain, Kashan, Kashaun, Kashen, Kashon

Kasib (Arabic) fertile.

Kasim (Arabic) a form of
Kaseem.
Kassim

Kasimir (Arabic) peace.
(Slavic) a form of Casimir.
Kasim, Kazimierz, Kazimir,
Kazio, Kazmer, Kazmér,
Kázmér

Kasiya (Nguni) separate.

Kasper (Persian) treasurer.
(German) a form of Casper.
Jasper, Kaspar, Kaspero

Kass (German) blackbird.
Kaese, Kasch, Kase

Kassidy (Irish) a form of
Cassidy.
Kassady, Kassie, Kassy

Kateb (Arabic) writer.

Kato (Runyankore) second of
twins.

Katungi (Runyankore) rich.

Kavan (Irish) handsome.
Cavan, Kavánagh, Kavaugn,
Kaven, Kavenaugh, Kavin,
Kavon, Kayvan

Kaveh (Persian) ancient hero.

Kavi (Hindi) poet.

Kavin, Kavon (Irish) forms of
Kavan.
Kaveon, Kavion, Kavone,
Kayvon, Kaywon

Kawika (Hawaiian) a form of
David.

Kay (Greek) rejoicing.
(German) fortified place.
Literature: one of King
Arthur's knights of the
Round Table.
Kai, Kaycee, Kaye, Kayson

Kayden (Arabic) a form of
Kadin.
Kayde, Kaydee, Kaydin, Kaydn,
Kaydon

Kayin (Nigerian) celebrated.
(Yoruba) long-hoped-for
child.

Kayle (Hebrew) faithful dog.
(Arabic) a short form of
Kahlil.
Kayl, Kayla, Kaylee

Kayleb (Hebrew) a form of
Caleb.
Kaylib, Kaylob, Kaylub

Kaylen (Irish) a form of
Kellen.
Kaylan, Kaylin, Kaylon,
Kaylyn, Kaylynn

Kayne (Hebrew) a form of
Cain.
Kaynan, Kaynen, Kaynon

Kayode (Yoruba) he brought
joy.

Kayonga (Runyankore) ash.

Kazio (Polish) a form of
Casimir, Kasimir. See also
Cassidy.

Kazuo (Japanese) man of
peace.

KC (American) a combination of the initials K. + C. See also Kacey.
Kc, K.C., Kcee, Kcey

Keagan (Irish) a form of Keegan.
Keagean, Keagen, Keaghan, Keagyn

Keahi (Hawaiian) flames.

Keaka (Hawaiian) a form of Jack.

Kealoha (Hawaiian) fragrant.
Ke'ala

Keanan (Irish) a form of Keenan.
Keanen, Keanna, Keannan, Keanon

Keandre (American) a combination of the prefix Ke + Andre.
Keandra, Keandray, Keandré, Keandree, Keandrell, Keondre

Keane (German) bold; sharp. (Irish) handsome. (English) a form of Keene.
Kean

Keanu (Irish) a form of Keenan.
Keaneu, Keani, Keanno, Keano, Keanue, Keeno, Keenu, Kianu

Kearn (Irish) a short form of Kearney.
Kearne

Kearney (Irish) a form of Carney.
Kar, Karney, Karny, Kearn, Kearny

Keary (Irish) a form of Kerry.
Kearie

Keaton (English) where hawks fly.
Keatan, Keaten, Keatin, Keatton, Keatyn, Keeton, Keetun

Keaven (Irish) a form of Kevin.
Keavan, Keavon

Keawe (Hawaiian) strand.

Keb (Egyptian) earth. Mythology: an ancient earth god, also known as Geb.

Kedar (Hindi) mountain lord. (Arabic) powerful. Religion: another name for the Hindu god Shiva.
Kadar, Kedaar, Keder

Keddy (Scottish) a form of Adam.
Keddie

Kedem (Hebrew) ancient.

Kedrick (English) a form of Cedric.
Keddrick, Kederick, Kedrek, Kedric, Kiedric, Kiedrick

Keefe (Irish) handsome; loved.

Keegan (Irish) little; fiery.
Kaegan, Kagan, Keagan,

*Keagen, Keeghan, Keegon,
Keegun, Kegan, Keigan*

Keelan (Irish) little; slender.
*Keelen, Keelin, Keelyn, Keilan,
Kelan*

Keeley (Irish) handsome.
*Kealey, Kealy, Keeli, Keelian,
Keelie, Keely*

Keenan (Irish) little Keene.
*Kaenan, Keanan, Keanu,
Keenen, Keennan, Keenon,
Kenan, Keynan, Kienan,
Kienon*

Keene (German) bold; sharp.
(English) smart. See also
Kane.
Kaene, Keane, Keen, Keenan

Keenen (Irish) a form of
Keenan.
Keenin, Kienen

Kees (Dutch) a form of
Kornelius.
Keese, Keesee, Keyes

Keevon (Irish) a form of
Kevin.
*Keevan, Keeven, Keevin,
Keewan, Keewin*

Kegan (Irish) a form of
Keegan.
Kegen, Keghan, Kegon, Kegun

Kehind (Yoruba) second-born
twin.
Kehinde

Keiffer (German) a form of
Cooper.
Keefer, Keifer, Kiefer

Keigan (Irish) a form of
Keegan.
Keighan, Keighen

Keiji (Japanese) cautious ruler.

Keilan (Irish) a form of
Keelan.
*Keilen, Keilin, Keillene,
Keillyn, Keilon, Keilynn*

Keir (Irish) a short form of
Kieran.

Keitaro (Japanese) blessed.
Keita

Keith (Welsh) forest. (Scottish)
battle place. See also Kika.
Keath, Keeth, Keithen

Keithen (Welsh, Scottish) a
form of Keith.
Keithan, Keitheon, Keithon

Keivan (Irish) a form of
Kevin.
Keiven, Keivn, Keivon, Keivone

Kekapa (Hawaiian) tapa cloth.

Kekipi (Hawaiian) rebel.

Kekoa (Hawaiian) bold,
courageous.

Kelby (German) farm by the
spring.
*Keelby, Kelbee, Kelbey, Kelbi,
Kellby*

Kele (Hopi) sparrow hawk.
(Hawaiian) a form of Jerry.
Kelle

Kelemen (Hungarian) gentle;
kind.
Kellman

Kelevi (Finnish) hero.

Keli (Hawaiian) a form of
Terry.

Keli'i (Hawaiian) chief.

Kelile (Ethiopian) protected.

Kell (Scandinavian) spring.

Kellan (Irish) a form of
Kellen.
Keillan

Kellen (Irish) mighty warrior.
*Kaelan, Kailen, Kalan, Kalen,
Kalin, Kallen, Kalon, Kalyn,
Kaylen, Keelan, Kelden, Kelin,
Kellan, Kelle, Kellin, Kellyn,
Kelyn, Kelynn*

Keller (Irish) little companion.

Kelly (Irish) warrior.
*Kelle, Kellen, Kelley, Kelli,
Kellie, Kely*

Kelmen (Basque) merciful.
Kelmin

Kelsey (Scandinavian) island
of ships.
*Kelcy, Kelse, Kelsea, Kelsi,
Kelsie, Kelso, Kelsy, Kesley,
Kesly*

Kelton (English) keel town;
port.
*Kelden, Keldon, Kelson,
Kelston, Kelten, Keltin,
Keltonn, Keltyn*

Kelvin (Irish, English) narrow
river. Geography: a river in
Scotland.
*Kelvan, Kelven, Kelvon,
Kelvyn, Kelwin, Kelwyn*

Kemal (Turkish) highest
honor.

Kemen (Basque) strong.

Kemp (English) fighter; champion.

Kempton (English) military
town.

Ken (Japanese) one's own
kind. (Scottish) a short form
of Kendall, Kendrick,
Kenneth.
Kena, Kenn, Keno

Kenan (Irish) a form of
Keenan.

Kenaz (Hebrew) bright.

Kendal (English) a form of
Kendall.
*Kendale, Kendali, Kendel,
Kendul, Kendyl*

Kendall (English) valley of the
river Kent.
*Ken, Kendal, Kendell, Kendrall,
Kendryll, Kendyll, Kyndall*

Kendarius (American) a combination of Ken + Darius.
Kendarious, Kendarrious, Kendarrius, Kenderious, Kenderius, Kenderyious

Kendell (English) a form of Kendall.
Kendelle, Kendrel, Kendrell

Kendrew (Scottish) a form of Andrew.

Kendrick (Irish) son of Henry. (Scottish) royal chieftain.
Ken, Kenderrick, Kendric, Kendrich, Kenedrick, Kendricks, Kendrik, Kendrix, Kendryck, Kenndrick, Keondric, Keondrick

Kenley (English) royal meadow.
Kenlea, Kenlee, Kenleigh, Kenlie, Kenly

Kenn (Scottish) a form of Ken.

Kennan (Scottish) little Ken.
Kenna, Kenan, Kenen, Kennen, Kennon

Kennard (Irish) brave chieftain.
Kenner

Kennedy (Irish) helmeted chief. History: John F. Kennedy was the thirty-fifth U.S. president.
Kenedy, Kenidy, Kennady, Kennedey

Kenneth (Irish) handsome. (English) royal oath.
Ken, Keneth, Kenneith, Kennet, Kennethen, Kennett, Kennieth, Kennith, Kennth, Kenny, Kennyth, Kenya

Kenny (Scottish) a familiar form of Kenneth.
Keni, Kenney, Kenni, Kennie, Kinnie

Kenrick (English) bold ruler; royal ruler.
Kenric, Kenricks, Kenrik

Kent (Welsh) white; bright. (English) a short form of Kenton. Geography: a region in England.

Kentaro (Japanese) big boy.

Kenton (English) from Kent, England.
Kent, Kenten, Kentin, Kentonn

Kentrell (English) king's estate.
Kenreal, Kentrel, Kentrelle

Kenward (English) brave; royal guardian.

Kenya (Hebrew) animal horn. (Russian) a form of Kenneth. Geography: a country in east-central Africa.
Kenyatta

Kenyatta (American) a form of Kenya.
Kenyata, Kenyatae, Kenyatee, Kenyatter, Kenyatti, Kenyotta

Kenyon (Irish) white haired, blond.
Kenyan, Kenynn, Keonyon

Kenzie (Scottish) wise leader. See also Mackenzie.
Kensie

Keoki (Hawaiian) a form of George.

Keola (Hawaiian) life.

Keon (Irish) a form of Ewan.
Keeon, Keion, Keionne, Keondre, Keone, Keonne, Keonte, Keony, Keyon, Kian, Kion

Keoni (Hawaiian) a form of John.

Keonte (American) a form of Keon.
Keonntay, Keonta, Keontae, Keontay, Keontaye, Keontez, Keontia, Keontis, Keontrae, Keontre, Keontrey, Keontrye

Kerbasi (Basque) warrior.

Kerel (Afrikaans) young.
Kerell

Kerem (Turkish) noble; kind.
Kereem

Kerey (Gypsy) homeward bound.
Ker

Kerman (Basque) from Germany.

Kermit (Irish) a form of Dermot.
Kermey, Kermie, Kermitt, Kermy

Kern (Irish) a short form of Kieran.
Kearn, Kerne

Kerr (Scandinavian) a form of Carr.
Karr

Kerrick (English) king's rule.

Kerry (Irish) dark; dark haired.
Keary, Keri, Kerrey, Kerri, Kerrie

Kers (Todas) Botany: an Indian plant.

Kersen (Indonesian) cherry.

Kerstan (Dutch) a form of Christian.

Kerwin (Irish) little; dark. (English) friend of the marshlands.
Kervin, Kervyn, Kerwinn, Kerwyn, Kerwynn, Kirwin, Kirwyn

Kesar (Russian) a form of Caesar.
Kesare

Keshawn (American) a combination of the prefix Ke + Shawn.
Keeshaun, Keeshawn, Keeshon, Kesean, Keshan, Keshane, Keshaun, Keshayne, Keshion,

Keshon, Keshone, Keshun,
Kishan

Kesin (Hindi) long-haired
beggar.

Kesse (Ashanti, Fante) chubby
baby.
Kessie

Kester (English) a form of
Christopher.

Kestrel (English) falcon.
Kes

Keung (Chinese) universe.

Kevan (Irish) a form of Kevin.
Kavan, Kewan, Kewane,
Kewaun, Keyvan, Kiwan,
Kiwane

Keven (Irish) a form of Kevin.
Keve, Keveen, Kiven

Kevin (Irish) handsome. See
also Cavan.
Kaiven, Keaven, Keevon,
Keivan, Kev, Kevan, Keven,
Keverne, Kevian, Kevien,
Kévin, Kevinn, Kevins, Kevis,
Kevn, Kevon, Kevvy, Kevyn,
Kyven

Kevon (Irish) a form of Kevin.
Keveon, Kevion, Kevone,
Kevonne, Kevontae, Kevonte,
Kevoyn, Kevron, Kewon,
Kewone, Keyvon, Kivon

Kevyn (Irish) a form of Kevin.
Kevyon

Key (English) key; protected.

Keyon (Irish) a form of Keon.
Keyan, Keyen, Keyin, Keyion

Keyshawn (American) a com-
bination of Key + Shawn.
Keyshan, Keyshaun, Keyshon,
Keyshun

Khachig (Armenian) small
cross.
Khachik

Khaim (Russian) a form of
Chaim.

Khaldun (Arabic) forever.
Khaldoon, Khaldoun

Khalfani (Swahili) born to
lead.
Khalfan

Khälid (Arabic) eternal.
Khaled, Khallid, Khalyd

Khalíl (Arabic) friend.
Kahlil, Kaleel, Kalil, Khahlil,
Khailil, Khailyl, Khalee,
Khaleel, Khaleil, Khali,
Khalial, Khaliel, Khalihl,
Khalill, Khaliyl

Khaliq (Arabic) creative.
Kaliq, Khalique

Khamisi (Swahili) born on
Thursday.
Kham

Khan (Turkish) prince.
Khanh

Kharald (Russian) a form of
Gerald.

Khayru (Arabic) benevolent.
Khiri, Khiry, Kiry

Khoury (Arabic) priest.
Khory

Khristian (Greek) a form of
Christian, Kristian.
*Khris, Khristan, Khristin,
Khriston, Khrystian*

Khristopher (Greek) a form
of Kristopher.
*Khristofer, Khristophar,
Khrystopher*

Khristos (Greek) a form of
Christos.
*Khris, Khristophe, Kristo,
Kristos*

Kibo (Uset) worldly; wise.

Kibuuka (Luganda) brave warrior. History: a Ganda warrior deity.

Kidd (English) child; young
goat.

Kiefer (German) a form of
Keifer.
*Kief, Kieffer, Kiefor, Kiffer,
Kiiefer*

Kiel (Irish) a form of Kyle.
Kiell

Kiele (Hawaiian) gardenia.

Kieran (Irish) little and dark;
little Keir.
*Keiran, Keiren, Keiron, Kiaron,
Kiarron, Kier, Kieren, Kierian,
Kierien, Kierin, Kiernan,*

*Kieron, Kierr, Kierre, Kierron,
Kyran*

Kiernan (Irish) a form of
Kieran.
Kern, Kernan, Kiernen

Kiet (Tai) honor.

Kifeda (Luo) only boy among
girls.

Kiho (Rutooro) born on a
foggy day.

Kijika (Native American)
quiet walker.

Kika (Hawaiian) a form of
Keith.

Kiki (Spanish) a form of
Henry.

Kile (Irish) a form of Kyle.
Kilee, Kilen, Kiley, Kiyl, Kiyle

Killian (Irish) little Kelly.
*Kilean, Kilian, Kilien, Killie,
Killien, Killiean, Killion, Killy*

Kim (English) a short form of
Kimball.
Kimie, Kimmy

Kimball (Greek) hollow ves-
sel. (English) warrior chief.
*Kim, Kimbal, Kimbel, Kimbell,
Kimble*

Kimo (Hawaiian) a form of
James.

Kimokeo (Hawaiian) a form
of Timothy.

Kin (Japanese) golden.

Kincaid (Scottish) battle chief.
Kincade, Kinkaid

Kindin (Basque) fifth.

King (English) king. A short
form of names beginning
with "King."

Kingsley (English) king's
meadow.
*King, Kings, Kingslea, Kingslie,
Kingsly, Kingzlee, Kinslea,
Kinslee, Kinsley, Kinslie, Kinsly*

Kingston (English) king's
estate.
King, Kinston

Kingswell (English) king's
well.
King

Kini (Hawaiian) a short form
of Iukini.

Kinnard (Irish) tall slope.

Kinsey (English) victorious
royalty.
Kinze, Kinzie

Kinton (Hindi) crowned.

Kion (Irish) a form of Keon.
Kione, Kionie, Kionne

Kioshi (Japanese) quiet.

Kipp (English) pointed hill.
*Kip, Kippar, Kipper, Kippie,
Kippy*

Kir (Bulgarian) a familiar form
of Cyrus.

Kiral (Turkish) king; supreme
leader.

Kiran (Sanskrit) beam of light.
Kyran

Kirby (Scandinavian) church
village. (English) cottage by
the water.
*Kerbey, Kerbie, Kerby, Kirbey,
Kirbie, Kirkby*

Kiri (Cambodian) mountain.

Kiril (Slavic) a form of Cyril.
Kirill, Kiryl, Kyrillos

Kiritan (Hindi) wearing a
crown.

Kirk (Scandinavian) church.
Kerk

Kirkland (English) church
land.
Kirklin, Kirklind, Kirklynd

Kirkley (English) church
meadow.

Kirklin (English) a form of
Kirkland.
*Kirklan, Kirklen, Kirkline,
Kirkloun, Kirklun, Kirklyn,
Kirklynn*

Kirkwell (English) church
well; church spring.

Kirkwood (English) church
forest.

Kirton (English) church town.

Kishan (American) a form of Keshawn.
Kishaun, Kishawn, Kishen, Kishon, Kyshon, Kyshun

Kistna (Hindi) sacred, holy. Geography: a sacred river in India.

Kistur (Gypsy) skillful rider.

Kit (Greek) a familiar form of Christian, Christopher, Kristopher.
Kitt, Kitts

Kito (Swahili) jewel; precious child.

Kitwana (Swahili) pledged to live.

Kiva (Hebrew) a short form of Akiva, Jacob.
Kiba, Kivi, Kiwa

Kiyoshi (Japanese) quiet; peaceful.

Kizza (Luganda) born after twins.
Kizzy

Kjell (Swedish) a form of Karl.
Kjel

Klaus (German) a short form of Nicholas. A form of Claus.
Klaas, Klaes, Klas, Klause

Klay (English) a form of Clay.

Klayton (English) a form of Clayton.

Kleef (Dutch) cliff.

Klement (Czech) a form of Clement.
Klema, Klemenis, Klemens, Klemet, Klemo, Klim, Klimek, Kliment, Klimka

Kleng (Norwegian) claw.

Knight (English) armored knight.
Knightly

Knoton (Native American) a form of Nodin.

Knowles (English) grassy slope.
Knolls, Nowles

Knox (English) hill.

Knute (Scandinavian) a form of Canute.
Knud, Knut

Koby (Polish) a familiar form of Jacob.
Kobby, Kobe, Kobey, Kobi, Kobia, Kobie

Kodi (English) a form of Kody.
Kode, Kodee, Kodie

Kody (English) a form of Cody.
Kodey, Kodi, Kodye, Koty

Kofi (Twi) born on Friday.

Kohana (Lakota) swift.

Koi (Choctaw) panther. (Hawaiian) a form of Troy.

Kojo (Akan) born on Monday.

Koka (Hawaiian) Scotsman.

Kokayi (Shona) gathered together.

Kolby (English) a form of Colby.
Kelby, Koalby, Koelby, Kohlbe, Kohlby, Kolbe, Kolbey, Kolbi, Kolbie, Kolebe, Koleby, Kollby

Kole (English) a form of Cole.
Kohl, Kohle

Koleman (English) a form of Coleman.
Kolemann, Kolemen

Kolin (English) a form of Colin.
Kolen, Kollen, Kollin, Kollyn, Kolyn

Kolton (English) a form of Colton.
Kolt, Koltan, Kolte, Kolten, Koltin, Koltn, Koltyn

Kolya (Russian) a familiar form of Nikolai, Nikolos.
Kola, Kolenka, Kolia, Kolja

Kona (Hawaiian) a form of Don.
Konala

Konane (Hawaiian) bright moonlight.

Kondo (Swahili) war.

Kong (Chinese) glorious; sky.

Konner (Irish) a form of Conner, Connor.
Konar, Koner

Konnor (Irish) a form of Connor.
Kohner, Kohnor, Konor

Kono (Moquelumnan) squirrel eating a pine nut.

Konrad (German) a form of Conrad.
Khonrad, Koen, Koenraad, Kon, Konn, Konney, Konni, Konnie, Konny, Konrád, Konrade, Konrado, Kord, Kort, Kunz

Konstantin (German, Russian) a form of Constantine. See also Dinos.
Konstancji, Konstadine, Konstadino, Konstandinos, Konstantinas, Konstantine, Konstantinos, Konstantio, Konstanty, Konstantyn, Konstanz, Konstatino, Kostadino, Kostadinos, Kostandino, Kostandinos, Kostantin, Kostantino, Kostas, Kostenka, Kostya, Kotsos

Kontar (Akan) only child.

Korb (German) basket.

Korbin (English) a form of Corbin.
Korban, Korben, Korbyn

Kordell (English) a form of Cordell.
Kordel

Korey (Irish) a form of Corey,
Kory.
Kore, Koree, Korei, Korio,
Korre, Korria, Korrye

Kornel (Latin) a form of
Cornelius, Kornelius.
Kees, Korneil, Kornél, Korneli,
Kornelisz, Kornell, Krelis, Soma

Kornelius (Latin) a form of
Cornelius. See also Kees,
Kornel.
Karnelius, Korneilius,
Korneliaus, Kornelious,
Kornellius

Korrigan (Irish) a form of
Corrigan.
Korigan, Korigan, Korrigon,
Korrigun

Kort (German, Dutch) a form
of Cort, Kurt.
Kourt

Kortney (English) a form of
Courtney.
Kortni, Kourtney

Korudon (Greek) helmeted
one.

Kory (Irish) a form of Corey.
Korey, Kori, Korie, Korrey,
Korri, Korrie, Korry

Kosey (African) lion.
Kosse

Kosmo (Greek) a form of
Cosmo.
Kosmy, Kozmo

Kostas (Greek) a short form
of Konstantin.

Kosti (Finnish) a form of
Gustave.

Kosumi (Moquelumnan) spear
fisher.

Koukalaka (Hawaiian) a form
of Douglas.

Kourtland (English) a form of
Courtland.
Kortlan, Kortland, Kortlend,
Kortlon, Kourtlin

Kovit (Tai) expert.

Kraig (Irish, Scottish) a form
of Craig.
Kraggie, Kraggy, Krayg, Kreg,
Kreig, Kreigh

Krikor (Armenian) a form of
Gregory.

Kris (Greek) a form of Chris.
A short form of Kristian,
Kristofer, Kristopher.
Kriss, Krys

Krischan (German) a form of
Christian.
Krishan, Krishaun, Krishawn,
Krishon, Krishun

Krishna (Hindi) delightful,
pleasurable. Religion: the
eighth and principal avatar of
the Hindu god Vishnu.
Kistna, Kistnah, Krisha,
Krishnah

Krispin (Latin) a form of Crispin.
Krispian, Krispino, Krispo

Krister (Swedish) a form of Christian.
Krist, Kristar

Kristian (Greek) a form of Christian, Khristian.
Kerstan, Khristos, Kit, Kris, Krischan, Krist, Kristan, Kristar, Kristek, Kristen, Krister, Kristien, Kristin, Kristine, Kristinn, Kristion, Kristjan, Kristo, Kristos, Krists, Krystek, Krystian, Khrystiyan

Kristo (Greek) a short form of Khristos.

Kristofer (Swedish) a form of Kristopher.
Kris, Kristafer, Kristef, Kristifer, Kristoff, Kristoffer, Kristofo, Kristofor, Kristofyr, Kristufer, Kristus, Krystofer

Kristoff (Greek) a short form of Kristofer, Kristopher.
Kristof, Kristóf

Kristophe (French) a form of Kristopher.

Kristopher (Greek) a form of Christopher. See also Topher.
Khristopher, Kit, Kris, Krisstopher, Kristapher, Kristepher, Kristfer, Kristfor, Kristo, Kristofer, Kristoff, Kristoforo, Kristoph, Kristophe, Kristophor, Kristos, Krists,
Krisus, Krystopher, Krystupas, Krzysztof

Kruz (Spanish) a form of Cruz.
Kruise, Kruize, Kruse, Kruze

Krystian (Polish) a form of Christian.
Krys, Krystek, Krystien, Krystin

Kuba (Czech) a form of Jacob.
Kubo, Kubus

Kueng (Chinese) universe.

Kugonza (Rutooro) love.

Kuiril (Basque) lord.

Kumar (Sanskrit) prince.

Kunle (Yoruba) home filled with honors.

Kuper (Yiddish) copper.

Kurt (Latin, German, French) a short form of Kurtis. A form of Curt.
Kirt, Kort, Kuno, Kurtt

Kurtis (Latin, French) a form of Curtis.
Kirtis, Kirtus, Kurt, Kurtes, Kurtez, Kurtice, Kurties, Kurtiss, Kurtus, Kurtys

Kuruk (Pawnee) bear.

Kuzih (Carrier) good speaker.

Kwabena (Akan) born on Tuesday.

Kwacha (Nguni) morning.

Kwako (Akan) born on
Wednesday.
Kwaka, Kwaku

Kwam (Zuni) a form of John.

Kwame (Akan) born on
Saturday.
Kwamen, Kwami, Kwamin

Kwan (Korean) strong.
Kwane

Kwasi (Akan) born on Sunday.
(Swahili) wealthy.
Kwasie, Kwazzi, Kwesi

Kwayera (Nguni) dawn.

Kwende (Nguni) let's go.

Kyele (Irish) a form of Kyle.

Kylan (Irish) a form of Kyle.
*Kyelen, Kyleen, Kylen, Kylin,
Kyline, Kylon, Kylun*

Kyle (Irish) narrow piece of
land; place where cattle
graze. (Yiddish) crowned
with laurels.
*Cyle, Kiel, Kilan, Kile, Kilen,
Kiley, Ky, Kye, Kyel, Kyele,
Kylan, Kylee, Kyler, Kyley,
Kylie, Kyll, Kylle, Kyrell*

Kyler (English) a form of
Kyle.
Kylar, Kylor

Kynan (Welsh) chief.

Kyndall (English) a form of
Kendall.
*Kyndal, Kyndel, Kyndell,
Kyndle*

Kyne (English) royal.

Kyran (Sanskrit) a form of
Kiran.
Kyren, Kyron, Kyrone

Kyros (Greek) master.

Kyven (American) a form of
Kevin.
*Kyvan, Kyvaun, Kyvon,
Kywon, Kywynn*

L

Laban (Hawaiian) white.
Labon, Lebaan, Leban, Liban

Labaron (American) a combi-
nation of the prefix La +
Baron.
*Labaren, Labarren, Labarron,
Labearon, Labron*

Labib (Arabic) sensible; intelligent.

Labrentsis (Russian) a form
of Lawrence.
Labhras, Labhruinn, Labrencis

Lachlan (Scottish) land of
lakes.
*Lache, Lachlann, Lachunn,
Lakelan, Lakeland*

Ladarian (American) a com-
bination of the prefix La +
Darian.
*Ladarien, Ladarin, Ladarion,
Ladarren, Ladarrian, Ladarrien,*

Ladarrin, Ladarrion, Laderion, Laderrian, Laderrion

Ladarius (American) a combination of the prefix La + Darius.
Ladarious, Ladaris, Ladarrius, Ladauris, Laderius, Ladirus

Ladarrius (American) a form of Ladarius.
Ladarrias, Ladarries, Ladarrious, Laderrious, Laderris

Ladd (English) attendant.
Lad, Laddey, Laddie, Laddy

Laderrick (American) a combination of the prefix La + Derrick.
Ladarrick, Ladereck, Laderic, Laderricks

Ladislav (Czech) a form of Walter.
Laco, Lada, Ladislaus

Lado (Fante) second-born son.

Lafayette (French) History: Marquis de Lafayette was a French soldier and politician who aided the American Revolution.
Lafaiete, Lafayett, Lafette, Laffyette

Laine (English) a form of Lane.
Lain

Laird (Scottish) wealthy landowner.

Lais (Arabic) lion.

Lajos (Hungarian) famous; holy.
Lajcsi, Laji, Lali

Lake (English) lake.
Lakan, Lakane, Lakee, Laken, Lakin

Lakota (Dakota) a tribal name.
Lakoda

Lal (Hindi) beloved.

Lamar (German) famous throughout the land. (French) sea, ocean.
Lamair, Lamario, Lamaris, Lamarr, Lamarre, Larmar, Lemar

Lambert (German) bright land.
Bert, Lambard, Lamberto, Lambirt, Lampard, Landbert

Lamond (French) world.
Lammond, Lamon, Lamonde, Lamondo, Lamondre, Lamund, Lemond

Lamont (Scandinavian) lawyer.
Lamaunt, Lamonta, Lamonte, Lamontie, Lamonto, Lamount, Lemont

Lance (German) a short form of Lancelot.
Lancy, Lantz, Lanz, Launce

Lancelot (French) attendant. Literature: the knight who loved King Arthur's wife, Queen Guinevere.
Lance, Lancelott, Launcelet, Launcelot

Landen (English) a form of
Landon.
Landenn

Lander (Basque) lion man.
(English) landowner.
Landers, Landor

Lando (Portuguese, Spanish) a
short form of Orlando,
Rolando.

Landon (English) open, grassy
meadow.
*Landan, Landen, Landin,
Landyn*

Landry (French, English)
ruler.
Landre, Landré, Landrue

Lane (English) narrow road.
Laine, Laney, Lanie, Layne

Lang (Scandinavian) tall man.
Lange

Langdon (English) long hill.
Landon, Langsdon, Langston

Langford (English) long ford.
Lanford, Lankford

Langley (English) long
meadow.
*Langlea, Langlee, Langleigh,
Langly*

Langston (English) long, narrow town.
Langsden, Langsdon

Langundo (Native American)
peaceful.

Lani (Hawaiian) heaven.

Lanny (American) a familiar
form of Lawrence, Laurence.
Lanney, Lannie, Lennie

Lanu (Moquelumnan) running
around the pole.

Lanz (Italian) a form of Lance.
Lanzo, Lonzo

Lao (Spanish) a short form of
Stanislaus.

Lap (Vietnamese) independent.

Lapidos (Hebrew) torches.
Lapidoth

Laquan (American) a combi-
nation of the prefix La +
Quan.
*Laquain, Laquann, Laquanta,
Laquantae, Laquante, Laquawn,
Laquawne, Laquin, Laquinn,
Laqun, Laquon, Laquone,
Laqwan, Laqwon*

Laquintin (American) a com-
bination of the prefix La +
Quintin.
*Laquentin, Laquenton,
Laquintas, Laquinten,
Laquintiss, Laquinton*

Laramie (French) tears of love.
Geography: a town in
Wyoming on the Overland
Trail.
Larami, Laramy, Laremy

Larenzo (Italian, Spanish) a
form of Lorenzo.
*Larenz, Larenza, Larinzo,
Laurenzo*

Larkin (Irish) rough; fierce.
Larklin

Larnell (American) a combination of Larry + Darnell.

Laron (French) thief.
Laran, La'ron, La Ron, Larone, Laronn, Larron, La Ruan

Larrimore (French) armorer.
Larimore, Larmer, Larmor

Larry (Latin) a familiar form of Lawrence.
Larrie, Lary

Lars (Scandinavian) a form of Lawrence.
Laris, Larris, Larse, Larsen, Larson, Larsson, Larz, Lasse, Laurans, Laurits, Lavrans, Lorens

LaSalle (French) hall.
Lasal, Lasalle, Lascell, Lascelles

Lash (Gypsy) a form of Louis.
Lashi, Lasho

Lashawn (American) a combination of the prefix La + Shawn.
Lasaun, Lasean, Lashajaun, Lashan, Lashane, Lashaun, Lashon, Lashun

Lashon (American) a form of Lashawn.
Lashone, Lashonne

Lasse (Finnish) a form of Nicholas.

László (Hungarian) famous ruler.
Laci, Lacko, Laslo, Lazlo

Lateef (Arabic) gentle; pleasant.
Latif, Letif

Latham (Scandinavian) barn.
(English) district.
Laith, Lathe, Lay

Lathan (American) a combination of the prefix La + Nathan.
Lathaniel, Lathen, Lathyn, Leathan

Lathrop (English) barn, farmstead.
Lathe, Lathrope, Lay

Latimer (English) interpreter.
Lat, Latimor, Lattie, Latty, Latymer

Latravis (American) a combination of the prefix La + Travis.
Latavious, Latavius, Latraveus, Latraviaus, Latravious, Latravius, Latrayvious, Latrayvous, Latrivis

Latrell (American) a combination of the prefix La + Kentrell.
Latreal, Latreil, Latrel, Latrelle, Letreal, Letrel, Letrell, Letrelle

Laudalino (Portuguese) praised.
Lino

Laughlin (Irish) servant of
Saint Secundinus.
Lanty, Lauchlin, Leachlainn

Laurence (Latin) crowned
with laurel. A form of
Lawrence. See also Rance,
Raulas, Raulo, Renzo.
*Lanny, Lauran, Laurance,
Laureano, Lauren, Laurencho,
Laurencio, Laurens, Laurent,
Laurentij, Laurentios, Laurentiu,
Laurentius, Laurentz,
Laurentzi, Laurie, Laurin,
Lauris, Laurits, Lauritz,
Laurnet, Lauro, Laurus,
Lavrenti, Lurance*

Laurencio (Spanish) a form of
Laurence.

Laurens (Dutch) a form of
Laurence.
Laurenz

Laurent (French) a form of
Laurence.
Laurente

Laurie (English) a familiar
form of Laurence.
Lauri, Laury, Lorry

Lauris (Swedish) a form of
Laurence.

Lauro (Filipino) a form of
Laurence.

LaValle (French) valley.
*Lavail, Laval, Lavalei, Lavalle,
Lavell*

Lavan (Hebrew) white.
*Lavane, Lavaughan, Laven,
Lavon, Levan*

Lavaughan (American) a form
of Lavan.
*Lavaughn, Levaughan,
Levaughn*

Lave (Italian) lava. (English)
lord.

Lavell (French) a form of
LaValle.
*Lavel, Lavele, Lavelle, Levele,
Levell, Levelle*

Lavi (Hebrew) lion.

Lavon (American) a form of
Lavan.
*Lavion, Lavone, Lavonn,
Lavonne, Lavont, Lavonte*

Lavrenti (Russian) a form of
Lawrence.
*Larenti, Lavrentij, Lavrusha,
Lavrik, Lavro*

Lawerence (Latin) a form of
Lawrence.
Lawerance

Lawford (English) ford on the
hill.
Ford, Law

Lawler (Irish) soft-spoken.
Lawlor, Lollar, Loller

Lawrence (Latin) crowned
with laurel. See also Brencis,
Chencho.
*Labrentsis, Laiurenty, Lanny,
Lanty, Larance, Laren, Larian,*

Larien, Laris, Larka, Larrance, Larrence, Larry, Lars, Larya, Laurence, Lavrenti, Law, Lawerence, Lawrance, Lawren, Lawrey, Lawrie, Lawron, Lawry, Lencho, Lon, Lóránt, Loreca, Loren, Loretto, Lorenzo, Lorne, Lourenco, Lowrance

Lawson (English) son of Lawrence.
Lawsen, Layson

Lawton (English) town on the hill.
Laughton, Law

Layne (English) a form of Lane.
Layn, Laynee

Layton (English) a form of Leighton.
Laydon, Layten, Layth, Laythan, Laython

Lazaro (Italian) a form of Lazarus.
Lazarillo, Lazarito, Lazzaro

Lazarus (Greek) a form of Eleazar. Bible: Lazarus was raised from the dead by Jesus.
Lazar, Lázár, Lazare, Lazarius, Lazaro, Lazaros, Lazorus

Leander (Greek) lion-man; brave as a lion.
Ander, Leandro

Leandro (Spanish) a form of Leander.
Leandra, Léandre, Leandrew, Leandros

Leben (Yiddish) life.
Laben, Lebon

Lebna (Ethiopian) spirit; heart.

Ledarius (American) a combination of the prefix Le + Darius.
Ledarrious, Ledarrius, Lederious, Lederris

Lee (English) a short form of Farley, Leonard, and names containing "lee."
Leigh

Leggett (French) one who is sent; delegate.
Legate, Legette, Leggitt, Liggett

Lei (Chinese) thunder. (Hawaiian) a form of Ray.

Leib (Yiddish) roaring lion.
Leibel

Leif (Scandinavian) beloved.
Laif, Leife, Lief

Leigh (English) a form of Lee.

Leighton (English) meadow farm.
Lay, Layton, Leigh, Leyton

Leith (Scottish) broad river.

Lek (Tai) small.

Lekeke (Hawaiian) powerful ruler.

Leks (Estonian) a familiar
form of Alexander.
Leksik, Lekso

Lel (Gypsy) taker.

Leland (English) meadowland;
protected land.
*Lealand, Lee, Leeland, Leigh,
Leighland, Lelan, Lelann,
Lelend, Lelund, Leyland*

Lemar (French) a form of
Lamar.
Lemario, Lemarr

Lemuel (Hebrew) devoted to
God.
Lem, Lemmie, Lemmy

Len (Hopi) flute. (German) a
short form of Leonard.

Lenard (German) a form of
Leonard.
Lennard

Lencho (Spanish) a form of
Lawrence.
Lenci, Lenzy

Lennart (Swedish) a form of
Leonard.
Lennerd

Lenno (Native American)
man.

Lennon (Irish) small cloak;
cape.
Lenon

Lennor (Gypsy) spring; summer.

Lennox (Scottish) with many
elms.
Lennix, Lenox

Lenny (German) a familiar
form of Leonard.
Leni, Lennie, Leny

Leo (Latin) lion. (German) a
short form of Leon, Leopold.
*Lavi, Leão, Lee, Leib, Leibel,
Leos, Leosko, Léo, Léocadie,
Leos, Leosoko, Lev, Lio, Lion,
Liutas, Lyon, Nardek*

Leobardo (Italian) a form of
Leonard.

Leon (Greek, German) a short
form of Leonard, Napoleon.
*Leo, Léon, Leonas, Léonce,
Leoncio, Leondris, Leone,
Leonek, Leonetti, Leoni, Leonid,
Leonidas, Leonirez, Leonizio,
Leonon, Leons, Leontes,
Leontios, Leontrae, Liutas*

Leonard (German) brave as a
lion.
*Leanard, Lee, Len, Lena,
Lenard, Lennart, Lenny, Leno,
Leobardo, Leon, Léonard,
Leonardis, Leonardo, Leonart,
Leonerd, Leonhard, Leonidas,
Leonnard, Leontes, Lernard,
Lienard, Linek, Lnard, Lon,
Londard, Lonnard, Lonya,
Lynnard*

Leonardo (Italian) a form of
Leonard.
Leonaldo, Lionardo

Leonel (English) little lion. See also Lionel.
Leonell

Leonhard (German) a form of Leonard.
Leonhards

Leonid (Russian) a form of Leonard.
Leonide, Lyonechka, Lyonya

Leonidas (Greek) a form of Leonard.
Leonida, Leonides

Leopold (German) brave people.
Leo, Leopoldo, Leorad, Lipót, Lopolda, Luepold, Luitpold, Poldi

Leopoldo (Italian) a form of Leopold.

Leor (Hebrew) my light.
Leory, Lior

Lequinton (American) a combination of the prefix Le + Quinton.
Lequentin, Lequenton, Lequinn

Leron (French) round, circle. (American) a combination of the prefix Le + Ron.
Leeron, Le Ron, Lerone, Liron, Lyron

Leroy (French) king. See also Delroy, Elroy.
Lee, Leeroy, LeeRoy, Leigh, Lerai, Leroi, LeRoi, LeRoy, Roy

Les (Scottish, English) a short form of Leslie, Lester.
Lessie

Lesharo (Pawnee) chief.

Leshawn (American) a combination of the prefix Le + Shawn.
Lashan, Lesean, Leshaun, Leshon, Leshun

Leslie (Scottish) gray fortress.
Lee, Leigh, Les, Leslea, Leslee, Lesley, Lesli, Lesly, Lezlie, Lezly

Lester (Latin) chosen camp. (English) from Leicester, England.
Leicester, Les

Lev (Hebrew) heart. (Russian) a form of Leo. A short form of Leverett, Levi.
Leb, Leva, Levka, Levko, Levushka

Leverett (French) young hare.
Lev, Leveret, Leverit, Leveritt

Levi (Hebrew) joined in harmony. Bible: the third son of Jacob; Levites are the priestly tribe of the Israelites.
Leavi, Leevi, Leevie, Lev, Levey, Levie, Levin, Levitis, Levy, Lewi, Leyvi

Levin (Hebrew) a form of Levi.
Levine, Levion

Levon (American) a form of
Lavon.
*Leevon, Levone, Levonn,
Levonne, Levonte, Lyvonne*

Lew (English) a short form of
Lewis.

Lewin (English) beloved
friend.

Lewis (Welsh) a form of
Llewellyn. (English) a form
of Louis.
Lew, Lewes, Lewie, Lewy

Lex (English) a short form of
Alexander.
Lexi, Lexie, Lexin

Lexus (Greek) a short form of
Alexander.
Lexis, Lexius, Lexxus

Leyati (Moquelumnan) shape
of an abalone shell.

Lí (Chinese) strong.

Liam (Irish) a form of
William.
Liem, Lliam, Lyam

Liang (Chinese) good, excellent.

Liban (Hawaiian) a form of
Laban.
Libaan, Lieban

Liberio (Portuguese) libera-
tion.
Liberaratore, Liborio

Lidio (Greek, Portuguese)
ancient.

Ligongo (Yao) who is this?

Likeke (Hawaiian) a form of
Richard.

Liko (Chinese) protected by
Buddha. (Hawaiian) bud.
Like

Lin (Burmese) bright. (English)
a short form of Lyndon.
Linh, Linn, Linny, Lyn, Lynn

Linc (English) a short form of
Lincoln.
Link

Lincoln (English) settlement
by the pool. History:
Abraham Lincoln was the
sixteenth U.S. president.
Linc, Lincon, Lyncoln

Lindberg (German) mountain
where linden grow.
Lindbergh, Lindburg, Lindy

Lindell (English) valley of the
linden.
*Lendall, Lendel, Lendell,
Lindall, Lindel, Lyndale,
Lyndall, Lyndel, Lyndell*

Linden (English) a form of
Lyndon.

Lindley (English) linden field.
*Lindlea, Lindlee, Lindleigh,
Lindly*

Lindon (English) a form of
Lyndon.
Lin, Lindan

Lindsay (English) a form of Lindsey.
Linsay

Lindsey (English) linden-tree island.
Lind, Lindsay, Lindsee, Lindsie, Lindsy, Lindzy, Linsey, Linzie, Linzy, Lyndsay, Lyndsey, Lyndsie, Lynzie

Linford (English) linden ford.
Lynford

Linfred (German) peaceful, calm.

Linley (English) flax meadow.
Linlea, Linlee, Linleigh, Linly

Linton (English) flax town.
Lintonn, Lynton, Lyntonn

Linu (Hindi) lily.

Linus (Greek) flaxen haired.
Linas, Linux

Linwood (English) flax wood.

Lio (Hawaiian) a form of Leo.

Lionel (French) lion cub. See also Leonel.
Lional, Lionell, Lionello, Lynel, Lynell, Lyonel

Liron (Hebrew) my song.
Lyron

Lise (Moquelumnan) salmon's head coming out of the water.

Lisimba (Yao) lion.
Simba

Lister (English) dyer.

Litton (English) town on the hill.
Liton

Liu (African) voice.

Liuz (Polish) light.
Lius

Livingston (English) Leif's town.
Livingstone

Liwanu (Moquelumnan) growling bear.

Llewellyn (Welsh) lionlike.
Lewis, Llewelin, Llewellen, Llewelleyn, Llewellin, Llewlyn, Llywellyn, Llywellynn, Llywelyn

Lloyd (Welsh) gray haired; holy. See also Floyd.
Loy, Loyd, Loyde, Loydie

Lobo (Spanish) wolf.

Lochlain (Irish, Scottish) land of lakes.
Laughlin, Lochlan, Lochlann, Lochlin, Locklynn

Locke (English) forest.
Lock, Lockwood

Loe (Hawaiian) a form of Roy.

Logan (Irish) meadow.
Llogan, Loagan, Loagen, Loagon, Logann, Logen, Loggan, Loghan, Logon, Logn, Logun, Logunn, Logyn

Lok (Chinese) happy.

Lokela (Hawaiian) a form of Roger.

Lokni (Moquelumnan) raining through the roof.

Lomán (Irish) bare. (Slavic) sensitive.

Lombard (Latin) long bearded.
Bard, Barr

Lon (Irish) fierce. (Spanish) a short form of Alonso, Alonzo, Leonard, Lonnie.
Lonn

Lonan (Zuni) cloud.

Lonato (Native American) flint stone.

London (English) fortress of the moon. Geography: the capital of the United Kingdom.
Londen, Londyn, Lunden, Lundon

Long (Chinese) dragon. (Vietnamese) hair.

Lonnie (German, Spanish) a familiar form of Alonso, Alonzo.
Lon, Loni, Lonie, Lonnell, Lonney, Lonni, Lonniel, Lonny

Lono (Hawaiian) Mythology: the god of learning and intellect.

Lonzo (German, Spanish) a short form of Alonso, Alonzo.
Lonso

Lootah (Lakota) red.

Lopaka (Hawaiian) a form of Robert.

Loránd (Hungarian) a form of Roland.

Lóránt (Hungarian) a form of Lawrence.
Lorant

Lorcan (Irish) little; fierce.

Lord (English) noble title.

Loren (Latin) a short form of Lawrence.
Lorin, Lorren, Lorrin, Loryn

Lorenzo (Italian, Spanish) a form of Lawrence.
Larenzo, Lerenzo, Lewrenzo, Lorenc, Lorence, Lorenco, Lorencz, Lorens, Lorenso, Lorentz, Lorenz, Lorenza, Loretto, Lorinc, Lörinc, Lorinzo, Loritz, Lorrenzo, Lorrie, Lorry, Lourenza, Lourenzo, Lowrenzo, Renzo, Zo

Loretto (Italian) a form of Lawrence.
Loreto

Lorimer (Latin) harness maker.
Lorrie, Lorrimer, Lorry

Loring (German) son of the famous warrior.
Lorrie, Lorring, Lorry

Loris (Dutch) clown.

Loritz (Latin, Danish) laurel.
Lauritz

Lorne (Latin) a short form of Lawrence.
Lorn, Lornie

Lorry (English) a form of Laurie.
Lori, Lorri, Lory

Lot (Hebrew) hidden, covered. Bible: Lot fled from Sodom, but his wife glanced back upon its destruction and was transformed into a pillar of salt.
Lott

Lothar (German) a form of Luther.
Lotaire, Lotarrio, Lothair, Lothaire, Lothario, Lotharrio

Lou (German) a short form of Louis.

Loudon (German) low valley.
Loudan, Louden, Loudin, Lowden

Louie (German) a familiar form of Louis.

Louis (German) famous warrior. See also Aloisio, Aloysius, Clovis, Luigi.
Lash, Lashi, Lasho, Lewis, Lou, Loudovicus, Louie, Louies,
Louise, Lucho, Lude, Ludek, Ludirk, Ludis, Ludko, Ludwig, Lughaidh, Lui, Luigi, Luis, Luiz, Luki, Lutek

Lourdes (French) from Lourdes, France. Religion: a place where the Virgin Mary was said to have appeared.

Louvain (English) Lou's vanity. Geography: a city in Belgium.
Louvin

Lovell (English) a form of Lowell.
Louvell, Lovel, Lovelle, Lovey

Lowell (French) young wolf. (English) beloved.
Lovell, Lowe, Lowel

Loyal (English) faithful, loyal.
Loy, Loyall, Loye, Lyall, Lyell

Lubomir (Polish) lover of peace.

Luboslaw (Polish) lover of glory.
Lubs, Lubz

Luc (French) a form of Luke.
Luce

Luca (Italian) a form of Lucius.
Lucca, Luka

Lucas (German, Irish, Danish, Dutch) a form of Lucius.
Lucais, Lucassie, Lucaus, Luccas, Luccus, Luckas, Lucus

Lucian (Latin) a form of Lucius.
Liuz, Lucan, Lucanus, Luciano, Lucianus, Lucias, Lucjan, Lukianos, Lukyan

Luciano (Italian) a form of Lucian.
Luca, Lucca, Lucino, Lucio

Lucien (French) a form of Lucius.

Lucio (Italian) a form of Lucius.

Lucius (Latin) light; bringer of light.
Loukas, Luc, Luca, Lucais, Lucanus, Lucas, Luce, Lucian, Lucien, Lucio, Lucious, Lucis, Luke, Lusio

Lucky (American) fortunate.
Luckee, Luckie, Luckson, Lucson

Ludlow (English) prince's hill.

Ludovic (German) a form of Ludwig.
Ludovick, Ludovico

Ludwig (German) a form of Louis. Music: Ludwig van Beethoven was a famous nineteenth-century German composer.
Ludovic, Ludvig, Ludvik, Ludwik, Lutz

Lui (Hawaiian) a form of Louis.

Luigi (Italian) a form of Louis.
Lui, Luiggi, Luigino, Luigy

Luis, Luiz (Spanish) forms of Louis.
Luise

Lukas, Lukus (Greek, Czech, Swedish) forms of Luke.
Loukas, Lukais, Lukash, Lukasha, Lukass, Lukasz, Lukaus, Lukkas

Luke (Latin) a form of Lucius. Bible: companion of Saint Paul and author of the third Gospel of the New Testament.
Luc, Luchok, Luck, Lucky, Luk, Luka, Lúkács, Lukas, Luken, Lukes, Lukus, Lukyan, Lusio

Lukela (Hawaiian) a form of Russel.

Luken (Basque) bringer of light.
Lucan, Lucane, Lucano, Luk

Luki (Basque) famous warrior.

Lukman (Arabic) prophet.
Luqman

Lulani (Hawaiian) highest point in heaven.

Lumo (Ewe) born facedown.

Lundy (Scottish) grove by the island.

Lunn (Irish) warlike.
Lon, Lonn

Lunt (Swedish) grove.

Lusila (Hindi) leader.

Lusio (Zuni) a form of Lucius.

Lutalo (Luganda) warrior.

Lutfi (Arabic) kind, friendly.

Luther (German) famous warrior. History: Martin Luther was one of the central figures of the Reformation.
Lothar, Lutero, Luthor

Lutherum (Gypsy) slumber.

Luyu (Moquelumnan) head shaker.

Lyall, Lyell (Scottish) loyal.

Lyle (French) island.
Lisle, Ly, Lysle

Lyman (English) meadow.
Leaman, Leeman, Lymon

Lynch (Irish) mariner.
Linch

Lyndal (English) valley of lime trees.
Lyndale, Lyndall, Lyndel, Lyndell

Lyndon (English) linden hill. History: Lyndon B. Johnson was the thirty-sixth U.S. president.
Lin, Linden, Lindon, Lyden, Lydon, Lyn, Lyndan, Lynden, Lynn

Lynn (English) waterfall; brook.
Lyn, Lynell, Lynette, Lynnard, Lynoll

Lyron (Hebrew) a form of Leron, Liron.

Lysander (Greek) liberator.
Lyzander, Sander

M

Maalik (Punjabi) a form of Malik.
Maalek, Maaliek

Mac (Scottish) son.
Macs

Macadam (Scottish) son of Adam.
MacAdam, McAdam

Macallister (Irish) son of Alistair.
Macalaster, Macalister, MacAlister, McAlister, McAllister

Macario (Spanish) a form of Makarios.

Macarthur (Irish) son of Arthur.
MacArthur, McArthur

Macaulay (Scottish) son of righteousness.
Macaulee, Macauley, Macaully, Macauly, Maccauley, Mackauly, Macualay, McCauley

Macbride (Scottish) son of a follower of Saint Brigid.
Macbryde, Mcbride, McBride

Maccoy (Irish) son of Hugh, Coy.
MacCoy, Mccoy, McCoy

Maccrea (Irish) son of grace.
MacCrae, MacCray, MacCrea, Macrae, Macray, Makray, Mccrea, McCrea

Macdonald (Scottish) son of Donald.
MacDonald, Mcdonald, McDonald, Mcdonna, Mcdonnell, McDonnell

Macdougal (Scottish) son of Dougal.
MacDougal, Mcdougal, McDougal, McDougall, Dougal

Mace (French) club. (English) a short form of Macy, Mason.
Macean, Maceo, Macer, Macey, Macie, Macy

Macgregor (Scottish) son of Gregor.
Macgreggor

Machas (Polish) a form of Michael.

Mack (Scottish) a short form of names beginning with "Mac" and "Mc."
Macke, Mackey, Mackie, Macklin, Macks, Macky

Mackenzie (Irish) son of Kenzie.
Mackensy, Mackenxo, Mackenze, Mackenzey, Mackenzi, MacKenzie,
Mackenzly, Mackenzy, Mackienzie, Mackinsey, Mackinzie, Makenzie, McKenzie, Mickenzie

Mackinnley (Irish) son of the learned ruler.
Mackinley, MacKinnley, Mackinnly, Mckinley

Macklain (Irish) a form of Maclean.
Macklaine, Macklane

Maclean (Irish) son of Leander.
Machlin, Macklain, MacLain, MacLean, Maclin, Maclyn, Makleen, McLaine, McLean

Macmahon (Irish) son of Mahon.
MacMahon, McMahon

Macmurray (Irish) son of Murray.
McMurray

Macnair (Scottish) son of the heir.
Macknair

Maco (Hungarian) a form of Emmanuel.

Macon (German, English) maker.

Macy (French) Matthew's estate.
Mace, Macey

Maddock (Welsh) generous.
Madoc, Madock, Madog

Maddox (Welsh, English)
benefactor's son.
Maddux, Madox

Madhar (Hindi) full of intoxi-
cation; relating to spring.

Madison (English) son of
Maude; good son.
*Maddie, Maddison, Maddy,
Madisen, Madisson, Madisyn,
Madsen, Son, Sonny*

Madongo (Luganda) uncir-
cumcised.

Madu (Ibo) people.

Magar (Armenian) groom's
attendant.
Magarious

Magee (Irish) son of Hugh.
MacGee, MacGhee, McGee

Magen (Hebrew) protector.

Magnar (Norwegian) strong;
warrior.
Magne

Magnus (Latin) great.
*Maghnus, Magnes, Manius,
Mayer*

Magomu (Luganda) younger
of twins.

Maguire (Irish) son of the
beige one.
MacGuire, McGuire, McGwire

Mahammed (Arabic) a form
of Muhammad.
Mahamad, Mahamed

Mahdi (Arabic) guided to the
right path.
Mahde, Mahdee, Mahdy

Mahesa (Hindi) great lord.
Religion: another name for
the Hindu god Shiva.

Mahi'ai (Hawaiian) a form of
George.

Mahir (Arabic, Hebrew) excellent; industrious.
Maher

Mahkah (Lakota) earth.

Mahmoud (Arabic) a form of
Muhammad.
*Mahamoud, Mahmmoud,
Mahmuod*

Mahmúd (Arabic) a form of
Muhammad.
Mahmed, Mahmood, Mahmut

Mahomet (Arabic) a form of
Muhammad.
Mehemet, Mehmet

Mahon (Irish) bear.

Mahpee (Lakota) sky.

Maimun (Arabic) lucky.
Maimon

Mairtin (Irish) a form of
Martin.
Martain, Martainn

Maitias (Irish) a form of
Mathias.
Maithias

Maitiú (Irish) a form of Matthew.

Maitland (English) meadowland.

Majid (Arabic) great, glorious.
Majd, Majde, Majdi, Majdy, Majed, Majeed

Major (Latin) greater; military rank.
Majar, Maje, Majer, Mayer, Mayor

Makaio (Hawaiian) a form of Matthew.

Makalani (Mwera) writer.

Makani (Hawaiian) wind.

Makarios (Greek) happy; blessed.
Macario, Macarios, Maccario, Maccarios

Makenzie (Irish) a form of Mackenzie.
Makensie, Makenzy

Makin (Arabic) strong.
Makeen

Makis (Greek) a form of Michael.

Makoto (Japanese) sincere.

Maks (Hungarian) a form of Max.
Makszi

Maksim (Russian) a form of Maximilian.
Maksimka, Maksym, Maxim

Maksym (Polish) a form of Maximilian.
Makimus, Maksim, Maksymilian

Makyah (Hopi) eagle hunter.

Mal (Irish) a short form of names beginning with "Mal."

Malachi (Hebrew) angel of God. Bible: the last canonical Hebrew prophet.
Maeleachlainn, Mal, Malachai, Malachia, Malachie, Malachy, Malakai, Malake, Malaki, Malchija, Malechy, Málik

Malachy (Irish) a form of Malachi.

Malajitm (Sanskrit) garland of victory.

Malcolm (Scottish) follower of Saint Columba who Christianized North Scotland. (Arabic) dove.
Mal, Malcalm, Malcohm, Malcolum, Malcom, Malkolm

Malcom (Scottish) a form of Malcolm.
Malcome, Malcum, Malkom, Malkum

Malden (English) meeting place in a pasture.
Mal, Maldon

Malek (Arabic) a form of Málik.
Maleak, Maleek, Maleik, Maleka, Maleke, Mallek

Maleko (Hawaiian) a form of Mark.

Málik (Punjabi) lord, master. (Arabic) a form of Malachi. *Maalik, Mailik, Malak, Malic, Malick, Malicke, Maliek, Maliik, Malik, Malike, Malikh, Maliq, Malique, Mallik, Malyk, Malyq*

Malin (English) strong, little warrior. *Mal, Mallin, Mallon*

Mallory (German) army counselor. (French) wild duck. *Lory, Mal, Mallery, Mallori, Mallorie, Malory*

Maloney (Irish) church going. *Malone, Malony*

Malvern (Welsh) bare hill. *Malverne*

Malvin (Irish, English) a form of Melvin. *Mal, Malvinn, Malvyn, Malvynn*

Mamo (Hawaiian) yellow flower; yellow bird.

Manchu (Chinese) pure.

Manco (Peruvian) supreme leader. History: a sixteenth-century Incan king.

Mandala (Yao) flowers. *Manda, Mandela*

Mandeep (Punjabi) mind full of light. *Mandieep*

Mandel (German) almond. *Mandell*

Mandek (Polish) a form of Armand, Herman. *Mandie*

Mander (Gypsy) from me.

Manford (English) small ford.

Manfred (English) man of peace. See also Fred. *Manfret, Manfrid, Manfried, Maniferd, Mannfred, Mannfryd*

Manger (French) stable.

Mango (Spanish) a familiar form of Emmanuel, Manuel.

Manheim (German) servant's home.

Manipi (Native American) living marvel.

Manius (Scottish) a form of Magnus. *Manus, Manyus*

Manley (English) hero's meadow. *Manlea, Manleigh, Manly*

Mann (German) man. *Manin*

Manning (English) son of the hero.

Mannix (Irish) monk. *Mainchin*

Manny (German, Spanish) a familiar form of Manuel.
Mani, Manni, Mannie, Many

Mano (Hawaiian) shark. (Spanish) a short form of Manuel.
Manno, Manolo

Manoj (Sanskrit) cupid.

Mansa (Swahili) king. History: a fourteenth-century king of Mali.

Mansel (English) manse; house occupied by a clergyman.
Mansell

Mansfield (English) field by the river; hero's field.

Man-Shik (Korean) deeply rooted.

Mansür (Arabic) divinely aided.
Mansoor, Mansour

Manton (English) man's town; hero's town.
Mannton, Manten

Manu (Hindi) lawmaker. History: the reputed writer of the Hindi compendium of sacred laws and customs. (Hawaiian) bird. (Ghanaian) second-born son.

Manuel (Hebrew) a short form of Emmanuel.
Maco, Mango, Mannuel, Manny, Mano, Manolón, Manual, Manuale, Manue,

Manuelli, Manuelo, Manuil, Manyuil, Minel

Manville (French) worker's village. (English) hero's village.
Mandeville, Manvel, Manvil

Man-Young (Korean) ten thousand years of prosperity.

Manzo (Japanese) third son.

Maona (Winnebago) creator, earth maker.

Mapira (Yao) millet.

Marc (French) a form of Mark.

Marcel (French) a form of Marcellus.
Marcell, Marsale, Marsel

Marcelino (Italian) a form of Marcellus.
Marceleno, Marcelin, Marcellin, Marcellino

Marcelo, Marcello (Italian) forms of Marcellus.
Marchello, Marsello, Marselo

Marcellus (Latin) a familiar form of Marcus.
Marceau, Marcel, Marceles, Marcelias, Marcelino, Marcelis, Marcelius, Marcellas, Marcelleous, Marcellis, Marcellous, Marcelluas, Marcelo, Marcelus, Marcely, Marciano, Marcilka, Marcsseau, Marquel, Marsalis

March (English) dweller by a boundary.

Marciano (Italian) a form of Martin.
Marci, Marcio

Marcilka (Hungarian) a form of Marcellus.
Marci, Marcilki

Marcin (Polish) a form of Martin.

Marco (Italian) a form of Marcus. History: Marco Polo was a thirteenth-century Venetian traveler who explored Asia.
Marcko, Marko

Marcos (Spanish) a form of Marcus.
Marckos, Marcous, Markos, Markose

Marcus (Latin) martial, war-like.
Marc, Marcas, Marcellus, Marcio, Marckus, Marco, Marcos, Marcous, Marcuss, Marcuus, Marcux, Marek, Mark, Markov, Markus

Marek (Slavic) a form of Marcus.

Maren (Basque) sea.

Mareo (Japanese) uncommon.

Marian (Polish) a form of Mark.

Mariano (Italian) a form of Mark.

Marid (Arabic) rebellious.

Marin (French) sailor.
Marine, Mariner, Marino, Marius, Marriner

Marino (Italian) a form of Marin.
Marinos, Marinus, Mario, Mariono

Mario (Italian) a form of Marino.
Marios, Marrio

Marion (French) bitter; sea of bitterness.
Mareon, Mariano

Marius (Latin) a form of Marin.
Marious

Mark (Latin) a form of Marcus. Bible: author of the second Gospel in the New Testament. See also Maleko.
Marc, Marek, Marian, Mariano, Marke, Markee, Markel, Markell, Markey, Marko, Markos, Márkus, Markusha, Marque, Martial, Marx

Markanthony (Italian) a combination of Mark + Anthony.

Marke (Polish) a form of Mark.

Markel, Markell (Latin) forms of Mark.
Markelle, Markelo

Markes (Portuguese) a form of Marques.
Markess, Markest

Markese (French) a form of Marquis.
Markease, Markeece, Markees, Markeese, Markei, Markeice, Markeis, Markeise, Markes, Markez, Markeze, Markice

Markham (English) homestead on the boundary.

Markis (French) a form of Marquis.
Markies, Markiese, Markise, Markiss, Markist

Marko (Latin) a form of Marco, Mark.
Markco

Markus (Latin) a form of Marcus.
Markas, Markcus, Markcuss, Markys, Marqus

Marland (English) lake land.

Marley (English) lake meadow.
Marlea, Marleigh, Marly, Marrley

Marlin (English) deep-sea fish.
Marlen, Marlion, Marlyn

Marlon (French) a form of Merlin.

Marlow (English) hill by the lake.
Mar, Marlo, Marlowe

Marmion (French) small.
Marmyon

Marnin (Hebrew) singer; bringer of joy.

Maro (Japanese) myself.

Marquan (American) a combination of Mark + Quan.
Marquane, Marquante

Marquel (American) a form of Marcellus.
Marqueal, Marquelis, Marquell, Marquelle, Marquellis, Marquiel, Marquil, Marquiles, Marquill, Marquille, Marquillus, Marqwel, Marqwell

Marques (Portuguese) nobleman.
Markes, Markqes, Markques, Markquese, Marqese, Marqesse, Marqez, Marqeze, Marquees, Marquese, Marquess, Marquesse, Marquest, Markqueus, Marquez, Marqus

Marquez (Portuguese) a form of Marques.
Marqueze, Marquiez

Marquice (American) a form of Marquis.
Marquaice, Marquece

Marquis, Marquise (French) nobleman.
Marcquis, Marcuis, Markis,

Markquis, Markquise, Markuis,
Marqise, Marquee, Marqui,
Marquice, Marquie, Marquies,
Marquiss, Marquist, Marquiz,
Marquize

Marquon (American) a com-
bination of Mark + Quon.
Marquin, Marquinn, Marqwan,
Marqwon, Marqwyn

Marr (Spanish) divine. (Arabic)
forbidden.

Mars (Latin) bold warrior.
Mythology: the Roman god
of war.

Marsalis (Italian) a form of
Marcellus.
Marsalius, Marsallis, Marsellis,
Marsellius, Marsellus

Marsden (English) marsh valley.
Marsdon

Marsh (English) swamp land.
(French) a short form of
Marshall.

Marshal (French) a form of
Marshall.
Marschal, Marshel

Marshall (French) caretaker of
the horses; military title.
Marsh, Marshal, Marshell

Marshawn (American) a com-
bination of Mark + Shawn.
Marshaine, Marshaun,
Marshauwn, Marshean,
Marshon, Marshun

Marston (English) town by
the marsh.

Martell (English) hammerer.
Martel, Martele, Martellis

Marten (Dutch) a form of
Martin.
Maarten, Martein

Martez (Spanish) a form of
Martin.
Martaz, Martaze, Martes,
Martese, Marteze, Martice,
Martiece, Marties, Martiese,
Martiez, Martis, Martise,
Martize

Marti (Spanish) a form of
Martin.
Martee, Martie

Martial (French) a form of
Mark.

Martin (Latin, French) a form
of Martinus. History: Martin
Luther King, Jr. led the Civil
Rights movement and won
the Nobel Peace Prize. See
also Tynek.
Maartin, Mairtin, Marciano,
Marcin, Marinos, Marius, Mart,
Martan, Marten, Martez,
Marti, Martijn, Martinas,
Martine, Martinez, Martinho,
Martiniano, Martinien,
Martinka, Martino, Martins,
Marto, Marton, Márton, Marts,
Marty, Martyn, Mattin, Mertin,
Morten, Moss

Martinez (Spanish) a form of
Martin.
Martines

Martinho (Portuguese) a form
of Martin.

Martino (Italian) a form of
Martin.
Martinos

Martins (Latvian) a form of
Martin.

Martinus (Latin) martial, warlike.
Martin

Marty (Latin) a familiar form
of Martin.
Martey, Marti, Martie

Marut (Hindi) Religion: the
Hindu god of the wind.

Marv (English) a short form of
Marvin.
Marve, Marvi, Marvis

Marvin (English) lover of the
sea.
*Marv, Marvein, Marven,
Marvion, Marvn, Marvon,
Marvyn, Marwin, Marwynn,
Mervin*

Marwan (Arabic) history per-
sonage.

Marwood (English) forest
pond.

Masaccio (Italian) twin.
Masaki

Masahiro (Japanese) broad-
minded.

Masamba (Yao) leaves.

Masao (Japanese) righteous.

Masato (Japanese) just.

Mashama (Shona) surprising.

Maska (Native American)
powerful. (Russian) mask.

Maslin (French) little Thomas.
Maslen, Masling

Mason (French) stone worker.
*Mace, Maison, Masson, Masun,
Masyn, Sonny*

Masou (Native American) fire
god.

Massey (English) twin.
Massi

Massimo (Italian) greatest.
Massimiliano

Masud (Arabic, Swahili) fortunate.
Masood, Masoud, Mhasood

Matai (Basque, Bulgarian) a
form of Matthew.
Máté, Matei

Matalino (Filipino) bright.

Mateo (Spanish) a form of
Matthew.
Matías, Matteo

Mateusz (Polish) a form of
Matthew.
Matejs, Mateus

Mathe (German) a short form of Matthew.

Mather (English) powerful army.

Matheu (German) a form of Matthew.
Matheau, Matheus, Mathu

Mathew (Hebrew) a form of Matthew.

Mathias, Matthias (German, Swedish) forms of Matthew.
Maitias, Mathi, Mathia, Mathis, Matías, Matthia, Matthieus, Mattia, Mattias, Matus

Mathieu, Matthieu (French) forms of Matthew.
Mathie, Mathieux, Mathiew, Matthiew, Mattieu, Mattieux

Matías (Spanish) a form of Mathias.
Mattias

Mato (Native American) brave.

Matope (Rhodesian) our last child.

Matoskah (Lakota) white bear.

Mats (Swedish) a familiar form of Matthew.
Matts, Matz

Matson (Hebrew) son of Matt.
Matison, Matsen, Mattison, Mattson

Matt (Hebrew) a short form of Matthew.
Mat

Matteen (Afghan) disciplined; polite.

Matteus (Scandinavian) a form of Matthew.

Matthew (Hebrew) gift of God. Bible: author of the first Gospel of the New Testament.
Mads, Makaio, Maitiú, Mata, Matai, Matek, Mateo, Mateusz, Matfei, Mathe, Matheson, Matheu, Mathew, Mathian, Mathias, Mathieson, Mathieu, Matro, Mats, Matt, Matteus, Matthaeus, Matthaios, Matthaus, Matthäus, Mattheus, Matthews, Mattmias, Matty, Matvey, Matyas, Mayhew

Matty (Hebrew) a familiar form of Matthew.
Mattie

Matus (Czech) a form of Mathias.

Matvey (Russian) a form of Matthew.
Matviy, Matviyko, Matyash, Motka, Motya

Matyas (Polish) a form of Matthew.
Mátyás

Mauli (Hawaiian) a form of Maurice.

Maurice (Latin) dark skinned; moor; marshland. See also Seymour.
Mauli, Maur, Maurance, Maureo, Mauricio, Maurids, Mauriece, Maurikas, Maurin, Maurino, Maurise, Mauritz, Maurius, Maurizio, Mauro, Maurrel, Maurtel, Maury, Maurycy, Meurig, Moore, Morice, Moritz, Morrel, Morrice, Morrie, Morrill, Morris

Mauricio (Spanish) a form of Maurice.
Mauriccio, Mauriceo, Maurico, Maurisio

Mauritz (German) a form of Maurice.

Maurizio (Italian) a form of Maurice.

Mauro (Latin) a short form of Maurice.
Maur, Maurio

Maury (Latin) a familiar form of Maurice.
Maurey, Maurie, Morrie

Maverick (American) independent.
Maverik, Maveryke, Mavric, Mavrick

Mawuli (Ewe) there is a God.

Max (Latin) a short form of Maximilian, Maxwell.
Mac, Mack, Maks, Maxe, Maxx, Maxy, Miksa

Maxfield (English) Mack's field.

Maxi (Czech, Hungarian, Spanish) a familiar form of Maximilian, Máximo.
Makszi, Maxey, Maxie, Maxis, Maxy

Maxim (Russian) a form of Maxime.

Maxime (French) most excellent.
Maxim, Maxyme

Maximilian (Latin) greatest.
Mac, Mack, Maixim, Maksim, Maksym, Max, Maxamillion, Maxemilian, Maxemilion, Maxi, Maximalian, Maximili, Maximilia, Maximiliano, Maximilianus, Maximilien, Maximillian, Máximo, Maximos, Maxmilian, Maxmillion, Maxon, Maxymilian, Maxymillian, Mayhew, Miksa

Maximiliano (Italian) a form of Maximilian.
Massimiliano, Maximiano, Maximino

Maximillian (Latin) a form of Maximilian.
Maximillan, Maximillano, Maximillien, Maximillion, Maxmillian, Maxximillian, Maxximillion

Máximo (Spanish) a form of Maximilian.
Massimo, Maxi, Maximiano,

Maximiliano, Maximino,
Máximo

Maximos (Greek) a form of
Maximilian.

Maxwell (English) great
spring.
Max, Maxwel, Maxwill,
Maxxwell, Maxy

Maxy (English) a familiar form
of Max, Maxwell.
Maxi

Mayer (Hebrew) a form of
Meir. (Latin) a form of
Magnus, Major.
Mahyar, Mayeer, Mayor, Mayur

Mayes (English) field.
Mayo, Mays

Mayhew (English) a form of
Matthew.

Maynard (English) powerful;
brave. See also Meinhard.
May, Mayne, Maynhard,
Maynor, Ménard

Mayo (Irish) yew-tree plain.
(English) a form of Mayes.
Geography: a county in
Ireland.

Mayon (Indian) person of
black complexion. Religion:
another name for the Indian
god Mal.

Mayonga (Luganda) lake
sailor.

Mazi (Ibo) sir.
Mazzi

Mazin (Arabic) proper.
Mazen, Mazinn, Mazzin

Mbita (Swahili) born on a
cold night.

Mbwana (Swahili) master.

McGeorge (Scottish) son of
George.
MacGeorge

Mckade (Scottish) son of
Kade.
Mccade

Mckay (Scottish) son of Kay.
Mackay, MacKay, Mckae,
Mckai, McKay

McKenzie (Irish) a form of
Mackenzie.
Mccenzie, Mckennzie,
Mckensey, Mckensie, Mckenson,
Mckensson, Mckenzi, Mckenzy,
Mckinzie

Mckinley (Irish) a form of
Mackinnley.
Mckinely, Mckinnely, Mckinnlee,
Mckinnley, McKinnley

Mead (English) meadow.
Meade, Meed

Medgar (German) a form of
Edgar.

Medwin (German) faithful
friend.

Mehetabel (Hebrew) who
God benefits.

Mehrdad (Persian) gift of the sun.

Mehtar (Sanskrit) prince.
Mehta

Meinhard (German) strong, firm. See also Maynard.
Meinhardt, Meinke, Meino, Mendar

Meinrad (German) strong counsel.

Meir (Hebrew) one who brightens, shines; enlightener. History: Golda Meir was the prime minister of Israel.
Mayer, Meyer, Muki, Myer

Meka (Hawaiian) eyes.

Mel (English, Irish) a familiar form of Melvin.

Melbourne (English) mill stream.
Melborn, Melburn, Melby, Milborn, Milbourn, Milbourne, Milburn, Millburn, Millburne

Melchior (Hebrew) king.
Meilseoir, Melchor, Melker, Melkior

Meldon (English) mill hill.
Melden

Melrone (Irish) servant of Saint Ruadhan.

Melvern (Native American) great chief.

Melville (French) mill town. Literature: Herman Melville was a well-known nineteenth-century American writer.
Milville

Melvin (Irish) armored chief. (English) mill friend; council friend. See also Vinny.
Malvin, Mel, Melvino, Melvon, Melvyn, Melwin, Melwyn, Melwynn

Menachem (Hebrew) comforter.
Menahem, Nachman

Menassah (Hebrew) cause to forget.
Menashe, Menashi, Menashia, Menashiah, Menashya, Manasseh

Mendel (English) repairman.
Mendeley, Mendell, Mendie, Mendy

Mengesha (Ethiopian) kingdom.

Menico (Spanish) a short form of Domenico.

Mensah (Ewe) third son.

Menz (German) a short form of Clement.

Mercer (English) storekeeper.
Merce

Mered (Hebrew) revolter.

Meredith (Welsh) guardian from the sea.
Meredyth, Merideth, Meridith, Merry

Merion (Welsh) from Merion,
Wales.
Merrion

Merle (French) a short form
of Merlin, Merrill.
Meryl

Merlin (English) falcon.
Literature: the magician who
served as counselor in King
Arthur's court.
*Marlon, Merle, Merlen,
Merlinn, Merlyn, Merlynn*

Merrick (English) ruler of the
sea.
*Merek, Meric, Merick, Merik,
Merric, Merrik, Meryk,
Meyrick, Myrucj*

Merrill (Irish) bright sea.
(French) famous.
*Meril, Merill, Merle, Merrel,
Merrell, Merril, Meryl*

Merritt (Latin, Irish) valuable;
deserving.
Merit, Meritt, Merrett

Merton (English) sea town.
Murton

Merv (Irish) a short form of
Mervin.

Merville (French) sea village.

Mervin (Irish) a form of
Marvin.
*Merv, Mervyn, Mervynn,
Merwin, Merwinn, Merwyn,
Murvin, Murvyn, Myrvyn,
Myrvynn, Myrwyn*

Meshach (Hebrew) artist.
Bible: one of Daniel's three
friends who emerged
unharmed from the fiery
furnace of Babylon.

Mesut (Turkish) happy.

Metikla (Moquelumnan)
reaching a hand underwater
to catch a fish.

Mette (Greek, Danish) pearl.
Almeta, Mete

Meurig (Welsh) a form of
Maurice.

Meyer (German) farmer.
Mayer, Meier, Myer

Mhina (Swahili) delightful.

Micah (Hebrew) a form of
Michael. Bible: a Hebrew
prophet.
*Mic, Micaiah, Michiah, Mika,
Mikah, Myca, Mycah*

Micha (Hebrew) a short form
of Michael.
Mica, Micha, Michah

Michael (Hebrew) who is like
God? See also Micah,
Miguel, Mika, Miles.
*Machael, Machas, Mahail,
Maichail, Maikal, Makael,
Makal, Makel, Makell, Makis,
Meikel, Mekal, Mekhail,
Mhichael, Micael, Micah,
Micahel, Mical, Micha,
Michaele, Michaell, Michail,
Michak, Michal, Michale,*

Michael *(cont.)*
Michalek, Michalel, Michau,
Micheal, Micheil, Michel,
Michele, Michelet, Michiel,
Micho, Michoel, Mick, Mickael,
Mickey, Mihail, Mihalje,
Mihkel, Mika, Mikael, Mikáele,
Mikal, Mike, Mikeal, Mikel,
Mikelis, Mikell, Mikhail,
Mikkel, Mikko, Miksa, Milko,
Miquel, Misael, Misi, Miska,
Mitchell, Mychael, Mychajlo,
Mychal, Mykal, Mykhas

Michail (Russian) a form of
Michael.
Mihas, Mikail, Mikale, Misha

Michal (Polish) a form of
Michael.
Michak, Michalek, Michall

Micheal (Irish) a form of
Michael.

Michel (French) a form of
Michael.
Michaud, Miche, Michee,
Michell, Michelle, Michon

Michelangelo (Italian) a com-
bination of Michael +
Angelo. Art: Michelangelo
Buonarroti was one of the
greatest Renaissance painters.
Michelange, Miguelangelo

Michele (Italian) a form of
Michael.

Michio (Japanese) man with
the strength of three thousand.

Mick (English) a short form of
Michael, Mickey.
Mickerson

Mickael (English) a form of
Michael.
Mickaele, Mickal, Mickale,
Mickeal, Mickel, Mickell,
Mickelle, Mickle

Mickenzie (Irish) a form of
Mackenzie.
Mickenze, Mickenzy, Mikenzie

Mickey (Irish) a familiar form
of Michael.
Mick, Micki, Mickie, Micky,
Miki, Mique

Micu (Hungarian) a form of
Nick.

Miguel (Portuguese, Spanish) a
form of Michael.
Migeel, Migel, Miguelly, Migui

Miguelangel (Spanish) a combination of Miguel + Angel.

Mihail (Greek, Bulgarian,
Romanian) a form of
Michael.
Mihailo, Mihal, Mihalis, Mikail

Mika (Ponca) raccoon.
(Hebrew) a form of Micah.
(Russian) a familiar form of
Michael.
Miika, Mikah

Mikael (Swedish) a form of
Michael.
Mikaeel, Mikaele

Mikáele (Hawaiian) a form of Michael.
Mikele

Mikal (Hebrew) a form of Michael.
Mekal, Mikahl, Mikale

Mikasi (Omaha) coyote.

Mike (Hebrew) a short form of Michael.
Mikey, Myk

Mikeal (Irish) a form of Michael.

Mikel (Basque) a form of Michael.
Mekel, Mikele, Mekell, Mikell, Mikelle

Mikelis (Latvian) a form of Michael.
Mikus, Milkins

Mikhail (Greek, Russian) a form of Michael.
Mekhail, Mihály, Mikhael, Mikhale, Mikhalis, Mikhalka, Mikhall, Mikhel, Mikhial, Mikhos

Miki (Japanese) tree.
Mikio

Mikkel (Norwegian) a form of Michael.
Mikkael, Mikle

Mikko (Finnish) a form of Michael.
Mikk, Mikka, Mikkohl, Mikkol, Miko, Mikol

Mikolaj (Polish) a form of Nicholas.
Mikolai

Mikolas (Greek) a form of Nicholas.
Miklós, Milek

Miksa (Hungarian) a form of Max.
Miks

Milan (Italian) northerner. Geography: a city in northern Italy.
Milaan, Milano, Milen, Millan, Millen, Mylan, Mylen, Mylon, Mylynn

Milap (Native American) giving.

Milborough (English) middle borough.
Milbrough

Milek (Polish) a familiar form of Nicholas.

Miles (Greek) millstone. (Latin) soldier. (German) merciful. (English) a short form of Michael.
Milas, Milles, Milo, Milson, Myles

Milford (English) mill by the ford.

Mililani (Hawaiian) heavenly caress.

Milko (Czech) a form of
Michael. (German) a familiar
form of Emil.
Milkins

Millard (Latin) caretaker of the
mill.
*Mill, Millar, Miller, Millward,
Milward, Myller*

Miller (English) miller; grain
grinder.
Mellar, Millard, Millen

Mills (English) mills.

Milo (German) a form of
Miles. A familiar form of
Emil.
Millo, Mylo

Milos (Greek, Slavic) pleasant.

Miloslav (Czech) lover of
glory.
Milda

Milt (English) a short form of
Milton.

Milton (English) mill town.
Milt, Miltie, Milty, Mylton

Mimis (Greek) a familiar form
of Demetrius.

Min (Burmese) king.
Mina

Mincho (Spanish) a form of
Benjamin.

Minel (Spanish) a form of
Manuel.

Miner (English) miner.

Mingan (Native American)
gray wolf.

Mingo (Spanish) a short form
of Domingo.

Minh (Vietnamese) bright.
*Minhao, Minhduc, Minhkhan,
Minhtong, Minhy*

Minkah (Akan) just, fair.

Minor (Latin) junior; younger.
Mynor

Minoru (Japanese) fruitful.

Mique (Spanish) a form of
Mickey.
Mequel, Mequelin, Miquel

Miron (Polish) peace.

Miroslav (Czech) peace; glory.
Mirek, Miroslaw, Miroslawy

Mirwais (Afghan) noble ruler.

Misael (Hebrew) a form of
Michael.
Mischael, Mishael, Missael

Misha (Russian) a short form
of Michail.
*Misa, Mischa, Mishael, Mishal,
Mishe, Mishenka, Mishka*

Miska (Hungarian) a form of
Michael.
Misi, Misik, Misko, Miso

Mister (English) mister.
Mistur

Misu (Moquelumnan) rippling
water.

Mitch (English) a short form of Mitchell.

Mitchel (English) a form of Mitchell.
Mitchael, Mitchal, Mitcheal, Mitchele, Mitchil, Mytchel

Mitchell (English) a form of Michael.
Mitch, Mitchall, Mitchel, Mitchelle, Mitchem, Mytch, Mytchell

Mitsos (Greek) a familiar form of Demetrius.

Modesto (Latin) modest.

Moe (English) a short form of Moses.
Mo

Mogens (Dutch) powerful.
Mohamad (Arabic) a form of Muhammad.
Mohamid

Mohamed (Arabic) a form of Muhammad.
Mohamd, Mohameed

Mohamet (Arabic) a form of Muhammad.
Mahomet, Mehemet, Mehmet

Mohammad (Arabic) a form of Muhammad.
Mahammad, Mohammadi, Mohammd, Mohammid, Mohanad, Mohmad

Mohammed (Arabic) a form of Muhammad.
Mahammed, Mahomet,
Mohammad, Mohaned, Mouhamed, Muhammad

Mohamud (Arabic) a form of Muhammad.
Mohammud, Mohamoud

Mohan (Hindi) delightful.

Moises (Portuguese, Spanish) a form of Moses.
Moices, Moise, Moisés, Moisey, Moisis

Moishe (Yiddish) a form of Moses.
Moshe

Mojag (Native American) crying baby.

Molimo (Moquelumnan) bear going under shady trees.

Momuso (Moquelumnan) yellow jackets crowded in their nests for the winter.

Mona (Moquelumnan) gathering jimsonweed seed.

Monahan (Irish) monk.
Monaghan, Monoghan

Mongo (Yoruba) famous.

Monroe (Irish) Geography: the mouth of the Roe River.
Monro, Munro, Munroe

Montague (French) pointed mountain.
Montagne, Montagu, Monte

Montana (Spanish) mountain.
Geography: a U.S. state.
Montaine, Montanna

Montaro (Japanese) big boy.
Montario, Monterio, Montero

Monte (Spanish) a short form
of Montgomery.
*Montae, Montaé, Montay,
Montea, Montee, Monti,
Montoya, Monty*

Montel (American) a form of
Montreal.
Montele, Montell, Montelle

Montez (Spanish) dweller in
the mountains.
*Monteiz, Monteze, Montezz,
Montisze*

Montgomery (English) rich
man's mountain.
Monte, Montgomerie, Monty

Montre (French) show.
*Montra, Montrae, Montray,
Montraz, Montres, Montrey,
Montrez, Montreze*

Montreal (French) royal
mountain. Geography: a city
in Quebec.
*Montel, Monterial, Monterrell,
Montrail, Montrale, Montrall,
Montreall, Montrell, Montrial*

Montrell (French) a form of
Montreal.
*Montral, Montrel, Montrele,
Montrelle*

Montsho (Tswana) black.

Monty (English) a familiar
form of Montgomery.

Moore (French) dark; moor;
marshland.
Moor, Mooro, More

Mordecai (Hebrew) martial,
warlike. Mythology: Marduk
was the Babylonian god of
war. Bible: wise counselor to
Queen Esther.
*Mord, Mordachai, Mordechai,
Mordie, Mordy, Mort*

Mordred (Latin) painful.
Literature: the bastard son of
King Arthur.
Modred

Morel (French) an edible
mushroom.
Morrel

Moreland (English) moor;
marshland.
Moorland, Morland

Morell (French) dark; from
Morocco.
*Moor, Moore, Morelle, Morelli,
Morill, Morrell, Morrill, Murrel,
Murrell*

Morey (Greek) a familiar form
of Moris. (Latin) a form of
Morrie.
Morrey, Morry

Morgan (Scottish) sea warrior.
*Morgen, Morghan, Morgin,
Morgon, Morgun, Morgunn,
Morgwn, Morgyn, Morrgan*

Morio (Japanese) forest.

Moris (Greek) son of the dark one. (English) a form of Morris.
Morey, Morisz, Moriz

Moritz (German) a form of Maurice, Morris.
Morisz

Morley (English) meadow by the moor.
Moorley, Moorly, Morlee, Morleigh, Morlon, Morly, Morlyn, Morrley

Morrie (Latin) a familiar form of Maurice, Morse.
Maury, Morey, Mori, Morie, Morry, Mory, Morye

Morris (Latin) dark skinned; moor; marshland. (English) a form of Maurice.
Moris, Moriss, Moritz, Morrese, Morrise, Morriss, Morry, Moss

Morse (English) son of Maurice.
Morresse, Morrie, Morrison, Morrisson

Mort (French, English) a short form of Morten, Mortimer, Morton.
Morte, Mortey, Mortie, Mortty, Morty

Morten (Norwegian) a form of Martin.
Mort

Mortimer (French) still water.
Mort, Mortymer

Morton (English) town near the moor.
Mort

Morven (Scottish) mariner.
Morvien, Morvin

Mose (Hebrew) a short form of Moses.

Moses (Hebrew) drawn out of the water. (Egyptian) son, child. Bible: the Hebrew law-giver who brought the Ten Commandments down from Mount Sinai.
Moe, Moise, Moïse, Moisei, Moises, Moishe, Mose, Mosese, Moshe, Mosiah, Mosie, Moss, Mosses, Mosya, Mosze, Moszek, Mousa, Moyses, Moze

Moshe (Hebrew, Polish) a form of Moses.
Mosheh

Mosi (Swahili) first-born.

Moss (Irish) a short form of Maurice, Morris. (English) a short form of Moses.

Moswen (African) light in color.

Motega (Native American) new arrow.

Mouhamed (Arabic) a form of Muhammad.
Mouhamad, Mouhamadou, Mouhammed, Mouhamoin

Mousa (Arabic) a form of
Moses.
Moussa

Moze (Lithuanian) a form of
Moses.
Mozes, Mózes

Mpasa (Nguni) mat.

Mposi (Nyakyusa) blacksmith.

Mpoza (Luganda) tax collector.

Msrah (Akan) sixth-born.

Mtima (Nguni) heart.

Muata (Moquelumnan) yellow jackets in their nest.

Mugamba (Runyoro) talks
too much.

Mugisa (Rutooro) lucky.
Mugisha, Mukisa

Muhammad (Arabic) praised.
History: the founder of the
Islamic religion. See also
Ahmad, Hamid, Yasin.
*Mahmoud, Mahmúd,
Mohamad, Mohamed,
Mohamet, Mohamud,
Mohammed, Mouhamed,
Muhamad, Muhamed,
Muhamet, Muhammadali,
Muhammed*

Muhannad (Arabic) sword.
Muhanad

Muhsin (Arabic) beneficent;
charitable.

Muhtadi (Arabic) rightly
guided.

Muir (Scottish) moor; marshland.

Mujahid (Arabic) fighter in
the way of Allah.

Mukasa (Luganda) God's chief
administrator.

Mukhtar (Arabic) chosen.
Mukhtaar

Mukul (Sanskrit) bud, blossom;
soul.

Mulogo (Musoga) wizard.

Mundan (Rhodesian) garden.

Mundo (Spanish) a short form
of Edmundo.

Mundy (Irish) from
Reamonn.

Mungo (Scottish) amiable.

Mun-Hee (Korean) literate;
shiny.

Munir (Arabic) brilliant; shining.

Munny (Cambodian) wise.

Muraco (Native American)
white moon.

Murali (Hindi) flute. Religion:
the instrument the Hindu
god Krishna is usually
depicted as playing.

Murat (Turkish) wish come
true.

Murdock (Scottish) wealthy sailor.
Murdo, Murdoch, Murtagh

Murphy (Irish) sea warrior.
Murfey, Murfy

Murray (Scottish) sailor.
Macmurray, Moray, Murrey, Murry

Murtagh (Irish) a form of Murdock.
Murtaugh

Musa (Swahili) child.

Musád (Arabic) untied camel.

Musoke (Rukonjo) born while a rainbow was in the sky.

Mustafa (Arabic) chosen; royal.
Mostafa, Mostaffa, Moustafa, Mustafaa, Mustafah, Mustafe, Mustaffa, Mustafo, Mustapha, Mustoffa, Mustofo

Mustapha (Arabic) a form of Mustafa.
Mostapha, Moustapha

Muti (Arabic) obedient.

Mwaka (Luganda) born on New Year's Eve.

Mwamba (Nyakyusa) strong.

Mwanje (Luganda) leopard.

Mwinyi (Swahili) king.

Mwita (Swahili) summoner.

Mychajlo (Latvian) a form of Michael.
Mykhaltso, Mykhas

Mychal (American) a form of Michael.
Mychall, Mychalo, Mycheal

Myer (English) a form of Meir.
Myers, Myur

Mykal, Mykel (American) forms of Michael.
Mykael, Mikele, Mykell

Myles (Latin) soldier. (German) a form of Miles.
Myels, Mylez, Mylles, Mylz

Mynor (Latin) a form of Minor.

Myo (Burmese) city.

Myron (Greek) fragrant ointment.
Mehran, Mehrayan, My, Myran, Myrone, Ron

Myung-Dae (Korean) right; great.

Mzuzi (Swahili) inventive.

N

Naaman (Hebrew) pleasant.

Nabiha (Arabic) intelligent.

Nabil (Arabic) noble.
Nabeel, Nabiel

Nachman (Hebrew) a short
form of Menachem.
Nachum, Nahum

Nada (Arabic) generous.

Nadav (Hebrew) generous;
noble.
Nadiv

Nadidah (Arabic) equal to
anyone else.

Nadim (Arabic) friend.
Nadeem

Nadir (Afghan, Arabic) dear,
rare.
Nader

Nadisu (Hindi) beautiful river.

Naeem (Arabic) benevolent.
Naem, Naim, Naiym, Nieem

Naftali (Hebrew) wreath.
Naftalie

Nagid (Hebrew) ruler; prince.

Nahele (Hawaiian) forest.

Nahma (Native American)
sturgeon.

Nailah (Arabic) successful.

Nairn (Scottish) river with
alder trees.
Nairne

Najee (Arabic) a form of Naji.
Najae, Najée, Najei, Najiee

Naji (Arabic) safe.
Najee, Najih

Najíb (Arabic) born to nobility.
Najib, Nejeeb

Najji (Muganda) second child.

Nakia (Arabic) pure.
*Nakai, Nakee, Nakeia, Naki,
Nakiah, Nakii*

Nakos (Arapaho) sage, wise.

Naldo (Spanish) a familiar
form of Reginald.

Nalren (Dene) thawed out.

Nam (Vietnamese) scrape off.

Namaka (Hawaiian) eyes.

Namid (Ojibwa) star dancer.

Namir (Hebrew) leopard.
Namer

Nandin (Hindi) Religion: a
servant of the Hindu god
Shiva.
Nandan

Nando (German) a familiar
form of Ferdinand.
Nandor

Nangila (Abaluhya) born
while parents traveled.

Nangwaya (Mwera) don't
mess with me.

Nansen (Swedish) son of
Nancy.

Nantai (Navajo) chief.

Nantan (Apache) spokesman.

Naoko (Japanese) straight, honest.

Napayshni (Lakota) he does not flee; courageous.

Napier (Spanish) new city.
Neper

Napoleon (Greek) lion of the woodland. (Italian) from Naples, Italy. History: Napoleon Bonaparte was a famous nineteenth-century French emperor.
Leon, Nap, Napolean, Napoléon, Napoleone, Nappie, Nappy

Naquan (American) a combination of the prefix Na + Quan.
Naqawn, Naquain, Naquen, Naquon

Narain (Hindi) protector. Religion: another name for the Hindu god Vishnu.
Narayan

Narcisse (French) a form of Narcissus.
Narcis, Narciso, Narkis, Narkissos

Narcissus (Greek) daffodil. Mythology: the youth who fell in love with his own reflection.
Narcisse

Nard (Persian) chess player.

Nardo (German) strong, hardy. (Spanish) a short form of Bernardo.

Narve (Dutch) healthy, strong.

Nashashuk (Fox, Sauk) loud thunder.

Nashoba (Choctaw) wolf.

Nasim (Persian) breeze; fresh air.
Naseem, Nassim

Nasser (Arabic) victorious.
Naseer, Naser, Nasier, Nasir, Nasr, Nassir, Nassor

Nat (English) a short form of Nathan, Nathaniel.
Natt, Natty

Natal (Spanish) a form of Noël.
Natale, Natalie, Natalino, Natalio, Nataly

Natan (Hebrew, Hungarian, Polish, Russian, Spanish) God has given.
Naten

Natanael (Hebrew) a form of Nathaniel.
Natanel, Nataniel

Nate (Hebrew) a short form of Nathan, Nathaniel.

Natesh (Hindi) destroyer. Religion: another name for the Hindu god Shiva.

Nathan (Hebrew) a short
form of Nathaniel. Bible: a
prophet during the reigns of
David and Solomon.
*Naethan, Nat, Nate, Nathann,
Nathean, Nathen, Nathian,
Nathin, Nathon, Nathyn,
Natthan, Naythan, Nethan*

Nathanael (Hebrew) gift of
God. Bible: one of the
Twelve Apostles. Also known
as Bartholomew.
*Nathanae, Nathanal,
Nathaneal, Nathaneil,
Nathanel, Nathaneol*

Nathanial (Hebrew) a form of
Nathaniel.
Nathanyal, Nathanual

Nathanie (Hebrew) a familiar
form of Nathaniel.
Nathania, Nathanni

Nathaniel (Hebrew) gift of
God. Bible: one of the
Twelve Apostles.
*Nat, Natanael, Nate, Nathan,
Nathanael, Nathanial,
Nathanie, Nathanielle,
Nathanil, Nathanile,
Nathanuel, Nathanyel,
Nathanyl, Natheal, Nathel,
Nathinel, Nethaniel, Thaniel*

Nathen (Hebrew) a form of
Nathan.

Nav (Gypsy) name.

Navarro (Spanish) plains.
Navarre

Navdeep (Sikh) new light.
Navdip

Navin (Hindi) new, novel.
Naveen, Naven

Nawat (Native American) left-
handed.

Nawkaw (Winnebago) wood.

Nayati (Native American)
wrestler.

Nayland (English) island
dweller.

Nazareth (Hebrew) born in
Nazareth, Israel.
*Nazaire, Nazaret, Nazarie,
Nazario, Nazerene, Nazerine*

Nazih (Arabic) pure, chaste.
*Nazeeh, Nazeem, Nazeer,
Nazieh, Nazim, Nazir, Nazz*

Ndale (Nguni) trick.

Neal (Irish) a form of Neil.
*Neale, Neall, Nealle, Nealon,
Nealy*

Neci (Latin) a familiar form of
Ignatius.

Nectarios (Greek) saint.
Religion: a saint in the
Greek Orthodox Church.

Ned (English) a familiar form
of Edward, Edwin.
Neddie, Neddym, Nedrick

Nehemiah (Hebrew) compassion of Jehovah. Bible: a Jewish leader.
Nahemiah, Nechemya, Nehemias, Nehemie, Nehemyah, Nehimiah, Nehmia, Nehmiah, Nemo, Neyamia

Nehru (Hindi) canal.

Neil (Irish) champion.
Neal, Neel, Neihl, Neile, Neill, Neille, Nels, Niall, Niele, Niels, Nigel, Nil, Niles, Nilo, Nils, Nyle

Neka (Native American) wild goose.

Nelek (Polish) a form of Cornelius.

Nellie (English) a familiar form of Cornelius, Cornell, Nelson.
Nell, Nelly

Nelius (Latin) a short form of Cornelius.

Nelo (Spanish) a form of Daniel.
Nello, Nilo

Nels (Scandinavian) a form of Neil, Nelson.
Nelse, Nelson, Nils

Nelson (English) son of Neil.
Nealson, Neilsen, Neilson, Nellie, Nels, Nelsen, Nilson, Nilsson

Nemesio (Spanish) just.
Nemi

Nemo (Greek) glen, glade. (Hebrew) a short form of Nehemiah.

Nen (Egyptian) ancient waters.

Neptune (Latin) sea ruler. Mythology: the Roman god of the sea.

Nero (Latin, Spanish) stern. History: a cruel Roman emperor.
Neron, Nerone, Nerron

Nesbit (English) nose-shaped bend in a river.
Naisbit, Naisbitt, Nesbitt, Nisbet, Nisbett

Nestor (Greek) traveler; wise.
Nester

Nethaniel (Hebrew) a form of Nathaniel.
Netanel, Netania, Netaniah, Netaniel, Netanya, Nethanel, Nethanial, Nethaniel, Nethanyal, Nethanyel

Neto (Spanish) a short form of Ernesto.

Nevada (Spanish) covered in snow. Geography: a U.S. state.
Navada, Nevade

Nevan (Irish) holy.
Nevean

Neville (French) new town.
Nev, Nevil, Nevile, Nevill, Nevyle

Nevin (Irish) worshiper of the saint. (English) middle; herb.
Nefen, Nev, Nevan, Neven, Nevins, Nevyn, Niven

Newbold (English) new tree.

Newell (English) new hall.
Newall, Newel, Newyle

Newland (English) new land.
Newlan

Newlin (Welsh) new lake.
Newlyn

Newman (English) newcomer.
Neiman, Neimann, Neimon, Neuman, Numan, Numen

Newton (English) new town.
Newt

Ngai (Vietnamese) herb.

Nghia (Vietnamese) forever.

Ngozi (Ibo) blessing.

Ngu (Vietnamese) sleep.

Nguyen (Vietnamese) a form of Ngu.

Nhean (Cambodian) self-knowledge.

Niall (Irish) a form of Neil. History: Niall of the Nine Hostages was a famous Irish king.
Nial, Nialle

Nibal (Arabic) arrows.
Nibel

Nibaw (Native American) standing tall.

Nicabar (Gypsy) stealthy.

Nicho (Spanish) a form of Dennis.

Nicholas (Greek) victorious people. Religion: Nicholas of Myra is a patron saint of children. See also Caelan, Claus, Cola, Colar, Cole, Colin, Colson, Klaus, Lasse, Mikolaj, Mikolas, Milek.
Niccolas, Nichalas, Nichelas, Nichele, Nichlas, Nichlos, Nichola, Nicholaas, Nicholaes, Nicholase, Nicholaus, Nichole, Nicholias, Nicholl, Nichollas, Nicholos, Nichols, Nicholus, Nick, Nickalus, Nicklaus, Nickolas, Nicky, Niclas, Niclasse, Nico, Nicola, Nicolai, Nicolas, Nicoles, Nicolis, Nicoll, Nicolo, Nikhil, Niki, Nikili, Nikita, Nikko, Niklas, Niko, Nikolai, Nikolas, Nikolaus, Nikolos, Nils, Nioclás, Niocol, Nycholas

Nicholaus (Greek) a form of Nicholas.
Nichalaus, Nichalous, Nichaolas, Nichlaus, Nichloas, Nichlous, Nicholaos, Nicholous

Nichols, Nicholson (English) son of Nicholas.
Nicholes, Nicholis, Nicolls, Nickelson, Nickoles

Nick (English) a short form of Dominic, Nicholas. See also Micu.
Nic, Nik

Nickalus (Greek) a form of Nicholas.
Nickalas, Nickalis, Nickalos, Nickelas, Nickelus

Nicklaus, Nicklas (Greek) forms of Nicholas.
Nickalaus, Nickalous, Nickelous, Nicklauss, Nicklos, Nicklous, Nicklus, Nickolau, Nickolaus, Nicolaus, Niklaus, Nikolaus

Nickolas (Greek) a form of Nicholas.
Nickolaos, Nickolis, Nickolos, Nickolus, Nickolys, Nickoulas

Nicky (Greek) a familiar form of Nicholas.
Nickey, Nicki, Nickie, Niki, Nikki

Nico (Greek) a short form of Nicholas.
Nicco

Nicodemus (Greek) conqueror of the people.
Nicodem, Nicodemius, Nikodem, Nikodema, Nikodemious, Nikodim

Nicola (Italian) a form of Nicholas. See also Cola.
Nicolá, Nikolah

Nicolai (Norwegian, Russian) a form of Nicholas.
Nicholai, Nickolai, Nicolaj,
Nicolau, Nicolay, Nicoly, Nikalai

Nicolas (Italian) a form of Nicholas.
Nico, Nicolaas, Nicolás, Nicolaus, Nicoles, Nicolis, Nicolus

Nicolo (Italian) a form of Nicholas.
Niccolo, Niccolò, Nicol, Nicolao, Nicollo

Niels (Danish) a form of Neil.
Niel, Nielsen, Nielson, Niles, Nils

Nien (Vietnamese) year.

Nigan (Native American) ahead.
Nigen

Nigel (Latin) dark night.
Niegel, Nigal, Nigale, Nigele, Nigell, Nigiel, Nigil, Nigle, Nijel, Nye, Nygel, Nyigel, Nyjil

Nika (Yoruba) ferocious.

Nike (Greek) victorious.
Nikka

Niki (Hungarian) a familiar form of Nicholas.
Nikia, Nikiah, Nikki, Nikkie, Nykei, Nykey

Nikita (Russian) a form of Nicholas.
Nakita, Nakitas, Nikula

Nikiti (Native American) round and smooth like an abalone shell.

Nikko, Niko (Hungarian) forms of Nicholas.
Nikoe, Nyko

Niklas (Latvian, Swedish) a form of Nicholas.
Niklaas, Niklaus

Nikola (Greek) a short form of Nicholas.
Nikolao, Nikolay, Nykola

Nikolai (Estonian, Russian) a form of Nicholas.
Kolya, Nikolais, Nikolaj, Nikolajs, Nikolay, Nikoli, Nikolia, Nikula, Nikulas

Nikolas (Greek) a form of Nicholas.
Nicanor, Nikalas, Nikalis, Nikalus, Nikholas, Nikolaas, Nikolaos, Nikolis, Nikolos, Nikos, Nilos, Nykolas, Nykolus

Nikolaus (Greek) a form of Nicholas.
Nikalous, Nikolaos

Nikolos (Greek) a form of Nicholas. See also Kolya.
Niklos, Nikolaos, Nikolò, Nikolous, Nikolus, Nikos, Nilos

Nil (Russian) a form of Neil.
Nilya

Nila (Hindi) blue.

Niles (English) son of Neil.
Nilesh, Nyles

Nilo (Finnish) a form of Neil.

Nils (Swedish) a short form of Nicholas.

Nimrod (Hebrew) rebel. Bible: a great-grandson of Noah.

Niño (Spanish) young child.

Niran (Tai) eternal.

Nishan (Armenian) cross, sign, mark.
Nishon

Nissan (Hebrew) sign, omen; miracle.
Nisan, Nissim, Nissin, Nisson

Nitis (Native American) friend.
Netis

Nixon (English) son of Nick.
Nixan, Nixson

Nizam (Arabic) leader.

Nkunda (Runyankore) loves those who hate him.

N'namdi (Ibo) his father's name lives on.

Noach (Hebrew) a form of Noah.

Noah (Hebrew) peaceful, restful. Bible: the patriarch who built the ark to survive the Flood.
Noach, Noak, Noe, Noé, Noi

Noam (Hebrew) sweet; friend.

Noble (Latin) born to nobility.
Nobe, Nobie, Noby

Nodin (Native American)
wind.
Knoton, Noton

Noe (Czech, French) a form
of Noah.

Noé (Hebrew, Spanish) quiet,
peaceful. See also Noah.

Noël (French) day of Christ's
birth. See also Natal.
*Noel, Noél, Noell, Nole, Noli,
Nowel, Nowell*

Nohea (Hawaiian) handsome.
Noha, Nohe

Nokonyu (Native American)
katydid's nose.
Noko, Nokoni

Nolan (Irish) famous; noble.
*Noland, Nolande, Nolane,
Nolen, Nolin, Nollan, Nolyn*

Nollie (Latin, Scandinavian) a
familiar form of Oliver.
Noll, Nolly

Norbert (Scandinavian) brilliant hero.
Bert, Norberto, Norbie, Norby

Norberto (Spanish) a form of
Norbert.

Norman (French) Norseman.
History: a name for the
Scandinavians who settled in
northern France in the tenth

century, and who later con-
quered England in 1066.
*Norm, Normand, Normen,
Normie, Normy*

Norris (French) northerner.
(English) Norman's horse.
*Norice, Norie, Noris, Norreys,
Norrie, Norry, Norrys*

Northcliff (English) northern
cliff.
*Northcliffe, Northclyff,
Northclyffe*

Northrop (English) north
farm.
North, Northup

Norton (English) northern
town.

Norville (French, English)
northern town.
*Norval, Norvel, Norvell, Norvil,
Norvill, Norvylle*

Norvin (English) northern
friend.
*Norvyn, Norwin, Norwinn,
Norwyn, Norwynn*

Norward (English) protector
of the north.
Norwerd

Norwood (English) northern
woods.

Notaku (Moquelumnan)
growing bear.

Nowles (English) a short form
of Knowles.

Nsoah (Akan) seventh-born.

Numa (Arabic) pleasant.

Numair (Arabic) panther.

Nuncio (Italian) messenger.
Nunzi, Nunzio

Nuri (Hebrew, Arabic) my fire.
*Nery, Noori, Nur, Nuris,
Nurism, Nury*

Nuriel (Hebrew, Arabic) fire of
the Lord.
Nuria, Nuriah, Nuriya

Nuru (Swahili) born in daylight.

Nusair (Arabic) bird of prey.

Nwa (Nigerian) son.

Nwake (Nigerian) born on
market day.

Nye (English) a familiar form
of Aneurin, Nigel.

Nyle (English) island. (Irish) a
form of Neil.
Nyal, Nyll

Oakes (English) oak trees.
Oak, Oakie, Oaks, Ochs

Oakley (English) oak-tree
field.
*Oak, Oakes, Oakie, Oaklee,
Oakleigh, Oakly, Oaks*

Oalo (Spanish) a form of Paul.

Oba (Yoruba) king.

Obadele (Yoruba) king arrives
at the house.

Obadiah (Hebrew) servant of
God.
*Obadias, Obed, Obediah, Obie,
Ovadiach, Ovadiah, Ovadya*

Obed (English) a short form
of Obadiah.

Oberon (German) noble;
bearlike. Literature: the king
of the fairies in the
Shakespearean play *A
Midsummer Night's Dream*.
See also Auberon, Aubrey.
Oberen, Oberron, Oeberon

Obert (German) wealthy;
bright.

Obie (English) a familiar form
of Obadiah.
Obbie, Obe, Obey, Obi, Oby

Ocan (Luo) hard times.

Octavio (Latin) eighth. See
also Tavey, Tavian.
*Octave, Octavia, Octavian,
Octaviano, Octavien, Octavious,
Octavius, Octavo, Octavous,
Octavus, Ottavio*

Octavious, Octavius (Latin)
forms of Octavio.
*Octavaius, Octaveous, Octaveus,
Octavias, Octaviaus, Octavis,
Octavous, Octavus*

Odakota (Lakota) friendly.
Oda

Odd (Norwegian) point.
Oddvar

Ode (Benin) born along the
road. (Irish, English) a short
form of Odell.
Odey, Odie, Ody

Oded (Hebrew) encouraging.

Odell (Greek) ode, melody.
(Irish) otter. (English)
forested hill.
Dell, Odall, Ode

Odin (Scandinavian) ruler.
Mythology: the Norse god
of wisdom and war.
Oden

Odion (Benin) first of twins.

Odo (Norwegian) a form of
Otto.

Odolf (German) prosperous
wolf.
Odolff

Odom (Ghanaian) oak tree.

Odon (Hungarian) wealthy
protector.
Odi

Odran (Irish) pale green.
*Odhrán, Oran, Oren, Orin,
Orran, Orren, Orrin*

Odysseus (Greek) wrathful.
Literature: the hero of
Homer's epic poem *Odyssey*.

Ofer (Hebrew) young deer.

Og (Aramaic) king. Bible: the
king of Basham.

Ogaleesha (Lakota) red shirt.

Ogbay (Ethiopian) don't take
him from me.

Ogbonna (Ibo) image of his
father.
Ogbonnia

Ogden (English) oak valley.
Literature: Ogden Nash
was a twentieth-century
American writer of light
verse.
Ogdan, Ogdon

Ogima (Chippewa) chief.

Ogun (Nigerian) Mythology:
the god of war.
*Ogunkeye, Ogunsanwo,
Ogunsheye*

Ohanko (Native American)
restless.

Ohannes (Turkish) a form of
John.

Ohanzee (Lakota) comforting
shadow.

Ohin (African) chief.
Ohan

Ohitekah (Lakota) brave.

Oistin (Irish) a form of
Austin.
Osten, Ostyn, Ostynn

OJ (American) a combination
of the initials O. + J.
O.J., Ojay

Ojo (Yoruba) difficult delivery.

Okapi (Swahili) an African
animal related to the giraffe
but having a short neck.

Oke (Hawaiian) a form of
Oscar.

Okechuku (Ibo) God's gift.

Okeke (Ibo) born on market
day.
Okorie

Okie (American) from
Oklahoma.
Okee, Okey

Oko (Ghanaian) older twin.
(Yoruba) god of war.

Okorie (Ibo) a form of
Okeke.

Okpara (Ibo) first son.

Okuth (Luo) born in a rain
shower.

Ola (Yoruba) wealthy, rich.

Olaf (Scandinavian) ancestor.
History: a patron saint and
king of Norway.
*Olaff, Olafur, Olav, Ole, Olef,
Olof, Oluf*

Olajuwon (Yoruba) wealth
and honor are God's gifts.
*Olajawon, Olajawun,
Olajowuan, Olajuan,
Olajuanne, Olajuawon,
Olajuwa, Olajuwan,
Olaujawon, Oljuwoun*

Olamina (Yoruba) this is my
wealth.

Olatunji (Yoruba) honor
reawakens.

Olav (Scandinavian) a form of
Olaf.
*Ola, Olave, Olavus, Ole, Olen,
Olin, Olle, Olov, Olyn*

Ole (Scandinavian) a familiar
form of Olaf, Olav.
Olay, Oleh, Olle

Oleg (Latvian, Russian) holy.
Olezka

Oleksandr (Russian) a form
of Alexander.
Olek, Olesandr, Olesko

Olés (Polish) a familiar form
of Alexander.

Olin (English) holly.
Olen, Olney, Olyn

Olindo (Italian) from
Olinthos, Greece.

Oliver (Latin) olive tree.
(Scandinavian) kind; affec-
tionate.
*Nollie, Oilibhéar, Oliverio,
Oliverios, Olivero, Olivier,
Oliviero, Oliwa, Ollie, Olliver,
Ollivor, Olvan*

Olivier (French) a form of
Oliver.

Oliwa (Hawaiian) a form of Oliver.

Ollie (English) a familiar form of Oliver.
Olie, Olle, Olley, Olly

Olo (Spanish) a short form of Orlando, Rolando.

Olubayo (Yoruba) highest joy.

Olufemi (Yoruba) wealth and honor favors me.

Olujimi (Yoruba) God gave me this.

Olushola (Yoruba) God has blessed me.

Omar (Arabic) highest; follower of the Prophet. (Hebrew) reverent.
Omair, Omari, Omarr, Omer, Umar

Omari (Swahili) a form of Omar.
Omare, Omaree, Omarey

Omer (Arabic) a form of Omar.
Omeer, Omero

Omolara (Benin) child born at the right time.

On (Burmese) coconut. (Chinese) peace.

Onan (Turkish) prosperous.

Onaona (Hawaiian) pleasant fragrance.

Ondro (Czech) a form of Andrew.
Ondra, Ondre, Ondrea, Ondrey

O'neil (Irish) son of Neil.
Oneal, O'neal, Oneil, O'neill, Onel, Oniel, Onil

Onkar (Hindi) God in his entirety.

Onofrio (German) a form of Humphrey.
Oinfre, Onfre, Onfrio, Onofre, Onofredo

Onslow (English) enthusiast's hill.
Ounslow

Onufry (Polish) a form of Humphrey.

Onur (Turkish) honor.

Ophir (Hebrew) faithful. Bible: an Old Testament people and country.

Opio (Ateso) first of twin boys.

Oral (Latin) verbal; speaker.

Oran (Irish) green.
Odhran, Odran, Ora, Orane, Orran

Oratio (Latin) a form of Horatio.
Orazio

Orbán (Hungarian) born in the city.

Ordell (Latin) beginning.
Orde

Oren (Hebrew) pine tree.
(Irish) light skinned, white.
*Oran, Orin, Oris, Orono,
Orren, Orrin*

Orestes (Greek) mountain
man. Mythology: the son of
the Greek leader
Agamemnon.
Aresty, Oreste

Ori (Hebrew) my light.
Oree, Orie, Orri, Ory

Orien (Latin) visitor from the
east.
*Orian, Orie, Orin, Oris, Oron,
Orono, Orrin, Oryan*

Orion (Greek) son of fire.
Mythology: a giant hunter
who was killed by Artemis.
See also Zorion.

Orji (Ibo) mighty tree.

Orlando (German) famous
throughout the land.
(Spanish) a form of Roland.
*Lando, Olando, Olo, Orlan,
Orland, Orlanda, Orlandas,
Orlandes, Orlandis, Orlandos,
Orlandus, Orlo, Orlondo,
Orlondon*

Orleans (Latin) golden.
Orlean, Orlin

Orman (German) mariner,
seaman. (Scandinavian) ser-
pent, worm.
Ormand

Ormond (English) bear
mountain; spear protector.
Ormande, Ormon, Ormonde

Oro (Spanish) golden.

Orono (Latin) a form of
Oren.
Oron

Orrick (English) old oak tree.
Orric

Orrin (English) river.
Orin, Oryn, Orynn

Orris (Latin) a form of
Horatio.
Oris, Orriss

Orry (Latin) from the Orient.
Oarrie, Orrey, Orrie

Orsino (Italian) a form of
Orson.

Orson (Latin) bearlike.
*Orscino, Orsen, Orsin, Orsini,
Orsino, Son, Sonny, Urson*

Orton (English) shore town.

Ortzi (Basque) sky.

Orunjan (Yoruba) born under
the midday sun.

Orval (English) a form of
Orville.
Orvel

Orville (French) golden village. History: Orville Wright
and his brother Wilbur were

the first men to fly an airplane.
Orv, Orval, Orvell, Orvie, Orvil

Orvin (English) spear friend.
Orwin, Owynn

Osahar (Benin) God hears.

Osayaba (Benin) God forgives.

Osaze (Benin) whom God likes.

Osbert (English) divine; bright.

Osborn (Scandinavian) divine bear. (English) warrior of God.
Osbern, Osbon, Osborne, Osbourn, Osbourne, Osburn, Osburne, Oz, Ozzie

Oscar (Scandinavian) divine spearman.
Oke, Oskar, Osker, Oszkar

Osei (Fante) noble.
Osee

Osgood (English) divinely good.

O'Shea (Irish) son of Shea.
Oshae, Oshai, Oshane, O'Shane, Oshaun, Oshay, Oshaye, Oshe, Oshea, Osheon

Osip (Russian, Ukrainian) a form of Joseph, Yosef. See also Osya.

Oskar (Scandinavian) a form of Oscar.
Osker, Ozker

Osman (Turkish) ruler. (English) servant of God.
Osmanek, Osmen, Osmin, Otthmor, Ottmar

Osmar (English) divine; wonderful.

Osmond (English) divine protector.
Osmand, Osmonde, Osmont, Osmund, Osmunde, Osmundo

Osric (English) divine ruler.
Osrick

Ostin (Latin) a form of Austin.
Ostan, Osten, Ostyn

Osvaldo (Spanish) a form of Oswald.
Osbaldo, Osbalto, Osvald, Osvalda

Oswald (English) God's power; God's crest. See also Waldo.
Osvaldo, Oswaldo, Oswall, Oswell, Oswold, Oz, Ozzie

Oswaldo (Spanish) a form of Oswald.

Oswin (English) divine friend.
Osvin, Oswinn, Oswyn, Oswynn

Osya (Russian) a familiar form of Osip.

Ota (Czech) prosperous.
Otik

Otadan (Native American) plentiful.

Otaktay (Lakota) kills many; strikes many.

Otek (Polish) a form of Otto.

Otello (Italian) a form of Othello.

Otem (Luo) born away from home.

Othello (Spanish) a form of Otto. Literature: the title character in the Shakespearean tragedy *Othello*.
Otello

Othman (German) wealthy.
Ottoman

Otis (Greek) keen of hearing. (German) son of Otto.
Oates, Odis, Otes, Otess, Otez, Otise, Ottis, Otys

Ottah (Nigerian) thin baby.

Ottar (Norwegian) point warrior; fright warrior.

Ottmar (Turkish) a form of Osman.
Otomars, Ottomar

Otto (German) rich.
Odo, Otek, Otello, Otfried, Othello, Otho, Othon, Otik, Otilio, Otman, Oto, Otón, Otton, Ottone

Ottokar (German) happy warrior.
Otokars, Ottocar

Otu (Native American) collecting seashells in a basket.

Ouray (Ute) arrow. Astrology: born under the sign of Sagittarius.

Oved (Hebrew) worshiper, follower.

Owen (Irish) born to nobility; young warrior. (Welsh) a form of Evan.
Owain, Owens, Owin, Uaine

Owney (Irish) elderly.
Oney

Oxford (English) place where oxen cross the river.
Ford

Oya (Moquelumnan) speaking of the jacksnipe.

Oystein (Norwegian) rock of happiness.
Ostein, Osten, Ostin, Øystein

Oz (Hebrew) a short form of Osborn, Oswald.

Ozturk (Turkish) pure; genuine Turk.

Ozzie (English) a familiar form of Osborn, Oswald.
Ossie, Ossy, Ozee, Ozi, Ozzi, Ozzy

P

Paavo (Finnish) a form of Paul.
Paaveli

Pablo (Spanish) a form of Paul.
Pable, Paublo

Pace (English) a form of Pascal.
Payce

Pacifico (Filipino) peaceful.

Paco (Italian) pack. (Spanish) a familiar form of Francisco. (Native American) bald eagle. See also Quico.
Pacorro, Panchito, Pancho, Paquito

Paddy (Irish) a familiar form of Padraic, Patrick.
Paddey, Paddi, Paddie

Paden (English) a form of Patton.

Padget (English) a form of Page.
Padgett, Paget, Pagett

Padraic (Irish) a form of Patrick.
Paddrick, Paddy, Padhraig, Padrai, Pádraig, Padraigh, Padreic, Padriac, Padric, Padron, Padruig

Page (French) youthful assistant.
Padget, Paggio, Paige, Payge

Paige (English) a form of Page.

Pakelika (Hawaiian) a form of Patrick.

Paki (African) witness.

Pal (Swedish) a form of Paul.

Pál (Hungarian) a form of Paul.
Pali, Palika

Palaina (Hawaiian) a form of Brian.

Palani (Hawaiian) a form of Frank.

Palash (Hindi) flowery tree.

Palben (Basque) blond.

Palladin (Native American) fighter.
Pallaton, Palleten

Palmer (English) palm-bearing pilgrim.
Pallmer, Palmar

Palti (Hebrew) God liberates.
Palti-el

Panas (Russian) immortal.

Panayiotis (Greek) a form of Peter.
Panagiotis, Panajotis, Panayioti, Panayoti, Panayotis

Pancho (Spanish) a familiar form of Francisco, Frank.
Panchito

Panos (Greek) a form of Peter.
Petros

Paolo (Italian) a form of Paul.

Paquito (Spanish) a familiar form of Paco.

Paramesh (Hindi) greatest. Religion: another name for the Hindu god Shiva.

Pardeep (Sikh) mystic light.
Pardip

Paris (Greek) lover. Geography: the capital of France. Mythology: the prince of Troy who started the Trojan War by abducting Helen.
Paras, Paree, Pares, Parese, Parie, Parris, Parys

Park (Chinese) cypress tree. (English) a short form of Parker.
Parke, Parkes, Parkey, Parks

Parker (English) park keeper.
Park

Parkin (English) little Peter.
Perkin

Parlan (Scottish) a form of Bartholomew. See also Parthalán.

Parnell (French) little Peter. History: Charles Stewart Parnell was a famous Irish politician.
Nell, Parle, Parnel, Parrnell, Pernell

Parr (English) cattle enclosure, barn.

Parrish (English) church district.
Parish, Parrie, Parrisch, Parrysh

Parry (Welsh) son of Harry.
Parrey, Parrie, Pary

Parth (Irish) a short form of Parthalán.
Partha, Parthey

Parthalán (Irish) plowman. See also Bartholomew.
Parlan, Parth

Parthenios (Greek) virgin. Religion: a Greek Orthodox saint.

Pascal (French) born on Easter or Passover.
Pace, Pascale, Pascalle, Paschal, Paschalis, Pascoe, Pascow, Pascual, Pasquale

Pascual (Spanish) a form of Pascal.
Pascul

Pasha (Russian) a form of Paul.
Pashenka, Pashka

Pasquale (Italian) a form of
Pascal.
*Pascuale, Pasqual, Pasquali,
Pasquel*

Pastor (Latin) spiritual leader.

Pat (Native American) fish.
(English) a short form of
Patrick.
Pattie, Patty

Patakusu (Moquelumnan) ant
biting a person.

Patamon (Native American)
raging.

Patek (Polish) a form of
Patrick.
Patick

Patric (Latin) a form of
Patrick.

Patrice (French) a form of
Patrick.

Patricio (Spanish) a form of
Patrick.
Patricius, Patrizio

Patrick (Latin) nobleman.
Religion: the patron saint of
Ireland. See also Fitzpatrick,
Ticho.
*Paddy, Padraic, Pakelika, Pat,
Patek, Patric, Patrice, Patricio,
Patrickk, Patrik, Patrique,
Patrizius, Patryk, Pats, Patsy,
Pattrick*

Patrin (Gypsy) leaf trail.

Patryk (Latin) a form of
Patrick.
Patryck

Patterson (Irish) son of Pat.
Patteson

Pattin (Gypsy) leaf.

Patton (English) warrior's
town.
*Paden, Paten, Patin, Paton,
Patten, Pattin, Patty, Payton,
Peyton*

Patwin (Native American)
man.

Patxi (Basque, Teutonic) free.

Paul (Latin) small. Bible: Saul,
later renamed Paul, was the
first to bring the teachings of
Christ to the Gentiles.
*Oalo, Paavo, Pablo, Pal, Pál,
Pall, Paolo, Pasha, Pasko, Pauli,
Paulia, Paulin, Paulino, Paulis,
Paulo, Pauls, Paulus, Pavel,
Pavlos, Pawel, Pol, Poul*

Pauli (Latin) a familiar form of
Paul.
Pauley, Paulie, Pauly

Paulin (German, Polish) a
form of Paul.

Paulino (Spanish) a form of
Paul.

Paulo (Portuguese, Swedish,
Hawaiian) a form of Paul.

Pavel (Russian) a form of Paul.
Paavel, Pasha, Pavils, Pavlik, Pavlo, Pavlusha, Pavlushenka, Pawl

Pavit (Hindi) pious, pure.

Pawel (Polish) a form of Paul.
Pawelek, Pawl

Pax (Latin) peaceful.
Paz

Paxton (Latin) peaceful town.
Packston, Pax, Paxon, Paxten, Paxtun

Payat (Native American) he is on his way.
Pay, Payatt

Payden (English) a form of Payton.
Paydon

Payne (Latin) from the country.
Paine, Paynn

Paytah (Lakota) fire.
Pay, Payta

Payton (English) a form of Patton.
Paiton, Pate, Payden, Peaton, Peighton, Peyton

Paz (Spanish) a form of Pax.

Pearce (English) a form of Pierce.
Pears, Pearse

Pearson (English) son of Peter. See also Pierson.
Pearsson, Pehrson, Peirson, Peterson

Peder (Scandinavian) a form of Peter.
Peadar, Pedey

Pedro (Spanish) a form of Peter.
Pedrin, Pedrín, Petronio

Peers (English) a form of Peter.
Peerus, Piers

Peeter (Estonian) a form of Peter.
Peet

Peirce (English) a form of Peter.
Peirs

Pekelo (Hawaiian) a form of Peter.
Pekka

Peleke (Hawaiian) a form of Frederick.

Pelham (English) tannery town.

Pelí (Latin, Basque) happy.

Pell (English) parchment.
Pall

Pello (Greek, Basque) stone.
Peru, Piarres

Pelton (English) town by a pool.

Pembroke (Welsh) headland.
(French) wine dealer.
(English) broken fence.
Pembrook

Peniamina (Hawaiian) a form
of Benjamin.
Peni

Penley (English) enclosed
meadow.

Penn (Latin) pen, quill.
(English) enclosure.
(German) a short form of
Penrod.
Pen, Penna, Penney, Pennie,
Penny

Penrod (German) famous
commander.
Penn, Pennrod, Rod

Pepa (Czech) a familiar form
of Joseph.
Pepek, Pepik

Pepe (Spanish) a familiar form
of José.
Pepillo, Pepito, Pequin, Pipo

Pepin (German) determined;
petitioner. History: Pepin the
Short was an eighth-century
king of the Franks.
Pepi, Peppie, Peppy

Peppe (Italian) a familiar form
of Joseph.
Peppi, Peppo, Pino

Per (Swedish) a form of Peter.

Perben (Greek, Danish) stone.

Percival (French) pierce the
valley. Literature: a knight of
the Round Table who first
appears in Chrétien de
Troyes's poem about the
quest for the Holy Grail.
Parsafal, Parsefal, Parsifal,
Parzival, Perc, Perce, Perceval,
Percevall, Percivall, Percy,
Peredur, Purcell

Percy (French) a familiar form
of Percival.
Pearcey, Pearcy, Percey, Percie,
Piercey, Piercy

Peregrine (Latin) traveler; pil-
grim; falcon.
Peregrin, Peregryne, Perine,
Perry

Pericles (Greek) just leader.
History: an Athenian statesman.

Perico (Spanish) a form of
Peter.
Pequin, Perequin

Perine (Latin) a short form of
Peregrine.
Perino, Perion, Perrin, Perryn

Perkin (English) little Peter.
Perka, Perkins, Perkyn, Perrin

Pernell (French) a form of
Parnell.
Perren, Perrnall

Perry (English) a familiar form
of Peregrine, Peter.
Parry, Perrie, Perrye

Perth (Scottish) thorn-bush thicket. Geography: a burgh in Scotland; a city in Australia.

Pervis (Latin) passage.
Pervez

Pesach (Hebrew) spared. Religion: another name for Passover.
Pessach

Petar (Greek) a form of Peter.

Pete (English) a short form of Peter.
Peat, Peet, Petey, Peti, Petie, Piet, Pit

Peter (Greek, Latin) small rock. Bible: Simon, renamed Peter, was the leader of the Twelve Apostles. See also Boutros, Ferris, Takis.
Panayiotos, Panos, Peadair, Peder, Pedro, Peers, Peeter, Peirce, Pekelo, Per, Perico, Perion, Perkin, Perry, Petar, Pete, Péter, Peterke, Peterus, Petr, Petras, Petros, Petru, Petruno, Petter, Peyo, Piaras, Pierce, Piero, Pierre, Pieter, Pietrek, Pietro, Piotr, Piter, Piti, Pjeter, Pyotr

Peterson (English) son of Peter.
Peteris, Petersen

Petiri (Shona) where we are.
Petri

Petr (Bulgarian) a form of Peter.

Petras (Lithuanian) a form of Peter.
Petra, Petrelis

Petros (Greek) a form of Peter.
Petro

Petru (Romanian) a form of Peter.
Petrukas, Petrus, Petruso

Petter (Norwegian) a form of Peter.

Peverell (French) piper.
Peverall, Peverel, Peveril

Peyo (Spanish) a form of Peter.

Peyton (English) a form of Patton, Payton.
Peyt, Peyten, Peython, Peytonn

Pharaoh (Latin) ruler. History: a title for the ancient kings of Egypt.
Faroh, Pharo, Pharoah, Pharoh

Phelan (Irish) wolf.

Phelipe (Spanish) a form of Philip.

Phelix (Latin) a form of Felix.

Phelps (English) son of Phillip.

Phil (Greek) a short form of Philip, Phillip.
Fil, Phill

Philander (Greek) lover of mankind.

Philbert (English) a form of
Filbert.
Philibert, Phillbert

Philemon (Greek) kiss.
*Phila, Philamina, Phileman,
Philémon, Philmon*

Philip (Greek) lover of horses.
Bible: one of the Twelve
Apostles. See also Felipe,
Felippo, Filip, Fillipp, Filya,
Fischel, Flip.
*Phelps, Phelipe, Phil, Philipp,
Philippe, Philippo, Phillip,
Phillipos, Phillp, Philly, Philp,
Phylip, Piers, Pilib, Pilipo, Pippo*

Philipp (German) a form of
Philip.
Phillipp

Philippe (French) a form of
Philip.
*Philipe, Phillepe, Phillipe,
Phillippe, Phillippee, Phyllipe*

Phillip (Greek) a form of
Philip.
*Phil, Phillipos, Phillipp, Phillips,
Philly, Phyllip*

Phillipos (Greek) a form of
Phillip.

Philly (American) a familiar
form of Philip, Phillip.
Phillie

Philo (Greek) love.

Phinean (Irish) a form of
Finian.
Phinian

Phineas (English) a form of
Pinchas.
Fineas, Phinehas, Phinny

Phirun (Cambodian) rain.

Phoenix (Latin) phoenix, a
legendary bird.
Phenix, Pheonix, Phynix

Phuok (Vietnamese) good.
Phuoc

Pias (Gypsy) fun.

Pickford (English) ford at the
peak.

Pickworth (English) wood
cutter's estate.

Pierce (English) a form of
Peter.
*Pearce, Peerce, Peers, Peirce,
Piercy, Piers*

Piero (Italian) a form of Peter.
Pero, Pierro

Pierre (French) a form of
Peter.
Peirre, Piere, Pierrot

Pierre-Luc (French) a combination of Pierre + Luc.
Piere Luc

Piers (English) a form of
Philip.

Pierson (English) son of Peter.
See also Pearson.
*Pierrson, Piersen, Piersson,
Piersun*

Pieter (Dutch) a form of
Peter.
Pietr

Pietro (Italian) a form of
Peter.

Pilar (Spanish) pillar.

Pili (Swahili) second born.

Pilipo (Hawaiian) a form of
Philip.

Pillan (Native American)
supreme essence.
Pilan

Pin (Vietnamese) faithful boy.

Pinchas (Hebrew) oracle.
(Egyptian) dark skinned.
*Phineas, Pincas, Pinchos, Pincus,
Pinkas, Pinkus, Pinky*

Pinky (American) a familiar
form of Pinchas.
Pink

Pino (Italian) a form of
Joseph.

Piñon (Tupi-Guarani)
Mythology: the hunter who
became the constellation
Orion.

Pio (Latin) pious.

Piotr (Bulgarian) a form of
Peter.
Piotrek

Pippin (German) father.

Piran (Irish) prayer. Religion:
the patron saint of miners.
Peran, Pieran

Pirro (Greek, Spanish) flaming
hair.

Pista (Hungarian) a familiar
form of István.
Pisti

Piti (Spanish) a form of Peter.

Pitin (Spanish) a form of
Felix.
Pito

Pitney (English) island of the
strong-willed man.
Pittney

Pitt (English) pit, ditch.

Placido (Spanish) serene.
*Placide, Placidus, Placyd,
Placydo*

Plato (Greek) broad
shouldered. History: a famous
Greek philosopher.
Platon

Platt (French) flatland.
Platte

Pol (Swedish) a form of Paul.
Pól, Pola, Poul

Poldi (German) a familiar
form of Leopold.
Poldo

Pollard (German) close-
cropped head.
Poll, Pollerd, Pollyrd

Pollock (English) a form of Pollux. Art: American artist Jackson Pollock was a leader of abstract expressionism.
Pollack, Polloch

Pollux (Greek) crown. Astronomy: one of the stars in the constellation Gemini.
Pollock

Polo (Tibetan) brave wanderer. (Greek) a short form of Apollo. Culture: a game played on horseback. History: Marco Polo was a thirteenth-century Venetian explorer who traveled throughout Asia.

Pomeroy (French) apple orchard.
Pommeray, Pommeroy

Ponce (Spanish) fifth. History: Juan Ponce de León of Spain searched for the Fountain of Youth in Florida.

Pony (Scottish) small horse.
Poni

Porfirio (Greek, Spanish) purple stone.
Porphirios, Prophyrios

Porter (Latin) gatekeeper.
Port, Portie, Porty

Poshita (Sanskrit) cherished.

Po Sin (Chinese) grand-father elephant.

Poul (Danish) a form of Paul.
Poulos, Poulus

Pov (Gypsy) earth.

Powa (Native American) wealthy.

Powell (English) alert.
Powel

Pramad (Hindi) rejoicing.

Pravat (Tai) history.

Prem (Hindi) love.

Prentice (English) apprentice.
Prent, Prentis, Prentiss, Printes, Printiss

Prescott (English) priest's cottage. See also Scott.
Prescot, Prestcot, Prestcott

Presley (English) priest's meadow. Music: Elvis Presley was an influential American rock 'n' roll singer.
Presleigh, Presly, Presslee, Pressley, Prestley, Priestley, Priestly

Preston (English) priest's estate.
Prestan, Presten, Prestin, Prestyn

Prewitt (French) brave little one.
Preuet, Prewet, Prewett, Prewit, Pruit, Pruitt

Price (Welsh) son of the ardent one.
Brice, Bryce, Pryce

Pricha (Tai) clever.

Primo (Italian) first; premier quality.
Preemo, Premo

Prince (Latin) chief; prince.
Prence, Prinz, Prinze

Princeton (English) princely town.
Prenston, Princeston, Princton

Proctor (Latin) official, administrator.
Prockter, Procter

Prokopios (Greek) declared leader.

Prosper (Latin) fortunate.
Prospero, Próspero

Pryor (Latin) head of the monastery; prior.
Prior, Pry

Pumeet (Sanskrit) pure.

Purdy (Hindi) recluse.

Purvis (French, English) providing food.
Pervis, Purves, Purviss

Putnam (English) dweller by the pond.
Putnem

Pyotr (Russian) a form of Peter.
Petenka, Petinka, Petrusha, Petya, Pyatr

Q

Qabil (Arabic) able.

Qadim (Arabic) ancient.

Qadir (Arabic) powerful.
Qaadir, Qadeer, Quaadir, Quadeer, Quadir

Qamar (Arabic) moon.
Quamar, Quamir

Qasim (Arabic) divider.
Quasim

Qimat (Hindi) valuable.

Quaashie (Ewe) born on Sunday.

Quadarius (American) a combination of Quan + Darius.
Quadara, Quadarious, Quadaris, Quandarious, Quandarius, Quandarrius, Qudarius, Qudaruis

Quade (Latin) fourth.
Quadell, Quaden, Quadon, Quadre, Quadrie, Quadrine, Quadrion, Quaid, Quayd, Quayde, Qwade

Quamaine (American) a combination of Quan + Jermaine.
Quamain, Quaman, Quamane, Quamayne, Quarmaine

Quan (Comanche) a short form of Quanah.

Quanah (Comanche) fragrant.
Quan

Quandre (American) a combination of Quan + Andre.
Quandrae, Quandré

Quant (Greek) how much?
Quanta, Quantae, Quantai, Quantas, Quantay, Quante, Quantea, Quantey, Quantez, Quantu

Quantavius (American) a combination of Quan + Octavius.
Quantavian, Quantavin, Quantavion, Quantavious, Quantavis, Quantavous, Quatavious, Quatavius

Quashawn (American) a combination of Quan + Shawn.
Quasean, Quashaan, Quashan, Quashaun, Quashaunn, Quashon, Quashone, Quashun, Queshan, Queshon, Qweshawn, Qyshawn

Qudamah (Arabic) courage.

Quenby (Scandinavian) a form of Quimby.

Quennell (French) small oak.
Quenell, Quennel

Quenten (Latin) a form of Quentin.
Quienten

Quentin (Latin) fifth. (English) queen's town.
Qeuntin, Quantin, Quent, Quentan, Quenten, Quentine, Quenton, Quentyn, Quentynn, Quientin, Quinten, Quintin, Quinton, Qwentin

Quenton (Latin) a form of Quentin.
Quienton

Quico (Spanish) a familiar form of many names.
Paco

Quigley (Irish) maternal side.
Quigly

Quillan (Irish) cub.
Quill, Quillen, Quillin, Quillon

Quimby (Scandinavian) woman's estate.
Quenby, Quinby

Quincy (French) fifth son's estate.
Quenci, Quency, Quince, Quincee, Quincey, Quinci, Quinn, Quinncy, Quinnsy, Quinsey, Quinzy

Quindarius (American) a combination of Quinn + Darius.
Quindarious, Quindarrius, Quinderious, Quinderus, Quindrius

Quinlan (Irish) strong; well shaped.
Quindlen, Quinlen, Quinlin, Quinn, Quinnlan, Quinnlin

Quinn (Irish) a short form of Quincy, Quinlan, Quinton.
Quin

Quintavius (American) a combination of Quinn + Octavius.
Quintavious, Quintavis, Quintavus, Quintayvious

Quinten (Latin) a form of Quentin.
Quinnten

Quintin (Latin) a form of Quentin.
Quinntin, Quintine, Quintyn

Quinton (Latin) a form of Quentin.
Quinn, Quinneton, Quinnton, Quint, Quintan, Quintann, Quintin, Quintion, Quintus, Quitin, Quito, Quiton, Qunton, Qwinton

Quiqui (Spanish) a familiar form of Enrique.
Quinto, Quiquin

Quitin (Latin) a short form of Quinton.
Quiten, Quito, Quiton

Quito (Spanish) a short form of Quinton.

Quon (Chinese) bright.

R

Raanan (Hebrew) fresh; luxuriant.

Rabi (Arabic) breeze.
Rabbi, Rabee, Rabeeh, Rabiah, Rabie, Rabih

Race (English) race.
Racel, Rayce

Racham (Hebrew) compassionate.
Rachaman, Rachamim, Rachim, Rachman, Rachmiel, Rachum, Raham, Rahamim

Rad (English) advisor. (Slavic) happy.
Raad, Radd, Raddie, Raddy, Rade, Radee, Radell, Radey, Radi

Radbert (English) brilliant advisor.

Radburn (English) red brook; brook with reeds.
Radborn, Radborne, Radbourn, Radbourne, Radburne

Radcliff (English) red cliff; cliff with reeds.
Radcliffe, Radclyffe

Radford (English) red ford; ford with reeds.

Radley (English) red meadow;
meadow of reeds.
*Radlea, Radlee, Radleigh,
Radly*

Radman (Slavic) joyful.
Radmen, Radusha

Radnor (English) red shore;
shore with reeds.

Radomil (Slavic) happy peace.

Radoslaw (Polish) happy
glory.
Radik, Rado, Radzmir, Slawek

Raekwon (American) a form
of Raquan.
*Raekwan, Raikwan, Rakwane,
Rakwon*

Raequan (American) a form
of Raquan.
*Raequon, Raeqwon, Raiquan,
Raiquen, Raiqoun*

Raeshawn (American) a form
of Rashawn.
*Raesean, Raeshaun, Raeshon,
Raeshun*

Rafael (Spanish) a form of
Raphael. See also Falito.
*Rafaelle, Rafaello, Rafaelo,
Rafal, Rafeal, Rafeé, Rafel,
Rafello, Raffael, Raffaelo,
Raffeal, Raffel, Raffiel, Rafiel*

Rafaele (Italian) a form of
Raphael.
Raffaele

Rafal (Polish) a form of
Raphael.

Rafe (English) a short form of
Rafferty, Ralph.
Raff

Rafer (Irish) a short form of
Rafferty.
Raffer

Rafferty (Irish) rich, prosper-
ous.
*Rafe, Rafer, Raferty, Raffarty,
Raffer*

Rafi (Arabic) exalted.
(Hebrew) a familiar form of
Raphael.
Raffe, Raffee, Raffi, Raffy, Rafi

Rafiq (Arabic) friend.
Raafiq, Rafeeq, Rafic, Rafique

Raghib (Arabic) desirous.
Raquib

Raghnall (Irish) wise power.

Ragnar (Norwegian) powerful
army.
*Ragnor, Rainer, Rainier,
Ranieri, Rayner, Raynor,
Reinhold*

Rago (Hausa) ram.

Raheem (Punjabi) compassionate God.
Rakeem

Rahim (Arabic) merciful.
*Raaheim, Rahaeim, Raheam,
Raheim, Rahiem, Rahiim,
Rahime, Rahium, Rakim*

Rahman (Arabic) compassionate.
Rahmatt, Rahmet

Rahul (Arabic) traveler.

Raíd (Arabic) leader.

Raiden (Japanese) Mythology:
the thunder god.
Raidan, Rayden

Raimondo (Italian) a form of
Raymond.
Raymondo, Reimundo

Raimund (German) a form of
Raymond.
Rajmund

Raimundo (Portuguese,
Spanish) a form of
Raymond.
*Mundo, Raimon, Raimond,
Raimonds, Raymundo*

Raine (English) lord; wise.
Rain, Raines, Rayne

Rainer (German) counselor.
*Rainar, Rainey, Rainier, Rainor,
Raynier, Reinier*

Rainey (German) a familiar
form of Rainer.
*Raine, Rainee, Rainie, Rainney,
Rainy, Reiny*

Raini (Tupi-Guaraní)
Religion: the god who created the world.

Raishawn (American) a form
of Rashawn.
Raishon, Raishun

Rajabu (Swahili) born in the
seventh month of the Islamic
calendar.

Rajah (Hindi) prince; chief.
*Raj, Raja, Rajaah, Rajae,
Rajahe, Rajan, Raje, Rajeh,
Raji*

Rajak (Hindi) cleansing.

Rajan (Hindi) a form of
Rajah.
Rajaahn, Rajain, Rajen, Rajin

Rakeem (Punjabi) a form of
Raheem.
Rakeeme, Rakeim, Rakem

Rakim (Arabic) a form of
Rahim.
Rakiim

Rakin (Arabic) respectable.
Rakeen

Raktim (Hindi) bright red.

Raleigh (English) a form of
Rawleigh.
Ralegh

Ralph (English) wolf coun-
selor.
*Radolphus, Rafe, Ralf,
Ralpheal, Ralphel, Ralphie,
Ralston, Raoul, Raul, Rolf*

Ralphie (English) a familiar
form of Ralph.
Ralphy

Ralston (English) Ralph's settlement.

Ram (Hindi) god; godlike. Religion: another name for the Hindu god Rama. (English) male sheep. A short form of Ramsey.
Rami, Ramie, Ramy

Ramadan (Arabic) ninth month of the Arabic year in the Islamic calendar.
Rama

Ramanan (Hindi) god; god-like.
Raman, Ramandeep, Ramanjit, Ramanjot

Rami (Hindi, English) a form of Ram. (Spanish) a short form of Ramiro.
Rame, Ramee, Ramey, Ramih

Ramiro (Portuguese, Spanish) supreme judge.
Ramario, Rameer, Rameir, Ramere, Rameriz, Ramero, Rami, Ramires, Ramirez, Ramos

Ramón (Spanish) a form of Raymond.
Ramon, Remon, Remone, Romone

Ramone (Dutch) a form of Raymond.
Raemon, Raemonn, Ramond, Ramonte, Remone

Ramsden (English) valley of rams.

Ramsey (English) ram's island.
Ram, Ramsay, Ramsee, Ramsie, Ramsy, Ramzee, Ramzey, Ramzi, Ramzy

Rance (English) a short form of Laurence. (American) a familiar form of Laurence.
Rancel, Rancell, Rances, Rancey, Rancie, Rancy, Ransel, Ransell

Rand (English) shield; warrior.
Randy

Randal (English) a form of Randall.
Randahl, Randale, Randel, Randl, Randle

Randall (English) a form of Randolph.
Randal, Randell, Randy, Randyll

Randolph (English) shield wolf.
Randall, Randol, Randolf, Randolfo, Randolpho, Randy, Ranolph

Randy (English) a familiar form of Rand, Randall, Randolph.
Randdy, Randee, Randey, Randi, Randie, Ranndy

Ranger (French) forest keeper.
Rainger, Range

Rangle (American) cowboy.
Rangler, Wrangle

Rangsey (Cambodian) seven kinds of colors.

Rani (Hebrew) my song; my joy.
Ranen, Ranie, Ranon, Roni

Ranieri (Italian) a form of Ragnar.
Raneir, Ranier, Rannier

Ranjan (Hindi) delighted; gladdened.

Rankin (English) small shield.
Randkin

Ransford (English) raven's ford.

Ransley (English) raven's field.

Ransom (Latin) redeemer. (English) son of the shield.
Rance, Ransome, Ranson

Raoul (French) a form of Ralph, Rudolph.
Raol, Raul, Raúl, Reuel

Raphael (Hebrew) God has healed. Bible: one of the archangels. Art: a prominent painter of the Renaissance. See also Falito, Rafi.
Rafael, Rafaele, Rafal, Rafel, Raphaél, Raphale, Raphaello, Rapheal, Raphel, Raphello, Raphiel, Ray, Rephael

Rapheal (Hebrew) a form of Raphael.
Rafel, Raphiel

Rapier (French) blade-sharp.

Raquan (American) a combination of the prefix Ra + Quan.
Raaquan, Rackwon, Racquan, Raekwon, Raequan, Rahquan, Raquané, Raquon, Raquwan, Raquwn, Raquwon, Raqwan, Raqwann

Rashaad (Arabic) a form of Rashad.

Rashaan (American) a form of Rashawn.
Rasaan, Rashan, Rashann

Rashad (Arabic) wise counselor.
Raashad, Rachad, Rachard, Raeshad, Raishard, Rashaad, Rashadd, Rashade, Rashaud, Rasheed, Rashid, Rashod, Reshad, Rhashad, Rishad, Roshad

Rashard (American) a form of Richard.
Rasharrd

Rashaud (Arabic) a form of Rashad.
Rachaud, Rashaude

Rashaun (American) a form of Rashawn.

Rashawn (American) a combination of the prefix Ra + Shawn.
Raashawn, Raashen, Raeshawn, Rahshawn, Raishawn, Rasaun, Rasawn, Rashaan, Rashaun, Rashaw,

Rashon, Rashun, Raushan,
Raushawn, Rhashan,
Rhashaun, Rhashawn

Rashean (American) a combi-
nation of the prefix Ra +
Sean.
Rahsaan, Rahsean, Rahseen,
Rasean, Rashane, Rasheen,
Rashien, Rashiena

Rasheed (Arabic) a form of
Rashad.
Rashead, Rashed, Rasheid,
Rhasheed

Rashid (Arabic) a form of
Rashad.
Rasheyd, Rashida, Rashidah,
Rashied, Rashieda, Raushaid

Rashida (Swahili) righteous.

Rashidi (Swahili) wise counselor.

Rashod (Arabic) a form of
Rashad.
Rashoda, Rashodd, Rashoud,
Rayshod, Rhashod

Rashon (American) a form of
Rashawn.
Rashion, Rashone, Rashonn,
Rashuan, Rashun, Rashunn

Rasmus (Greek, Danish) a
short form of Erasmus.

Raul (French) a form of
Ralph.

Raulas (Lithuanian) a form of
Laurence.

Raulo (Lithuanian) a form of
Laurence.
Raulas

Raven (English) a short form
of Ravenel.
Ravan, Ravean, Raveen, Ravin,
Ravine, Ravon, Ravyn, Reven,
Rhaven

Ravenel (English) raven.
Raven, Ravenell, Revenel

Ravi (Hindi) sun.
Ravee, Ravijot

Ravid (Hebrew) a form of
Arvid.

Raviv (Hebrew) rain, dew.

Ravon (English) a form of
Raven.
Raveon, Ravion, Ravone,
Ravonn, Ravonne, Rayvon,
Revon

Rawdon (English) rough hill.

Rawleigh (English) deer
meadow.
Raleigh, Rawle, Rawley,
Rawling, Rawly, Rawylyn

Rawlins (French) a form of
Roland.
Rawlings, Rawlinson, Rawson

Ray (French) kingly, royal.
(English) a short form of
Rayburn, Raymond. See also
Lei.
Rae, Raye

Rayan (Irish) a form of Ryan.
Rayaun

Rayburn (English) deer brook.
*Burney, Raeborn, Raeborne,
Raebourn, Ray, Raybourn,
Raybourne, Rayburne*

Rayce (English) a form of
Race.

Rayden (Japanese) a form of
Raiden.
Raidin, Raydun, Rayedon

Rayhan (Arabic) favored by
God.
Rayhaan

Rayi (Hebrew) my friend, my
companion.

Raymon (English) a form of
Raymond.
*Rayman, Raymann, Raymen,
Raymone, Raymun, Reamonn*

Raymond (English) mighty;
wise protector. See also
Aymon.
*Radmond, Raemond,
Raimondo, Raimund,
Raimundo, Ramón, Ramond,
Ramonde, Ramone, Ray,
Raymand, Rayment, Raymon,
Raymont, Raymund,
Raymunde, Raymundo,
Redmond, Reymond,
Reymundo*

Raymundo (Spanish) a form
of Raymond.
*Raemondo, Raimondo,
Raimundo, Raymondo*

Raynaldo (Spanish) a form of
Reynold.
Raynal, Raynald, Raynold

Raynard (French) a form of
Renard, Reynard.
Raynarde

Rayne (English) a form of
Raine.
Raynee, Rayno

Raynor (Scandinavian) a form
of Ragnar.
*Rainer, Rainor, Ranier, Ranieri,
Raynar, Rayner*

Rayshawn (American) a com-
bination of Ray + Shawn.
*Raysean, Rayshaan, Rayshan,
Rayshaun, Raysheen, Rayshon,
Rayshone, Rayshonn, Rayshun,
Rayshunn*

Rayshod (American) a form
of Rashad.
*Raychard, Rayshad, Rayshard,
Rayshaud*

Rayvon (American) a form of
Ravon.
*Rayvan, Rayvaun, Rayven,
Rayvone, Reyven, Reyvon*

Razi (Aramaic) my secret.
Raz, Raziel, Raziq

Read (English) a form of
Reed, Reid.
*Raed, Raede, Raeed, Reaad,
Reade*

Reading (English) son of the red wanderer.
Redding, Reeding, Reiding

Reagan (Irish) little king. History: Ronald Wilson Reagan was the fortieth U.S. president.
Raegan, Reagen, Reaghan, Reegan, Reegen, Regan, Reigan, Reighan, Reign, Rheagan

Rebel (American) rebel.
Reb

Red (American) red, redhead.
Redd

Reda (Arabic) satisfied.
Ridha

Redford (English) red river crossing.
Ford, Radford, Reaford, Red, Redd

Redley (English) red meadow; meadow with reeds.
Radley, Redlea, Redleigh, Redly

Redmond (German) protecting counselor. (English) a form of Raymond.
Radmond, Radmund, Reddin, Redmund

Redpath (English) red path.

Reece (Welsh) enthusiastic; stream.
Reace, Rece, Reese, Reice, Reyes, Rhys, Rice, Ryese

Reed (English) a form of Reid.
Raeed, Read, Reyde, Rheed

Reese (Welsh) a form of Reece.
Rease, Rees, Reis, Reise, Reiss, Rhys, Riese, Riess

Reeve (English) steward.
Reave, Reaves, Reeves

Reg (English) a short form of Reginald.

Regan (Irish) a form of Reagan.
Regen

Reggie (English) a familiar form of Reginald.
Regi, Regie

Reginal (English) a form of Reginald.
Reginale, Reginel

Reginald (English) king's advisor. A form of Reynold. See also Naldo.
Reg, Reggie, Regginald, Reggis, Reginal, Reginaldo, Reginalt, Reginauld, Reginault, Reginold, Reginuld, Regnauld, Ronald

Regis (Latin) regal.

Rehema (Swahili) second-born.

Rei (Japanese) rule, law.

Reid (English) redhead.
Read, Reed, Reide, Reyd, Ried

Reidar (Norwegian) nest warrior.

Reilly (Irish) a form of Riley.
Reiley, Reilley, Reily, Rielly

Reinaldo (Spanish) a form of Reynold.

Reinhart (German) a form of Reynard.
Rainart, Rainhard, Rainhardt, Rainhart, Reinart, Reinhard, Reinhardt, Renke

Reinhold (Swedish) a form of Ragnar.
Reinold

Reku (Finnish) a form of Richard.

Remi, Rémi (French) forms of Remy.
Remie, Remmie

Remington (English) raven estate.
Rem, Reminton, Tony

Remus (Latin) speedy, quick. Mythology: Remus and his twin brother, Romulus, founded Rome.

Remy (French) from Rheims, France.
Ramey, Remee, Remi, Rémi, Remmy

Renaldo (Spanish) a form of Reynold.
Raynaldo, Reynaldo, Rinaldo

Renard (French) a form of Reynard.
Ranard, Raynard, Reinard, Rennard

Renardo (Italian) a form of Reynard.

Renato (Italian) reborn.

Renaud (French) a form of Reynard, Reynold.
Renauld, Renauldo, Renault, Renould

Rendor (Hungarian) policeman.

René (French) reborn.
Renat, Renato, Renatus, Renault, Renay, Renee, Renny

Renfred (English) lasting peace.

Renfrew (Welsh) raven woods.

Renjiro (Japanese) virtuous.

Renny (Irish) small but strong. (French) a familiar form of René.
Ren, Renn, Renne, Rennie

Reno (American) gambler. Geography: a city in Nevada known for gambling.
Renos, Rino

Renshaw (English) raven woods.
Renishaw

Renton (English) settlement of the roe deer.

Renzo (Latin) a familiar form
of Laurence. (Italian) a short
form of Lorenzo.
Renz, Renzy, Renzzo

Reshad (American) a form of
Rashad.
*Reshade, Reshard, Resharrd,
Reshaud, Reshawd, Reshead,
Reshod*

Reshawn (American) a com-
bination of the prefix Re +
Shawn.
*Reshaun, Reshaw, Reshon,
Reshun*

Reshean (American) a combi-
nation of the prefix Re +
Sean.
*Resean, Reshae, Reshane,
Reshay, Reshayne, Reshea,
Resheen, Reshey*

Reuben (Hebrew) behold a
son.
*Reuban, Reubin, Reuven,
Rheuben, Rhuben, Rube,
Ruben, Rubey, Rubin, Ruby,
Rueben*

Reuven (Hebrew) a form of
Reuben.
Reuvin, Rouvin, Ruvim

Rex (Latin) king.
Rexx

Rexford (English) king's ford.

Rexton (English) king's town.

Rey (Spanish) a short form of
Reynaldo, Reynard,
Reynold.

Reyes (English) a form of
Reece.
Reyce

Reyhan (Arabic) favored by
God.
Reyham

Reymond (English) a form of
Raymond.
Reymon. Reymound, Reymund

Reymundo (Spanish) a form
of Raymond.
*Reimond, Reimonde, Reimundo,
Reymon*

Reynaldo (Spanish) a form of
Reynold.
Renaldo, Rey, Reynauldo

Reynard (French) wise; bold,
courageous.
*Raynard, Reinhard, Reinhardt,
Reinhart, Renard, Renardo,
Renaud, Rennard, Rey,
Reynardo, Reynaud*

Reynold (English) king's advi-
sor. See also Reginald.
*Rainault, Rainhold, Ranald,
Raynald, Raynaldo, Reinald,
Reinaldo, Reinaldos, Reinhart,
Reinhold, Reinold, Reinwald,
Renald, Renaldi, Renaldo,
Renaud, Renauld, Rennold,
Renold, Rey, Reynald,
Reynaldo, Reynaldos, Reynol,
Reynolds, Rinaldo, Ronald*

Réz (Hungarian) copper; red-head.
Rezsö

Rhett (Welsh) a form of Rhys. Literature: Rhett Butler was the hero of Margaret Mitchell's novel *Gone with the Wind*.
Rhet

Rhodes (Greek) where roses grow. Geography: an island of southeast Greece.
Rhoads, Rhodas, Rodas

Rhyan (Irish) a form of Rian.
Rhian

Rhys (Welsh) a form of Reece, Reese.
Rhett, Rhyce, Rhyse, Rice

Rian (Irish) little king.
Rhyan

Ric (Italian, Spanish) a short form of Rico.
Ricca, Ricci, Ricco

Ricardo (Portuguese, Spanish) a form of Richard.
Racardo, Recard, Ricaldo, Ricard, Ricardoe, Ricardos, Riccardo, Riccarrdo, Ricciardo, Richardo

Rice (English) rich, noble. (Welsh) a form of Reece.
Ryce

Rich (English) a short form of Richard.
Ritch

Richard (English) a form of Richart. See also Aric, Dick, Juku, Likeke.
Rashard, Reku, Ricardo, Rich, Richar, Richards, Richardson, Richart, Richaud, Richer, Richerd, Richie, Richird, Richshard, Rick, Rickard, Rickert, Rickey, Ricky, Rico, Rihardos, Rihards, Rikard, Riocard, Riócard, Risa, Risardas, Rishard, Ristéard, Ritchard, Rostik, Rye, Rysio, Ryszard

Richart (German) rich and powerful ruler.

Richie (English) a familiar form of Richard.
Richey, Richi, Richy, Rishi, Ritchie

Richman (English) powerful.

Richmond (German) powerful protector.
Richmon, Richmound

Rick (German, English) a short form of Cedric, Frederick, Richard.
Ric, Ricke, Rickey, Ricks, Ricky, Rik, Riki, Rykk

Rickard (Swedish) a form of Richard.

Ricker (English) powerful army.

Rickey (English) a familiar form of Richard, Rick, Riqui.

Rickie (English) a form of
Ricky.
Rickee, Ricki

Rickward (English) mighty
guardian.
Rickwerd, Rickwood

Ricky (English) a familiar form
of Richard, Rick.
*Ricci, Rickie, Riczi, Riki,
Rikki, Rikky, Riqui*

Rico (Spanish) a familiar form
of Richard. (Italian) a short
form of Enrico.
Ric, Ricco

Rida (Arabic) favor.

Riddock (Irish) smooth field.
Riddick

Rider (English) horseman.
Ridder, Ryder

Ridge (English) ridge of a
cliff.
Ridgy, Rig, Rigg

Ridgeley (English) meadow
near the ridge.
*Ridgeleigh, Ridglea, Ridglee,
Ridgleigh, Ridgley*

Ridgeway (English) path along
the ridge.

Ridley (English) meadow of
reeds.
*Rhidley, Riddley, Ridlea,
Ridleigh, Ridly*

Riel (Spanish) a short form of
Gabriel.

Rigby (English) ruler's valley.

Rigel (Arabic) foot.
Astronomy: one of the stars
in the constellation Orion.

Rigg (English) ridge.
Rigo

Rigoberto (German) splendid;
wealthy.
Rigobert

Rikard (Scandinavian) a form
of Richard.
Rikárd

Riki (Estonian) a form of
Rick.
Rikkey, Rikki, Riks, Riky

Riley (Irish) valiant.
*Reilly, Rhiley, Rhylee, Rhyley,
Rieley, Rielly, Riely, Rilee,
Rilley, Rily, Rilye, Rylee, Ryley*

Rinaldo (Italian) a form of
Reynold.
Rinald, Rinaldi

Ring (English) ring.
Ringo

Ringo (Japanese) apple.
(English) a familiar form of
Ring.

Rio (Spanish) river.
Geography: Rio de Janeiro is
a city in Brazil.

Riordan (Irish) bard, royal
poet.
Rearden, Reardin, Reardon

Rip (Dutch) ripe; full grown. (English) a short form of Ripley.
Ripp

Ripley (English) meadow near the river.
Rip, Ripleigh, Ripply

Riqui (Spanish) a form of Rickey.

Rishad (American) a form of Rashad.
Rishaad

Rishawn (American) a combination of the prefix Ri + Shawn.
Rishan, Rishaun, Rishon, Rishone

Rishi (Hindi) sage.

Risley (English) meadow with shrubs.
Rislea, Rislee, Risleigh, Risly, Wrisley

Risto (Finnish) a short form of Christopher.

Riston (English) settlement near the shrubs.
Wriston

Ritchard (English) a form of Richard.
Ritcherd, Ritchyrd, Ritshard, Ritsherd

Ritchie (English) a form of Richie.
Ritchy

Rithisak (Cambodian) powerful.

Ritter (German) knight; chivalrous.
Rittner

River (English) river; riverbank.
Rivers, Riviera, Rivor

Riyad (Arabic) gardens.
Riad, Riyaad, Riyadh, Riyaz, Riyod

Roald (Norwegian) famous ruler.

Roan (English) a short form of Rowan.
Rhoan

Roar (Norwegian) praised warrior.
Roary

Roarke (Irish) famous ruler.
Roark, Rorke, Rourke, Ruark

Rob (English) a short form of Robert.
Robb, Robe

Robbie (English) a familiar form of Robert.
Robie, Robbi

Robby (English) a familiar form of Robert.
Rhobbie, Robbey, Robhy, Roby

Robert (English) famous brilliance. See also Bobek, Dob, Lopaka.
Bob, Bobby, Rab, Rabbie, Raby,

Riobard, Riobart, Rob, Robars,
Robart, Robbie, Robby, Rober,
Roberd, Robers, Roberte,
Roberto, Roberts, Robin,
Robinson, Roibeárd, Rosertas,
Rubert, Ruberto, Rudbert,
Rupert

Roberto (Italian, Portuguese, Spanish) a form of Robert.

Roberts, Robertson (English) son of Robert.
Roberson, Robertson, Robeson,
Robinson, Robson

Robin (English) a short form of Robert.
Robben, Robbin, Robbins,
Robbyn, Roben, Robinet,
Robinn, Robins, Robyn, Roibín

Robinson (English) a form of Roberts.
Robbinson, Robens, Robenson,
Robson, Robynson

Robyn (English) a form of Robin.

Rocco (Italian) rock.
Rocca, Rocio, Rocko, Rocky,
Roko, Roque

Rochester (English) rocky fortress.
Chester, Chet

Rock (English) a short form of Rockwell.
Roch, Rocky

Rockford (English) rocky ford.

Rockland (English) rocky land.

Rockledge (English) rocky ledge.

Rockley (English) rocky field.
Rockle

Rockwell (English) rocky spring. Art: Norman Rockwell was a well-known twentieth-century American illustrator.
Rock

Rocky (American) a familiar form of Rocco, Rock.
Rockey, Rockie

Rod (English) a short form of Penrod, Roderick, Rodney.
Rodd

Rodas (Greek, Spanish) a form of Rhodes.

Roddy (English) a familiar form of Roderick.
Roddie, Rody

Roden (English) red valley. Art: Auguste Rodin was an innovative French sculptor.
Rodin

Roderich (German) a form of Roderick.

Roderick (German) famous ruler. See also Broderick.
Rhoderick, Rod, Rodderick,
Roddy, Roderic, Roderich,
Roderigo, Roderik, Roderrick,
Roderyck, Rodgrick, Rodrick,
Rodricki, Rodrigo, Rodrigue,

Roderick *(cont.)*
Rodrugue, Roodney, Rory,
Rurik, Ruy

Rodger (German) a form of
Roger.
Rodge, Rodgy

Rodman (German) famous
man, hero.
Rodmond

Rodney (English) island clear-
ing.
Rhodney, Rod, Rodnee, Rodnei,
Rodni, Rodnie, Rodnne, Rodny

Rodolfo (Spanish) a form of
Rudolph.
Rodolpho, Rodulfo

Rodrick (German) a form of
Roderick.
Roddrick, Rodric, Rodrich,
Rodrik, Rodrique, Rodryck,
Rodryk

Rodrigo (Italian, Spanish) a
form of Roderick.

Rodriguez (Spanish) son of
Rodrigo.
Roddrigues, Rodrigues,
Rodriquez

Rodrik (German) famous
ruler.

Rodriquez (Spanish) a form of
Rodriguez.
Rodrigquez, Rodriques,
Rodriquiez

Roe (English) roe deer.
Row, Rowe

Rogan (Irish) redhead.
Rogein, Rogen

Rogelio (Spanish) famous
warrior.
Rojelio

Roger (German) famous spear-
man. See also Lokela.
Rodger, Rog, Rogelio, Rogerick,
Rogerio, Rogers, Rogiero, Rojelio,
Rüdiger, Ruggerio, Rutger

Rogerio (Portuguese, Spanish)
a form of Roger.
Rogerios

Rohan (Hindi) sandalwood.

Rohin (Hindi) upward path.

Rohit (Hindi) big and beautiful fish.

Roi (French) a form of Roy.

Roja (Spanish) red.
Rojay

Roland (German) famous
throughout the land.
Loránd, Orlando, Rawlins, Rolan,
Rolanda, Rolando, Rolek,
Rolland, Rolle, Rollie, Rollin,
Rollo, Rowe, Rowland, Ruland

Rolando (Portuguese, Spanish)
a form of Roland.
Lando, Olo, Roldan, Roldán,
Rolondo

Rolf (German) a form of
Ralph. A short form of
Rudolph.
Rolfe, Rolle, Rolph, Rolphe

Rolle (Swedish) a familiar form of Roland, Rolf.

Rollie (English) a familiar form of Roland.
Roley, Rolle, Rolli, Rolly

Rollin (English) a form of Roland.
Rolin, Rollins

Rollo (English) a familiar form of Roland.
Rolla, Rolo

Rolon (Spanish) famous wolf.

Romain (French) a form of Roman.
Romaine, Romane, Romanne

Roman (Latin) from Rome, Italy.
Roma, Romain, Romann, Romanos, Romman, Romochka, Romy

Romanos (Greek) a form of Roman.
Romano

Romario (Italian) a form of Romeo.
Romar, Romarius, Romaro, Romarrio

Romel (Latin) a short form of Romulus.
Romele, Romell, Romello, Rommel

Romello (Italian) of Romel.
Romelo, Rommello

Romeo (Italian) pilgrim to Rome; Roman. Literature: the title character of the Shakespearean play *Romeo and Juliet.*
Romario, Roméo, Romero

Romero (Latin) a form of Romeo.
Romario, Romeiro, Romer, Romere, Romerio, Romeris, Romeryo

Romney (Welsh) winding river.
Romoney

Romulus (Latin) citizen of Rome. Mythology: Romulus and his twin brother, Remus, founded Rome.
Romel, Romolo, Romono, Romulo

Romy (Italian) a familiar form of Roman.
Rommie, Rommy

Ron (Hebrew) a short form of Aaron, Ronald.
Ronn

Ronald (Scottish) a form of Reginald.
Ranald, Ron, Ronal, Ronaldo, Ronnald, Ronney, Ronnie, Ronnold, Ronoldo

Ronaldo (Portuguese) a form of Ronald.

Rónán (Irish) seal.
Renan, Ronan, Ronat

Rondel (French) short poem.
*Rondal, Rondale, Rondall,
Rondeal, Rondell, Rondey,
Rondie, Rondrell, Rondy, Ronel*

Ronel (American) a form of
Rondel.
*Ronell, Ronelle, Ronnel,
Ronnell, Ronyell*

Roni (Hebrew) my song; my
joy.
*Rani, Roneet, Roney, Ronit,
Ronli, Rony*

Ronnie (Scottish) a familiar
form of Ronald.
Roni, Ronie, Ronnie, Ronny

Ronny (Scottish) a form of
Ronnie.
Ronney

Ronson (Scottish) son of
Ronald.
Ronaldson

Ronté (American) a combination of Ron + the suffix Te.
Rontae, Rontay, Ronte, Rontez

Rooney (Irish) redhead.

Roosevelt (Dutch) rose field.
History: Theodore and
Franklin D. Roosevelt were
the twenty-sixth and thirty-
second U.S. presidents,
respectively.
Roosvelt, Rosevelt

Roper (English) rope maker.

Rory (German) a familiar
form of Roderick. (Irish) red
king.
Rorey, Rori, Rorrie, Rorry

Rosalio (Spanish) rose.
Rosalino

Rosario (Portuguese) rosary.

Roscoe (Scandinavian) deer
forest.
Rosco

Roshad (American) a form of
Rashad.
Roshard

Roshean (American) a combi-
nation of the prefix Ro +
Sean.
*Roshain, Roshan, Roshane,
Roshaun, Roshawn, Roshay,
Rosheen, Roshene*

Rosito (Filipino) rose.

Ross (Latin) rose. (Scottish)
peninsula. (French) red.
*Rosse, Rossell, Rossi, Rossie,
Rossy*

Rosswell (English) springtime
of roses.
Rosvel

Rostislav (Czech) growing
glory.
Rosta, Rostya

Roswald (English) field of
roses.
Ross, Roswell

Roth (German) redhead.

Rothwell (Scandinavian) red spring.

Rover (English) traveler.

Rowan (English) tree with red berries.
Roan, Rowe, Rowen, Rowney, Rowyn

Rowell (English) roe-deer well.

Rowland (English) rough land. (German) a form of Roland.
Rowlando, Rowlands, Rowlandson

Rowley (English) rough meadow.
Rowlea, Rowlee, Rowleigh, Rowly

Rowson (English) son of the redhead.

Roxbury (English) rook's town or fortress.
Roxburghe

Roy (French) king. A short form of Royal, Royce. See also Conroy, Delroy, Fitzroy, Leroy, Loe.
Rey, Roi, Roye, Ruy

Royal (French) kingly, royal.
Roy, Royale, Royall, Royell

Royce (English) son of Roy.
Roice, Roy, Royz

Royden (English) rye hill.
Royd, Roydan

Ruben (Hebrew) a form of Reuben.
Ruban, Rube, Rubean, Rubens, Rubin, Ruby

Rubert (Czech) a form of Robert.

Ruby (Hebrew) a familiar form of Reuben, Ruben.

Rudd (English) a short form of Rudyard.

Ruda (Czech) a form of Rudolph.
Rude, Rudek

Rudi (Spanish) a familiar form of Rudolph.
Ruedi

Rudo (Shona) love.

Rudolf (German) a form of Rudolph.
Rodolf, Rodolfo, Rudolfo

Rudolph (German) famous wolf. See also Dolf.
Raoul, Rezsó, Rodolfo, Rodolph, Rodolphe, Rolf, Ruda, Rudek, Rudi, Rudolf, Rudolpho, Rudolphus, Rudy

Rudolpho (Italian) a form of Rudolph.

Rudy (English) a familiar form of Rudolph.
Roody, Ruddy, Ruddie, Rudey, Rudi, Rudie

Rudyard (English) red enclosure.
Rudd

Rueben (Hebrew) a form of Reuben.
Rueban, Ruebin

Ruff (French) redhead.

Rufin (Polish) redhead.
Rufino

Ruford (English) red ford; ford with reeds.
Rufford

Rufus (Latin) redhead.
Rayfus, Rufe, Ruffis, Ruffus, Rufino, Rufo, Rufous

Rugby (English) rook fortress. History: a famous British school after which the sport of Rugby was named.

Ruggerio (Italian) a form of Roger.
Rogero, Ruggero, Ruggiero

Ruhakana (Rukiga) argumentative.

Ruland (German) a form of Roland.
Rulan, Rulon, Rulondo

Rumford (English) wide river crossing.

Runako (Shona) handsome.

Rune (German, Swedish) secret.

Runrot (Tai) prosperous.

Rupert (German) a form of Robert.
Ruperth, Ruperto, Ruprecht

Ruperto (Italian) a form of Rupert.

Ruprecht (German) a form of Rupert.

Rush (French) redhead. (English) a short form of Russell.
Rushi

Rushford (English) ford with rushes.

Rusk (Spanish) twisted bread.

Ruskin (French) redhead.
Rush, Russ

Russ (French) a short form of Russell.

Russel (French) a form of Russell.

Russell (French) redhead; fox colored. See also Lukela.
Roussell, Rush, Russ, Russel, Russelle, Rusty

Rusty (French) a familiar form of Russell.
Ruste, Rusten, Rustie, Rustin, Ruston, Rustyn

Rutger (Scandinavian) a form of Roger.
Ruttger

Rutherford (English) cattle ford.
Rutherfurd

Rutland (Scandinavian) red land.

Rutledge (English) red ledge.

Rutley (English) red meadow.

Ruy (Spanish) a short form of Roderick.
Rui

Ryan (Irish) little king.
Rayan, Rhyan, Rhyne, Ryane, Ryann, Ryen, Ryian, Ryiann, Ryin, Ryne, Ryon, Ryuan, Ryun, Ryyan

Rycroft (English) rye field.
Ryecroft

Ryder (English) a form of Rider.
Rydder, Rye

Rye (English) a short form of Ryder. A grain used in cereal and whiskey. (Gypsy) gentleman.
Ry.

Ryen (Irish) a form of Ryan.
Ryein, Ryien

Ryerson (English) son of Rider, Ryder.

Ryese (English) a form of Reece.
Reyse, Ryez, Ryse

Ryker (American) a surname used as a first name.
Riker, Ryk

Rylan (English) land where rye is grown.
Ryland, Rylean, Rylen, Rylin, Rylon, Rylyn, Rylynn

Ryland (English) a form of Rylan.
Ryeland, Rylund

Ryle (English) rye hill.
Ryal, Ryel

Rylee (Irish) a form of Riley.
Ryeleigh, Ryleigh, Rylie, Rillie

Ryley (Irish) a form of Riley.
Ryely

Ryman (English) rye seller.

Ryne (Irish) a form of Ryan.
Rynn

Ryon (Irish) a form of Ryan.

S

Sabastian (Greek) a form of Sebastian.
Sabastain, Sabastiano, Sabastien, Sabastin, Sabastion, Sabaston, Sabbastiun, Sabestian

Saber (French) sword.
Sabir, Sabre

Sabin (Basque) ancient tribe of central Italy.
Saban, Saben, Sabian, Sabien, Sabino

Sabiti (Rutooro) born on Sunday.

Sabola (Nguni) pepper.

Saburo (Japanese) third-born son.

Sacha (Russian) a form of Sasha.
Sascha

Sachar (Russian) a form of Zachary.

Saddam (Arabic) powerful ruler.

Sadiki (Swahili) faithful.
Saadiq, Sadeek, Sadek, Sadik, Sadiq, Sadique

Sadler (English) saddle maker.
Saddler

Safari (Swahili) born while traveling.
Safa, Safarian

Safford (English) willow river crossing.

Sage (English) wise. Botany: an herb.
Sagen, Sager, Saige, Saje

Sahale (Native American) falcon.
Sael, Sahal, Sahel, Sahil

Sahen (Hindi) above.
Sahan

Sahil (Native American) a form of Sahale.
Saheel, Sahel

Sahir (Hindi) friend.

Sa'id (Arabic) happy.
Sa'ad, Saaid, Saed, Sa'eed, Saeed, Sahid, Saide, Sa'ied, Saied, Saiyed, Saiyeed, Sajid, Sajjid, Sayed, Sayeed, Sayid, Seyed, Shahid

Sajag (Hindi) watchful.

Saka (Swahili) hunter.

Sakeri (Danish) a form of Zachary.
Sakarai, Sakari

Sakima (Native American) king.

Sakuruta (Pawnee) coming sun.

Sal (Italian) a short form of Salvatore.

Salam (Arabic) lamb.
Salaam

Salamon (Spanish) a form of Solomon.
Saloman, Salomón

Salaun (French) a form of Solomon.

Sálih (Arabic) right, good.
Saleeh, Saleh, Salehe

Salim (Swahili) peaceful.

Salím (Arabic) peaceful, safe.
Saleem, Salem, Saliym, Salman

Salmalin (Hindi) taloned.

Salman (Czech) a form of
Salím, Solomon.
Salmaan, Salmaine, Salmon

Salomon (French) a form of
Solomon.
Salomone

Salton (English) manor town;
willow town.

Salvador (Spanish) savior.
Salvadore

Salvatore (Italian) savior. See
also Xavier.
*Sal, Salbatore, Sallie, Sally,
Salvator, Salvattore, Salvidor,
Sauveur*

Sam (Hebrew) a short form of
Samuel.
*Samm, Sammy, Sem, Shem,
Shmuel*

Sambo (American) a familiar
form of Samuel.
Sambou

Sameer (Arabic) a form of
Samír.

Sami, Samy (Hebrew) forms
of Sammy.
*Sameeh, Sameh, Samie, Samih,
Sammi*

Samír (Arabic) entertaining
companion.
Sameer

Samman (Arabic) grocer.
Saman, Sammon

Sammy (Hebrew) a familiar
form of Samuel.
*Saamy, Samey, Sami, Sammee,
Sammey, Sammie, Samy*

Samo (Czech) a form of
Samuel.
Samho, Samko

Samson (Hebrew) like the
sun. Bible: a judge and pow-
erful warrior betrayed by
Delilah.
*Sampson, Sansao, Sansom,
Sansón, Shem, Shimshon*

Samual (Hebrew) a form of
Samuel.
Samuael, Samuail

Samuel (Hebrew) heard God;
asked of God. Bible: a
famous Old Testament
prophet and judge. See also
Kamuela, Zamiel, Zanvil.
*Sam, Samael, Samaru,
Samauel, Samaul, Sambo,
Sameul, Samiel, Sammail,
Sammel, Sammuel, Sammy,
Samo, Samouel, Samu, Samual,
Samuele, Samuelis, Samuell,
Samuello, Samuil, Samuka,
Samule, Samuru, Samvel,
Sanko, Saumel, Schmuel, Shem,
Shmuel, Simão, Simuel,
Somhairle, Zamuel*

Samuele (Italian) a form of
Samuel.
Samulle

Samuru (Japanese) a form of
Samuel.

Sanat (Hindi) ancient.

Sanborn (English) sandy brook.
Sanborne, Sanbourn, Sanbourne, Sanburn, Sanburne, Sandborn, Sandbourne

Sanchez (Latin) a form of Sancho.
Sanchaz, Sancheze

Sancho (Latin) sanctified; sincere. Literature: Sancho Panza was Don Quixote's squire.
Sanchez, Sauncho

Sandeep (Punjabi) enlightened.
Sandip

Sander (English) a short form of Alexander, Lysander.
Sandor, Sándor, Saunder

Sanders (English) son of Sander.
Sanderson, Saunders, Saunderson

Sándor (Hungarian) a short form of Alexander.
Sanyi

Sandro (Greek, Italian) a short form of Alexander.
Sandero, Sandor, Sandre, Saundro, Shandro

Sandy (English) a familiar form of Alexander.
Sande, Sandey, Sandi, Sandie

Sanford (English) sandy river crossing.
Sandford

Sani (Hindi) the planet Saturn. (Navajo) old.

Sanjay (American) a combination of Sanford + Jay.
Sanjaya, Sanje, Sanjey, Sanjo

Sanjiv (Hindi) long lived.
Sanjeev

Sankar (Hindi) a form of Shankara, another name for the Hindu god Shiva.

Sansón (Spanish) a form of Samson.
Sanson, Sansone, Sansun

Santana (Spanish) History: Antonio López de Santa Anna was a Mexican general and political leader.
Santanna

Santiago (Spanish) a form of James.

Santino (Spanish) a form of Santonio.
Santion

Santo (Italian, Spanish) holy.
Santos

Santon (English) sandy town.

Santonio (Spanish) Geography: a short form of San Antonio, a city in Texas.
Santino, Santon, Santoni

Santos (Spanish) saint.
Santo

Santosh (Hindi) satisfied.

Sanyu (Luganda) happy.

Saqr (Arabic) falcon.

Saquan (American) a combination of the prefix Sa + Quan.
Saquané, Saquin, Saquon, Saqwan, Saqwone

Sarad (Hindi) born in the autumn.

Sargent (French) army officer.
Sargant, Sarge, Sarjant, Sergeant, Sergent, Serjeant

Sarito (Spanish) a form of Caesar.
Sarit

Sariyah (Arabic) clouds at night.

Sarngin (Hindi) archer; protector.

Sarojin (Hindi) like a lotus.
Sarojun

Sasha (Russian) a short form of Alexander.
Sacha, Sash, Sashenka, Sashka, Sashok, Sausha

Sasson (Hebrew) joyful.
Sason

Satchel (French) small bag.
Satch

Satordi (French) Saturn.
Satori

Saul (Hebrew) asked for, borrowed. Bible: in the Old Testament, a king of Israel and the father of Jonathan; in the New Testament, Saint Paul's original name was Saul.
Saül, Shaul, Sol, Solly

Saverio (Italian) a form of Xavier.

Saville (French) willow town.
Savelle, Savil, Savile, Savill, Savylle, Seville, Siville

Savon (Spanish) a treeless plain.
Savan, Savaughn, Saveion, Saveon, Savhon, Saviahn, Savian, Savino, Savion, Savo, Savone, Sayvon, Sayvone

Saw (Burmese) early.

Sawyer (English) wood worker.
Sawyere

Sax (English) a short form of Saxon.
Saxe

Saxon (English) swordsman. History: the Roman name for the Teutonic raiders who ravaged the Roman British coasts.
Sax, Saxen, Saxsin, Saxxon

Sayer (Welsh) carpenter.
Say, Saye, Sayers, Sayr, Sayre, Sayres

Sayyid (Arabic) master.
Sayed, Sayid, Sayyad, Sayyed

Scanlon (Irish) little trapper.
Scanlan, Scanlen

Schafer (German) shepherd.
Schaefer, Schaffer, Schiffer, Shaffar, Shäffer

Schmidt (German) blacksmith.
Schmid, Schmit, Schmitt, Schmydt

Schneider (German) tailor.
Schnieder, Snider, Snyder

Schön (German) handsome.
Schoen, Schönn, Shon

Schuyler (Dutch) sheltering.
Schuylar, Schyler, Scoy, Scy, Skuyler, Sky, Skylar, Skyler, Skylor

Schyler (Dutch) a form of Schuyler.
Schylar, Schylre, Schylur

Scorpio (Latin) dangerous, deadly. Astronomy: a southern constellation near Libra and Sagittarius. Astrology: the eighth sign of the zodiac.
Scorpeo

Scott (English) from Scotland. A familiar form of Prescott.
Scot, Scottie, Scotto, Scotty

Scottie (English) a familiar form of Scott.
Scotie, Scotti

Scotty (English) a familiar form of Scott.
Scottey

Scoville (French) Scott's town.

Scully (Irish) town crier.

Seabert (English) shining sea.
Seabright, Sebert, Seibert

Seabrook (English) brook near the sea.

Seamus (Irish) a form of James.
Seamas, Seumas, Shamus

Sean (Hebrew) God is gracious. (Irish) a form of John.
Seaghan, Séan, Seán, Seanán, Seane, Seann, Shaan, Shaine, Shane, Shaun, Shawn, Shayne, Shon, Sión

Searlas (Irish, French) a form of Charles.
Séarlas, Searles, Searlus

Searle (English) armor.

Seasar (Latin) a form of Caesar.
Seasare, Seazar, Sesar, Sesear, Sezar

Seaton (English) town near the sea.
Seeton, Seton

Sebastian (Greek) venerable. (Latin) revered.
Bastian, Sabastian, Sabastien,

Sebashtian, Sebastain, Sebastiane, Sebastiano, Sebastien, Sébastien, Sebastin, Sebastine, Sebastion, Sebbie, Sebestyén, Sebo, Sepasetiano

Sebastien, Sébastien (French) forms of Sebastian. *Sebasten, Sebastyen*

Sebastion (Greek) a form of Sebastian.

Sedgely (English) sword meadow. *Sedgeley, Sedgly*

Sedric (Irish) a form of Cedric. *Seddrick, Sederick, Sedrick, Sedrik, Sedriq*

Seeley (English) blessed. *Sealey, Seely, Selig*

Sef (Egyptian) yesterday. Mythology: one of the two lions that make up the Akeru, guardian of the gates of morning and night.

Sefton (English) village of rushes.

Sefu (Swahili) sword.

Seger (English) sea spear; sea warrior. *Seager, Seeger, Segar*

Segun (Yoruba) conqueror.

Segundo (Spanish) second.

Seibert (English) bright sea. *Seabert, Sebert*

Seif (Arabic) religion's sword.

Seifert (German) a form of Siegfried.

Sein (Basque) innocent.

Sekaye (Shona) laughter.

Selby (English) village by the mansion. *Selbey, Shelby*

Seldon (English) willow tree valley. *Selden, Sellden*

Selig (German) a form of Seeley. *Seligman, Seligmann, Zelig*

Selwyn (English) friend from the palace. *Selvin, Selwin, Selwinn, Selwynn, Selwynne, Wyn*

Semanda (Luganda) cow clan.

Semer (Ethiopian) a form of George. *Semere, Semier*

Semon (Greek) a form of Simon. *Semion*

Sempala (Luganda) born in prosperous times.

Sen (Japanese) wood fairy. *Senh*

Sener (Turkish) bringer of joy.

Senior (French) lord.

Sennett (French) elderly.
Sennet

Senon (Spanish) living.

Senwe (African) dry as a grain stalk.

Sepp (German) a form of Joseph.
Seppi

Septimus (Latin) seventh.

Serafino (Portuguese) a form of Seraphim.

Seraphim (Hebrew) fiery, burning. Bible: the highest order of angels, known for their zeal and love.
Saraf, Saraph, Serafim, Serafin, Serafino, Seraphimus, Seraphin

Sereno (Latin) calm, tranquil.

Serge (Latin) attendant.
Seargeoh, Serg, Sergei, Sergio, Sergios, Sergius, Sergiusz, Serguel, Sirgio, Sirgios

Sergei (Russian) a form of Serge.
Sergey, Sergeyuk, Serghey, Sergi, Sergie, Sergo, Sergunya, Serhiy, Serhiyko, Serjiro, Serzh

Sergio (Italian) a form of Serge.
Serginio, Serigo, Serjio

Servando (Spanish) to serve.
Servan, Servio

Seth (Hebrew) appointed. Bible: the third son of Adam.
Set, Sethan, Sethe, Shet

Setimba (Luganda) river dweller. Geography: a river in Uganda.

Seumas (Scottish) a form of James.
Seaumus

Severiano (Italian) a form of Séverin.

Séverin (French) severe.
Seve, Sevé, Severan, Severian, Severiano, Severo, Sevien, Sevrin, Sevryn

Severn (English) boundary.
Sevearn, Sevren, Sevrnn

Sevilen (Turkish) beloved.

Seward (English) sea guardian.
Sewerd, Siward

Sewati (Moquelumnan) curved bear claws.

Sexton (English) church official; sexton.

Sextus (Latin) sixth.
Sixtus

Seymour (French) prayer. Religion: name honoring Saint Maur. See also Maurice.
Seamor, Seamore, Seamour, See

Shabouh (Armenian) king, noble. History: a fourth-century Persian king.

Shad (Punjabi) happy-go-lucky.
Shadd

Shadi (Arabic) singer.
Shadde, Shaddi, Shaddy, Shade, Shadee, Shadeed, Shadey, Shadie, Shady, Shydee, Shydi

Shadrach (Babylonian) god; godlike. Bible: one of three companions who emerged unharmed from the fiery furnace of Babylon.
Shad, Shadrack, Shadrick, Sheddrach, Shedrach, Shedrick

Shadwell (English) shed by a well.

Shah (Persian) king. History: a title for rulers of Iran.

Shaheem (American) a combination of Shah + Raheem.
Shaheim, Shahiem, Shahm

Shahid (Arabic) a form of Sa'id.
Shahed, Shaheed

Shai (Hebrew) a short form of Yeshaya.
Shaie

Shaiming (Chinese) life; sunshine.

Shaine (Irish) a form of Sean.
Shain

Shaka (Zulu) founder, first. History: Shaka Zulu was the founder of the Zulu empire.

Shakeel (Arabic) a form of Shaquille.
Shakeil, Shakel, Shakell, Shakiel, Shakil, Shakille, Shakyle

Shakir (Arabic) thankful.
Shaakir, Shakeer, Shakeir, Shakur

Shakur (Arabic) a form of Shakir.
Shakuur

Shalom (Hebrew) peace.
Shalum, Shlomo, Sholem, Sholom

Shalya (Hindi) throne.

Shaman (Sanskrit) holy man, mystic, medicine man.
Shamaine, Shamaun, Shamin, Shamine, Shammon, Shamon, Shamone

Shamar (Hebrew) a form of Shamir.
Shamaar, Shamare, Shamari

Shamir (Hebrew) precious stone.
Shahmeer, Shahmir, Shamar, Shameer, Shamyr

Shamus (American) slang for detective.
Shamas, Shames, Shamos, Shemus

Shan (Irish) a form of Shane.
Shann, Shanne

Shanahan (Irish) wise, clever.

Shandy (English) rambunctious.
Shandey, Shandie

Shane (Irish) a form of Sean.
Shan, Shayn, Shayne

Shangobunni (Yoruba) gift from Shango.

Shanley (Irish) small; ancient.
Shaneley, Shannley

Shannon (Irish) small and wise.
Shanan, Shannan, Shannen, Shannin, Shannone, Shanon

Shantae (French) a form of Chante.
Shant, Shanta, Shantai, Shante, Shantell, Shantelle, Shanti, Shantia, Shantie, Shanton, Shanty

Shap (English) a form of Shep.

Shaquan (American) a combination of the prefix Sha + Quan.
Shaqaun, Shaquand, Shaquane, Shaquann, Shaquaunn, Shaquawn, Shaquen, Shaquian, Shaquin, Shaqwan

Shaquell (American) a form of Shaquille.
Shaqueal, Shaqueil, Shaquel, Shaquelle, Shaquiel, Shaquiell, Shaquielle

Shaquille (Arabic) handsome.
Shakeel, Shaquell, Shaquil, Shaquile, Shaquill, Shaqul

Shaquon (American) a combination of the prefix Sha + Quon.
Shaikwon, Shaqon, Shaquoin, Shaquoné

Sharad (Pakistani) autumn.
Sharod

Sharif (Arabic) honest; noble.
Shareef, Sharef, Shareff, Shareif, Sharief, Sharife, Shariff, Shariyf, Sharrif, Sharyif

Sharod (Pakistani) a form of Sharad.
Sharrod

Sharron (Hebrew) flat area, plain.
Sharon, Sharone, Sharonn, Sharonne

Shattuck (English) little shad fish.

Shaun (Irish) a form of Sean.
Shaughan, Shaughn, Shaugn, Shauna, Shaunahan, Shaune, Shaunn, Shaunne

Shavar (Hebrew) comet.
Shavit

Shavon (American) a combination of the prefix Sha + Yvon.
Shauvan, Shauvon, Shavan, Shavaughn, Shaven, Shavin,

Shavone, Shawan, Shawon,
Shawun

Shaw (English) grove.

Shawn (Irish) a form of Sean.
Shawen, Shawne, Shawnee,
Shawnn, Shawon

Shawnta (American) a combi-
nation of Shawn + the suffix
Ta.
Shawntae, Shawntel, Shawnti

Shay (Irish) a form of Shea.
Shae, Shai, Shaya, Shaye, Shey

Shayan (Cheyenne) a form of
Cheyenne.
Shayaan, Shayann, Shayon

Shayne (Hebrew) a form of
Sean.
Shayn, Shaynne, Shean

Shea (Irish) courteous.
Shay

Shedrick (Babylonian) a form
of Shadrach.
Shadriq, Shederick, Shedric,
Shedrique

Sheehan (Irish) little; peaceful.
Shean

Sheffield (English) crooked
field.
Field, Shef, Sheff, Sheffie, Sheffy

Shel (English) a short form of
Shelby, Sheldon, Shelton.

Shelby (English) ledge estate.
Shel, Shelbe, Shelbey, Shelbie,
Shell, Shellby, Shelley, Shelly

Sheldon (English) farm on
the ledge.
Shel, Sheldan, Shelden, Sheldin,
Sheldyn, Shell, Shelley, Shelly,
Shelton

Shelley (English) a familiar
form of Shelby, Sheldon,
Shelton. Literature: Percy
Bysshe Shelley was a nine-
teenth-century British poet.
Shell, Shelly

Shelton (English) town on a
ledge.
Shel, Shelley, Shelten

Shem (Hebrew) name; reputa-
tion. (English) a short form
of Samuel. Bible: Noah's oldest son.

Shen (Egyptian) sacred
amulet. (Chinese) medita-
tion.

Shep (English) a short form of
Shepherd.
Shap, Ship, Shipp

Shepherd (English) shepherd.
Shep, Shepard, Shephard, Shepp,
Sheppard, Shepperd

Shepley (English) sheep
meadow.
Sheplea, Sheplee, Shepply,
Shipley

Sherborn (English) clear
brook.
Sherborne, Sherbourn, Sherburn,
Sherburne

Sheridan (Irish) wild.
*Dan, Sheredan, Sheriden,
Sheridon, Sherridan*

Sherill (English) shire on a
hill.
Sheril, Sherril, Sherrill

Sherlock (English) light
haired. Literature: Sherlock
Holmes is a famous British
detective character, created
by Sir Arthur Conan Doyle.
Sherlocke, Shurlock, Shurlocke

Sherman (English) sheep
shearer; resident of a shire.
*Scherman, Schermann, Sherm,
Shermain, Shermaine,
Shermann, Shermie, Shermon,
Shermy*

Sherrod (English) clearer of
the land.
*Sherod, Sherrad, Sherrard,
Sherrodd*

Sherwin (English) swift run-
ner, one who cuts the wind.
*Sherveen, Shervin, Sherwan,
Sherwind, Sherwinn, Sherwyn,
Sherwynd, Sherwynne, Win*

Sherwood (English) bright
forest.
Sherwoode, Shurwood, Woody

Shihab (Arabic) blaze.

Shìlín (Chinese) intellectual.
Shilan

Shiloh (Hebrew) God's gift.
*Shi, Shile, Shiley, Shilo, Shiloe,
Shy, Shyle, Shylo, Shyloh*

Shimon (Hebrew) a form of
Simon.
Shymon

Shimshon (Hebrew) a form
of Samson.
Shimson

Shing (Chinese) victory.
Shingae, Shingo

Shipton (English) sheep village; ship village.

Shiquan (American) a combi-
nation of the prefix Shi +
Quan.
*Shiquane, Shiquann, Shiquawn,
Shiquoin, Shiqwan*

Shiro (Japanese) fourth-born
son.

Shiva (Hindi) life and death.
Religion: the most common
name for the Hindu god of
destruction and reproduc-
tion.
Shiv, Shivan, Siva

Shlomo (Hebrew) a form of
Solomon.
*Shelmu, Shelomo, Shelomoh,
Shlomi, Shlomot*

Shmuel (Hebrew) a form of
Samuel.
*Shem, Shemuel, Shmelke,
Shmiel, Shmulka*

Shneur (Yiddish) senior.
Shneiur

Shon (German) a form of
Schön. (American) a form of
Sean.
*Shoan, Shoen, Shondae,
Shondale, Shondel, Shone,
Shonn, Shonntay, Shontae,
Shontarious, Shouan, Shoun*

Shunnar (Arabic) pheasant.

Si (Hebrew) a short form of
Silas, Simon.
Sy

Sid (French) a short form of
Sidney.
Cyd, Siddie, Siddy, Sidey, Syd

Siddel (English) wide valley.
Siddell

Siddhartha (Hindi) History:
Siddhartha Gautama was the
original name of Buddha, the
founder of Buddhism.
*Sida, Siddartha, Siddhaarth,
Siddhart, Siddharth, Sidh,
Sidharth, Sidhartha, Sidhdharth*

Sidney (French) from Saint-
Denis, France.
*Cydney, Sid, Sidnee, Sidny,
Sidon, Sidonio, Sydney, Sydny*

Sidonio (Spanish) a form of
Sidney.

Sidwell (English) wide stream.

Siegfried (German) victorious
peace. See also Zigfrid,
Ziggy.
*Seifert, Seifried, Siegfred, Siffre,
Sig, Sigfrid, Sigfried, Sigfroi,
Sigfryd, Siggy, Sigifredo, Sigvard,
Singefrid, Sygfried, Szygfrid*

Sierra (Irish) black. (Spanish)
saw-toothed.
Siera

Sig (German) a short form of
Siegfried, Sigmund.

Sigifredo (German) a form of
Siegfried.
Sigefriedo, Sigfrido, Siguefredo

Siggy (German) a familiar
form of Siegfried, Sigmund.

Sigmund (German) victorious
protector. See also Ziggy,
Zsigmond, Zygmunt.
*Siegmund, Sig, Siggy,
Sigismond, Sigismondo,
Sigismund, Sigismundo,
Sigismundus, Sigmond,
Sigsmond, Szygmond*

Sigurd (German,
Scandinavian) victorious
guardian.
Sigord, Sjure, Syver

Sigwald (German) victorious
leader.

Silas (Latin) a short form of
Silvan.
Si, Sias, Sylas

Silvan (Latin) forest dweller.
Silas, Silvain, Silvano, Silvaon,
Silvie, Silvio, Sylvain, Sylvan,
Sylvanus, Sylvio

Silvano (Italian) a form of
Silvan.
Silvanos, Silvanus, Silvino

Silvester (Latin) a form of
Sylvester.
Silvestr, Silvestre, Silvestro, Silvy

Silvestro (Italian) a form of
Sylvester.

Silvio (Italian) a form of
Silvan.

Simão (Portuguese) a form of
Samuel.

Simba (Swahili) lion. (Yao) a
short form of Lisimba.
Sim

Simcha (Hebrew) joyful.
Simmy

Simeon (French) a form of
Simon.
Simione, Simone

Simms (Hebrew) son of
Simon.
Simm, Sims

Simmy (Hebrew) a familiar
form of Simcha, Simon.
Simmey, Simmi, Simmie,
Symmy

Simon (Hebrew) he heard.
Bible: one of the Twelve
Disciples. See also

Symington, Ximenes.
Saimon, Samien, Semon,
Shimon, Si, Sim, Simao, Simen,
Simeon, Simion, Simm,
Simmon, Simmonds, Simmons,
Simms, Simmy, Simonas,
Simone, Simson, Simyon,
Síomón, Symon, Szymon

Simpson (Hebrew) son of
Simon.
Simonson, Simson

Sinclair (French) prayer.
Religion: name honoring
Saint Clair.
Sinclare, Synclair

Singh (Hindi) lion.
Sing

Sinjon (English) saint, holy
man. Religion: name honoring Saint John.
Sinjin, Sinjun, Sjohn, Syngen,
Synjen, Synjon

Sipatu (Moquelumnan) pulled
out.

Sipho (Zulu) present.

Siraj (Arabic) lamp, light.

Siseal (Irish) a form of Cecil.

Sisi (Fante) born on Sunday.

Siva (Hindi) a form of Shiva.
Siv

Sivan (Hebrew) ninth month
of the Jewish year.

Siwatu (Swahili) born during a time of conflict.
Siwazuri

Siwili (Native American) long fox's tail.

Skah (Lakota) white.
Skai

Skee (Scandinavian) projectile.
Ski, Skie

Skeeter (English) swift.
Skeat, Skeet, Skeets

Skelly (Irish) storyteller.
Shell, Skelley, Skellie

Skelton (Dutch) shell town.

Skerry (Scandinavian) stony island.

Skip (Scandinavian) a short form of Skipper.

Skipper (Scandinavian) shipmaster.
Skip, Skipp, Skippie, Skipton

Skiriki (Pawnee) coyote.

Skule (Norwegian) hidden.

Skye (Dutch) a short form of Skylar, Skyler, Skylor.
Sky

Skylar (Dutch) a form of Schuyler.
Skilar, Skkylar, Skye, Skyelar, Skylaar, Skylare, Skylarr, Skylayr

Skyler (Dutch) a form of Schuyler.
Skieler, Skiler, Skye, Skyeler, Skylee, Skyller

Skylor (Dutch) a form of Schuyler.
Skye, Skyelor, Skyloer, Skylore, Skylour, Skylur, Skylyr

Slade (English) child of the valley.
Slaide, Slayde

Slane (Czech) salty.
Slan

Slater (English) roof slater.
Slader, Slate, Slayter

Slava (Russian) a short form of Stanislav, Vladislav, Vyacheslav.
Slavik, Slavoshka

Slawek (Polish) a short form of Radoslaw.

Slevin (Irish) mountaineer.
Slaven, Slavin, Slawin

Sloan (Irish) warrior.
Sloane, Slone

Smedley (English) flat meadow.
Smedleigh, Smedly

Smith (English) blacksmith.
Schmidt, Smid, Smidt, Smitt, Smitty, Smyth, Smythe

Snowden (English) snowy hill.
Snowdon

Socrates (Greek) wise, learned. History: a famous ancient Greek philosopher.
Socratis, Sokrates, Sokratis

Sofian (Arabic) devoted.

Sohrab (Persian) ancient hero.

Soja (Yoruba) soldier.

Sol (Hebrew) a short form of Saul, Solomon.
Soll, Sollie, Solly

Solly (Hebrew) a familiar form of Saul, Solomon.
Sollie, Zollie, Zolly

Solomon (Hebrew) peaceful. Bible: a king of Israel famous for his wisdom. See also Zalman.
Salamen, Salamon, Salamun, Salaun, Salman, Salomo, Salomon, Selim, Shelomah, Shlomo, Sol, Solamh, Solaman, Solly, Solmon, Soloman, Solomonas, Sulaiman

Solon (Greek) wise. History: a noted ancient Athenian law-maker.

Somerset (English) place of the summer settlers. Literature: William Somerset Maugham was a well-known British writer.
Sommerset, Sumerset, Summerset

Somerville (English) summer village.
Somerton, Summerton, Summerville

Son (Vietnamese) mountain. (Native American) star. (English) son, boy. A short form of Madison, Orson.
Sonny

Songan (Native American) strong.
Song

Sonny (English) a familiar form of Grayson, Madison, Orson, Son.
Soni, Sonnie, Sony

Sono (Akan) elephant.

Sören (Danish) thunder; war.
Sorren

Sorrel (French) reddish brown.
Sorel, Sorell, Sorrell

Soroush (Persian) happy.

Soterios (Greek) savior.
Soteris, Sotero

Southwell (English) south well.

Sovann (Cambodian) gold.

Sowande (Yoruba) wise healer sought me out.

Spalding (English) divided field.
Spaulding

Spangler (German) tinsmith.
Spengler

Spark (English) happy.
Sparke, Sparkie, Sparky

Spear (English) spear carrier.
Speare, Spears, Speer, Speers,
Spiers

Speedy (English) quick; successful.
Speed

Spence (English) a short form
of Spencer.
Spense

Spencer (English) dispenser of
provisions.
Spence, Spencre, Spenser

Spenser (English) a form of
Spencer. Literature: Edmund
Spenser was the British poet
who wrote *The Faerie*
Queene.
Spanser, Spense

Spike (English) ear of grain;
long nail.
Spyke

Spiro (Greek) round basket;
breath.
Spiridion, Spiridon, Spiros,
Spyridon, Spyros

Spoor (English) spur maker.
Spoors

Sproule (English) energetic.
Sprowle

Spurgeon (English) shrub.

Spyros (Greek) a form of
Spiro.

Squire (English) knight's assistant; large landholder.

Stacey, Stacy (English) familiar forms of Eustace.
Stace, Stacee

Stafford (English) riverbank
landing.
Staffard, Stafforde, Staford

Stamford (English) a form of
Stanford.

Stamos (Greek) a form of
Stephen.
Stamatis, Stamatos

Stan (Latin, English) a short
form of Stanley.

Stanbury (English) stone for-
tification.
Stanberry, Stanbery, Stanburghe,
Stansbury

Stancio (Spanish) a form of
Constantine.
Stancy

Stancliff (English) stony cliff.
Stanclife, Stancliffe

Standish (English) stony park-
land. History: Miles Standish
was a leader in colonial
America.

Stane (Slavic) a short form of
Stanislaus.

Stanfield (English) stony field.
Stansfield

Stanford (English) rocky ford.
Sandy, Stamford, Stan,
Standford, Stanfield

Stanislaus (Latin) stand of
glory. See also Lao, Tano.
Slavik, Stana, Standa, Stane,
Stanislao, Stanislas, Stanislau,
Stanislav, Stanislus, Stannes,
Stano, Stasik, Stasio

Stanislav (Slavic) a form of
Stanislaus. See also Slava.
Stanislaw

Stanley (English) stony
meadow.
Stan, Stanely, Stanlea, Stanlee,
Stanleigh, Stanly

Stanmore (English) stony
lake.

Stannard (English) hard as
stone.

Stanton (English) stony farm.
Stan, Stanten, Staunton

Stanway (English) stony road.

Stanwick (English) stony village.
Stanwicke, Stanwyck

Stanwood (English) stony
woods.

Starbuck (English) challenger
of fate. Literature: a character
in Herman Melville's novel
Moby-Dick.

Stark (German) strong, vigorous.
Starke, Stärke, Starkie

Starling (English) bird.
Sterling

Starr (English) star.
Star, Staret, Starlight, Starlon,
Starwin

Stasik (Russian) a familiar
form of Stanislaus.
Stas, Stash, Stashka, Stashko,
Stasiek

Stasio (Polish) a form of
Stanislaus.
Stas, Stasiek, Stasiu, Staska,
Stasko

Stavros (Greek) a form of
Stephen.

Steadman (English) owner of
a farmstead.
Steadmann, Stedman, Stedmen,
Steed

Steel (English) like steel.
Steele

Steen (German, Danish)
stone.
Steenn, Stein

Steeve (Greek) a short form
of Steeven.

Steeven (Greek) a form of
Steven.
Steaven, Steavin, Steavon,
Steevan, Steeve, Steevn

Stefan (German, Polish, Swedish) a form of Stephen.
Steafan, Steafeán, Stefaan, Stefane, Stefanson, Stefaun, Stefawn, Steffan

Stefano (Italian) a form of Stephen.
Stefanos, Steffano

Stefanos (Greek) a form of Stephen.
Stefans, Stefos, Stephano, Stephanos

Stefen (Norwegian) a form of Stephen.
Steffen, Steffin, Stefin

Steffan (Swedish) a form of Stefan.
Staffan

Stefon (Polish) a form of Stephon.
Staffon, Steffon, Steffone, Stefone, Stefonne

Stein (German) a form of Steen.
Steine, Steiner

Steinar (Norwegian) rock warrior.

Stepan (Russian) a form of Stephen.
Stepa, Stepane, Stepanya, Stepka, Stipan

Steph (English) a short form of Stephen.

Stephan (Greek) a form of Stephen.
Stepfan, Stephanas, Stephano, Stephanos, Stephanus, Stephaun

Stéphane (French) a form of Stephen.
Stefane, Stepháne, Stephanne

Stephen (Greek) crowned.
See also Estéban, Estebe, Estevan, Estevao, Étienne, István, Szczepan, Tapani, Teb, Teppo, Tiennot.
Stamos, Stavros, Stefan, Stefano, Stefanos, Stefen, Stenya, Stepan, Stepanos, Steph, Stephan, Stephanas, Stéphane, Stephens, Stephenson, Stephfan, Stephin, Stephon, Stepven, Steve, Steven, Stevie

Stephon (Greek) a form of Stephen.
Stefon, Stepfon, Stepfone, Stephfon, Stephion, Stephone, Stephonne

Sterling (English) valuable; silver penny. A form of Starling.
Sterlen, Sterlin, Stirling

Stern (German) star.

Sterne (English) austere.
Stearn, Stearne, Stearns

Stetson (Danish) stepson.
Steston, Steton, Stetsen, Stetzon

Stevan (Greek) a form of Steven.
Stevano, Stevanoe, Stevaughn, Stevean

Steve (Greek) a short form of Stephen, Steven.
Steave, Stevie, Stevy

Steven (Greek) a form of Stephen.
Steeven, Steiven, Stevan, Steve, Stevens, Stevie, Stevin, Stevon, Stiven

Stevens (English) son of Steven.
Stevenson, Stevinson

Stevie (English) a familiar form of Stephen, Steven.
Stevey, Stevy

Stevin, Stevon (Greek) forms of Steven.
Stevieon, Stevion, Stevyn

Stewart (English) a form of Stuart.
Steward, Stu

Stian (Norwegian) quick on his feet.

Stig (Swedish) mount.

Stiggur (Gypsy) gate.

Stillman (English) quiet.
Stillmann, Stillmon

Sting (English) spike of grain.

Stockman (English) tree-stump remover.

Stockton (English) tree-stump town.

Stockwell (English) tree-stump well.

Stoddard (English) horse keeper.

Stoffel (German) a short form of Christopher.

Stoker (English) furnace tender.
Stoke, Stokes, Stroker

Stone (English) stone.
Stoen, Stoner, Stoney, Stonie, Stonie, Stoniy, Stony

Storm (English) tempest, storm.
Storme, Stormey, Stormi, Stormmie, Stormy

Storr (Norwegian) great.
Story

Stover (English) stove tender.

Stowe (English) hidden; packed away.

Strahan (Irish) minstrel.
Strachan

Stratford (English) bridge over the river. Literature: Stratford-upon-Avon was Shakespeare's birthplace.
Stradford

Stratton (Scottish) river valley town.
Straten, Straton

Strephon (Greek) one who turns.

Strom (Greek) bed, mattress. (German) stream.

Strong (English) powerful.

Stroud (English) thicket.

Struthers (Irish) brook.

Stu (English) a short form of Stewart, Stuart.
Stew

Stuart (English) caretaker, steward. History: a Scottish and English royal family.
Stewart, Stu, Stuarrt

Studs (English) rounded nail heads; shirt ornaments; male horses used for breeding. History: Louis "Studs" Terkel is a famous American journalist.
Stud, Studd

Styles (English) stairs put over a wall to help cross it.
Stiles, Style, Stylz

Subhi (Arabic) early morning.

Suck Chin (Korean) unshakable rock.

Sudi (Swahili) lucky.
Su'ud

Sued (Arabic) master, chief.
Suede

Suffield (English) southern field.

Sugden (English) valley of sows.

Suhail (Arabic) gentle.
Sohail, Sohayl, Souhail, Suhael, Sujal

Suhuba (Swahili) friend.

Sukru (Turkish) grateful.

Sulaiman (Arabic) a form of Solomon.
Sulaman, Sulay, Sulaymaan, Sulayman, Suleiman, Suleman, Suleyman, Sulieman, Sulman, Sulomon, Sulyman

Sullivan (Irish) black eyed.
Sullavan, Sullevan, Sully

Sully (Irish) a familiar form of Sullivan. (French) stain, tarnish. (English) south.
Sulleigh, Sulley

Sultan (Swahili) ruler.
Sultaan

Sum (Tai) appropriate.

Summit (English) peak, top.
Sumeet, Sumit, Summet, Summitt

Sumner (English) church officer; summoner.
Summer

Sundeep (Punjabi) light; enlightened.
Sundip

Sunny (English) sunny, sunshine.
Sun, Sunni

Sunreep (Hindi) pure.
Sunrip

Sutcliff (English) southern cliff.
Sutcliffe

Sutherland (Scandinavian) southern land.
Southerland, Sutherlan

Sutton (English) southern town.

Sven (Scandinavian) youth.
Svein, Svend, Svenn, Swen, Swenson

Swaggart (English) one who sways and staggers.
Swaggert

Swain (English) herdsman; knight's attendant.
Swaine, Swane, Swanson, Swayne

Swaley (English) winding stream.
Swail, Swailey, Swale, Swales

Sweeney (Irish) small hero.
Sweeny

Swinbourne (English) stream used by swine.
Swinborn, Swinborne, Swinburn, Swinburne, Swinbyrn, Swynborn

Swindel (English) valley of the swine.
Swindell

Swinfen (English) swine's mud.

Swinford (English) swine's crossing.
Swynford

Swinton (English) swine town.

Sy (Latin) a short form of Sylas, Symon.
Si

Sydney (French) a form of Sidney.
Syd, Sydne, Sydnee, Syndey

Syed (Arabic) happy.
Syeed, Syid

Sying (Chinese) star.

Sylas (Latin) a form of Silas.
Sy, Syles, Sylus

Sylvain (French) a form of Silvan, Sylvester.
Sylvan, Sylvian

Sylvester (Latin) forest dweller.
Silvester, Silvestro, Sly, Syl, Sylvain, Sylverster, Sylvestre

Symington (English) Simon's town, Simon's estate.

Symon (Greek) a form of Simon.
Sy, Syman, Symeon, Symion, Symms, Symon, Symone

Szczepan (Polish) a form of Stephen.

Szygfrid (Hungarian) a form
of Siegfried.
Szigfrid

Szymon (Polish) a form of
Simon.

T

Taaveti (Finnish) a form of
David.
Taavi, Taavo

Tab (German) shining, brilliant. (English) drummer.
Tabb, Tabbie, Tabby

Tabari (Arabic) he remembers.
*Tabahri, Tabares, Tabarious,
Tabarius, Tabarus, Tabur*

Tabib (Turkish) physician.
Tabeeb

Tabo (Spanish) a short form of
Gustave.

Tabor (Persian) drummer.
(Hungarian) encampment.
*Tabber, Taber, Taboras, Taibor,
Tayber, Taybor, Taver*

Tad (Welsh) father. (Greek,
Latin) a short form of
Thaddeus.
Tadd, Taddy, Tade, Tadek, Tadey

Tadan (Native American)
plentiful.
Taden

Tadarius (American) a combi-
nation of the prefix Ta +
Darius.
*Tadar, Tadarious, Tadaris,
Tadarrius*

Taddeo (Italian) a form of
Thaddeus.
Tadeo

Taddeus (Greek, Latin) a form
of Thaddeus.
*Taddeous, Taddeusz, Taddius,
Tadeas, Tades, Tadeusz, Tadio,
Tadious*

Tadi (Omaha) wind.

Tadzi (Carrier) loon.

Tadzio (Polish, Spanish) a
form of Thaddeus.
Taddeusz

Taffy (Welsh) a form of David.
(English) a familiar form of
Taft.

Taft (English) river.
Taffy, Tafton

Tage (Danish) day.
Tag

Taggart (Irish) son of the
priest.
Tagart, Taggert

Tahír (Arabic) innocent, pure.
Taheer

Tai (Vietnamese) weather;
prosperous; talented.

Taima (Native American)
born during a storm.

Taishawn (American) a combination of Tai + Shawn.
Taisen, Taishaun, Taishon

Tait (Scandinavian) a form of Tate.
Taite, Taitt

Taiwan (Chinese) island; island dweller. Geography: a country off the coast of China.
Taewon, Tahwan, Taivon, Taiwain, Tawain, Tawan, Tawann, Tawaun, Tawon, Taywan, Tywan

Taiwo (Yoruba) first-born of twins.

Taj (Urdu) crown.
Taje, Tajee, Tajeh, Tajh, Taji

Tajo (Spanish) day.
Taio

Tajuan (American) a combination of the prefix Ta + Juan.
Taijuan, Taijun, Taijuon, Tájuan, Tajwan, Taquan, Tyjuan

Takeo (Japanese) strong as bamboo.
Takeyo

Takis (Greek) a familiar form of Peter.
Takias, Takius

Takoda (Lakota) friend to everyone.

Tal (Hebrew) dew; rain.
Tali, Talia, Talley, Talor, Talya

Talbert (German) bright valley.

Talbot (French) boot maker.
Talbott, Tallbot, Tallbott, Tallie, Tally

Talcott (English) cottage near the lake.

Tale (Tswana) green.

Talen (English) a form of Talon.
Talin, Tallen

Talib (Arabic) seeker.

Taliesin (Welsh) radiant brow.
Tallas, Tallis

Taliki (Hausa) fellow.

Talli (Delaware) legendary hero.

Talmadge (English) lake between two towns.
Talmage

Talmai (Aramaic) mound; furrow.
Telem

Talman (Aramaic) injured; oppressed.
Talmon

Talon (French, English) claw, nail.
Taelon, Taelyn, Talen, Tallin, Tallon, Talyn

Talor (English) a form of Tal, Taylor.
Taelor, Taelur

Tam (Vietnamese) number eight. (Hebrew) honest. (English) a short form of Thomas.
Tama, Tamas, Tamás, Tameas, Tamlane, Tammany, Tammas, Tammen, Tammy

Taman (Slavic) dark, black.
Tama, Tamann, Tamin, Tamon, Tamone

Tamar (Hebrew) date; palm tree.
Tamarie, Tamario, Tamarr, Timur

Tambo (Swahili) vigorous.

Tamir (Arabic) tall as a palm tree.
Tameer

Tammy (English) a familiar form of Thomas.
Tammie

Tamson (Scandinavian) son of Thomas.
Tamsen

Tan (Burmese) million. (Vietnamese) new.
Than

Tanek (Greek) immortal. See also Atek.

Taneli (Finnish) God is my judge.
Taneil, Tanell, Tanella

Taner (English) a form of Tanner.
Tanar

Tanguy (French) warrior.

Tani (Japanese) valley.

Tanmay (Sanskrit) engrossed.

Tanner (English) leather worker; tanner.
Tan, Taner, Tanery, Tann, Tannar, Tannir, Tannor, Tanny

Tannin (English) tan colored; dark.
Tanin, Tannen, Tannon, Tanyen, Tanyon

Tanny (English) a familiar form of Tanner.
Tana, Tannee, Tanney, Tannie, Tany

Tano (Spanish) camp glory. (Ghanaian) Geography: a river in Ghana. (Russian) a short form of Stanislaus.
Tanno

Tanton (English) town by the still river.

Tapan (Sanskrit) sun; summer.

Tapani (Finnish) a form of Stephen.
Tapamn, Teppo

Täpko (Kiowa) antelope.

Taquan (American) a combination of the prefix Ta + Quan.
Taquann, Taquawn, Taquon, Taqwan

Tarak (Sanskrit) star; protector.

Taran (Sanskrit) heaven.
Tarran

Tarek (Arabic) a form of
Táriq.
Tareek, Tareke

Tarell (German) a form of
Terrell.
Tarelle, Tarrel, Tarrell, Taryl

Taren (American) a form of
Taron.
Tarren, Tarrin

Tarif (Arabic) uncommon.
Tareef

Tarik (Arabic) a form of Táriq.
*Taric, Tarick, Tariek, Tarikh,
Tarrick, Tarrik, Taryk*

Táriq (Arabic) conqueror.
History: Tariq bin Ziyad was
the Muslim general who
conquered Spain.
*Tareck, Tarek, Tarik, Tarique,
Tarreq, Tereik*

Tarleton (English) Thor's settlement.
Tarlton

Taro (Japanese) first-born
male.

Taron (American) a combina-
tion of Tad + Ron.
*Taeron, Tahron, Taren, Tarone,
Tarrion, Tarron, Taryn*

Tarrant (Welsh) thunder.
Terrant

Tarun (Sanskrit) young, youth.
Taran

Tarver (English) tower; hill;
leader.
Terver

Taryn (American) a form of
Taron.
Tarryn, Taryon

Tas (Gypsy) bird's nest.

Tashawn (American) a combi-
nation of the prefix Ta +
Shawn.
*Tashaan, Tashan, Tashaun,
Tashon, Tashun*

Tass (Hungarian) ancient
mythology name.

Tasunke (Dakota) horse.

Tate (Scandinavian, English)
cheerful. (Native American)
long-winded talker.
Tait, Tayte

Tatius (Latin) king, ruler.
History: a Sabine king.
Tatianus, Tazio, Titus

Tatum (English) cheerful.

Tau (Tswana) lion.

Tauno (Finnish) a form of
Donald.

Taurean (Latin) strong; force-
ful. Astrology: born under the
sign of Taurus.
*Tauraun, Taurein, Taurin,
Taurion, Taurone, Taurus*

Taurus (Latin) Astrology: the second sign of the zodiac.
Taurice, Tauris

Tavares (Aramaic) a form of Tavor.
Tarvarres, Tavarres, Taveress

Tavaris (Aramaic) a form of Tavor.
Tarvaris, Tavar, Tavaras, Tavari, Tavarian, Tavarious, Tavarius, Tavarous, Tavarri, Tavarris, Tavars, Tavarse, Tavarus, Tevaris, Tevarius, Tevarus

Tavey (Latin) a familiar form of Octavio.

Tavi (Aramaic) good.

Tavian (Latin) a form of Octavio.
Taveon, Taviann, Tavien, Tavieon, Tavin, Tavio, Tavion, Tavionne, Tavon, Tayvon

Tavish (Scottish) a form of Thomas.
Tav, Tavi, Tavis

Tavo (Slavic) a short form of Gustave.

Tavon (American) a form of Tavian.
Tavonn, Tavonne, Tavonni

Tavor (Aramaic) misfortune.
Tarvoris, Tavares, Tavaris, Tavores, Tavorious, Tavoris, Tavorise, Tavorres, Tavorris, Tavuris

Tawno (Gypsy) little one.
Tawn

Tayib (Hindi) good; delicate.

Tayler (English) a form of Taylor.
Tailer, Taylar, Tayller, Teyler

Taylor (English) tailor.
Tailor, Talor, Tayler, Tayllor, Taylour, Taylr, Teylor

Tayshawn (American) a combination of Taylor + Shawn.
Taysean, Tayshan, Tayshun, Tayson

Tayvon (American) a form of Tavian.
Tayvan, Tayvaughn, Tayven, Tayveon, Tayvin, Tayvohn, Taywon

Taz (Arabic) shallow ornamental cup.
Tazz

Tazio (Italian) a form of Tatius.

Teagan (Irish) a form of Teague.
Teagen, Teagun, Teegan

Teague (Irish) bard, poet.
Teag, Teagan, Teage, Teak, Tegan, Teige

Tearence (Latin) a form of Terrence.
Tearance, Tearnce, Tearrance

Tearlach (Scottish) a form of Charles.

Tearle (English) stern, severe.

Teasdale (English) river dweller. Geography: a river in England.

Teb (Spanish) a short form of Stephen.

Ted (English) a short form of Edward, Edwin, Theodore.
Tedd, Tedek, Tedik, Tedson

Teddy (English) a familiar form of Edward, Theodore.
Teddey, Teddie, Tedy

Tedmund (English) protector of the land.
Tedman, Tedmond

Tedorik (Polish) a form of Theodore.
Teodoor, Teodor, Teodorek

Tedrick (American) a combination of Ted + Rick.
Teddrick, Tederick, Tedric

Teetonka (Lakota) big lodge.

Tefere (Ethiopian) seed.

Tegan (Irish) a form of Teague.
Teghan, Teigan, Tiegan

Tej (Sanskrit) light; lustrous.

Tejas (Sanskrit) sharp.

Tekle (Ethiopian) plant.

Telek (Polish) a form of Telford.

Telem (Hebrew) mound; furrow.
Talmai, Tel

Telford (French) iron cutter.
Telek, Telfer, Telfor, Telfour

Teller (English) storyteller.
Tell, Telly

Telly (Greek) a familiar form of Teller, Theodore.

Telmo (English) tiller, cultivator.

Telutci (Moquelumnan) bear making dust as it runs.

Telvin (American) a combination of the prefix Te + Melvin.
Tellvin, Telvan

Tem (Gypsy) country.

Teman (Hebrew) on the right side; southward.

Tembo (Swahili) elephant.

Tempest (French) storm.

Temple (Latin) sanctuary.

Templeton (English) town near the temple.
Temp, Templeten

Tennant (English) tenant, renter.
Tenant, Tennent

Tennessee (Cherokee) mighty warrior. Geography: a southern U.S. state.
Tennesee, Tennesy, Tennysee

Tennyson (English) a form of Dennison. Literature: Alfred, Lord Tennyson was a nine-

teenth-century British poet.
Tenney, Tenneyson, Tennie,
Tennis, Tennison, Tenny, Tenson

Teo (Vietnamese) a form of
Tom.

Teobaldo (Italian, Spanish) a
form of Theobald.

Teodoro (Italian, Spanish) a
form of Theodore.
Teodore, Teodorico

Teppo (French) a familiar
form of Stephen.

Tequan (American) a combination of the prefix Te + Quan.
Tequinn, Tequon

Terance (Latin) a form of
Terrence.
Terriance

Terell (German) a form of
Terrell.
Tarell, Tereall, Terel, Terelle, Tyrel

Teremun (Tiv) father's accept-
ance.
Terence (Latin) a form of
Terrence.
Teren, Teryn

Terencio (Spanish) a form of
Terrence.

Terran (Latin) a short form of
Terrance.
Teran, Teren, Terran, Terren

Terrance (Latin) a form of
Terrence.
Tarrance, Terran

Terrell (German) thunder
ruler.
Terell, Terrail, Terral, Terrale,
Terrall, Terreal, Terrel, Terrelle,
Terrill, Terryal, Terryel, Tirel,
Tirrel, Tirrell, Turrell, Tyrel,
Tyrell

Terrence (Latin) smooth.
Tarrance, Tearence, Terance,
Terence, Terencio, Terrance, Terren,
Terrin, Terry, Torrence, Tyreese

Terrick (American) a combi-
nation of the prefix Te +
Derrick.
Teric, Terick, Terik, Teriq, Terric,
Terrik, Tirek, Tirik

Terrill (German) a form of
Terrell.
Teriel, Teriell, Terril, Terryl,
Terryll, Teryll, Teryl, Tyrill

Terrin (Latin) a short form of
Terrence.
Terin, Terrien, Terryn, Teryn,
Tiren

Terris (Latin) son of Terry.

Terron (American) a form of
Tyrone.
Tereon, Terion, Terione, Teron,
Terone, Terrion, Terrione,
Terriyon, Terrone, Terronn,
Terryon, Tiron

Terry (English) a familiar form
of Terrence. See also Keli.
Tarry, Terrey, Terri, Terrie, Tery

Tertius (Latin) third.

Teshawn (American) a combination of the prefix Te + Shawn.
Tesean, Teshaun, Teshon

Teva (Hebrew) nature.

Tevan (American) a form of Tevin.
Tevaughan, Tevaughn, Teven, Tevvan

Tevel (Yiddish) a form of David.

Tevin (American) a combination of the prefix Te + Kevin.
Teavin, Teivon, Tevan, Tevien, Tevinn, Tevon, Tevvin, Tevyn

Tevis (Scottish) a form of Thomas.
Tevish

Tevon (American) a form of Tevin.
Tevion, Tevohn, Tevone, Tevonne, Tevoun, Teyvon

Tewdor (German) a form of Theodore.

Tex (American) from Texas.
Tejas

Thabit (Arabic) firm, strong.

Thad (Greek, Latin) a short form of Thaddeus.
Thadd, Thade, Thadee, Thady

Thaddeus (Greek) courageous. (Latin) praiser. Bible: one of the Twelve Apostles. See also Fadey.
Tad, Taddeo, Taddeus, Thaddis, Thadeaus, Tadzio, Thad, Thaddaeus, Thaddaus, Thaddeau, Thaddeaus, Thaddeo, Thaddeous, Thaddiaus, Thaddius, Thadeaou, Thadeous, Thadeus, Thadieus, Thadious, Thadius, Thadus

Thady (Irish) praise.
Thaddy

Thai (Vietnamese) many, multiple.

Thaman (Hindi) god; godlike.

Than (Burma) million.
Tan, Thanh

Thane (English) attendant warrior.
Thain, Thaine, Thayne

Thang (Vietnamese) victorious.

Thanh (Vietnamese) finished.

Thaniel (Hebrew) a short form of Nathaniel.

Thanos (Greek) nobleman; bear-man.
Athanasios, Thanasis

Thatcher (English) roof thatcher, repairer of roofs.
Thacher, Thatch, Thaxter

Thaw (English) melting ice.

Thayer (French) nation's army.
Thay

Thel (English) upper story.

Thenga (Yao) bring him.

Theo (English) a short form of Theodore.

Theobald (German) people's prince. See also Dietbald.
Teobaldo, Thebault, Theòbault, Thibault, Tibalt, Tibold, Tiebold, Tiebout, Toiboid, Tybald, Tybalt, Tybault

Theodore (Greek) gift of God. See also Feodor, Fyodor.
Téadóir, Téador, Ted, Teddy, Tedor, Tedorek, Tedorik, Telly, Teodomiro, Teodoro, Teodus, Teos, Tewdor, Theo, Theodor, Theódor, Theodors, Theodorus, Theodosios, Theodrekr, Tivadar, Todor, Tolek, Tudor

Theodoric (German) ruler of the people. See also Dedrick, Derek, Dirk.
Teodorico, Thedric, Thedrick, Thierry, Till

Theophilus (Greek) loved by God.
Teofil, Théophile, Theophlous, Theopolis

Theron (Greek) hunter.
Theran, Theren, Thereon, Therin, Therion, Therrin, Therron, Theryn, Theryon

Thian (Vietnamese) smooth.
Thien

Thibault (French) a form of Theobald.
Thibaud, Thibaut

Thierry (French) a form of Theodoric.
Theirry, Theory

Thom (English) a short form of Thomas.
Thomy

Thoma (German) a form of Thomas.

Thomas (Greek, Aramaic) twin. Bible: one of the Twelve Apostles. See also Chuma, Foma, Maslin.
Tam, Tammy, Tavish, Tevis, Thom, Thoma, Thomason, Thomaz, Thomeson, Thomison, Thommas, Thompson, Thomson, Tom, Toma, Tomas, Tomás, Tomasso, Tomcy, Tomey, Tomey, Tomi, Tommy, Toomas

Thompson (English) son of Thomas.
Thomason, Thomison, Thomsen, Thomson

Thor (Scandinavian) thunder. Mythology: the Norse god of thunder.
Thorin, Tor, Tyrus

Thorald (Scandinavian) Thor's follower.
Terrell, Terrill, Thorold, Torald

Thorbert (Scandinavian) Thor's brightness.
Torbert

Thorbjorn (Scandinavian)
Thor's bear.
Thorburn, Thurborn, Thurburn

Thorgood (English) Thor is
good.

Thorleif (Scandinavian) Thor's
beloved.
Thorlief

Thorley (English) Thor's
meadow.
*Thorlea, Thorlee, Thorleigh,
Thorly, Torley*

Thorndike (English) thorny
embankment.
*Thorn, Thorndyck, Thorndyke,
Thorne*

Thorne (English) a short form
of names beginning with
"Thorn."
Thorn, Thornie, Thorny

Thornley (English) thorny
meadow.
*Thorley, Thorne, Thornlea,
Thornleigh, Thornly*

Thornton (English) thorny
town.
Thorne

Thorpe (English) village.
Thorp

Thorwald (Scandinavian)
Thor's forest.
Thorvald

Thuc (Vietnamese) aware.

Thurlow (English) Thor's hill.
Thurlo

Thurmond (English) defended
by Thor.
Thormond, Thurmund

Thurston (Scandinavian)
Thor's stone.
*Thorstan, Thorstein, Thorsten,
Thurstain, Thurstan, Thursten,
Torsten, Torston*

Tiago (Spanish) a form of
Jacob.

Tiberio (Italian) from the
Tiber River region.
*Tiberias, Tiberious, Tiberiu,
Tiberius, Tibius, Tyberious,
Tyberius, Tyberrius*

Tibor (Hungarian) holy place.
Tiburcio

Tichawanna (Shona) we shall
see.

Ticho (Spanish) a short form
of Patrick.

Tieler (English) a form of
Tyler.
Tielar, Tielor, Tielyr

Tiennot (French) a form of
Stephen.
Tien

Tiernan (Irish) lord.

Tierney (Irish) lordly.
Tiarnach, Tiernan

Tige (English) a short form of
Tiger.
*Ti, Tig, Tighe, Ty, Tyg, Tyge,
Tygh, Tyghe*

Tiger (American) tiger; powerful and energetic.
Tige, Tigger, Tyger

Tiimu (Moquelumnan) caterpillar coming out of the
ground.

Tilden (English) tilled valley.
Tildon

Tiktu (Moquelumnan) bird
digging up potatoes.

Tilford (English) prosperous
ford.

Till (German) a short form of
Theodoric.
*Thilo, Til, Tillman, Tilman,
Tillmann, Tilson*

Tilton (English) prosperous
town.

Tim (Greek) a short form of
Timothy.
Timmie, Timmy

Timin (Arabic) born near the
sea.

Timmothy (Greek) a form of
Timothy.
*Timmathy, Timmithy, Timmoty,
Timmthy*

Timmy (Greek) a familiar
form of Timothy.
Timmie

Timo (Finnish) a form of
Timothy.
Timio

Timofey (Russian) a form of
Timothy.
Timofei, Timofej, Timofeo

Timon (Greek) honorable.

Timoteo (Portuguese, Spanish)
a form of Timothy.

Timothy (Greek) honoring
God. See also Kimokeo.
*Tadhg, Taidgh, Tiege, Tim, Tima,
Timithy, Timka, Timkin,
Timmothy, Timmy, Timo,
Timofey, Timok, Timon,
Timontheo, Timonthy, Timót,
Timote, Timotei, Timoteo,
Timoteus, Timothé, Timothée,
Timotheo, Timotheos, Timotheus,
Timothey, Timothie, Timthie,
Tiomóid, Tisha, Tomothy,
Tymon, Tymothy*

Timur (Hebrew) a form of
Tamar. (Russian) conqueror.
Timour

Tin (Vietnamese) thinker.

Tino (Spanish) venerable,
majestic. (Italian) small. A
familiar form of Antonio.
(Greek) a short form of
Augustine.
Tion

Tinsley (English) fortified
field.

Tiquan (American) a combination of the prefix Ti + Quan.
Tiquawn, Tiquine, Tiquon, Tiquwan, Tiqwan

Tisha (Russian) a form of Timothy.
Tishka

Tishawn (American) a combination of the prefix Ti + Shawn.
Tishaan, Tishaun, Tishean, Tishon, Tishun

Tito (Italian) a form of Titus.
Titas, Titis, Titos

Titus (Greek) giant. (Latin) hero. A form of Tatius. History: a Roman emperor.
Tite, Titek, Tito, Tytus

Tivon (Hebrew) nature lover.

TJ (American) a combination of the initials T. + J.
Teejay, Tj, T.J., T Jae, Tjayda

Tobal (Spanish) a short form of Christopher.
Tabalito

Tobar (Gypsy) road.

Tobi (Yoruba) great.

Tobias (Hebrew) God is good.
Tobia, Tobiah, Tobiás, Tobiath, Tobin, Tobit, Toby, Tobyas, Tuvya

Tobin (Hebrew) a form of Tobias.
Toben, Tobian, Tobyn, Tovin

Toby (Hebrew) a familiar form of Tobias.
Tobbie, Tobby, Tobe, Tobee, Tobey, Tobie

Todd (English) fox.
Tod, Toddie, Toddy

Todor (Basque, Russian) a form of Theodore.
Teodor, Todar, Todas, Todos

Toft (English) small farm.

Tohon (Native American) cougar.

Tokala (Dakota) fox.

Toland (English) owner of taxed land.
Tolan

Tolbert (English) bright tax collector.

Toller (English) tax collector.

Tom (English) a short form of Tomas, Thomas.
Teo, Thom, Tommey, Tommie, Tommy

Toma (Romanian) a form of Thomas.
Tomah

Tomas (German) a form of Thomas.
Tom, Tomaisin, Tomaz, Tomcio, Tome, Tomek, Tomelis, Tomico,

Tomik, Tomislav, Tommas, Tomo,
Tomson

Tomás (Irish, Spanish) a form
of Thomas.
Tomas, Tómas, Tomasz

Tomasso (Italian) a form of
Thomas.
Tomaso, Tommaso

Tombe (Kakwa) northerners.

Tomey (Irish) a familiar form
of Thomas.
Tome, Tomi, Tomie, Tomy

Tomi (Japanese) rich.
(Hungarian) a form of
Thomas.

Tomlin (English) little Tom.
Tomkin, Tomlinson

Tommie (Hebrew) a form of
Tommy.
Tommi

Tommy (Hebrew) a familiar
form of Thomas.
Tommie, Tomy

Tonda (Czech) a form of
Tony.
Tonek

Tong (Vietnamese) fragrant.

Toni (Greek, German, Slavic) a
form of Tony.
Tonee, Tonie, Tonio, Tonis, Tonnie

Tonio (Portuguese) a form of
Tony. (Italian) a short form of
Antonio.
Tono, Tonyo

Tony (Greek) flourishing.
(Latin) praiseworthy.
(English) a short form of
Anthony. A familiar form of
Remington.
Tonda, Tonek, Toney, Toni,
Tonik, Tonio, Tonny

Tooantuh (Cherokee) spring
frog.

Toomas (Estonian) a form of
Thomas.
Toomis, Tuomas, Tuomo

Topher (Greek) a short form
of Christopher, Kristopher.
Tofer, Tophor

Topo (Spanish) gopher.

Topper (English) hill.

Tor (Norwegian) thunder.
(Tiv) royalty, king.
Thor

Torian (Irish) a form of Torin.
Toran, Torean, Toriano, Toriaun,
Torien, Torrian, Torrien, Torryan

Torin (Irish) chief.
Thorfin, Thorstein, Torian,
Torion, Torrin, Toryn

Torkel (Swedish) Thor's caul-
dron.

Tormey (Irish) thunder spirit.
Tormé, Tormee

Tormod (Scottish) north.

Torn (Irish) a short form of
Torrence.
Toran

Torquil (Danish) Thor's kettle.
Torkel

Torr (English) tower.
Tory

Torrance (Irish) a form of
Torrence.
Torance

Torren (Irish) a short form of
Torrence.
Torehn, Toren

Torrence (Irish) knolls. (Latin)
a form of Terrence.
*Tawrence, Toreence, Torence,
Torenze, Torey, Torin, Torn, Torr,
Torrance, Torren, Torreon, Torrin,
Torry, Tory, Torynce, Tuarence,
Turance*

Torrey (English) a form of Tory.
*Toreey, Torie, Torre, Torri, Torrie,
Torry*

Toru (Japanese) sea.

Tory (English) familiar form
of Torr, Torrence.
Torey, Tori, Torrey

Toshi-Shita (Japanese) junior.

Tovi (Hebrew) good.
Tov

Townley (English) town
meadow.
*Townlea, Townlee, Townleigh,
Townlie, Townly*

Townsend (English) town's
end.
*Town, Townes, Towney, Townie,
Townsen, Townshend, Towny*

Trace (Irish) a form of Tracy.
Trayce

Tracey (Irish) a form of Tracy.
Traci

Tracy (Greek) harvester.
(Latin) courageous. (Irish)
battler.
Trace, Tracey, Tracie, Treacy

Trader (English) well-trodden
path; skilled worker.

Trae (English) a form of Trey.
Trai, Traie, Tre, Trea

Trahern (Welsh) strong as
iron.
Traherne, Tray

Tramaine (Scottish) a form of
Tremaine, Tremayne.
*Tramain, Traman, Tramane,
Tramayne, Traymain, Traymon*

Traquan (American) a combi-
nation of Travis + Quan.
*Traequan, Traqon, Traquon,
Traqwan, Traqwaun, Trayquan,
Trayquane, Trayqwon*

Trashawn (American) a com-
bination of Travis + Shawn.
*Trasen, Trashaun, Trasean,
Trashon, Trashone, Trashun,
Trayshaun, Trayshawn*

Traugott (German) God's
truth.

Travaris (French) a form of
Travers.
*Travares, Travaress, Travarious,
Travarius, Travarous, Travarus,
Travauris, Traveress, Traverez,
Traverus, Travoris, Travorus*

Travell (English) traveler.
*Travail, Travale, Travel, Travelis,
Travelle, Trevel, Trevell, Trevelle*

Traven (American) a form of
Trevon.
Travin, Travine, Trayven

Travers (French) crossroads.
Travaris, Traver, Travis

Travion (American) a form of
Trevon.
*Traveon, Travian, Travien,
Travione, Travioun*

Travis (English) a form of
Travers.
*Travais, Travees, Traves, Traveus,
Travious, Traviss, Travius,
Travous, Travus, Travys, Trayvis,
Trevais, Trevis*

Travon (American) a form of
Trevon.
*Traevon, Traivon, Travone,
Travonn, Travonne*

Tray (English) a form of Trey.
Traye

Trayton (English) town full of
trees.
Trayten

Trayvon (American) a combi-
nation of Tray + Von.
*Trayveon, Trayvin, Trayvion,
Trayvond, Trayvone, Trayvonne,
Trayvyon*

Treavon (American) a form of
Trevon.
Treavan, Treavin, Treavion

Tredway (English) well-worn
road.
Treadway

Tremaine, Tremayne
(Scottish) house of stone.
*Tramaine, Tremain, Tremane,
Treymaine, Trimaine*

Trent (Latin) torrent, rapid
stream. (French) thirty.
Geography: a city in northern Italy.
Trente, Trentino, Trento, Trentonio

Trenton (Latin) town by the
rapid stream. Geography: the
capital of New Jersey.
*Trendon, Trendun, Trenten,
Trentin, Trentton, Trentyn,
Trinten, Trintin, Trinton*

Trequan (American) a combi-
nation of Trey + Quan.
*Trequanne, Trequaun, Trequian,
Trequon, Treqwon, Treyquane*

Treshawn (American) a com-
bination of Trey + Shawn.
*Treshaun, Treshon, Treshun,
Treysean, Treyshawn, Treyshon*

Treston (Welsh) a form of Tristan.
Trestan, Trestin, Trestton, Trestyn

Trev (Irish, Welsh) a short form of Trevor.

Trevaughn (American) a combination of Trey + Vaughn.
Trevaughan, Trevaugn, Trevaun, Trevaune, Trevaunn, Treyvaughn

Trevelyan (English) Elian's homestead.

Trevin (American) a form of Trevon.
Trevian, Trevien, Trevine, Trevinne, Trevyn, Treyvin

Trevion (American) a form of Trevon.
Trevione, Trevionne, Trevyon, Treyveon, Treyvion

Trevis (English) a form of Travis.
Treves, Trevez, Treveze, Trevius

Trevon (American) a combination of Trey + Von.
Traven, Travion, Travon, Tre, Treavon, Trévan, Treveyon, Trevin, Trevion, Trevohn, Trevoine, Trévon, Trevone, Trevonn, Trevonne, Treyvon

Trevor (Irish) prudent. (Welsh) homestead.
Travor, Treavor, Trebor, Trefor, Trev, Trevar, Trevares, Trevarious, Trevaris, Trevarius, Trevaros, Trevarus, Trever, Trevore, Trevores,

Trevoris, Trevorus, Trevour, Trevyr, Treyvor

Trey (English) three; third.
Trae, Trai, Tray, Treye, Tri, Trie

Treyvon (American) a form of Trevon.
Treyvan, Treyven, Treyvenn, Treyvone, Treyvonn, Treyvun

Trigg (Scandinavian) trusty.

Trini (Latin) a short form of Trinity.

Trinity (Latin) holy trinity.
Trenedy, Trini, Trinidy

Trip, Tripp (English) traveler.

Tristan (Welsh) bold. Literature: a knight in the Arthurian legends who fell in love with his uncle's wife.
Treston, Tris, Trisan, Tristain, Tristano, Tristen, Tristian, Tristin, Triston, Tristyn, Trystan

Tristano (Italian) a form of Tristan.

Tristen (Welsh) a form of Tristan.
Trisden, Trissten

Tristin (Welsh) a form of Tristan.
Tristian, Tristinn

Triston (Welsh) a form of Tristan.

Tristram (Welsh) sorrowful. Literature: the title character in Laurence Sterne's eigh-

teenth-century novel *Tristram Shandy*.
Tristam

Tristyn (Welsh) a form of Tristan.
Tristynne

Trot (English) trickling stream.

Trowbridge (English) bridge by the tree.

Troy (Irish) foot soldier. (French) curly haired. (English) water. See also Koi.
Troi, Troye, Troyton

True (English) faithful, loyal.
Tru

Truesdale (English) faithful one's homestead.

Truitt (English) little and honest.
Truett

Truman (English) honest. History: Harry S. Truman was the thirty-third U.S. president.
Trueman, Trumain, Trumaine, Trumann

Trumble (English) strong; bold.
Trumball, Trumbell, Trumbull

Trustin (English) trustworthy.
Trustan, Trusten, Truston

Trygve (Norwegian) brave victor.

Trystan (Welsh) a form of Tristan.
Tryistan, Trysten, Trystian, Trystin, Trystn, Tryston, Trystyn

Tsalani (Nguni) good-bye.

Tse (Ewe) younger of twins.

Tu (Vietnamese) tree.

Tuaco (Ghanaian) eleventh-born.

Tuan (Vietnamese) goes smoothly.

Tucker (English) fuller, tucker of cloth.
Tuck, Tuckie, Tucky, Tuckyr

Tudor (Welsh) a form of Theodore. History: an English ruling dynasty.
Todor

Tug (Scandinavian) draw, pull.
Tugg

Tuketu (Moquelumnan) bear making dust as it runs.

Tukuli (Moquelumnan) caterpillar crawling down a tree.

Tulio (Italian, Spanish) lively.
Tullio

Tullis (Latin) title, rank.
Tullius, Tullos, Tully

Tully (Irish) at peace with God. (Latin) a familiar form of Tullis.
Tull, Tulley, Tullie, Tullio

Tumaini (Mwera) hope.

Tumu (Moquelumnan) deer thinking about eating wild onions.

Tung (Vietnamese) stately, dignified. (Chinese) everyone.

Tungar (Sanskrit) high; lofty.

Tupi (Moquelumnan) pulled up.

Tupper (English) ram raiser.

Turi (Spanish) a short form of Arthur.
Ture

Turk (English) from Turkey.

Turner (Latin) lathe worker; wood worker.

Turpin (Scandinavian) Finn named after Thor.

Tut (Arabic) strong and courageous. History: a short form of Tutankhamen, an Egyptian king.
Tutt

Tutu (Spanish) a familiar form of Justin.

Tuvya (Hebrew) a form of Tobias.
Tevya, Tuvia, Tuviah

Tuwile (Mwera) death is inevitable.

Tuyen (Vietnamese) angel.

Twain (English) divided in two. Literature: Mark Twain (whose real name was Samuel Langhorne Clemens) was one of the most prominent nineteenth-century American writers.
Tawine, Twaine, Twan, Twane, Tway, Twayn, Twayne

Twia (Fante) born after twins.

Twitchell (English) narrow passage.
Twytchell

Twyford (English) double river crossing.

Txomin (Basque) like the Lord.

Ty (English) a short form of Tyler, Tyrone, Tyrus.
Tye

Tyee (Native American) chief.

Tyger (English) a form of Tiger.
Tige, Tyg, Tygar

Tylar (English) a form of Tyler.
Tyelar, Tylarr

Tyler (English) tile maker.
Tieler, Tiler, Ty, Tyel, Tyeler, Tyelor, Tyhler, Tylar, Tyle, Tylee, Tylere, Tyller, Tylor, Tylyr

Tylor (English) a form of Tyler.
Tylour

Tymon (Polish) a form of Timothy. (Greek) a form of Timon.
Tymain, Tymaine, Tymane, Tymeik, Tymek, Tymen

Tymothy (English) a form of
Timothy.
*Tymithy, Tymmothy, Tymoteusz,
Tymothee, Timothi*

Tynan (Irish) dark.
Ty

Tynek (Czech) a form of
Martin.
Tynko

Tyquan (American) a combi-
nation of Ty + Quan.
*Tykwan, Tykwane, Tykwon,
Tyquaan, Tyquane, Tyquann,
Tyquine, Tyquinn, Tyquon,
Tyquone, Tyquwon, Tyqwan*

Tyran (American) a form of
Tyrone.
Tyraine, Tyrane

Tyree (Scottish) island dweller.
Geography: Tiree is an island
off the west coast of
Scotland.
*Tyra, Tyrae, Tyrai, Tyray, Tyre,
Tyrea, Tyrée*

Tyreese (American) a form of
Terrence.
*Tyreas, Tyrease, Tyrece, Tyreece,
Tyreice, Tyres, Tyrese, Tyresse,
Tyrez, Tyreze, Tyrice, Tyriece,
Tyriese*

Tyrel, Tyrell (American) forms
of Terrell.
Tyrelle, Tyrrel, Tyrrell

Tyrick (American) a combination of Ty + Rick.
Tyreck, Tyreek, Tyreik, Tyrek,

*Tyreke, Tyric, Tyriek, Tyrik,
Tyriq, Tyrique*

Tyrin (American) a form of
Tyrone.
Tyrinn, Tyrion, Tyrrin, Tyryn

Tyron (American) a form of
Tyrone.
*Tyrohn, Tyronn, Tyronna,
Tyronne*

Tyrone (Greek) sovereign.
(Irish) land of Owen.
*Tayron, Tayrone, Teirone, Terron,
Ty, Tyerone, Tyhrone, Tyran,
Tyrin, Tyron, Tyroney, Tyronne,
Tyroon, Tyroun*

Tyrus (English) a form of
Thor.
Ty, Tyruss, Tyryss

Tyshawn (American) a combi-
nation of Ty + Shawn.
*Tyshan, Tyshaun, Tyshauwn,
Tyshian, Tyshinn, Tyshion,
Tyshon, Tyshone, Tyshonne,
Tyshun, Tyshunn, Tyshyn*

Tyson (French) son of Ty.
*Tison, Tiszon, Tyce, Tycen,
Tyesn, Tyeson, Tysen, Tysie,
Tysin, Tysne, Tysone*

Tytus (Polish) a form of Titus.
Tyus

Tyvon (American) a combina-
tion of Ty + Von.
*Tyvan, Tyvin, Tyvinn, Tyvone,
Tyvonne*

Tywan (Chinese) a form of Taiwan.
Tywain, Tywaine, Tywane, Tywann, Tywaun, Tywen, Tywon, Tywone, Tywonne

Tzadok (Hebrew) righteous.
Tzadik, Zadok

Tzion (Hebrew) sign from God.
Zion

Tzuriel (Hebrew) God is my rock.
Tzuriya

Tzvi (Hebrew) deer.
Tzevi, Zevi

U

Uaine (Irish) a form of Owen.

Ubadah (Arabic) serves God.

Ubaid (Arabic) faithful.

Uberto (Italian) a form of Hubert.

Uche (Ibo) thought.

Uday (Sanskrit) to rise.

Udell (English) yew-tree valley.
Dell, Eudel, Udale, Udall, Yudell

Udit (Sanskrit) grown; shining.

Udo (Japanese) ginseng plant. (German) a short form of Udolf.

Udolf (English) prosperous wolf.
Udo, Udolfo, Udolph

Ugo (Italian) a form of Hugh, Hugo.

Ugutz (Basque) a form of John.

Uilliam (Irish) a form of William.
Uileog, Uilleam, Ulick

Uinseann (Irish) a form of Vincent.

Uistean (Irish) intelligent.
Uisdean

Uja (Sanskrit) growing.

Uku (Hawaiian) flea, insect; skilled ukulele player.

Ulan (African) first-born twin.

Ulbrecht (German) a form of Albert.

Ulf (German) wolf.

Ulfred (German) peaceful wolf.

Ulger (German) warring wolf.

Ulises (Latin) a form of Ulysses.
Ulishes, Ulisse, Ulisses

Ullock (German) sporting wolf.

Ulmer (English) famous wolf.
Ullmar, Ulmar

Ulmo (German) from Ulm, Germany.

Ulric (German) a form of Ulrich.
Ullric

Ulrich (German) wolf ruler; ruler of all. See also Alaric.
Uli, Ull, Ulric, Ulrick, Ulrik, Ulrike, Ulu, Ulz, Uwe

Ultman (Hindi) god; godlike.

Ulyses (Latin) a form of Ulysses.
Ulysee, Ulysees

Ulysses (Latin) wrathful. A form of Odysseus.
Eulises, Ulick, Ulises, Ulyses, Ulysse, Ulyssees, Ulysses, Ulyssius

Umang (Sanskrit) enthusiastic.
Umanga

Umar (Arabic) a form of Omar.
Umair, Umarr, Umayr, Umer

Umberto (Italian) a form of Humbert.
Uberto

Umi (Yao) life.

Umit (Turkish) hope.

Unai (Basque) shepherd.
Una

Uner (Turkish) famous.

Unika (Lomwe) brighten.

Unique (Latin) only, unique.
Uneek, Unek, Unikque, Uniqué, Unyque

Unwin (English) nonfriend.
Unwinn, Unwyn

Upshaw (English) upper wooded area.

Upton (English) upper town.

Upwood (English) upper forest.

Urban (Latin) city dweller; courteous.
Urbain, Urbaine, Urbane, Urbano, Urbanus, Urvan, Urvane

Urbane (English) a form of Urban.

Urbano (Italian) a form of Urban.

Uri (Hebrew) a short form of Uriah.
Urie

Uriah (Hebrew) my light. Bible: a soldier and the husband of Bathsheba. See also Yuri.
Uri, Uria, Urias, Urijah

Urian (Greek) heaven.
Urihaan

Uriel (Hebrew) God is my light.
Urie

Urson (French) a form of
Orson.
Ursan, Ursus

Urtzi (Basque) sky.

Usamah (Arabic) like a lion.
Usama

Useni (Yao) tell me.
Usene, Usenet

Usi (Yao) smoke.

Ustin (Russian) a form of
Justin.

Utatci (Moquelumnan) bear
scratching itself.

Uthman (Arabic) companion
of the Prophet.
Usman, Uthmaan

Uttam (Sanskrit) best.

Uwe (German) a familiar form
of Ulrich.

Uzi (Hebrew) my strength.
Uzzia

Uziel (Hebrew) God is my
strength; mighty force.
Uzie, Uzziah, Uzziel

Uzoma (Nigerian) born during a journey.

Uzumati (Moquelumnan)
grizzly bear.

V

Vachel (French) small cow.
Vache, Vachell

Vaclav (Czech) wreath of
glory.
Vasek

Vadin (Hindi) speaker.
Vaden

Vail (English) valley.
Vaile, Vaill, Vale, Valle

Val (Latin) a short form of
Valentin.

Valborg (Swedish) mighty
mountain.

Valdemar (Swedish) famous
ruler.

Valentin (Latin) strong;
healthy.
*Val, Valencio, Valenté, Valentijn,
Valentine, Valentino, Valenton,
Valentyn, Velentino*

Valentino (Italian) a form of
Valentin.

Valerian (Latin) strong;
healthy.
Valeriano, Valerii, Valerio, Valeryn

Valerii (Russian) a form of
Valerian.
*Valera, Valerie, Valerij, Valerik,
Valeriy, Valery*

Valfrid (Swedish) strong peace.

Valin (Hindi) a form of Balin.
Mythology: a tyrannical
monkey king.

Vallis (French) from Wales.
Valis

Valter (Lithuanian, Swedish) a
form of Walter.
Valters, Valther, Valtr, Vanda

Van (Dutch) a short form of
Vandyke.
Vander, Vane, Vann, Vanno

Vance (English) thresher.

Vanda (Lithuanian) a form of
Walter.
Vander

Vandyke (Dutch) dyke.
Van

Vanya (Russian) a familiar
form of Ivan.
*Vanechka, Vanek, Vanja, Vanka,
Vanusha, Wanya*

Vardon (French) green knoll.
*Vardaan, Varden, Verdan, Verdon,
Verdun*

Varian (Latin) variable.

Varick (German) protecting
ruler.
Varak, Varek, Warrick

Vartan (Armenian) rose pro-
ducer; rose giver.

Varun (Hindi) rain god.
Varron

Vasant (Sanskrit) spring.
Vasanth

Vashawn (American) a combi-
nation of the prefix Va +
Shawn.
*Vashae, Vashan, Vashann,
Vashaun, Vashawnn, Vashon,
Vashun, Vishon*

Vasilis (Greek) a form of Basil.
*Vas, Vasaya, Vaselios, Vashon,
Vasil, Vasile, Vasileior, Vasileios,
Vasilios, Vasilius, Vasilos, Vasilus,
Vasily, Vassilios, Vasylko, Vasyltso,
Vazul*

Vasily (Russian) a form of
Vasilis.
*Vasilek, Vasili, Vasilii, Vasilije,
Vasilik, Vasiliy, Vassili, Vassilij,
Vasya, Vasyenka*

Vasin (Hindi) ruler, lord.

Vasu (Sanskrit) wealth.

Vasyl (German, Slavic) a form
of William.
*Vasos, Vassily, Vassos, Vasya,
Vasyuta, VaVaska, Wassily*

Vaughn (Welsh) small.
*Vaughan, Vaughen, Vaun, Vaune,
Von, Voughn*

Veasna (Cambodian) lucky.

Ved (Sanskrit) sacred knowledge.

Vedie (Latin) sight.

Veer (Sanskrit) brave.

Vegard (Norwegian) sanctuary; protection.

Velvel (Yiddish) wolf.

Vencel (Hungarian) a short form of Wenceslaus.
Venci, Vencie

Venedictos (Greek) a form of Benedict.
Venedict, Venediktos, Venka, Venya

Veniamin (Bulgarian) a form of Benjamin.
Venyamin, Verniamin

Venkat (Hindi) god; godlike. Religion: another name for the Hindu god Vishnu.

Venya (Russian) a familiar form of Benedict.
Venedict, Venka

Vere (Latin, French) true.

Vered (Hebrew) rose.

Vergil (Latin) a form of Virgil. Literature: a Roman poet best known for his epic poem *Aenid*.
Verge

Vern (Latin) a short form of Vernon.
Verna, Vernal, Verne, Verneal, Vernel, Vernell, Vernelle, Vernial, Vernine, Vernis, Vernol

Vernados (German) courage of the bear.

Verner (German) defending army.
Varner

Verney (French) alder grove.
Vernie

Vernon (Latin) springlike; youthful.
Vern, Varnan, Vernen, Verney, Vernin

Verrill (German) masculine. (French) loyal.
Verill, Verrall, Verrell, Verroll, Veryl

Vian (English) full of life.

Vic (Latin) a short form of Victor.
Vick, Vicken, Vickenson

Vicente (Spanish) a form of Vincent.
Vicent, Visente

Vicenzo (Italian) a form of Vincent.

Victoir (French) a form of Victor.

Victor (Latin) victor, conqueror.
Vic, Victa, Victer, Victoir, Victoriano, Victorien, Victorin, Victorio, Viktor, Vitin, Vittorio, Vitya, Wikoli, Wiktor, Witek

Victorio (Spanish) a form of Victor.
Victorino

Vidal (Spanish) a form of Vitas.
Vida, Vidale, Vidall, Videll

Vidar (Norwegian) tree warrior.

Vidor (Hungarian) cheerful.

Vidur (Hindi) wise.

Viho (Cheyenne) chief.

Vijay (Hindi) victorious.

Vikas (Hindi) growing.
Vikash, Vikesh

Vikram (Hindi) valorous.
Vikrum

Vikrant (Hindi) powerful.
Vikran

Viktor (German, Hungarian, Russian) a form of Victor.
Viktoras, Viktors

Vilhelm (German) a form of William.
Vilhelms, Vilho, Vilis, Viljo, Villem

Vili (Hungarian) a short form of William.
Villy, Vilmos

Viliam (Czech) a form of William.
Vila, Vilek, Vilém, Viliami, Viliamu, Vilko, Vilous

Viljo (Finnish) a form of William.

Ville (Swedish) a short form of William.

Vimal (Hindi) pure.

Vin (Latin) a short form of Vincent.
Vinn

Vinay (Hindi) polite.

Vince (English) a short form of Vincent.
Vence, Vint

Vincent (Latin) victor, conqueror. See also Binkentios, Binky.
Uinseann, Vencent, Vicente, Vicenzo, Vikent, Vikenti, Vikesha, Vin, Vince, Vincence, Vincens, Vincente, Vincentius, Vincents, Vincenty, Vincenzo, Vinci, Vincien, Vincient, Vinciente, Vincint, Vinny, Vinsent, Vinsint, Wincent

Vincente (Spanish) a form of Vincent.
Vencente

Vincenzo (Italian) a form of Vincent.
Vincenz, Vincenza, Vincenzio, Vinchenzo, Vinzenz

Vinci (Hungarian, Italian) a familiar form of Vincent.
Vinci, Vinco, Vincze

Vinny (English) a familiar form of Calvin, Melvin, Vincent.
Vinnee, Vinney, Vinni, Vinnie

Vinod (Hindi) happy, joyful.
Vinodh, Vinood

Vinson (English) son of
Vincent.
Vinnis

Vipul (Hindi) plentiful.

Viraj (Hindi) resplendent.

Virat (Hindi) very big.

Virgil (Latin) rod bearer, staff
bearer.
*Vergil, Virge, Virgial, Virgie,
Virgilio*

Virgilio (Spanish) a form of
Virgil.
Virjilio

Virote (Tai) strong, powerful.

Vishal (Hindi) huge; great.
Vishaal

Vishnu (Hindi) protector.

Vitas (Latin) alive, vital.
Vidal, Vitus

Vito (Latin) a short form of
Vittorio.
*Veit, Vidal, Vital, Vitale, Vitalis,
Vitas, Vitin, Vitis, Vitus, Vitya,
Vytas*

Vittorio (Italian) a form of
Victor.
*Vito, Vitor, Vitorio, Vittore,
Vittorios*

Vitya (Russian) a form of
Victor.
Vitenka, Vitka

Vivek (Hindi) wisdom.
Vivekinan

Vladimir (Russian) famous
prince. See also Dima,
Waldemar, Walter.
*Bladimir, Vimka, Vlad,
Vladamir, Vladik, Vladimar,
Vladimeer, Vladimer, Vladimere,
Vladimire, Vladimyr, Vladjimir,
Vladka, Vladko, Vladlen,
Vladmir, Volodimir, Volodya,
Volya, Vova, Wladimir*

Vladislav (Slavic) glorious
ruler. See also Slava.
*Vladik, Vladya, Vlas, Vlasislava,
Vyacheslav, Wladislav*

Vlas (Russian) a short form of
Vladislav.

Volker (German) people's
guard.
Folke

Volney (German) national
spirit.

Von (German) a short form of
many German names.

Vova (Russian) a form of Walter.
Vovka

Vuai (Swahili) savior.

Vyacheslav (Russian) a form
of Vladislav. See also Slava.

Waban (Ojibwa) white.
Wabon

Wade (English) ford; river
crossing.
*Wad, Wadesworth, Wadi, Wadie,
Waed, Waid, Waide, Wayde,
Waydell, Whaid*

Wadley (English) ford
meadow.
Wadleigh, Wadly

Wadsworth (English) village
near the ford.
Waddsworth

Wagner (German) wagoner,
wagon maker. Music:
Richard Wagner was a
famous nineteenth-century
German composer.
Waggoner

Wahid (Arabic) single; exclu-
sively unequaled.
Waheed

Wahkan (Lakota) sacred.

Wahkoowah (Lakota) charg-
ing.

Wain (English) a short form of
Wainwright. A form of
Wayne.

Wainwright (English) wagon
maker.
*Wain, Wainright, Wayne,
Wayneright, Waynewright,
Waynright, Wright*

Waite (English) watchman.
Waitman, Waiton, Waits, Wayte

Wakefield (English) wet field.
Field, Wake

Wakely (English) wet meadow.

Wakeman (English) watchman.
Wake

Wakiza (Native American)
determined warrior.

Walcott (English) cottage by
the wall.
Wallcot, Wallcott, Wolcott

Waldemar (German) powerful; famous. See also Vladimir.
Valdemar, Waldermar, Waldo

Walden (English) wooded val-
ley. Literature: Henry David
Thoreau made Walden Pond
famous with his book
Walden.
Waldi, Waldo, Waldon, Welti

Waldo (German) a familiar
form of Oswald, Waldemar,
Walden.
Wald, Waldy

Waldron (English) ruler.

Waleed (Arabic) newborn.
Waled, Walid

Walerian (Polish) strong;
brave.

Wales (English) from Wales.
Wael, Wail, Wali, Walie, Waly

Walford (English) Welshman's
ford.

Walfred (German) peaceful
ruler.
Walfredo, Walfried

Wali (Arabic) all-governing.

Walker (English) cloth walker; cloth cleaner.
Wallie, Wally

Wallace (English) from Wales.
Wallach, Wallas, Wallie, Wallis, Wally, Walsh, Welsh

Wallach (German) a form of Wallace.
Wallache

Waller (German) powerful. (English) wall maker.

Wally (English) a familiar form of Walter.
Walli, Wallie

Walmond (German) mighty ruler.

Walsh (English) a form of Wallace.
Welch, Welsh

Walt (English) a short form of Walter, Walton.
Waltey, Waltli, Walty

Walter (German) army ruler, general. (English) woodsman. See also Gautier, Gualberto, Gualtiero, Gutierre, Ladislav, Vladimir.
Valter, Vanda, Vova, Walder, Wally, Walt, Waltli, Walther, Waltr, Wat, Waterio, Watkins Watson, Wualter

Walther (German) a form of Walter.

Walton (English) walled town.
Walt

Waltr (Czech) a form of Walter.

Walworth (English) fenced-in farm.

Walwyn (English) Welsh friend.
Walwin, Walwinn, Walwynn, Walwynne, Welwyn

Wamblee (Lakota) eagle.

Wang (Chinese) hope; wish.

Wanikiya (Lakota) savior.

Wanya (Russian) a form of Vanya.
Wanyai

Wapi (Native American) lucky.

Warburton (English) fortified town.

Ward (English) watchman, guardian.
Warde, Warden, Worden

Wardell (English) watchman's hill.

Wardley (English) watchman's meadow.
Wardlea Wardleigh

Ware (English) wary, cautious.

Warfield (English) field near the weir or fish trap.

Warford (English) ford near the weir or fish trap.

Warley (English) meadow near the weir or fish trap.

Warner (German) armed defender. (French) park keeper.
Werner

Warren (German) general; warden; rabbit hutch.
Ware, Waring, Warrenson, Warrin, Warriner, Worrin

Warton (English) town near the weir or fish trap.

Warwick (English) buildings near the weir or fish trap.
Warick, Warrick

Washburn (English) overflowing river.

Washington (English) town near water. History: George Washington was the first U.S. president.
Wash

Wasili (Russian) a form of Basil.
Wasyl

Wasim (Arabic) graceful; good-looking.
Waseem, Wasseem, Wassim

Watende (Nyakyusa) there will be revenge.

Waterio (Spanish) a form of Walter.
Gualtiero

Watford (English) wattle ford; dam made of twigs and sticks.

Watkins (English) son of Walter.
Watkin

Watson (English) son of Walter.
Wathson, Whatson

Waverly (English) quaking aspen-tree meadow.
Waverlee, Waverley

Wayland (English) a form of Waylon.
Weiland, Weyland

Waylon (English) land by the road.
Wallen, Walon, Way, Waylan, Wayland, Waylen, Waylin, Weylin

Wayman (English) road man; traveler.
Waymon

Wayne (English) wagon maker. A short form of Wainwright.
Wain, Wanye, Wayn, Waynell, Waynne, Wene, Whayne

Wazir (Arabic) minister.

Webb (English) weaver.
Web, Weeb

Weber (German) weaver.
Webber, Webner

Webley (English) weaver's
meadow.
Webbley, Webbly, Webly

Webster (English) weaver.

Weddel (English) valley near
the ford.

Wei-Quo (Chinese) ruler of
the country.
Wei

Welborne (English) spring-fed
stream.
*Welborn, Welbourne, Welburn,
Wellborn, Wellborne, Wellbourn,
Wellburn*

Welby (German) farm near
the well.
Welbey, Welbie, Wellbey, Wellby

Weldon (English) hill near the
well.
Weldan

Welfel (Yiddish) a form of
William.
Welvel

Welford (English) ford near
the well.

Wells (English) springs.
Welles

Welsh (English) a form of
Wallace, Walsh.
Welch

Welton (English) town near
the well.

Wemilat (Native American) all
give to him.

Wemilo (Native American) all
speak to him.

Wen (Gypsy) born in winter.

Wenceslaus (Slavic) wreath of
honor.
*Vencel, Wenceslao, Wenceslas,
Wenzel, Wenzell, Wiencyslaw*

Wendell (German) wanderer.
(English) good dale, good
valley.
*Wandale, Wendall, Wendel,
Wendle, Wendy*

Wene (Hawaiian) a form of
Wayne.

Wenford (English) white ford.
Wynford

Wentworth (English) pale
man's settlement.

Wenutu (Native American)
clear sky.

Werner (English) a form of
Warner.
Wernhar, Wernher

Wes (English) a short form of
Wesley.
Wess

Wesh (Gypsy) woods.

Wesley (English) western
meadow.
*Wes, Weseley, Wesle, Weslee,
Wesleyan, Weslie, Wesly, Wessley,
Westleigh, Westley, Wezley*

West (English) west.

Westbrook (English) western
  brook.
  Brook, West, Westbrooke

Westby (English) western
  farmstead.

Westcott (English) western
  cottage.
  Wescot, Wescott, Westcot

Westley (English) a form of
  Wesley.
  Westlee, Westly

Weston (English) western town.
  West, Westen, Westin

Wetherby (English) wether-
  sheep farm.
  *Weatherbey, Weatherbie,
  Weatherby, Wetherbey, Wetherbie*

Wetherell (English) wether-
  sheep corner.

Wetherly (English) wether-
  sheep meadow.

Weylin (English) a form of
  Waylon.
  Weylan, Weylyn

Whalley (English) woods near
  a hill.
  Whaley

Wharton (English) town on
  the bank of a lake.
  Warton

Wheatley (English) wheat
  field.
  *Whatley, Wheatlea, Wheatleigh,
  Wheatly*

Wheaton (English) wheat
  town.

Wheeler (English) wheel
  maker; wagon driver.

Whistler (English) whistler,
  piper.

Whit (English) a short form of
  Whitman, Whitney.
  Whitt, Whyt, Whyte, Wit, Witt

Whitby (English) white house.

Whitcomb (English) white
  valley.
  Whitcombe, Whitcumb

Whitelaw (English) small hill.
  Whitlaw

Whitey (English) white
  skinned; white haired.

Whitfield (English) white
  field.

Whitford (English) white
  ford.

Whitley (English) white
  meadow.
  Whitlea, Whitlee, Whitleigh

Whitman (English) white-
  haired man.
  Whit

Whitmore (English) white
  moor.
  *Whitmoor, Whittemore,
  Witmore, Wittemore*

Whitney (English) white
island; white water.
Whit, Whittney, Widney, Widny

Whittaker (English) white field.
Whitacker, Whitaker, Whitmaker

Wicasa (Dakota) man.

Wicent (Polish) a form of
Vincent.
Wicek, Wicus

Wichado (Native American)
willing.

Wickham (English) village
enclosure.
Wick

Wickley (English) village
meadow.
Wilcley

Wid (English) wide.

Wies (German) renowned
warrior.

Wikoli (Hawaiian) a form of
Victor.

Wiktor (Polish) a form of
Victor.

Wilanu (Moquelumnan) pour-
ing water on flour.

Wilbert (German) brilliant;
resolute.
Wilberto, Wilburt

Wilbur (English) wall fortifica-
tion; bright willows.
*Wilber, Wilburn, Wilburt,
Willbur, Wilver*

Wilder (English) wilderness,
wild.
Wylder

Wildon (English) wooded hill.
Wilden, Willdon

Wile (Hawaiian) a form of
Willie.

Wiley (English) willow
meadow; Will's meadow.
Whiley, Wildy, Willey, Wylie

Wilford (English) willow-tree
ford.
Wilferd

Wilfred (German) determined
peacemaker.
*Wilferd, Wilfredo, Wilfrid,
Wilfride, Wilfried, Wilfryd, Will,
Willfred, Willfried, Willie, Willy*

Wilfredo (Spanish) a form of
Wilfred.
*Fredo, Wifredo, Wilfrido,
Willfredo*

Wilhelm (German)
determined guardian.
Wilhelmus, Willem

Wiliama (Hawaiian) a form of
William.
Pila, Wile

Wilkie (English) a familiar
form of Wilkins.
Wikie, Wilke

Wilkins (English) William's kin.
*Wilkens, Wilkes, Wilkie, Wilkin,
Wilks, Willkes, Willkins*

Wilkinson (English) son of
little William.
Wilkenson, Willkinson

Will (English) a short form of
William.
Wil, Wilm, Wim

Willard (German) determined
and brave.
Williard

Willem (German) a form of
William.
Willim

William (English) a form of
Wilhelm. See also Gilamu,
Guglielmo, Guilherme,
Guillaume, Guillermo,
Gwilym, Liam, Uilliam,
Wilhelm.
*Bill, Billy, Vasyl, Vilhelm, Vili,
Viliam, Viljo, Ville, Villiam,
Welfel, Wilek, Wiliam, Wiliama,
Wiliame, Wiliame, Will, Willaim,
Willam, Willeam, Willem,
Williams, Willie, Willil, Willis,
Willium, Williu, Willyam, Wim*

Williams (German) son of
William.
*Wilams, Willaims, Williamson,
Wuliams*

Willie (German) a familiar
form of William.
Wile, Wille, Willi, Willia, Willy

Willis (German) son of Willie.
Willice, Wills, Willus, Wyllis

Willoughby (English) willow
farm.
Willoughbey, Willoughbie

Wills (English) son of Will.

Willy (German) a form of
Willie.
Willey, Wily

Wilmer (German) determined
and famous.
*Willimar, Willmer, Wilm,
Wilmar, Wylmar, Wylmer*

Wilmot (Teutonic) resolute
spirit.
*Willmont, Willmot, Wilm,
Wilmont*

Wilny (Native American) eagle
singing while flying.

Wilson (English) son of Will.
*Wilkinson, Willson, Wilsen,
Wolson*

Wilt (English) a short form of
Wilton.

Wilton (English) farm by the
spring.
Will, Wilt

Wilu (Moquelumnan) chicken
hawk squawking.

Win (Cambodian) bright.
(English) a short form of
Winston and names ending
in "win."
Winn, Winnie, Winny

Wincent (Polish) a form of Vincent.
Wicek, Wicenty, Wicus, Wince, Wincenty

Winchell (English) bend in the road; bend in the land.

Windsor (English) riverbank with a winch. History: the surname of the British royal family.
Wincer, Winsor, Wyndsor

Winfield (English) friendly field.
Field, Winfred, Winfrey, Winifield, Winnfield, Wynfield, Wynnfield

Winfried (German) friend of peace.

Wing (Chinese) glory.
Wing-Chiu, Wing-Kit

Wingate (English) winding gate.

Wingi (Native American) willing.

Winslow (English) friend's hill.

Winston (English) friendly town; victory town.
Win, Winsten, Winstin, Winstonn, Winton, Wynstan, Wynston

Winter (English) born in winter.
Winterford, Wynter

Winthrop (English) victory at the crossroads.

Winton (English) a form of Winston.
Wynten, Wynton

Winward (English) friend's guardian; friend's forest.

Wit (Polish) life. (English) a form of Whit. (Flemish) a short form of DeWitt.
Witt, Wittie, Witty

Witek (Polish) a form of Victor.

Witha (Arabic) handsome.

Witter (English) wise warrior.

Witton (English) wise man's estate.

Wladislav (Polish) a form of Vladislav.
Wladislaw

Wolcott (English) cottage in the woods.

Wolf (German, English) a short form of Wolfe, Wolfgang.
Wolff, Wolfie, Wolfy

Wolfe (English) wolf.
Wolf, Woolf

Wolfgang (German) wolf quarrel. Music: Wolfgang Amadeus Mozart was a famous eighteenth-century Austrian composer.
Wolf, Wolfegang, Wolfgans

Wood (English) a short form of Elwood, Garwood, Woodrow.
Woody

Woodfield (English) forest meadow.

Woodford (English) ford through the forest.

Woodrow (English) passage in the woods. History: Thomas Woodrow Wilson was the twenty-eighth U.S. president.
Wood, Woodman, Woodroe, Woody

Woodruff (English) forest ranger.

Woodson (English) son of Wood.
Woods, Woodsen

Woodward (English) forest warden.
Woodard

Woodville (English) town at the edge of the woods.

Woody (American) a familiar form of Elwood, Garwood, Woodrow.
Wooddy, Woodie

Woolsey (English) victorious wolf.

Worcester (English) forest army camp.

Wordsworth (English) wolf-guardian's farm. Literature: William Wordsworth was a famous British poet.
Worth

Worie (Ibo) born on market day.

Worth (English) a short form of Wordsworth.
Worthey, Worthington, Worthy

Worton (English) farm town.

Wouter (German) powerful warrior.

Wrangle (American) a form of Rangle.
Wrangler

Wray (Scandinavian) corner property. (English) crooked.
Wreh

Wren (Welsh) chief, ruler. (English) wren.

Wright (English) a short form of Wainwright.

Wrisley (English) a form of Risley.
Wrisee, Wrislie, Wrisly

Wriston (English) a form of Riston.
Wryston

Wuliton (Native American) will do well.

Wunand (Native American) God is good.

Wuyi (Moquelumnan) turkey vulture flying.

Wyatt (French) little warrior.
*Wiatt, Wyat, Wyatte, Wye,
Wyeth, Wyett, Wyitt, Wytt*

Wybert (English) battle
bright.

Wyborn (Scandinavian) war
bear.

Wyck (Scandinavian) village.

Wycliff (English) white cliff;
village near the cliff.
Wyckliffe, Wycliffe

Wylie (English) charming.
Wiley, Wye, Wyley, Wyllie, Wyly

Wyman (English) fighter, warrior.

Wymer (English) famous in
battle.

Wyn (Welsh) light skinned;
white. (English) friend. A
short form of Selwyn.
Win, Wyne, Wynn, Wynne

Wyndham (Scottish) village
near the winding road.
Windham, Wynndham

Wynono (Native American)
first-born son.

Wythe (English) willow tree.

Xabat (Basque) savior.

Xaiver (Basque) a form of
Xavier.
Xajavier, Xzaiver

Xan (Greek) a short form of
Alexander.
Xane

Xander (Greek) a short form
of Alexander.
Xande, Xzander

Xanthus (Latin) golden
haired.
Xanthos

Xarles (Basque) a form of
Charles.

Xavier (Arabic) bright.
(Basque) owner of the new
house. See also Exavier,
Javier, Salvatore, Saverio.
*Xabier, Xaiver, Xavaeir, Xaver,
Xavian, Xaviar, Xavior, Xavon,
Xavyer, Xever, Xizavier,
Xxavier, Xzavier, Zavier*

Xenophon (Greek) strange
voice.
Xeno, Zennie

Xenos (Greek) stranger; guest.
Zenos

Xerxes (Persian) ruler. History:
a king of Persia.
Zerk

Ximenes (Spanish) a form of
Simon.
*Ximenez, Ximon, Ximun,
Xymenes*

Xylon (Greek) forest.

Xzavier (Basque) a form of
Xavier.
*Xzavaier, Xzaver, Xzavion,
Xzavior, Xzvaier*

Y

Yadid (Hebrew) friend;
beloved.
Yedid

Yadon (Hebrew) he will
judge.
Yadean, Yadin, Yadun

Yael (Hebrew) a form of Jael.

Yafeu (Ibo) bold.

Yagil (Hebrew) he will rejoice.

Yago (Spanish) a form of
James.

Yahto (Lakota) blue.

Yahya (Arabic) living.
Yahye

Yair (Hebrew) he will
enlighten.
Yahir

Yakecen (Dene) sky song.

Yakez (Carrier) heaven.

Yakov (Russian) a form of
Jacob.
*Yaacob, Yaacov, Yaakov, Yachov,
Yacoub, Yacov, Yakob, Yashko*

Yale (German) productive.
(English) old.

Yan, Yann (Russian) forms of
John.
Yanichek, Yanick, Yanka, Yannick

Yana (Native American) bear.

Yancy (Native American)
Englishman, Yankee.
*Yan, Yance, Yancey, Yanci, Yansey,
Yansy, Yantsey, Yauncey, Yauncy,
Yency*

Yanick, Yannick (Russian)
familiar forms of Yan.
*Yanic, Yanik, Yannic, Yannik,
Yonic, Yonnik*

Yanka (Russian) a familiar
form of John.
Yanikm

Yanni (Greek) a form of John.
*Ioannis, Yani, Yannakis, Yannis,
Yanny, Yiannis, Yoni*

Yanton (Hebrew) a form of
Johnathon, Jonathon.

Yao (Ewe) born on Thursday.

Yaphet (Hebrew) a form of
Japheth.
Yapheth, Yefat, Yephat

Yarb (Gypsy) herb.

Yardan (Arabic) king.

Yarden (Hebrew) a form of
Jordan.

Yardley (English) enclosed meadow.
Lee, Yard, Yardlea, Yardlee, Yardleigh, Yardly

Yarom (Hebrew) he will raise up.
Yarum

Yaron (Hebrew) he will sing; he will cry out.
Jaron, Yairon

Yasashiku (Japanese) gentle; polite.

Yash (Hindi) victorious; glory.

Yasha (Russian) a form of Jacob, James.
Yascha, Yashka, Yashko

Yashwant (Hindi) glorious.

Yasin (Arabic) prophet.
Yasine, Yasseen, Yassin, Yassine, Yazen

Yasir (Afghan) humble; takes it easy. (Arabic) wealthy.
Yasar, Yaser, Yashar, Yasser

Yasuo (Japanese) restful.

Yates (English) gates.
Yeats

Yatin (Hindi) ascetic.

Yavin (Hebrew) he will understand.
Jabin

Yawo (Akan) born on Thursday.

Yazid (Arabic) his power will increase.
Yazeed, Yazide

Yechiel (Hebrew) God lives.

Yedidya (Hebrew) a form of Jedidiah. See also Didi.
Yadai, Yedidia, Yedidiah, Yido

Yegor (Russian) a form of George. See also Egor, Igor.
Ygor

Yehoshua (Hebrew) a form of Joshua.
Yeshua, Yeshuah, Yoshua, Y'shua, Yushua

Yehoyakem (Hebrew) a form of Joachim, Joaquín.
Yakim, Yehayakim, Yokim, Yoyakim

Yehudi (Hebrew) a form of Judah.
Yechudi, Yechudit, Yehuda, Yehudah, Yehudit

Yelutci (Moquelumnan) bear walking silently.

Yeoman (English) attendant; retainer.
Yoeman, Youman

Yeremey (Russian) a form of Jeremiah.
Yarema, Yaremka, Yeremy, Yerik

Yervant (Armenian) king, ruler. History: an Armenian king.

Yeshaya (Hebrew) gift. See also Shai.

Yeshurun (Hebrew) right way.

Yeska (Russian) a form of Joseph.
Yesya

Yestin (Welsh) just.

Yevgenyi (Russian) a form of Eugene.
Gena, Yevgeni, Yevgenij, Yevgeniy

Yigal (Hebrew) he will redeem.
Yagel, Yigael

Yirmaya (Hebrew) a form of Jeremiah.
Yirmayahu

Yishai (Hebrew) a form of Jesse.

Yisrael (Hebrew) a form of Israel.
Yesarel, Yisroel

Yitro (Hebrew) a form of Jethro.

Yitzchak (Hebrew) a form of Isaac. See also Itzak.
Yitzak, Yitzchok, Yitzhak

Yngve (Swedish) ancestor; lord, master.

Yo (Cambodian) honest.

Yoakim (Slavic) a form of Jacob.
Yoackim

Yoan (German) a form of Johan, Johann.
Yoann

Yoav (Hebrew) a form of Joab.

Yochanan (Hebrew) a form of John.
Yohanan

Yoel (Hebrew) a form of Joel.

Yogesh (Hindi) ascetic. Religion: another name for the Hindu god Shiva.

Yohance (Hausa) a form of John.

Yohan, Yohann (German) forms of Johan, Johann.
Yohane, Yohanes, Yohanne, Yohannes, Yohans, Yohn

Yonah (Hebrew) a form of Jonah.
Yona, Yonas

Yonatan (Hebrew) a form of Jonathan.
Yonathan, Yonathon, Yonaton, Yonattan

Yong (Chinese) courageous.
Yonge

Yong-Sun (Korean) dragon in the first position; courageous.

Yoni (Greek) a form of Yanni.
Yonis, Yonnas, Yonny, Yony

Yoofi (Akan) born on Friday.

Yooku (Fante) born on Wednesday.

Yoram (Hebrew) God is high.
Joram

Yorgos (Greek) a form of
George.
Yiorgos, Yorgo

York (English) boar estate;
yew-tree estate.
*Yorick, Yorke, Yorker, Yorkie,
Yorrick*

Yorkoo (Fante) born on
Thursday.

Yosef (Hebrew) a form of
Joseph. See also Osip.
*Yoceph, Yoosuf, Yoseff, Yoseph,
Yosief, Yosif, Yosuf, Yosyf, Yousef,
Yusif*

Yóshi (Japanese) adopted son.
Yoshiki, Yoshiuki

Yoshiyahu (Hebrew) a form
of Josiah.
*Yoshia, Yoshiah, Yoshiya,
Yoshiyah, Yosiah*

Yoskolo (Moquelumnan)
breaking off pine cones.

Yosu (Hebrew) a form of
Jesus.

Yotimo (Moquelumnan) yellow jacket carrying food to
its hive.

Yottoko (Native American)
mud at the water's edge.

Young (English) young.
Yung

Young-Jae (Korean) pile of
prosperity.

Young-Soo (Korean) keeping
the prosperity.

Youri (Russian) a form of
Yuri.

Yousef (Yiddish) a form of
Joseph.
*Yousaf, Youseef, Yousef, Youseph,
Yousif, Youssef, Yousseff, Yousuf*

Youssel (Yiddish) a familiar
form of Joseph.
Yussel

Yov (Russian) a short form of
Yoakim.

Yovani (Slavic) a form of
Jovan.
*Yovan, Yovanni, Yovanny, Yovany,
Yovni*

Yoyi (Hebrew) a form of
George.

Yrjo (Finnish) a form of
George.

Ysidro (Greek) a short form
of Isidore.

Yu (Chinese) universe.
Yue

Yudell (English) a form of
Udell.
Yudale, Yudel

Yuki (Japanese) snow.
Yukiko, Yukio, Yuuki

Yul (Mongolian) beyond the horizon.

Yule (English) born at Christmas.

Yuli (Basque) youthful.

Yuma (Native American) son of a chief.

Yunus (Turkish) a form of Jonah.

Yurcel (Turkish) sublime.

Yuri (Russian, Ukrainian) a form of George. (Hebrew) a familiar form of Uriah.
Yehor, Youri, Yura, Yure, Yuric, Yurii, Yurij, Yurik, Yurko, Yurri, Yury, Yusha

Yusif (Russian) a form of Joseph.
Yuseph, Yusof, Yussof, Yusup, Yuzef, Yuzep

Yustyn (Russian) a form of Justin.
Yusts

Yusuf (Arabic, Swahili) a form of Joseph.
Yusef, Yusuff

Yutu (Moquelumnan) coyote out hunting.

Yuval (Hebrew) rejoicing.

Yves (French) a form of Ivar, Ives.
Yvens, Yvon, Yyves

Yvon (French) a form of Ivar, Yves.
Ivon, Yuvon, Yvan, Yvonne

Z

Zac (Hebrew) a short form of Zachariah, Zachary.
Zacc

Zacarias (Portuguese, Spanish) a form of Zachariah.
Zacaria, Zacariah

Zacary (Hebrew) a form of Zachary.
Zac, Zacaras, Zacari, Zacariah, Zacarias, Zacarie, Zacarious, Zacery, Zacory, Zacrye

Zaccary (Hebrew) a form of Zachary.
Zac, Zaccaeus, Zaccari, Zaccaria, Zaccariah, Zaccary, Zaccea, Zaccharie, Zacchary, Zacchery, Zaccury

Zaccheus (Hebrew) innocent, pure.
Zacceus, Zacchaeus, Zacchious

Zach (Hebrew) a short form of Zachariah, Zachary.

Zachari (Hebrew) a form of Zachary.
Zacheri

Zacharia (Hebrew) a form of Zachary.
Zacharya

Zachariah (Hebrew) God remembered.
Zac, Zacarias, Zacarius, Zacary, Zaccary, Zach, Zacharias, Zachary, Zacharyah, Zachory, Zachury, Zack, Zakaria, Zako, Zaquero, Zecharia, Zechariah, Zecharya, Zeggery, Zeke, Zhachory

Zacharias (German) a form of Zachariah.
Zacarías, Zacharais, Zachariaus, Zacharius, Zackarias, Zakarias, Zecharias, Zekarias

Zacharie (Hebrew) a form of Zachary.
Zachare, Zacharee, Zachurie, Zecharie

Zachary (Hebrew) a familiar form of Zachariah. History: Zachary Taylor was the twelfth U.S. president. See also Sachar, Sakeri.
Xachary, Zac, Zacary, Zaccary, Zach, Zacha, Zachaery, Zachaios, Zacharay, Zacharey, Zachari, Zacharia, Zacharias, Zacharie, Zacharry, Zachaury, Zachery, Zachory, Zachrey, Zachry, Zachuery, Zachury, Zack, Zackary, Zackery, Zackory, Zakaria, Zakary, Zakery, Zakkary, Zechary, Zechery, Zeke

Zachery (Hebrew) a form of Zachary.
Zacheray, Zacherey, Zacheria, Zacherias, Zacheriah, Zacherie, Zacherius, Zackery

Zachory (Hebrew) a form of Zachary.

Zachry (Hebrew) a form of Zachary.
Zachre, Zachrey, Zachri

Zack (Hebrew) a short form of Zachariah, Zachary.
Zach, Zak, Zaks

Zackary (Hebrew) a form of Zachary.
Zack, Zackari, Zacharia, Zackare, Zackaree, Zackariah, Zackarie, Zackery, Zackhary, Zackie, Zackree, Zackrey, Zackry

Zackery (Hebrew) a form of Zachery.
Zackere, Zackeree, Zackerey, Zackeri, Zackeria, Zackeriah, Zackerie, Zackerry

Zackory (Hebrew) a form of Zachary.
Zackoriah, Zackorie, Zacorey, Zacori, Zacory, Zacry, Zakory

Zadok (Hebrew) a short form of Tzadok.
Zaddik, Zadik, Zadoc, Zaydok

Zadornin (Basque) Saturn.

Zafir (Arabic) victorious.
Zafar, Zafeer, Zafer, Zaffar

Zahid (Arabic) self-denying, ascetic.
Zaheed

Zahir (Arabic) shining, bright.
*Zahair, Zahar, Zaheer, Zahi,
Zair, Zaire, Zayyir*

Zahur (Swahili) flower.

Zaid (Arabic) increase, growth.
Zaied, Zaiid, Zayd

Zaide (Hebrew) older.

Zaim (Arabic) brigadier general.

Zain (English) a form of Zane.
Zaine

Zakaria (Hebrew) a form of
Zachariah.
*Zakaraiya, Zakareeya,
Zakareeyah, Zakariah,
Zakariya, Zakeria, Zakeriah*

Zakariyya (Arabic) prophet.
Religion: an Islamic prophet.

Zakary (Hebrew) a form of
Zachery.
*Zak, Zakarai, Zakare, Zakaree,
Zakari, Zakarias, Zakarie,
Zakarius, Zakariye, Zake,
Zakhar, Zaki, Zakir, Zakkai,
Zako, Zakqary, Zakree, Zakri,
Zakris, Zakry*

Zakery (Hebrew) a form of
Zachary.
Zakeri, Zakerie, Zakiry

Zaki (Arabic) bright; pure.
(Hausa) lion.
*Zakee, Zakia, Zakie, Zakiy,
Zakki*

Zakia (Swahili) intelligent.

Zakkary (Hebrew) a form of
Zachary.
*Zakk, Zakkari, Zakkery,
Zakkyre*

Zako (Hungarian) a form of
Zachariah.

Zale (Greek) sea strength.
Zayle

Zalmai (Afghan) young.

Zalman (Yiddish) a form of
Solomon.
Zaloman

Zamiel (German) a form of
Samuel.
Zamal, Zamuel

Zamir (Hebrew) song; bird.
Zameer

Zan (Italian) clown.
*Zann, Zanni, Zannie, Zanny,
Zhan*

Zander (Greek) a short form
of Alexander.
*Zandore, Zandra, Zandrae,
Zandy*

Zane (English) a form of
John.
Zain, Zayne, Zhane

Zanis (Latvian) a form of
Janis.
Zannis

Zanvil (Hebrew) a form of
Samuel.
Zanwill

Zaquan (American) a combination of the prefix Za + Quan.
Zaquain, Zaquon, Zaqwan

Zareb (African) protector.

Zared (Hebrew) ambush.
Zaryd

Zarek (Polish) may God protect the king.
Zarik, Zarrick, Zerek, Zerick, Zerric, Zerrick

Zavier (Arabic) a form of Xavier.
Zavair, Zaverie, Zavery, Zavierre, Zavior, Zavyr, Zayvius, Zxavian

Zayit (Hebrew) olive.

Zayne (English) a form of Zane.
Zayan, Zayin, Zayn

Zdenek (Czech) follower of Saint Denis.

Zeb (Hebrew) a short form of Zebediah, Zebulon.
Zev

Zebediah (Hebrew) God's gift.
Zeb, Zebadia, Zebadiah, Zebedee, Zebedia, Zebidiah, Zedidiah

Zebedee (Hebrew) a familiar form of Zebediah.
Zebadee

Zebulon (Hebrew) exalted, honored; lofty house.
Zabulan, Zeb, Zebulan, Zebulen, Zebulin, Zebulun, Zebulyn, Zev, Zevulon, Zevulun, Zhebulen, Zubin

Zechariah (Hebrew) a form of Zachariah.
Zecharia, Zecharian, Zecheriah, Zechuriah, Zekariah, Zekarias, Zeke, Zekeria, Zekeriah, Zekerya

Zed (Hebrew) a short form of Zedekiah.

Zedekiah (Hebrew) God is mighty and just.
Zed, Zedechiah, Zedekias, Zedikiah

Zedidiah (Hebrew) a form of Zebediah.

Zeeman (Dutch) seaman.

Zeév (Hebrew) wolf.
Zeévi, Zeff, Zif

Zeheb (Turkish) gold.

Zeke (Hebrew) a short form of Ezekiel, Zachariah, Zachary, Zechariah.

Zeki (Turkish) clever, intelligent.
Zeky

Zelgai (Afghan) heart.

Zelig (Yiddish) a form of Selig.
Zeligman, Zelik

Zelimir (Slavic) wishes for peace.

Zemar (Afghan) lion.

Zen (Japanese) religious. Religion: a form of Buddhism.

Zenda (Czech) a form of Eugene.
Zhek

Zeno (Greek) cart; harness. History: a Greek philosopher.
Zenan, Zenas, Zenon, Zino, Zinon

Zephaniah (Hebrew) treasured by God.
Zaph, Zaphania, Zeph, Zephan

Zephyr (Greek) west wind.
Zeferino, Zeffrey, Zephery, Zephire, Zephram, Zephran, Zephrin

Zero (Arabic) empty, void.

Zeroun (Armenian) wise and respected.

Zeshawn (American) a combination of the prefix Ze + Shawn.
Zeshan, Zeshaun, Zeshon, Zishaan, Zishan, Zshawn

Zesiro (Luganda) older of twins.

Zeus (Greek) living. Mythology: chief god of the Greek pantheon.

Zeusef (Portuguese) a form of Joseph.

Zev (Hebrew) a short form of Zebulon.

Zevi (Hebrew) a form of Tzvi.
Zhvie, Zhvy, Zvi

Zhek (Russian) a short form of Evgeny.
Zhenechka, Zhenka, Zhenya

Zhìxin (Chinese) ambitious.
Zhi, Zhìhuán, Zhipeng, Zhi-yang, Zhìyuan

Zhuàng (Chinese) strong.

Zhora (Russian) a form of George.
Zhorik, Zhorka, Zhorz, Zhurka

Zia (Hebrew) trembling; moving. (Arabic) light.
Ziah

Zigfrid (Latvian, Russian) a form of Siegfried.
Zegfrido, Zigfrids, Ziggy, Zygfryd, Zygi

Ziggy (American) a familiar form of Siegfried, Sigmund.
Ziggie

Zigor (Basque) punishment.

Zikomo (Nguni) thank-you.

Zilaba (Luganda) born while sick.
Zilabamuzale

Zimra (Hebrew) song of praise.
Zemora, Zimrat, Zimri, Zimria, Zimriah, Zimriya

Zimraan (Arabic) praise.

Zinan (Japanese) second son.

Zindel (Yiddish) a form of Alexander.
Zindil, Zunde

Zion (Hebrew) sign, omen; excellent. Bible: the name used to refer to Israel and to the Jewish people.
Tzion, Zyon

Ziskind (Yiddish) sweet child.

Ziv (Hebrew) shining brightly. (Slavic) a short form of Ziven.

Ziven (Slavic) vigorous, lively.
Zev, Ziv, Zivka, Zivon

Ziyad (Arabic) increase.
Zayd, Ziyaad

Zlatan (Czech) gold.
Zlatek, Zlatko

Zohar (Hebrew) bright light.
Zohair

Zollie, Zolly (Hebrew) forms of Solly.
Zoilo

Zoltán (Hungarian) life.

Zorba (Greek) live each day.

Zorion (Basque) a form of Orion.
Zoran, Zoren, Zorian, Zoron, Zorrine, Zorrion

Zorya (Slavic) star; dawn.

Zotikos (Greek) saintly, holy. Religion: a saint in the Eastern Orthodox Church.

Zotom (Kiowa) a biter.

Zsigmond (Hungarian) a form of Sigmund.
Ziggy, Zigmund, Zsiga

Zuberi (Swahili) strong.

Zubin (Hebrew) a short form of Zebulon.
Zubeen

Zuhayr (Arabic) brilliant, shining.
Zyhair, Zuheer

Zuka (Shona) sixpence.

Zuriel (Hebrew) God is my rock.

Zygmunt (Polish) a form of Sigmund.

Also from Meadowbrook Press

✦ **The Best Baby Shower Book**
The number one baby shower planner has been updated for the new millennium. This contemporary guide for planning baby showers is full of helpful hints, recipes, decorating ideas, and activities that are fun without being juvenile.

✦ **Busy Books**
The Children's Busy Book, The Toddler's Busy Book, The Preschooler's Busy Book, and *The Arts and Crafts Busy Book* each contain 365 activities (one for each day of the year) for your children using items found around the home. The books offer parents and child-care providers fun reading, math, and science activities that will stimulate a child's natural curiosity. They also provide great activities for indoor play during even the longest stretches of bad weather! All four show you how to save money by making your own paints, play dough, craft clays, glue, paste, and other arts-and-crafts supplies.

✦ **Pregnancy, Childbirth, and the Newborn**
More complete and up-to-date than any other pregnancy guide, this remarkable book is the "bible" for childbirth educators. Now revised with a greatly expanded treatment of pregnancy tests, complications, and infections; an expanded list of drugs and medications (plus advice for uses); and a brand-new chapter on creating a detailed birth plan.